COLORECTAL CANCER - FROM PATHOGENESIS TO TREATMENT

Edited by **Luis Rodrigo**

Colorectal Cancer - From Pathogenesis to Treatment
http://dx.doi.org/10.5772/61359
Edited by Luis Rodrigo

Contributors
Krassimir Ivanov, Dilyan Petrov, Georgi Ivanov, Alexander Zlatarov, Anton Tonev, Valentin Ignatov, Nikola Kolev, Deniz Tural, Rumeysa Ciftci, Soichiro Murata, Fatma Sen, Kezban Nur Pilanci, Shteryu Shterev, Tanya Kirilova, Yumi Zuhanis Has-Yun Hashim, Chris Gill, Nigel Ternan, Phirdaous Abbas, Cheryl Latimer, Martha Robles-Flores, Dora M. Velázquez, Maria Cristina Castañeda-Patlán, Mario Guerrieri, Monica Ortenzi, Roberto Ghiselli, Giovanni Lezoche, Josefa Leon, Jorge Casado, Sandra Ríos-Arrabal, Sergio Manuel Jimenez-Ruiz, Francisco Artacho-Cordon, Jose Antonio Muñoz-Gamez, Lorelei Irina Brasoveanu, Marinela Bostan, Camelia Hotnog, Mirela Mihaila, Viviana Roman, Gabriela Anton, Coralia Bleotu, Zodwa Dlamini, Rodney Hull, Mpho Choene, Thandeka Khoza, Shahid Ahmed, Selliah Kanthan, Nayyer Iqbal, Adnan Zaidi, Duc Le, Kamal Haider, Abbas Tahir, Timothy Jay Price, Amanda Townsend, Louisa Lo, Joanne Young, Gabriel Mak, Hendrik-Tobias Arkenau, Michele Moschetta, Serife Koc, Melek Nihal Esin, Aysun Ardic, Paul Mitrut, Ivan Donev, Assia Konsoulova, Elitza Encheva, Plamena Drenakova, Radu Badea, Diana Florian, Cosmin Caraiani

Published by InTech
Janeza Trdine 9, 51000 Rijeka, Croatia

Publishing Process Manager Iva Lipovic
Technical Editor SPi Global
Cover InTech Design team

First published September, 2016
Printed in Croatia

Additional hard copies can be obtained from orders@intechopen.com

Colorectal Cancer - From Pathogenesis to Treatment, Edited by Luis Rodrigo
p. cm.
Print ISBN 978-953-51-2544-0
Online ISBN 978-953-51-2545-7

For EU product safety concerns:
IN TECH d.o.o., Prolaz Marije Krucifikse Kozulić 3, 51000 Rijeka, Croatia,
info@intechopen.com or visit our website at intechopen.com.

Meet the editor

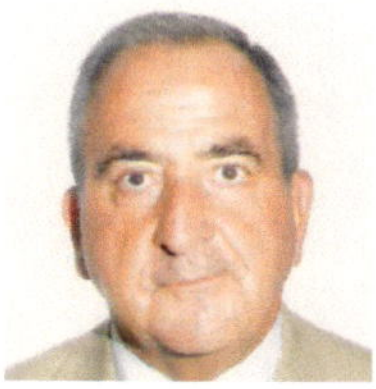

Dr. Luis Rodrigo, PhD, is currently Emeritus Professor at the University of Oviedo, Spain. He studied in the School of Medicine of Madrid University and obtained his PhD in Medicine in 1975. He has been the Head of Gastroenterology at the University Hospital Central of Asturias since 1996, Titular Professor at the Oviedo University since 1983, and Full-Time Professor since 2010. He has published a total of 255 scientific papers in English and 282 in Spanish. His total Impact Factor is 1581.96, total citation numbers are 5696, and the h-index is 39. He has written a total of 58 chapters and eight edited books about "Treatment in gastroenterological diseases" and the other digestive and liver diseases. He has participated in 50 clinical trials, in 15 as main investigator.

Contents

Preface

Colorectal carcinoma (CRC) is one of the most common malignancies found in the Western countries. In frequency, it ranked the third place in men (preceded only by the lung and prostate cancers) and the second place in women (after breast cancer). Its incidence increases with age, especially in people over the age of 50 years. The average presentation time is around 70 years, although there are few reported in individuals from 25 to 30 years of age. Cases appearing at younger ages tend to have an increased genetic predisposition. Its development is influenced by many factors related to the diet, lifestyle, and other environmental factors, constituting the so-called "sporadic" forms, representing more than 70% of the total CRC cases.

It is well established that the effect of hereditary factors appears in a minor proportion, representing the remaining 30% of cases, which includes several entities such as Lynch syndrome (LS), the so-called "hereditary non-polyposis CRC" (HNPCRC) forms, and the "familial adenomatous polyposis" (FAP) syndrome, as well as other several multiple polyposis syndromes of the colon. In even fewer, less than 1% of the cases, CRC is associated to an inflammatory bowel disease of long-lasting evolution. For all these hereditary forms, it is applied the global term of "family CRC."

A very important proportion of chapters explains the different pathogenetic mechanisms involved in their pathogenesis and evolution. There are three ways of well-characterized carcinogenesis, with allelic gains and losses on the CRC, through suppressive or chromosomal instability, through mutator or microsatellite instability, and methylation CpG phenotype (island methylator phenotype). Of these, through suppressive is the most common way.

In this book, the authors present the last advances related to early diagnosis, several modalities of treatment, and prognosis in the different types of tumors and also in advanced stages. The treatment of choice is surgery, if possible, elective and laparoscopically. Surgery robots are being introduced slowly and progressively. Chemotherapy and radiation therapy are complementary treatments, especially in advanced cases, and actually are considered very effective in the resection of liver metastases and also distant organs.

Finally, I want to thank all the authors for their wonderful contributions, as well as the speed and efficiency in the delivery of their chapters. A special gratitude mention to all the excellent team members from the Editorial InTech also for their continued support and final condition of this book.

Prof. Luis Rodrigo MD
Emeritus Professor of Medicine
University of Oviedo
Oviedo, Spain

Section 1

Pathogenesis

Chapter 1

Molecular Mechanisms Involved in the Acquisition of Resistance to Treatment of Colon Cancer Cells

Dora M. Velázquez,
María Cristina Castañeda-Patlán and
Martha Robles-Flores

Additional information is available at the end of the chapter

http://dx.doi.org/10.5772/63524

Abstract

Cancer cells are remarkably resilient to therapies aimed at their elimination. The exploration of pathways that sustain cancer cells and that allow cancer cells to become resistant has revealed new avenues for chemotherapeutic development, as well as rational approaches to combination therapies based on existing treatment options. Several signaling pathways, such as Wnt, phosphoinositide 3-kinase (PI3K), and Ras-Raf-MEK, constitute integrated networks that work together to maintain cellular homeostasis under basal conditions and to drive cell-mass accumulation and cell cycle progression in the presence of appropriate mitogenic stimuli. During cancer development, these pathways are corrupted in malignant cells to maintain viability and proliferative activity under environmentally stressful conditions such as limited growth factors, oxygen, and nutrients that drive normal cells into quiescence or death. Importantly, dysfunction within any one of these pathways results in compensatory responses from the other networks. Thus, biological research is gradually shifting toward more general approaches that target entire pathways rather than isolated components and integrate those pathways into biological networks.

Keywords: cancer resistance, autophagy, hypoxia, survival signaling pathways, colon cancer

INTECH
open science | open minds

1. Introduction

The inherent or developed resistance of many cancer cells to chemotherapy, targeted types of therapy, and irradiation is the primary cause for treatment failure in clinical oncology. Through basic research efforts aimed at gaining a better understanding of the mechanisms responsible for these effects, it is hoped that more effective strategies to manage this disease will be developed.

Wnt signaling has been recognized as one of the most important contributors to malignant transformation in many types of solid tumors. Canonical Wnt signaling is altered in most cases of colorectal cancer (CRC). Indeed, a great amount of experimental evidence has shown that mutations in the adenomatous polyposis coli (APC) gene, a key negative modulator of canonical Wnt signaling, trigger the molecular pathogenesis of this type of cancer [1, 2]. The Wnt pathway has also been demonstrated to play an important role in the regulation of adult stem cell systems, and canonical Wnt signaling regulates the self-renewal and maintenance of both stem and cancer stem cells (CSCs). Cross talk has been reported between canonical Wnt signaling and hypoxia-inducible factor (HIF) signaling in tumor progression and metastasis [3]. However, the molecular mechanisms involved in this cross talk remain poorly understood.

Diminished oxygen availability (hypoxia) with the hypoxia-inducible factors (HIFs) mediating adaptation to it causes autophagy establishment, particularly in RAS-driven and BRAF-driven cancers, such as in most colorectal carcinomas. However, the relevance of the relation between HIFs and autophagy in drug resistance is not well understood. We have examined the effects of stable knockdown of HIF-1α or HIF-2α expression on malignant phenotype maintenance and in the canonical Wnt activation (β-catenin dependent). Our results indicated that although both HIF-1α and HIF-2α are essential for stemness and malignancy maintenance, these two proteins exert different effects and play opposing roles in canonical Wnt signaling [3]. We have also examined the effects of HIFs silencing on autophagy and drug resistance displayed by cancer cells. In agreement with other groups, we have observed that cancer cells exhibit high basal levels of autophagy and co-expression of HIF-1α and HIF-2α, compared with control nonmalignant cells and that the combination of mTOR inhibition with the autophagy inhibitor hydroxychloroquine (HCQ) dramatically induced cell death via apoptosis [4].

In addition, it has been demonstrated recently that challenging cancer cells with stresses that they would typically encounter during tumor progression or as a part of a therapeutic regiment to treat or manage the disease, including chemotherapeutic agents, gamma irradiation, and hypoxic and serum-limiting conditions, increase the rate of microvesicles (MVs, referred also as oncosomes) formation and shedding by cells [5, 6]. These MVs are secreted from numerous types of cells and function in intercellular communication by transporting intracellular contents, such as protein, mRNA, and microRNAs (miRNAs) [7]. Oncosomes secreted by cancer cells may play an important role in cancer progression by promoting angiogenesis, neutrophil infiltration, and the education of bone marrow-derived cells [8]. Indeed, recent findings suggest that MVs can promote cell survival and contribute to drug resistance.

In this review we focus on the molecular mechanisms whereby cancer cells develop resistance to antineoplastic drugs, particularly focused in the cell signaling pathways involved. A better understanding of the mechanisms that drive such resistance would enable the development of approaches to overcome it.

2. Survival signaling pathways: highly integrated cellular networks

Targeted blockade of aberrantly activated signaling pathways is an attractive therapeutic strategy for solid tumors, but drug resistance is common. Several selective inhibitors, particularly against kinases and receptor tyrosine kinases (RTKs), have shown promising initial efficacy [9]; however, with few exceptions, the duration of response is limited; drug resistance rapidly emerges. This underscores the difficulty of successfully treating an adept, heterogeneous disease with a single targeted therapy and highlights the fact that monotherapy is often not a tractable long-term therapeutic approach.

Resistance mechanisms can include alterations in the drug target itself, the pathway in which the target signals, or a parallel pathway that can alleviate the pressure on the cell due to blockade of the target [10]. Alternatively, drug resistance may be mediated by epigenetic reprogramming [11], by epithelial-to-mesenchymal transition (EMT) [12], or by emergence of a less differentiated, progenitor cell type [13]. Inducers of EMT, such as growth factors, transforming growth factor beta (TGFβ), and Wnt ligands, induces the expression of a gene program that leads to the suppression of the expression of the cell adhesion protein E-cadherin via the expression of transcriptional repressors such as Snail, Slug, Zeb1, Zeb2, and Twist. Besides these genes, other typical markers of EMT are N-cadherin, vimentin, and fibronectin-1, which are usually expressed in mesenchymal cells [3].

The emergence of acquired resistance to targeted therapy against cancer is very common and the most frequent cause of treatment failure in cancer patients. This resistance can be mediated by signaling pathway reactivation [14] or by genetic or epigenetic events occurring within cancer cells [10]. Ultimately, these events lead to the activation of growth and survival signaling pathways within cancer cells that enable them to survive the stressful conditions. However, for most drugs, the identities of potential resistance pathways are unknown. The signaling pathways more frequently associated with cancer resistance to treatment are the following:

2.1. The PI3K signaling network

The phosphoinositide 3-kinase (PI3K) signaling pathway, which lies downstream of various growth factor receptor tyrosine kinases, including the EGFR, is often aberrantly activated in human cancers. It plays critical roles in the regulation of cell growth, proliferation, differentiation, motility, survival, and intracellular trafficking. When deregulated, it is a major driver of tissue hyperplasia, oncogenesis [15], and is implicated in many aspects of tumorigenesis, including inappropriate cellular proliferation, angiogenesis, metastasis, and resistance to cell death.

There are three classes of PI3K enzymes: the Class I PI3Ks play a central role in the transmission of regulatory signals through the metabolism-signaling supernetwork [15]. Class I PI3Ks are expressed as heterodimers consisting of four p110 catalytic subunits and one of two p85 regulatory subunits and are activated primarily by tyrosine kinase signaling pathways and heterotrimeric G protein-coupled signaling pathways. Upon activation, Class I PI3Ks preferentially phosphorylate PI-4,5-P2 to yield the second messenger PI-3,4,5-P3 [15]. The activation of PI3K activation is dampened by the lipid phosphatase PTEN, which dephosphorylates PI-3,4,5-P3 to regenerate PI-4,5-P2, thereby disengaging the proximal signaling proteins from the network. The local accumulation of PI-3,4,5-P3 at the inner leaflet of the plasma membrane attracts proteins containing pleckstrin homology (PH) domains, which bind PI-3,4,5-P3 and PI-3,4-P2 to act as proximal signal transducers in the PI3K pathway [15] (**Figure 1**).

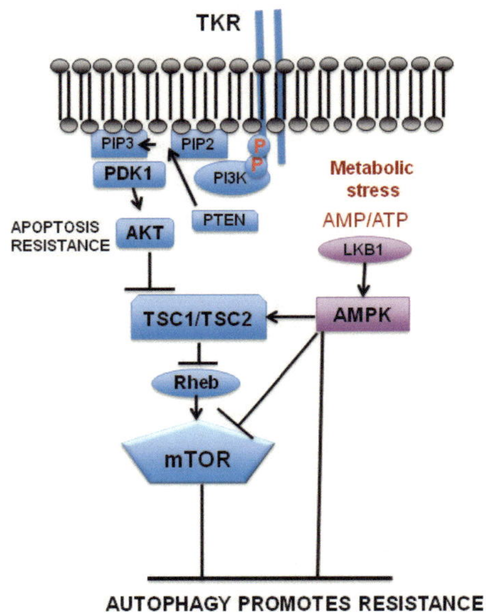

Figure 1. The PI3K and AMPK pathways are shown. Different members of the PI3K pathway increase apoptosis resistance. AMPK also regulates cellular metabolism by phosphorylating directly the tumor suppressor tuberous sclerosis 1 and 2 complex (TSC1/TSC2) to activate mTOR via Rheb GTPase.

The best-studied member of this set of PH domain-containing proteins is the serine-threonine kinase AKT, which is juxtaposed with its upstream activating protein kinase, PDK1. AKT is activated through phosphorylation of its threonine 308 residue by PDK1 and of serine 473 by mTOR complex 2 to mediate many PI3K responses, including growth, metabolism, survival, and glucose homeostasis [16]. AKT promotes apoptosis resistance by phosphorylating and thereby inhibiting proapoptotic substrates and profoundly influences cellular metabolism through its direct effects on metabolic enzymes and, more indirectly, through the stimulation of mTOR complex 1 (mTORC1) activity (**Figure 1**).

The PI3K-AKT pathway is central to the integration of growth factor-derived signals and nutrient availability with anabolic metabolism, growth, and cell cycle progression in multicellular organisms. In diseases such as cancer, this pathway is reprogrammed to fuel stress resistance and uncontrolled growth and couples growth factors and other hormonal stimuli to the metabolic and autophagy networks.

2.2. The Wnt pathway

Wnt signaling is a key pathway in embryonic development and adult homeostasis and aberrant activation of this pathway plays an important role in the development of many human cancer types [1, 2]. Indeed, aberrant Wnt signaling is a hallmark of the majority of colorectal cancers and it is implicated in maintenance of tumor-initiating cells, drug resistance, tumor progression, and metastasis.

Canonical Wnt signals are transduced through Frizzled family receptors and LRP5/LRP6 co-receptor to regulate the phosphorylation and degradation of the transcription co-activator β-catenin (**Figure 2**). Noncanonical Wnt signals are transduced independently of β-catenin through Frizzled family receptors and ROR2/RYK co-receptors to the Rho family guanosine triphosphatases, c-jun-NH_2-terminal kinase, or the Ca^{2+}-dependent signaling cascades.

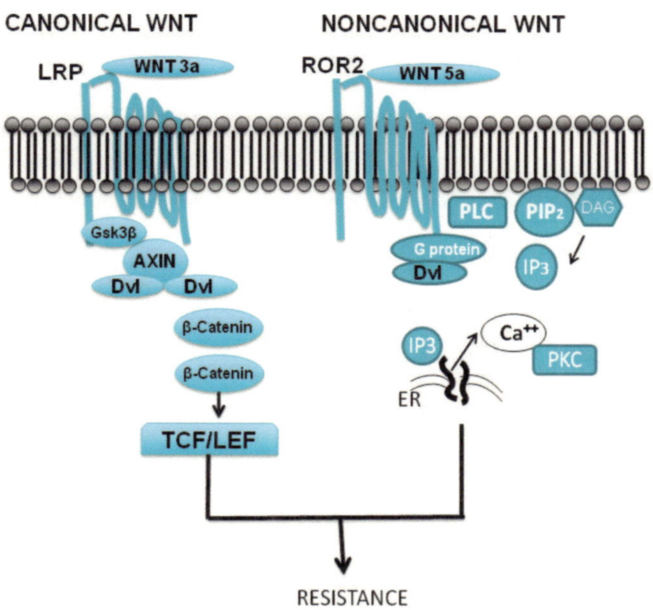

Figure 2. The canonical Wnt pathway shown controls β-catenin intracellular levels and localization. When it is activated, β-catenin is stabilized and translocated to the nucleus to bind TCF transcription factor and activate Wnt-responsive genes. Noncanonical Wnt pathway transduces signals in a β-catenin-independent manner and its activation has been associated with aggressive malignant phenotype.

In the absence of Wnt ligands, β-catenin is assembled into the so-called destruction complex assembled by adenomatous polyposis coli (APC) tumor suppressor, axin, glycogen synthase kinase-3β (GSK-3β), and casein kinase 1 (CK1). This complex promotes phosphorylation of β-catenin that targets it for ubiquitination and subsequent proteolysis via the proteasome [2, 3]. Upon Wnt stimulation β-catenin breakdown is inhibited, thereby causing its accumulation and entry to the nucleus, to activate Wnt target genes [2]. In noncanonical Wnt pathways, Wnt signals are transduced independently of β-catenin. The best-studied noncanonical Wnt pathways are planar cell polarity (PCP) pathway and Ca^{2+} pathway, which play central roles in developmental morphogenesis, cell polarity, and cell migration. In Wnt/Ca^{2+} pathway, Wnt-Frizzled (Fzd) binding activates phospholipase C (PLC) via G proteins, producing an increase of intracellular Ca^{2+} concentration and the activation of downstream effectors including protein kinase C, as it can be seen in **Figure 2** [1].

A great effort in developing selective drugs to target components of the Wnt pathway, particularly the β-catenin-dependent pathway, with anticancer activity, is underway but only a few of them have reached phase I clinical trials. In this respect, in models of KRAS-mutant colorectal cancer, it has been found by RNA-Seq data analysis for differential expression of canonical Wnt target genes that resistant cells display increased Wnt-β-catenin transcriptional activity [10], but there is also evidence, using this technique, that activation of noncanonical Wnt signaling exists in cancer-resistant cells and in different subsets of circulating tumor cells (CTCs) obtained from patients [17].

2.3. Ras-Raf-MEK signaling pathway

As mentioned before, oncogenic drivers often elicit a strong tumor dependence on the pathway that the driver controls, leading to the so-called pathway addiction. One such oncogenic driver that elicits a pathway addiction is mutant KRAS which is directly implicated in the simplified linear RAS-RAF-MEK ERK (extracellular signal-regulated kinase) signaling axis, as well as the

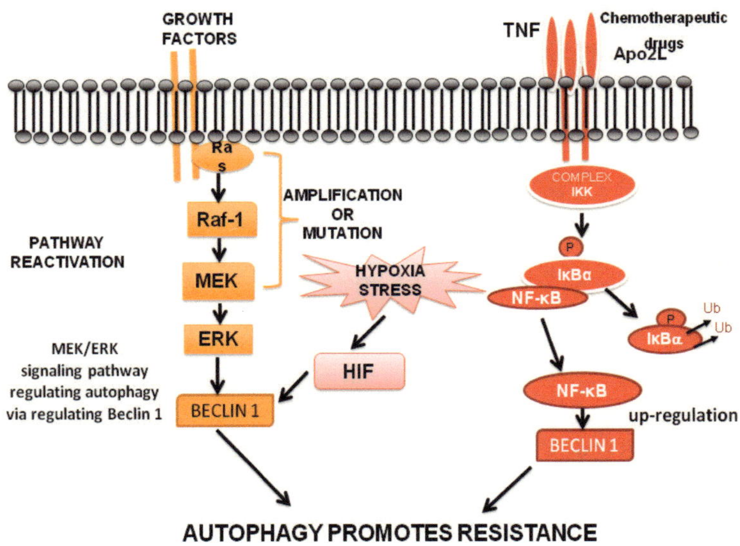

Figure 3. The Ras-Raf-MEK and NF-kB signaling pathways promote resistance. Mutations and amplification of Ras-Raf-MEK are frequently found in colorectal cancer allowing the development of resistance to treatment via autophagy activation. NF-kB upregulates Beclin 1 expression allowing positive regulation of autophagy. On the other hand, HIF-1α also modulates Beclin 1. IKK can promote the autophagy in an NF-kB-dependent manner.

PI3K-mTOR axis [10]. Mutations within RAS-Raf-Mex pathway have frequently detected in colorectal cancer, being BRAFV660E the most frequently found (**Figure 3**).

Little et al. [18] and Corcoran et al. [19] examined the mechanisms whereby colorectal cancers develop resistance. Both studies focused on the effects produced by inhibition of MEK (mitogen-activated or extracellular signal-regulated protein kinase kinase), which is a downstream effector of the oncogene BRAF or KRAS [9]. Both groups found that resistance arose through amplification of the driving oncogene (BRAF or KRAS) rather than through amplification or mutation of the targeted kinase itself (MEK).

There is also evidence that *BRAF* oncogene induces the expression of key autophagic markers, like microtubule-associated protein 1 light chain 3 (LC3) and Beclin 1 (BECN1) in colorectal tumor cells. Goulielmaki et al. [20] provided strong evidence that pretreatment with the autophagy inhibitor 3-methyl adenine (3-MA) followed by its combination with BRAFV600E targeting drug PLX4720 can synergistically sensitize resistant colorectal tumors.

2.4. LKB1/AMPK pathway

AMPK is the central metabolic sensor activated by elevated AMP/ATP ratios. LKB1 is a human tumor suppressor kinase that is a crucial upstream molecule for the activation of AMPK and hence links cell metabolism to growth control and cell polarity [21]. During nutrient and energy depletion, ATP becomes depleted while the AMP/ATP ratio rises, activating the energy-sensing kinase, LKB1, which consequently activates AMPK. The AMPK regulates mTORC1 by direct phosphorylation of the tumor suppressor tuberous sclerosis complex 2 (TSC2) to activate mTORC1 via Rheb GTPase (**Figure 1**).

2.5. Nuclear factor-kB

Aberrant activation of the nuclear factor kappa B (NF-kB) family of dimeric transcription factors has been linked to most cellular processes in tumor evolution including inflammation, transformation, proliferation, invasion, metastasis, and chemoresistance [22]. The most common constitutively active form reported in human malignancies is the p50/RelA dimer, but other forms, such as p50/p50, p52/p52, p52/RelA, p50/c-Rel, c-Rel/c-Rel, p52/RelB, and p50/RelB, have also been identified [22]. In normal inactivated state, this transcription factor is sequestered in the cytoplasm by its inhibitor IkB (**Figure 3**). In order to be activated, IkB must be phosphorylated by the IkB kinase (IKK) complex and degraded via proteasome, causing the liberation and translocation of NF-kB into the nucleus where it modulates gene expression.

Experimental evidence demonstrates that NF-kB can positively regulate autophagy (**Figure 3**). For instance, RelA upregulates Beclin 1 expression through direct binding to the NF-kB-binding site on the Beclin 1 gene promoter to induce autophagy [23]. The multilevel control of autophagy by the IKK/IkB/NF-kB axis is also highlighted by the finding that IKK may also promote the autophagic pathway in a manner independent of NF-kB. All these findings support the idea that NF-kB activation promotes autophagy.

3. Metabolic stress resistance

Metabolism is the process by which cells convert relatively simple extracellular nutrients into energy and building blocks necessary for their growth and survival. In cancer cells, metabolism is dramatically altered compared with normal cells.

Metabolic stress in tumors arises from multiple factors, including cell growth and proliferation in the setting of fluctuating supplies of oxygen and nutrients. Lack of adequate blood supply leads to several stress types in tumors: hypoxia, nutrient deprivation, and the accumulation of metabolic waste products [15]. These stress types are relieved in part by the over-expression of hypoxia-inducible factors (HIFs) to release proangiogenic factors for the construction of a tumor-associated vasculature. Persistent metabolic stress in tumors provokes the rewiring of the metabolic network to accommodate the stressful tumor microenvironment [17].

Metabolic reprogramming is a hallmark of cancer cells and is used by them for growth and survival. Their metabolism is highly dependent on glycolysis instead of mitochondrial oxidative phosphorylation, regardless of oxygen availability, a process termed as Warburg effect [15]. Glycolysis alone, although relatively inefficient means to produce ATP, provides a mechanism for rapid energy generation and a source of carbon for macromolecular synthesis. In addition, the shift to glycolytic metabolism allows rapidly proliferating cells to support both energy production and biosynthesis [15]. In addition, the glycolytic pathway generates metabolites that can be efficiently diverted into pathways that support nucleotide and amino acid biosynthesis in cycling cells [15].

One interesting facet, from a chemotherapeutic point of view, is that, in a large number of cases, cells undergoing a Warburg effect exhibit a marked dependence upon glutamine, to the extent that these cells are referred to as being "glutamine addicted" [24]. Glutamine addiction arises from the need for extracellular glutamine to be consumed for anaplerotic input in the citric acid cycle, which accounts for the majority of the bioenergetic needs of normal (non-transformed) cells. Cancer cells rely heavily on glutamine as a source of carbon and nitrogen for the synthesis of ATP, proteins, lipids, nucleic acids, and the antioxidant glutathione. Expression of the Wnt target MYC proto-oncogene increases glutamine uptake by stimulating expression of the glutamine transporters. At the same time, MYC increases the levels of glutaminase 1 (GLS1), the enzyme that converts glutamine to glutamate [15, 24].

During oncogenesis, the survival signaling pathways such as PI3K, intermediate metabolism, and autophagy constitute the metabolism-signaling supernetwork reprogrammed in ways that support aberrant cell growth, proliferation, and stress resistance. Indeed, emerging evidence suggests that autophagy is an important source of amino acids that supports the stressed cell's biosynthetic and bioenergetic needs.

4. Hypoxia and drug resistance

Diminished oxygen availability (hypoxia) is a hallmark of the tumor microenvironment. A major regulator of cellular adaptation to hypoxia is the hypoxia-inducible factor (HIF) family of transcription factors, which play key roles in many crucial aspects of cancer biology including angiogenesis, stem cell maintenance, metabolic reprogramming, resistance to apoptosis, autocrine growth factor signaling, the epithelial-mesenchymal transition (EMT) program, genetic instability, invasion, metastasis, and radiation resistance [25] (**Figure 4**). HIFs also cause autophagy establishment, particularly in RAS-driven and BRAF-driven cancers, such as most colorectal carcinomas (**Figure 4**). However, the relevance of the relation between HIFs and autophagy in drug resistance is not well understood.

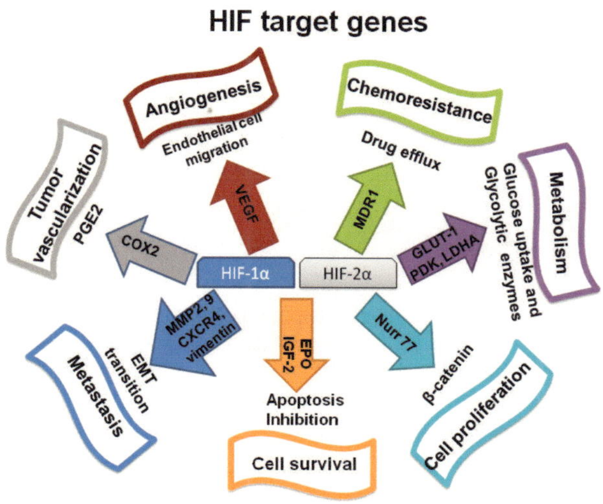

Figure 4. HIF target genes. The cellular processes regulated by HIF-1α and HIF-2α genes are indicated and also the target genes for each one.

HIFs are heterodimeric transcription factors consisting of an O_2-sensitive subunit HIF-α and a stable subunit HIF-β (or ARNT) that are expressed constitutively at the transcriptional and translational levels (**Figure 5**). In mammals, three HIF-α isoforms have been identified but HIF-1α and HIF-2α are the two best-studied members of the HIF-α family. Under normoxic conditions, the cellular stability and activity of HIF-α subunits are highly dependent on oxygen supply. Prolyl hydroxylases hydroxylate key proline residues on HIFs, which allows them to interact with the von Hippel-Lindau (pVHL) tumor suppressor, which is a component of an E3 ubiquitin ligase complex that targets HIF-α for proteasomal degradation (**Figure 5**). Hypoxic conditions stabilize HIF-α by inhibiting its hydroxylation and proteasomal degradation, making HIF-α capable to translocate to the nucleus and dimerize with ARNT activating the transcription of hypoxia-associated genes [25, 26]. Importantly, high levels of HIFs expression have also been detected in tumor cells in the absence of hypoxia (**Figure 5**) because the sustained oncogenic signaling mediated by growth factors in cancer cells can induce HIF-α expression through O_2-independent mechanisms, including increased transcription and/or translation of HIF-α mRNA [27, 28]. In this respect, we have reported that colon carcinoma cells co-express HIF-1α and HIF-2α under normoxic conditions, in contrast to nonmalignant colon cells, which do not express these factors under these conditions [3].

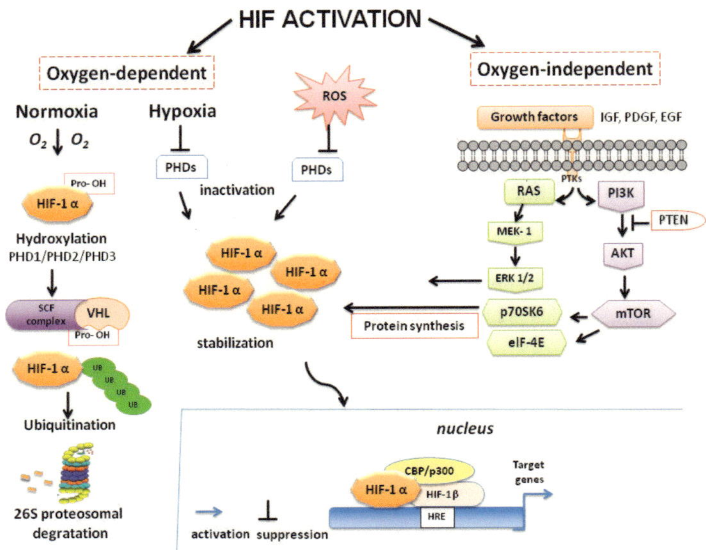

Figure 5. HIF activation. HIFs are heterodimeric transcription factors subjected to O_2-sensitive or O_2-independent mode of activation, as indicated in the figure. Both types of regulation converge in HIF protein stabilization, which can enter to the nucleus to bind HIF-1β at HIF-responsive elements (HRE) to activate target genes.

Hypoxia can lead to therapeutic resistance through diverse mechanisms [29, 30]: (1) direct effects due to the requirement of some drugs and radiation of lack of oxygen in order to be maximally cytotoxic, (2) indirect effects by altering cellular metabolism to decrease drug cytotoxicity, and (3) enhanced genetic instability which in turn leads to more rapid induction of drug resistance in tumor cells [29, 30]. HIF-1α and to a lesser extent HIF-2α have been associated with radio- and chemotherapy failure for decades [30] and interference with HIF function holds great promise to improve future anticancer therapy.

4.1. Hypoxia-induced drug resistance through metabolic alteration

One of the possible mechanisms of resistance to anticancer therapy in hypoxic tumor is the switching of cellular metabolism from oxidative phosphorylation to aerobic glycolysis (Warburg effect), a hallmark of cancer cells. As a result, cancer cells eventually develop a system that uses cytoplasmic glycolysis to generate ATP instead of mitochondrial oxidative respiration, even in the presence of oxygen. Several reports have indicated that activation of the HIF-1α signaling pathway under glucose deprivation induces resistance to cell death by apoptosis in human colon cancer cells and that targeting the HIF-1α signaling pathway may provide an effective way to treat resistant cancers to conventional therapy [31].

4.2. Hypoxia-induced drug resistance through increased drug efflux

HIF-1α upregulation has been shown to induce expression of drug efflux transporters, to alter the activity of DNA repair mechanisms, and to shift the balance between pro- and antiapoptotic factors toward cell survival [32].

Drug efflux is an important mechanism to chemoresistance in many solid tumors, including colon cancer. The multidrug resistance 1 (MDR1) gene, encoding the membrane-resident P-glycoprotein (P-gp) that belongs to a family of ATP-binding cassette (ABC) transporters, has been found to be a HIF-1α target gene [33]. The multidrug resistance-associated protein 1 (MRP1) is another ABC transporter encoded by the *ABCC1/MRP1* gene that confers cellular resistance to a broad range of structurally and functionally chemotherapeutic agents. Recently, it has been demonstrated that MRP1 is a downstream target gene of HIF-1α in human colon cancer LoVo cells. Genetic inhibition of HIF-1α by siRNA and dominant-negative HIF-1α reduced the expression of MRP1, which provides a potential novel mechanism for HIF-1α-mediated drug resistance [34].

4.3. Hypoxia-induced drug resistance through inhibition of apoptotic pathways and induction of autophagy

Defective apoptosis and/or changes in cell cycle regulation represent pivotal causes for drug resistance [35]. It has been proposed that increased cell survival, due to a shift favoring antiapoptotic pathways, is a primary mechanism of hypoxia-induced drug resistance [36]. In the vast majority of transformed cells, HIF-1α functions as a suppressor of apoptosis and functional interference with HIF-1α results in enhanced cell death upon treatment with chemotherapeutic agents in tumors of different origins [26]. Through the inhibition of proapoptotic and induction of antiapoptotic genes, HIF-1α can inhibit apoptosis and promote tumor cell survival in chemotherapy-treated cancer cells.

In colorectal cancer, the combination therapy of rapamycin, inhibitor of mTOR which regulates autophagy, and irinotecan, which is able to inhibit the accumulation of HIF-1α, has been reported to induce massive death of colon cancer cells under hypoxic, but not normoxic conditions in vitro, and a great reduction of tumor volume in vivo [37].

Enhanced autophagy has been associated with the elevated level of HIF-1α in several cancer types. In this regard, it has been observed that hypoxia-mediated failure of cytotoxic treatment in vitro can be conferred via HIF-1α-dependent induction of autophagy [14], but the relevance of the intriguing relation between HIF-1α and autophagy for drug resistance is still not known.

5. Role of autophagy in stress resistance

Autophagy is a term derived from the Greek words "auto" (self) and "phagy" (to eat) and refers to a multistep lysosomal degradation process in which a cell degrades damaged organelles and longlived proteins to maintain cellular homeostasis, particularly during exposure to stressful conditions. Three forms of autophagy have been identified based upon the mode of delivery to the lysosome, namely, macroautophagy, microautophagy, and chaperone-mediated autophagy. Macroautophagy (autophagy), the best characterized, is a major regulated catabolic process that involves the delivery of cytoplasmic cargo sequestered inside double-membrane vesicles to the lysosome [38]. The other two forms, microautophagy and chaperone-mediated autophagy, involve a direct membrane invagination to engulf damaged proteins and the translocation of soluble cytosolic proteins by chaperone-dependent selection across the lysosomal membrane, respectively [39]. Thirty-six genes (ATGs for AuTophaGy), have been identified that are required for the autophagy process to occur. Dysregulation of autophagy, which alters the rate of protein degradation and the metabolic state of the cells, has severe consequences and is associated with several pathophysiological conditions, such as cancer.

The best-characterized regulator of autophagy is mTOR, which integrates growth factor and nutrient signals to influence protein synthesis, growth, autophagy, and ribosomal biogenesis. M-TOR occurs in two multiprotein complexes, mTORC1, containing the specific binding proteins raptor and PRAS40, and mTORC2 containing rictor and other binding partners [38]. When nutrients are available, mTORC1 phosphorylates Unc-51-like kinase (ULK1) and ATG13 to block autophagy initiation. When nutrients are scarce, mTORC1 dissociates from the ULK1 complex, initiating the autophagy process [15, 40]. The initiation of autophagy occurs with the assembly of the double-membrane phagophore, the precursor of the autophagosome. This requires the formation of a protein complex constituted by Class III phosphatidylinositol 3-kinase (PtdIns3K) and the proteins VPS34, p150, ATG14, and BECLIN 1. In tumors, autophagy is stimulated by metabolic stress (e.g., nutrient/growth factor deprivation, hypoxia, and acidosis), cellular damage, or inhibition of pro-survival signals caused by anticancer therapies [41]. Through autophagy, cancer cells utilize a highly plastic and dynamic mechanism to either repress initial steps of carcinogenesis or support the survival and growth of established tumors [42, 43].

In multicellular organisms, autophagy also clears ubiquitinated or malfunctioning aggregated proteins. This selective degradative process is mediated through the recognition of ubiquitin-tagged cargos by the autophagy receptor p62/sequestosome 1 [44]. This protein directs them to the autophagosome through concomitant binding to the LC3 (microtubule associated protein 1 light chain 3) molecules localized at the inner and outer autophagosome membranes. Autophagy is responsible for the degradation of p62, and therefore, when autophagy is inhibited, p62 accumulates in mammalian cells.

Autophagy facilitates cancer cell resistance to chemotherapy treatment, and the inhibition of autophagy may potentiate the resensitization of therapeutic-resistant cancer cells to anticancer drugs. Chemotherapy treatment conferred resistance by triggering key autophagy signaling molecules in malignant cells. For example, in response to irinotecan, pro-survival autophagy was induced by activating MAPK14/p38 signaling, which lead to drug resistance [45]. It is likely that protective autophagy in 5-Fluouracil (5-FU) resistance occurs through c-Jun N-terminal Kinase (JNK) activation [46]. Given the propensity of PI3K-mTOR inhibition to robustly induce autophagy, increased autophagic flux is a suspect contributor to the modest efficacy of PI3K inhibitors. Several recent studies have provided evidence that combined inhibition of autophagy and PI3K inhibitors or a combination therapy with a mTORC1 inhibitor (temsirolimus) and autophagy inhibitor [hydroxychloroquine (HCQ)] can sensitize cells to chemotherapeutic agents [15, 47]. Several other trials that combine HCQ with radiation therapy or chemotherapeutic agents have also been used on the basis of the accumulating preclinical evidence supporting the notion that increased autophagy promotes therapy-induced resistance in tumor cells.

Examining the role of autophagy in RAS- and BRAF-induced transformation in colon cancer cell lines, Goulielmaki et al. [20] found that the MEK/ERK pathway can increase the protein levels of LC3, unlike the AKT/MTOR pathway, which has been shown to abolish the autophagic process. They showed that using specific autophagy inhibitors not only cancer cell proliferation rate can be reduced, but the otherwise resistant mutant BRAF colon cell lines to targeted BRAF agents, like PLX4720 (Vemurafenib), can be sensitized to apoptosis in a synergistic manner. This study proposed a promising rational combinatorial treatment using BRAF and autophagy inhibitors that will potentially provide efficient therapeutic protocols for these otherwise untreatable tumors.

6. Contribution of stem cells to resistance

The intestinal epithelium is an example of self-renewing tissue on expense of stem cells that reside at the crypt bottom. Tumor growth is sustained by a subpopulation of highly malignant cancer stem cells (CSCs) or tumor-initiating cells, which are characterized by a life-long capacity to self-renew, are multipotent, and can reversibly enter quiescent or even dormant states and resist cytotoxic drugs [48]. Successful treatment is thus dependent on the selective elimination of these highly resistant subpopulations, instead of only the main tumor mass. Over the past decade, several cell surface markers have been identified in these cell populations. CD133, Lgr5, and CD44 are the most frequently proposed stem cell markers in colorectal cancer, but their distribution differs between patients and tumor cell lines [48, 49].

CD133 (also called prominin-1) is a pentaspan transmembrane glycoprotein identified as cell surface stem cell marker that has been associated with tumorigenicity and progression of colon cancer [50], but its precise role and functions are unknown. CD44 is a transmembrane glycoprotein involved in cell-cell and cell-matrix adhesion through its affinity for hyaluronic acid. CD44 is encoded by a single gene, including 20 exons. The standard form, expressed in normal adult stem cells (referred to as CD44), consists of exons 1–5 and 15–20. Importantly, it has been demonstrated that cancer cells express different exon variants, such as CD44v6, produced by alternative splicing mRNA processing [48]. Thus, universal targeting of CD44 might be deleterious for patients and they can be avoided targeting different isoforms of CD44.

Several studies have implicated the potential contribution of a subpopulation of stem-like progenitor cells in resistance to both chemotherapeutic and targeted therapies [51]. Various groups have characterized the drug-resistant aspects of such stem-like subpopulations, including a quiescent state refractory to agents targeting rapidly dividing cells, enhanced DNA damage repair mechanisms, and decreased apoptotic machinery [52]. Recent studies have implicated a potential mechanistic link between EGFR activation and the acquisition of stem-like properties including the increase in known stem cell markers and enhanced spheroid formation [53]; however, the role of EGFR in promoting stem cell properties in CRC has not been fully characterized.

The radioresistance of cancer stems cells has been supported by several research groups in glioma and head and neck, breast, pancreatic, and colorectal cancer [48, 54]. Radiation itself has also been shown to increase the expression of AKT and CD133 and reduce the expression of CD44 in colorectal cancer cells [55]. Sahlberg et al. [48] found that cells with a CD44high/CD133high expression demonstrated a higher radioresistance compared to CD44low/CD133low cells and that different AKT isoforms have varying effects on the expression of cancer stem cell markers, which is an important consideration when targeting AKT in a clinical setting.

There is experimental evidence that hypoxia is associated with the maintenance and formation of CSCs, promoting their phenotype and tumorigenesis [56]. It has also been shown that hypoxia, by means of HIF-1α activation, is capable of maintaining CSCs phenotype in colon cancer cells [57]. However, it has been recognized that the resident microenvironment of cancer cells, also known as a "niche," plays an important role in the genetic instability, metastasis, and therapeutic resistance of CSCs [25]. Mao et al. [58] demonstrated that most CD133+ colon CSCs are located in a hypoxic niche, where oxaliplatin, rather than 5-FU, inhibits proliferation of these colon CSC cells. Recently several drugs have discovered to be selective against CSC. Examples of them are microbe-derived and plant-derived biomolecules; small inhibitors that target key signaling pathways of CSCs such as metformin, tranilast, and thioridazine; and also antibodies directed against CSC-specific cell surface molecules, such as the CD44, CD47, EpCAM, CD123, GD2, Lgr5, IGF-IR, Dll4, and FZD receptors [59].

7. Microvesicles: devices of intercellular communication

It has been demonstrated recently that challenging cancer cells with stresses that they would typically encounter during tumor progression, or as a part of a therapeutic regiment to treat or manage the disease, increase the rate of microvesicles (MVs referred also as oncosomes or exosomes), formation, and shedding by cells [5–7]. Interestingly, the noncanonical Wnt signaling pathways PCP and Wnt/Ca^{2+} appear to be involved in the regulation of MV biogenesis and budding in human cancer cells, since one of their downstream effectors, the Rho subfamily GTPase, that induce cell spreading and migration, has been demonstrated to promote the rearrangements of the actin cytoskeleton to stimulate MV budding [60, 61].

MVs generally range in size from 0.1 to 2 μm in diameter. In addition to containing conventional paracrine signaling molecules, such as growth factors and pro-inflammatory cytokines, MVs also contain membrane-associated, cytosolic, and nuclear molecules not normally released by normal cells such as metabolic enzymes, metalloproteases, molecular chaperones, and miRNAs and RNA transcripts [6, 7]. The uptake of MVs by cells has the potential to protect them from a variety of apoptotic challenges by up-regulating the expression and/or activation of proteins that work to counter the actions of cell death machinery. That is why recent findings suggesting that MVs can promote cell survival and contribute to drug resistance are possibly of significant value.

In addition, because cancer cell-derived MVs often contain oncogenic proteins that reflect their cell of origin, and their abundance and protein concentration correlate with the tumor grade/aggressiveness, they have been converted in the focus for searching cancer biomarkers and/or for monitoring tumor progression.

8. Concluding remarks

Mammalian cells coordinate cell metabolism and growth with environmentally induced stress. In cancer cells, survival signaling cascades, metabolism, and autophagy are corrupted and work in a highly integrated network to cope with stressful conditions such as hypoxia, limited nutrients, and drugs, in order to maintain viability and proliferative activity.

Understanding the signaling networks that contribute to cancer cell survival and how the changes in those networks allow cells to adapt in the presence of drugs that target key components implicated in cancer cell survival and proliferation is the challenge. Thus, we are hopeful that a better understanding of the signaling pathways involved and the development of strategies to inhibit autophagy and/or hypoxia represent a new approach to enhance the efficacy of cancer therapy to overcome therapeutic resistance in cancer cells.

Author details

Dora M. Velázquez, María Cristina Castañeda-Patlán and Martha Robles-Flores*

*Address all correspondence to: rmartha@unam.mx

Department of Biochemistry, Faculty of Medicine, National Autonomous University of Mexico (UNAM), Mexico City, Mexico

References

[1] Behrens J. Everything you would like to know about Wnt signaling. Sci Signal 2013, 6:pe17

[2] Clevers H, Nusse R. Wnt/β-catenin signaling and disease. Cell 2012, 149:1182–1205.

[3] Santoyo-Ramos P, Likhatcheva M, Castañeda-Patlán MC, García-Zepeda E, Robles-Flores M. Hypoxia-inducible factors modulate the stemness and malignancy of colon cancer cells by playing opposite roles in canonical Wnt signaling. PLoS One 2014, 9(11):e112580.

[4] Xie X, White EP, Mehnert JM. Coordinate autophagy and mTOR pathway inhibition enhances cell death in melanoma. PLoS One 2013; 8 (1): e55096

[5] Antonyak MA, Li B, Boroughs LK, et al. Cancer cell-derived microvesicles induce transformation by transferring tissue transglutaminase and fibronectin to recipient cells. Proc Natl Acad Sci U S A 2011, 108:4852–4857

[6] Peinado H, Aleckovic M, Lavotshkin S, et al. Melanoma exosomes educate bone marrow progenitor cells toward a pro-metastatic phenotype through MET. Nat Med 2012, 18:883–891.

[7] D'Souza-Schorey C, Clancy JW. Tumor-derived microvesicles: shedding light on novel microenvironment modulators and prospective cancer biomarkers. Genes Dev 2012, 26:1287–1299.

[8] Ono M, Kosaka N, Tominaga N, Yoshida Y, Tsuda H, Tamura K, Ochiya T. Exosomes from bone marrow mesenchymal stem cells contain a microRNA that promotes dormancy in metastatic breast cancer cells. Sci Signal 2014, 7(332):ra63. doi: 10.1126/scisignal.2005231.

[9] Adler EM, Gough NR. Focus issue: rendering resistance futile. Sci Signal 2011, 4(166); eg3.

[10] Belmont PJ, Jiang P, McKee TD, Xie T, Isaacson J, Baryla NE, Roper J, Sinnamon MJ, Lee NV, Kan JLC, Guicherit O, Wouters VG, O'Brien CA, Shields D, Olson P, Van Arsdale T, Weinrich SL, Rejto P, Christensen JG, Fantin VR, Hung KE, Martin ES. Resistance to dual blockade of the kinases PI3K and mTOR in KRAS-mutant colorectal cancer models results in combined sensitivity to inhibition of the receptor tyrosine kinase EGFR. Sci Signal 2014, 7(351):ra107.

[11] Crea F, Nobili S, Paolicchi E, Perrone G, Napoli C, Landini I, Danesi R, Mini E. Epigenetics and chemoresistance in colorectal cancer: an opportunity for treatment tailoring and novel therapeutic strategies. Drug Resist Updat 2011, 14:280–296

[12] Yang AD, Fan F, Camp ER, van Buren G, Liu W, Somcio R, Gray MJ, Cheng H, Hoff PM, Ellis LM. Chronic oxaliplatin resistance induces epithelial-to-mesenchymal transition in colorectal cancer cell lines. Clin Cancer Res 2006, 12:4147–4153.

[13] Singh A, Settleman J, EMT, cancer stem cells and drug resistance: an emerging axis of evil in the war on cancer. Oncogene 2010, 29:4741–4751.

[14] Martz CA, Ottina KA, Singleton KR, Jasper JS, Wardell SE, Peraza-Penton A, Anderson GR, Winter PS, Wang T, Alley HM, Kwong LN, Cooper ZA, Tetzlaff M, Chen PL, Rathmell JC, Flaherty KT, Wargo JA, McDonnell DP, Sabatini DM, Wood KC. Systematic identification of signaling pathways with potential to confer anticancer drug resistance. Sci Signal 2014, 7(357); ra121.

[15] Shanware NP, Bray K, Abraham RT. The PI3K, metabolic, and autophagy networks: interactive partners in cellular health and disease. Annu Rev Pharmacol Toxicol 2013, 53:89–106

[16] Manning BD, Cantley LC. AKT/PKB signaling: navigating downstream. Cell 2007, 129:1261–1274

[17] Miyamoto DT, Zheng Y, Wittner BS, Lee RJ, Zhu H, Broderick KT, Desai R, Fox DB, Brannigan BW, Trautwein J, Arora KS, Desai N, Dahl DM, Sequist LV, Smith MR, Kapur R, Wu CH, Shioda K, Ramaswamy S, Ting DT, Toner M, Maheswaran S, Haber DA. RNA-Seq of single prostate CTCs implicates noncanonical Wnt signaling in antiandrogen resistance. Sci Signal 2015, 349(6254):1351–1356.

[18] Little AS, Balmanno K, Sale MJ, Newman S, Dry JR, Hampson M, Edwards PAW, Smith PD, Cook SJ. Amplification of the driving oncogene, KRAS or BRAF, underpins acquired resistance to MEK1/2 inhibitors in colorectal cáncer cells. Sci Signal 2011, 4:ra17.

[19] Corcoran RB, Dias-Santagata D, Bergethon K, Iafrate AJ, Settleman J, Engelman JA. BRAF gene amplification can promote acquired resistance to MEK inhibitors in cancer cells harboring the BRAF V600E mutation. Sci Signal 2010, 3:ra84.

[20] Goulielmaki M, Koustas E, Moysidou E, Vlassi M, Sasazuki T, Shirasawa S, Zografos G, Oikonomou E, Pintzas A. BRAF associated autophagy exploitation: BRAF and autophagy inhibitors synergise to efficiently overcome resistance of BRAF mutant colorectal cancer cells. Oncotarget 2016, 7(8):9188–9221.

[21] Shackelford DB, Shaw RJ. The LKB1–AMPK pathway: metabolism and growth control in tumour suppression. Nat Rev Cancer 2009, 9:563–575.

[22] Chen F, Castranova V. Nuclear factor-kappaB, an unappreciated tumor suppressor. Cancer Res 2007, 67:11093–11098.

[23] Copetti T, Bertoli C, Dalla E, Demarchi F, Schneider C. p65/RelA modulates BECN1 transcription and autophagy. Mol Cell Biol 2009, 29:2594–2608.

[24] Katt WP, Cerione RA. Glutaminase regulation in cancer cells: a druggable chain of events. Drug Discov Today 2014, 19(4):450–457.

[25] Semenza, G.L. Defining the role of hypoxia-inducible factor 1 in cancer biology and therapeutics. Oncogene 2010, 29:625–634.

[26] Rohwer N, Cramer T. Hypoxia-mediated drug resistance: novel insights on the functional interaction of HIFs and cell death pathways. Drug Resist Updat 2011, 14:191–201.

[27] Koh MY, Powis G. HAF: the new player in oxygen-independent HIF-1α degradation. Cell Cycle 2009, 8: 1359–1366.

[28] Richard DE, Berra E, Gothié E, Roux D, Pouysségur J. P42/P44 mitogen activated protein kinases phosphorylate hypoxia-inducible factor 1 alpha and enhance the transcriptional activity of HIF-1. J Biol Chem 1999, 274:32631–32637.

[29] Teicher, B.A. Hypoxia and drug resistance. Cancer Metastasis Rev 1994, 13:139–168.

[30] Mimeault M, Batra S. Hypoxia-inducing factors as master regulators of stemness properties and altered metabolism of cancer- and metastasis-initiating cells. J Cell Mol Med 2013, 17:30–54.

[31] Nishimoto A, Kugimiya N, Hosoyama T, Enoki T, Li T-S, Hamano K. HIF-1α activation under glucose deprivation plays a central role in the acquisition of anti-apoptosis in human colon cancer cells. Int J Oncol 2014, 44:2077–2084.

[32] Semenza GL. HIF-1 mediates metabolic responses to intratumoral hypoxia and oncogenic mutations. J Clin Invest 2013, 123:3664–3671.

[33] Comerford KM, Wallace TJ, Karhausen J, Louis NA, Montalto MC, Colgan SP. Hypoxia-inducible factor-1-dependent regulation of the multidrug resistance (MDR1) gene. Cancer Res 2002, 62:3387–3394.

[34] Lv Y, Zhao S, Han J, Zheng L, Yang Z, Zhao L. Hypoxia-inducible factor-1α induces multidrug resistance protein in colon cancer. Onco Targets Ther 2015, 5:1941–1948.

[35] Brown JM, Attardi LD. The role of apoptosis in cancer development and treatment response. Nat Rev Cancer 2005, 5:231–237.

[36] Erler, J.T., Cawthorne, C.J., Williams, K.J., Koritzinsky, M., Wouters, B.G., Wilson, C. Hypoxia-mediated down-regulation of Bid and Bax in tumors occurs via hypoxia-inducible factor 1-dependent and -independent mechanisms and contributes to drug resistance. Mol Cell Biol 2004, 24:2875–2889.

[37] Pencreach E, Guerin E, Nicolet C, Lelong-Rebel I, Voegeli AC, Oudet P, Larsen AK, Gaub MP and Guenot D. Marked activity of irinotecan and rapamycin combination toward colon cancer cells in vivo and in vitro is mediated through cooperative modulation of the mammalian target of rapamycin/hypoxia-inducible factor-1alpha axis. Clin Cancer Res 2009, 15:1297–1307.

[38] Mizushima N, Komatsu M. Autophagy: renovation of cells and tissues. Cell 2011, 147:728–741.

[39] Klionsky DJ. The molecular machinery of autophagy: unanswered questions. J Cell Sci 2005, 118:7–18.

[40] Xie CM, Liu XY, Sham KW, Lai JM, Cheng CH. Silencing of EEF2K (eukaryotic elongation factor-2 kinase) reveals AMPK–ULK1-dependent autophagy in colon cancer cells. Autophagy 2014, 10:1495–1508.

[41] Simonsen A, Tooze SA. Coordination of membrane events during autophagy by multiple class III PI3-kinase complexes. J Cell Biol 2009, 186:773–782.

[42] Geng J, Klionsky DJ. The Atg8 and Atg12 ubiquitin-like conjugation systems in macroautophagy. EMBO Rep 2008, 9:859–864.

[43] Kabeya Y, Mizushima N, Ueno T, Yamamoto A, Kirisako T, Noda T, Kominami E, et al. LC3, a mammalian homologue of yeast Apg8p, is localized in autophagosome membranes after processing. EMBO J 2000, 19:5720–5728.

[44] Pankiv S, Clausen TH, Lamark T, Brech A, Bruun JA, Outzen H, et al. p62/SQSTM1 binds directly to Atg8/LC3 to facilitate degradation of ubiquitinated protein aggregates by autophagy. J Biol Chem 2007, 282:24131–24145.

[45] Paillas S, Causse A, Marzi L, de Medina P, Poirot M, Denis V, et al. MAPK14/p38 confers irinotecan resistance to TP53-defective cells by inducing survival autophagy. Autophagy 2012, 8:1098–1112

[46] Sui X, Kong N, Wang X, Fang Y, Hu X, Xu Y, et al. JNK confers 5-fluorouracil resistance in p53-deficient and mutant p53-expressing colon cancer cells by inducing survival autophagy. Sci Rep 2014, 4:4694.

[47] Li J, Hou N, Faried A, Tsutsumi S, Kuwano H. Inhibition of autophagy augments 5-fluorouracil chemotherapy in human colon cancer in vitro and in vivo model. Eur J Cancer 2010, 46:1900–1909.

[48] Sahlberg SH, Spiegelberg D, Glimelius B, Stenerlo B , Nestor M. Evaluation of cancer stem cell markers CD133, CD44, CD24: association with AKT isoforms and radiation resistance in colon cancer cells. PLoS One 2014, 9(4):e94621

[49] Chu P, Clanton DJ, Snipas TS, Lee J, Mitchell E, et al. Characterization of a subpopulation of colon cancer cells with stem cell-like properties. Int J Cancer 2009, 124:1312–1321.

[50] Horst D, Scheel SK, Liebmann S, Neumann J, Maatz S, et al. The cáncer stem cell marker CD133 has high prognostic impact but unknown functional relevance for the metastasis of human colon cancer. J Pathol 2009, 219:427–434.

[51] Dallas NA, Xia L, Fan F, Gray MJ, Gaur P, van Buren Jr.G, Samuel S, Kim MP, Lim SJ, Ellis LM. Chemoresistant colorectal cancer cells, the cancer stem cell phenotype, and increased sensitivity to insulin-like growth factor-I receptor inhibition. Cancer Res 2009, 69:1951–1957.

[52] Dean M, Fojo T, Bates S. Tumour stem cells and drug resistance. Nat Rev Cancer 2005, 5:275–284.

[53] Abhold EL, Kiang A, Rahimy E, Kuo SZ, Wang-Rodriguez J, Lopez JP, Blair KJ, Yu MA, Haas M, Brumund KT, Altuna X, Patel A, Weisman RA, Ongkeko WM. EGFR kinase promotes acquisition of stem cell-like properties: a potential therapeutic target in head and neck squamous cell carcinoma stem cells. PLoS One 2012, 7:e32459.

[54] Saigusa S, Tanaka K, Toiyama Y, Yokoe T, Okugawa Y, et al. Immunohistochemical features of CD133 expression: association with resistance to chemoradiotherapy in rectal cancer. Oncol Rep 2010, 24:345–350.

[55] Kawamoto A, Tanaka K, Saigusa S, Toiyama Y, Morimoto Y, et al. Clinical significance of radiation-induced CD133 expression in residual rectal cancer cells after chemoradiotherapy. Exp Ther Med 2012, 3:403–409.

[56] Mohyeldin A, Garzon-Muvdi T, Quinones-Hinojosa A. Oxygen in stem cell biology: a critical component of the stem cell niche. Cell Stem Cell 2010, 7:150–161.

[57] Yeung TM, Gandhi SC, Bodmer WF. Hypoxia and lineage specification of cell line-derived colorectal cancer stem cells. Proc Natl Acad Sci U S A 2011, 108: 4382–4387.

[58] Mao Q, Zhang Y, Fu X, Xue J, Guo W, Meng M, Zhou Z, Mo X, and Lu Y. A tumor hypoxic niche protects human colon cancer stem cells from chemotherapy. J Cancer Res Clin Oncol 2013, 139:211–222

[59] Garza-Treviño EN, Said-Fernández SL, Martínez-Rodríguez HG. Understanding the colon cancer stem cells and perspectives on treatment. Cancer Cell Int 2015, 15:2. doi: 10.1186/s12935-015-0163-7.

[60] Antonyak MA, Wilson KF, Cerione RA. R(h)oads to microvesicles. Small GTPases 2012, 3:219–224.

[61] Li B, Antonyak MA, Zhang J et al. RhoA triggers a specific signaling pathway that generates transforming microvesicles in cancer cells. Oncogene 2012, 31:4740-4749.

Chapter 2

Circadian Regulation of Colon Cancer Stem Cells: Implications for Therapy

Sandra Ríos-Arrabal, José Antonio Muñoz-Gámez, Sergio Manuel Jiménez-Ruíz, Jorge Casado-Ruíz, Francisco Artacho-Cordón and Josefa León-López

Additional information is available at the end of the chapter

http://dx.doi.org/10.5772/62323

Abstract

The presence of cancer stem cells (CSCs) in colorectal cancer (CRC) has been associated with tumor initiation, metastasis, relapse, and resistance to chemotherapy and radiotherapy. Therefore, a better knowledge of the molecular mechanisms involved in the regulation of CSCs is required to develop treatments that are more effective. Like normal cells, cancer cells contain molecular clocks that generate circadian rhythms in gene expression and metabolic activity. Disruption of circadian rhythms has been linked to increased cancer risk, chemoresistance, and progression in CRC. CSCs also generate rhythms, which could be exploited with a chronopharmacological approach. Although the regulation of the expression of circadian rhythm genes appears to be mediated mainly by transcription–translation feedback loops, the existence of forms of nontranscriptional regulation has been demonstrated. Particularly, microRNAs (miRNA) and SIRT1 are significant players in regulating various aspects of the circadian clock function. Furthermore, miRNA acts as a regulator of cancer progression by regulating the CSC characteristics through SIRT1. These findings led us to hypothesize that there is a circadian rhythm of CSC markers regulated by miRNAs in CRC with SIRT1 acting as a mediator of miRNA activity. The pharmacological regulation of SIRT1, and therefore of the circadian machinery, could result in antiproliferative effects and increased sensitivity to antitumor treatments in CRC.

Keywords: circadian rhythms, cancer stem cells, SIRT1, redox homeostasis, melatonin

1. Introduction

Cancer is a major health burden and one of the leading causes of death worldwide. There are more than 200 known types of cancer, being CRC one of the most common cancers. In men, CRC is the third most common, after lung and prostate cancer. In women, CRC is the second most common cancer behind breast cancer [1].

Cancer begins with the transformation of a normal cell into a tumor cell through a multistage process. In this process, the changes are the result of the interaction between the genetic factors of the patient and external agents, including physical, chemical, or biological agents. Aging is another fundamental factor in the development of cancer. The coming years will see an increase in the total number of cancer cases [2]. This will be caused by the dramatic increase in average life expectancy during the last century in the industrialized world and by the fact that about 5% of the population in the developed countries is predicted to have more than 85 years by 2050 [3].

CRC is an excellent example of the increased cell malignancy with age; according to the Centers for Control and Prevention of Diseases, the incidence rate of CRC increases progressively with age. In 2007, the Surveillance, Epidemiology, and End Results Program registry reported that CRC incidence was 74.5/100,000 in persons aged 50–64 years, 186.0/100,000 in persons aged 65–74 years, and 290.1/100,000 in persons aged ≥75 years [4].

Little is known about the precise biochemical mechanisms responsible for the rise in CRC rates with aging. Some authors have proposed cancer stem cells/stem-like cells (CSCs/CSLCs) as the main factor associated with age-related rise in CRCs [5]. CSCs are a small subpopulation of cells that might play a critical role in CRC progression and resistance to chemotherapy and radiotherapy. Because of these resistances, CSCs play an important role in the processes of tumor recurrence and metastasis [6–8]. Therefore, it is increasingly likely that therapies that specifically target CSCs will be needed for the complete eradication of the tumor [7] because these cells are responsible for the morbidity and mortality associated with this type of cancer [9].

2. CSCs and CRC

CSCs, also known as tumor-initiating cells, were first identified by John Dick in acute myeloid leukemia in the late 1990s. Since then, they have been an intense focus of cancer research. CSCs have recently been identified in several solid tumors, including breast [10], colon [11], head and neck [12], lung [13], pancreas [14], and central nervous system cancer [15]. CSCs are defined as cancer cells that possess characteristics associated with normal stem cells, specifically the ability to self-renew and differentiate into multiple cell types, in particular into all the heterogeneous cell types found in a particular cancer sample [16] (**Figure 1**).

http://dx.doi.org/10.5772/62323

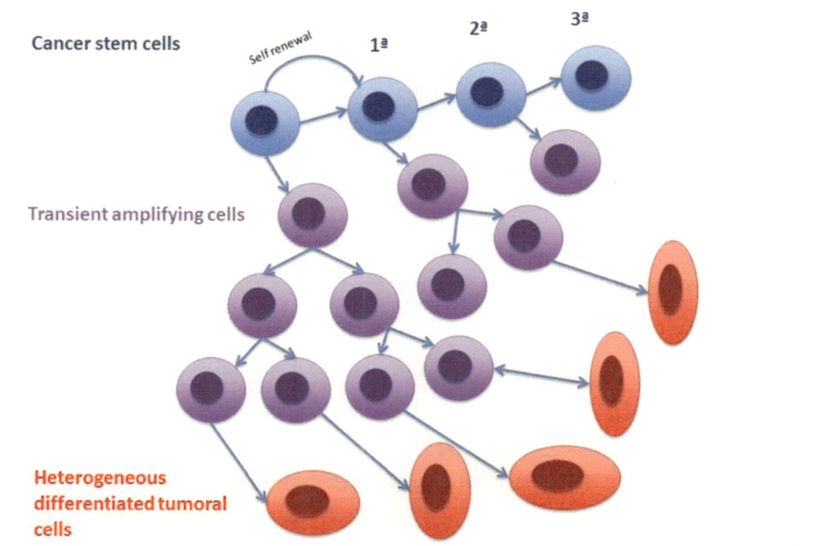

Figure 1. The cancer stem cells (CSCs) theory suggests that tumors grow like normal tissues of the body. In this way, the CSCs are able to both self-renew extensively, copying to them, and to produce the tissue grow (cancer tissue). In this process, the CSCs produce transit amplifying cells that have the capacity to divide a certain number of times, and then, they can differentiate into specialized heterogeneous tumor cells that do not have the skill to divide and therefore do not contribute to tumor growth.

Little is known about the origin of CSCs. Several proposals have been made regarding the origin of CSCs and probably several answers are possible depending on the tumor type and the tumor phenotype. In brief, CSC can arise if there are mutations in a developing stem or progenitor cells, in adult stem cells or adult progenitor cells, or in differentiated cells that acquire stem-like attributes [17]. Some data pointed to adult stem cells as origin of CSC in CRC. In this way, according to the most accepted model of CRC progression [18], four to five mutations in tumor suppressor genes or oncogenes are required and this takes about 8–12 years. As the colonic mucosa is a highly dynamic tissue, the mucosal cells are constantly replaced with cells derived from crypt stem cells. Therefore, only the long-lived cells (stem cells) may serve as reservoirs for accumulation of such mutations and epigenetic modifications.

In CRC, the presence of CSC has been correlated to tumor initiation, progression, metastasis, relapse, and resistance to chemotherapy and radiotherapy. [19]. CSCs have been isolated from CRC and are identified by the expression of specific surface markers and by their functional characteristics: CD44, CD166, CD133, ALDH1 (aldehyde dehydrogenase isoform 1), and ESA (epithelial-specific antigen, also known as EpCAM) [20]. Moreover, CSCs have been involved in the transition from adenoma to carcinoma, and this issue is age-dependent. In addition, an age-related rise in CSC has been observed in normal colonic mucosa and in premalignant adenomatous polyps. Moreover, the CSCs found showed an increased expression of CD44,

CD166, ALDH1, miR-21, and oncogenic miRNA, which suggests a predisposition of the organ to developing colorectal cancer [21]. Another characteristic of CSCs is that they can undergo epithelial–mesenchymal transition [22]. The fact that CSCs are resistant to conventional therapies has important implications in the development of novel strategies, such as CSCs-targeted treatments. It makes sense that eradication of CSCs or, alternatively, the attenuation of their malignant and stemness properties can lead us to achieve more effective therapeutic approaches. Therefore, development of specific CSCs-targeted therapies holds hope for improvement in the survival and quality of life of cancer patients, especially in patients with metastatic disease.

3. Epigenetic phenomena associated with CRC: miRNA regulatory network

Epigenetic processes are potentially reversible genetic modifications that lead to genomic instability and malfunction but that do not involve changes in DNA sequence. Epigenetic changes include (a) altered DNA methylation, (b) chromatin remodeling, and (c) small non-coding RNA (miRNAs). Notable changes in epigenetics have been reported for several age-related diseases, including CRC [23]. miRNAs are a small non-coding RNAs with 18–25 nucleotides found in plants, animals, and some viruses that are involved in RNA silencing and regulation of gene expression at the post-transcriptional level. miRNAs bind to the 3′-untranslated region (3′-UTR) of the protein-coding messenger RNAs (mRNAs). A single miRNA may regulate multiple mRNA targets and these small molecules are predicted to regulate approximately 60% of the human genes [24].

miRNAs are involved in different biological processes, including embryogenesis and the maintenance of stem cell characteristics, cell proliferation, metabolism, and transduction signals as in resistance to cancer treatments, including chemo- and radiotherapy [25, 26]. The presence of certain miRNAs has been associated with tumor development, tumor cell invasion, and cancer metastasis, and they may be of value as biomarkers for tumor detection and prognosis [27]. In addition, evidences show that miRNAs participate as oncogenic or tumor suppressors in the developmental and physiological processes of several human cancers, including CRC.

3.1. miRNA regulatory network in CRC

Approximately 450 unique miRNAs have been associated with CRC. In this disease, the aberrant expression of miRNAs has been associated with initiation and progression of CRC. Of special interest is miRNA involvement in the invasion, migration, and progression of disease through epithelial–mesenchymal transition into metastases. This event occurred due to IL6/STAT3 mediation and/or TP53 inactivation [28]. miRNAs are also involved in resistance to radio-chemotherapy [29].

Furthermore, miRNAs might regulate cell proliferation and apoptosis by targeting mitogen receptor tyrosine kinases and cell cycle regulators, such as cyclin-dependent kinases

(CDKs), reciprocal miRNA interactions with MYC (v-myc avian myelocytomatosis viral oncogene homolog) and TP53, and by regulating the proapoptotic and antiapoptotic mRNAs [30].

Moreover, due to the altered expression of miRNAs in tumor development, they have been proposed as tissue and circulation biomarkers (blood derivates and feces). They might play a role in the prognostic and predictive diagnosis of CRC [31]. **Table 1** shows the potential roles of miRNA in CRC. Additionally, miRNA-related polymorphisms might disrupt their binding sites, miRNA processing, and expression. In this way, the single-nucleotide polymorphism (SNP) and other genetic abnormalities might be of utility in the study of the risk and prognosis of CRC.

	Role in CRC	**miRNA**
Oncogene	Proliferation	miR-21, miR-92a, miR-96, miR-135a, miR-135b
	Apoptosis	miR-21
	DNA damage response	miR-155
	Invasion	miR-21, miR-92a
	Epithelial–mesenchymal transition	miR-92a
	Metastasis	miR-224
	Inflammation	miR-224
Tumor suppressor	Proliferation	let-7, miR-7, miR-18a, miR-26b, miR-27b, miR-143, miR-144, miR-145, miR-194, miR-320a
	Apoptosis	miR-26b, miR-34a, miR-194, miR-195, miR-365, miR-491
	Angiogenesis	miR-27b, miR-145, miR-101, miR-126
	Invasion	miR-26b, miR-145, miR-194
	Migration	miR-26b, miR-145, miR-194
Circulatory biomarkers	Diagnosis	miR-21, miR-31, miR-34a, miR-92a, miR-143, miR-145, miR-601, miR-760
	Prognosis/survival	miR-21, miR-124-5p, miR-141, miR-155, miR-182, miR-200c
	Chemotherapy	miR-17-5p, miR-19a, miR-20a, miR-27b, miR-126, miR-130, miR-140, miR-145, miR-192, miR-216, miR-200c

Table 1. MiRNAs described in CRC

MiRNA has also been described with high potential as therapeutic target. According to Schetter et al., the two strategies for miRNA-based therapies are (a) to inhibit oncogenic miRNAs and (b) to restore tumor suppressor miRNAs. Some preclinical models have shown that both strategies might be effective in the treatment of CRC cancers [29].

3.2. miRNA regulation of CSC in CRC

Many studies have reported that miRNAs are key players in the regulation of CSCs [32]. Bitarte et al. [33] have described that miR-451 is involved in the self-renewal, tumorigenicity, and chemoresistance of CRC stem cells. Up-regulation of miR-451 resulted in reduction of colon sphere formation and growth, inhibition of tumorigenicity in vivo, and sensitization to the active metabolite of irinotecan, SN38. This metabolite might be related to miR-451–mediated down-regulation of cyclooxygenase-2 (COX-2) and WNT (Wingless-type MMTV integration site family) pathway, essential to maintain cell stemness. On the other hand, Bitarte et al. also described that the regulation of expression of ATP-binding cassette (ABCB1) by miR-451 could decrease SN38 resistance.

Moreover, it has been suggested that miR-215 and miR-140 could control the slow proliferation and the chemoresistance of CSCs in the colon. In this respect, Jones et al. [34] described miRNA-215 (miR-215) as a direct transcriptional target of CDX1 in CRC stem cell differentiation. Song et al. [35] suggested miR-215 as molecular modulator of chemoresistance in CSC in CRC. Moreover, Yu et al. [36] have reported that miR-93 suppresses proliferation and colony formation of human CRC stem cells.

4. Circadian rhythms and CSC in CRC

Circadian rhythms are daily rhythms that take the form of a sine wave with high or active and low or quiet periods over the 24-hour clock. Many biological processes are temporally coordinated so that groups of genes called "clock genes" and their products are expressed at different critical times of the day, being likewise coordinated in circadian time [37]. A master clock in the suprachiasmatic nucleus (SCN) of the hypothalamus organizes the circadian system in a hierarchical manner. The SCN receives photic input through direct retinal innervation that initiates gene expression in the SCN [38]. In this way, light exposure synchronizes the SCN clock to solar time, adapting the oscillator to exact 24-hour cycle. The master clock of the SCN communicates day-night information to the rest of the body. The SCN receives light input from the retina and then conveys the photic information into neural or humoral signals. This information is then sent to peripheral circadian clocks that exist in almost all cells of the body and synchronize them to the same phase [39]. Whereas light is the dominant rhythmic signal for the SCN oscillator, the peripheral clocks respond to other environmental signal, such as body temperature, hunger, and hormone secretion cycles, and modify their phase accordingly [40, 41].

4.1. Regulation of circadian rhythms in mammals

In mammals, these daily rhythms are maintained by autoregulatory transcriptional and translational feedback and feed-forward loops (TTFLs) [42]. The core clock genes are BMAL1 (brain and muscle aryl-hydrocarbon receptor nuclear translocator-like 1), CLOCK (circadian locomotor output cycles kaput), PER (period homolog), and CRY (cryptochrome) [41]. BMAL1 heterodimerizes with either CLOCK or NPAS2 (neuronal PAS domain protein 2) and binds to E-box elements in PER (PER1-3) and CRY (CRY1-2) promoter regions and activates their transcription. Upon accumulation in the cytoplasm, PER and CRY proteins translocate to the nucleus where they repress the BMAL1: CLOCK/NPAS2 regulatory complex, thereby shutting down their own transcription. The PER and CRY heterodimers are progressively degraded, allowing the circuit to start again. This negative feedback leads to a cycle in gene expression that takes approximately 24 hours to complete (**Figure 2**) [43].

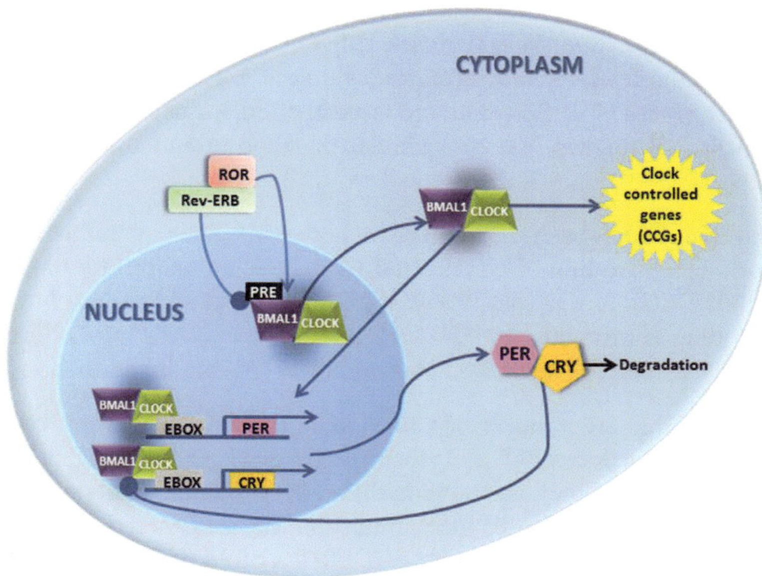

Figure 2. Schematic representation of the core circadian clock. (Adapted from Robinson and Reddy [52]. Copyright ©2014). BMAL1 and CLOCK transcription products translocate to the cytoplasm and dimerize. They then return to the nucleus and bind to E-box regions and promote Period (PER) and Cryptochrome (CRY) transcription. PER and CRY translocate to the cytoplasm, dimerize, and return to the nucleus and inhibit the binding of the CLOCK/BMAL complex. PER and CRY are subsequently degraded. REV-ERB inhibits the transcription of Bmal1, whereas ROR promotes BMAL1 expression. The clock-controlled genes REV-ERBα (REV-ERB) and RORα (ROR) generate additional circadian control by modulating the expression of BMAL1.

Post-transcriptional and post-translational modifications, such as phosphorylation, acetylation, methylation, sumoylation, and ubiquitination, are crucial to the clock molecular mechanism [44]. Post-translational modifications of the proteins of the circuit generate the essential time delay that maintains the period of the cycle at approximately 24 hours. Additional feedback pathways involving nuclear receptors, such as RORα (retinoid-related orphan receptor alpha), REV-ERBα (NR1D1, nuclear receptor subfamily 1, group D, member 1), PPARγ (peroxisome proliferator–activated receptor gamma), and PGC-1α (peroxisome proliferator–activated receptor gamma coactivator 1-alpha) provide further robustness to the circuit [45, 46]. Additionally, these clock genes control numerous target genes (termed clock controlled genes, CCGs) and they regulate the circadian rhythms of various biochemical and physiological processes [47].

4.2. Redox regulation of circadian rhythms

The possible relation between circadian rhythm and redox state has been long known but it was unclear whether redox oscillations are a driver of the clock or a biomarker of cellular time. The discovery that circadian redox oscillations appear to be conserved throughout evolution, and that circadian oscillations in redox parameters persist in the absence of transcriptional system, has consolidated the interplay between metabolic processes and the molecular clock [48]. In mammals, nearly 10,000 genes are known to be under circadian control [49]. Several studies have investigated circadian oscillations in gene expression in metabolic tissues, including brown fat, liver, and skeletal muscle [50]. Certain metabolic enzymes are rhythmically expressed in the liver, such as aconitase, aldolase 2, enolase 1, ketohexokinase, and succinate dehydrogenase 1 [51]. Since numerous metabolic diseases appear to have a circadian-related dysfunction, it follows that core cellular metabolism and the clock are intimately connected [52].

The redox state of a cell has been shown to be an integral component in the regulation of the molecular clock. DNA binding of NPAS2 and CLOCK is influenced by the redox state of NAD(H) and NHAP(H). NADP inhibits NPAS2:BMAL1 binding to DNA, but, on the other hand, DNA binding is promoted by NADPH. At a ratio of NADP:NADP(H) of over 75% NPAS2:BMAL1 DNA binding increases, whereas below 75% binding decreases [53].

Peroxiredoxins (PRDXs) are a family of antioxidants that help to prevent cellular damage resulting from the production of ROS and work by reducing H_2O_2 to water. Six PRDX isoforms are known (PRDX 1–6), and they are found in different cellular localizations: isoforms 1, 2, 5, and 6 in the cytosol, isoforms 3 and 5 in the mitochondria, isoform 5 in the peroxisome, and isoform 4 in the endoplasmic reticulum [54, 55]. PRDXs could have one or two redox active cysteine residues that bind H_2O_2 forming a sulfenic acid. In mammals, there are five two-Cysperoxiredoxins (PRDX 1–5) and a single one-Cysperoxiredoxin (PRDX 6) [56]. In most cases, a homodimer is formed by a resolving cysteine at the C terminus forming a disulphide bond with the cysteine sulfenic acid. This bond can then be 'resolved' by thioredoxin, enabling further catabolism of peroxide by PRDX [57].

The cycle of PRDX had been shown to follow a circadian rhythm, with two forms of PRDX6 oscillating in antiphase in the liver, emphasizing a role of post-translational modification in circadian rhythmicity [51]. While the core clockwork use TTFLs, many works suggest the redox state of PRDXs is driven by the metabolic state of the cell, but it is independent of transcription [58]. However, the reciprocal influence between the TTFL and the PRDX-based metabolic clock has not fully addressed yet.

4.3. Epigenetic regulation of circadian rhythms by miRNAs

Some miRNAs have regulatory functions contributing to the control over circadian protein expression [59]. The influences of the circadian clock function on miRNA expression or vice versa have been well established. Experimental evidence suggests that up to 30% of core clock genes are under the control of miRNA. Recently, miR-132 and miR-219 seem to be directly involved in the clock system and regulate light response [60].

Other studies examine the role of extracellular miRNAs in the regulation of molecular components and modulation of rhythmicity in peripheral cellular clocks. The studies revealed that exposure to miR-142-3p– and miR-494–enriched conditioned medium increases intracellular expression of these miRNAs and results in functional effects in recipient cells [59].

4.4. Circadian rhythms and CRC

In carcinogenesis, the levels of expression of many proteins may be dependent directly or indirectly on the circadian cycle. Investigations on the relation between the circadian clock and DNA damage response have revealed that DNA damage checkpoints, nucleotide excision repair, and apoptosis are appreciably influenced by the clock [61]. Changes in the circadian rhythm of cell division are considered important component in neoplastic transformation. The presence of DNA damage is usually associated with cell cycle arrest for attempted repairs or induction of apoptosis. The mechanism of repair happens before the S-phase of the cell cycle, and although there are post-replication mechanisms for induction of cell cycle arrest, the G1/S checkpoint is usually the most stringent cell cycle checkpoint and this event will take place at night for adjustment of the circadian rhythm [61]. On the other hand, disruptions of the circadian rhythm genes are associated with increased susceptibility to cancers [62].

Some experimental studies have showed the role of the disruption of the molecular clock work in colorectal carcinogenesis and CRC progression [63]. One example is seen in human cancer cells lines when PER1 is overexpressed. In this experiment, it was observed a reduced colony formation and clonogenic expansion, in sensitization to radiation-induced apoptosis, and in altered expression of transcriptional target genes, such as c-MYC and p21 [64]. In contrast, PER2-null mice showed an increase in hyperplasia and neoplasia in response to γ-radiation [65]. In line with this work, restoring CLOCK expression in a human colon adenocarcinoma cell line derived from a primary colon cancer, in response to ionizing radiation, conferred protection against ultraviolet (UV)-induced apoptosis and decreased G2/M arrest [66].

On the other hand, one study that used CRC tumor tissue from patients demonstrated that PER2 expression was higher in well-differentiated cancer cells when compared to poorly differentiated ones. Associations of decreased PER2 levels with patient age, histological grade, TNM (for tumors/nodes/metastases) stage, and expression of nuclear proliferation-related antigen Ki67 were also observed [67]. In addition, down-regulation of PER3 associated with various clinicopathological factors, including tumor location, differentiation, and stage, as well as poorer survival was seen in CRC tissues, thus suggesting an important role in CRC progression [68].

The efficacy of many drugs and the intensity of their effects depend on the time of day when they are administered (chronochemotherapy), and they are therefore associated with the circadian rhythm. The clock acts as a modulator of the pharmacokinetics and pharmacodynamics of chemotherapeutic drugs and of the activity of the DNA-repair enzymes that repair the DNA damage caused by anticancer drugs [61]. Some studies have demonstrated that chronomodulated chemotherapy has better tolerability and antitumor activity compared with conventional chemotherapy. A good example is the treatment of advanced stage CRC where oxaliplatin is administered in the afternoon and 5-FU and leucovorin are delivered late at night (chronoFLO4) [69]. Other authors have observed that 5-FU administration during the sleeping time before radiotherapy could have an advantage as a chronotherapy and also as a radiosensitizer [70].

4.5. Regulation of stemness by the circadian machinery

Numerous studies are demonstrating the importance of coherent circadian oscillations for a variety of homeostatic functions of tissues. One example is the timed activation and differentiation of stem and progenitor cells, and how perturbation of this temporal coordination leads to pathologies, including obesity and neurological diseases, aging, and cancer [71].

Like normal cells, cancer cells contain molecular clocks that generate circadian rhythms in gene expression and metabolic activity [72]. The circadian rhythms not only regulate the cell cycle in normal differentiated cells but there could also be a functional relation between circadian rhythm gene expression and the intrinsic control of the proliferation of CSCs and progenitor cells in different tissues [73]. In rodents and humans, all the hematopoietic stem and progenitor cells exhibit a predictable circadian variation [74, 75]. Some authors have shown that there is an increase in circadian rhythm gene expression of highly differentiated stem cell cultures. In both cancer and normal cells, a rhythmic nuclear translocation of PER2 and other critical clock proteins is an essential part of a clock timing mechanism based on transcriptional–translational feedback loops and rhythmic chromatin modification [73, 76].

The malignant phenotype depends not only on the characteristics of the cancer cell itself but also on the tumor microenvironment. CSCs have to survive for a long time in the body to generate the highly tumorigenic cells responsible for the clinical manifestations of cancer. During this period, the niche helps to shelter CSCs from different types of insults, such as the immune response and chemotherapy-induced genotoxic stress [77, 78]. This suggests that the niche may also play a protective role for CSCs, thus increasing the risk of cancer. In fact, BMAL1 suppresses cancer cell invasion by blocking the phosphoinositide 3-kinase-Akt-Matrix metalloproteinase-2 (MMP-2) signaling pathway [79]. Other authors have reported circadian oscillations in the levels of MMP-9 [80].

5. SIRT1 and the circadian regulation of CSCs by miRNAs

The silent information regulator (SIRT) 2 family of proteins, known as sirtuins, is a class III of histone deacetylases or NAD+–dependent deacetylases and is conserved from bacteria to humans. The requirement for NAD+ links the activity of sirtuins directly to the metabolic state of the cell, since the deacetylase activity of these proteins is controlled by the cellular NAD+/NADH ratio. There are seven sirtuins (SIRT1–7) in mammals. They have different specific substrates and biological functions and are found in various cell compartments [81].

http://dx.doi.org/10.5772/62323

The role of sirtuin activation in mammals is to regulate the progression of aging and age-associated disorders, including neurodegeneration, diabetes, cardiovascular diseases, and many types of cancer [82]. The best characterized and well-studied among the human sirtuins is SIRT1. It can be found in the nucleus and in the cytoplasm of the cells [83].

5.1. Sirt1 in cancer biology

SIRT1 is overexpressed in some types of human cancer tissues, such as ovary, liver, breast, stomach, pancreas and prostate, and down expressed in skin cancer. In CRC, SIRT1 is also overexpressed. However, other investigations have revealed pronounced SIRT1 expression in both normal colon and tumor tissues, although its expression is substantially reduced in higher grade CRC tumors [84].

SIRT1 has a dual role in tumorigenesis, where it can function as either a tumor promoter or a tumor suppressor. Its function in malignancy varies with concentration, cellular location, temporal and spatial distribution, and regulation by upstream and downstream factors [85].

The initial connection of sirtuins to cancer was made when SIRT1 was found to deacetylate and repress the activity of the tumor suppressor p53 [86, 87]. SIRT1-mediated deacetylation suppresses the functions of other tumor suppressors, including p73, hypermethylated in cancer 1 (HIC1), E2F transcription factor 1(E2F1, also known as retinoblastoma-associated protein 1), retinoblastoma protein (Rb), and phosphatase and tensin homologue deleted in chromosome 10 (PTEN), thus suggesting that SIRT1 acts as a promoter in tumor development and progression [88–93]. Other reports showed SIRT1 as a downstream of the oncoprotein BCR-ABL tyrosine kinase (Abelson murine leukemia viral oncogene homolog 1), implicated in the development of chronic myelogenous leukemia (CML)-like myeloproliferative disease [94].

Autophagy is a self-degradative process that plays a role by eliminating damaged organelles and misfolded or aggregated proteins through the lysosomal degradation pathway. Autophagy initially serves as a protective process to prevent cancer initiation; however, after neoplastic transformation, it can promote tumor cell survival and maintenance [95]. Autophagy can also affect chemotherapeutic and immunotherapeutic response in cancer cells making it an attractive target for development of anticancer drugs [96, 97]. SIRT1 forms a molecular complex with the genes related to autophagy and autophagosome formation, Atg5, Atg7, and Atg8. Loss of SIRT1 activity results in the acetylation of those factors thus leading to defects in the process of autophagy [98].

Consistent with a tumor-suppressor role, SIRT1 deacetylates and decreases the stability of the oncogene c-MYC [99]. In addition, the activity of SIRT1 can be increased by some tumor-suppressors, for example BRCA1 (breast cancer 1) [99]. SIRT1 exerts anticarcinogenic effects through multiple mechanisms [83]. SIRT1 can counteract various genotoxic insults, including oxidative DNA damage, thereby blocking initiation of carcinogenesis. SIRT1 deacetylates and inhibits proapoptotic p53 and PARP-1 (poly (ADP-ribose) polymerase 1) under stressful conditions, conferring cell survival [86, 100]. SIRT1 is also required for DNA repair processes to maintain genomic stability [101, 102].

SIRT1 inhibits the mediators involved in aberrantly amplified proinflammatory signaling during promotion and progression of carcinogenesis [103–105]. The anti-inflammatory effect of SIRT1 might be achieved by inhibition of several transcription factors related to inflammation, nuclear factor κB (NF-κB), signal transducer and activator of transcription 3 (STAT3), and the c-Jun and fos elements of transcription factor activator protein 1 (AP-1) [106–108]. Mainly through NF-κB and AP-1 pathways, SIRT1 was engaged in macrophage and T-cell activation [105, 109]. SIRT1 also regulates the differentiation and function of iTreg (induced Treg helper cells) [110]. Interestingly, SIRT1 translates metabolic cues during regulation of the immune responses, which would bring new insights into both pathogenesis and potential therapeutic strategies of a variety of immune-related diseases, such as cancer [111].

5.2. SIRT1 and stem cells

SIRT1 is considered an old multifaceted enzyme with an important role in the maintenance of pluripotency in various types of stem cells. Most of the in vivo data suggest that Sirt1 acts in early development as a modulatory molecule on basic developmental processes [112]. In cancer, SIRT1 has been implicated in the regulation of CSCs survival and differentiation. SIRT1 has been found to regulate the growth and survival of leukemia stem cells (LSCs) and confer resistance against chemotherapy [113], stimulate endometrial cell tumor growth through lipogenesis [114], maintain neural stem cells and promote oncogenic transformation [115], and foster hepatocellular carcinoma [116]. As a result, SIRT1 and agents that modulate SIRT1 activity may represent new therapeutic strategies against tumorigenesis.

One of the more intriguing hypotheses about aging and age-related disease is that age-associated phenotypic alterations derive from the inability of resident stem cells to maintain tissue structure and function [117]. This suggests that the aging process could arise from loss or malfunction of self-renewal and/or differentiation potential in adult stem cell populations. SIRT1 has a positive role in stemness by aiding in the silencing of differentiation genes, which suggests new potential explanations of its ability to extend lifespan and to avoid cell and organism senescence [112, 118].

5.3. SIRT1 and miRNAs

Expression of SIRT1 is controlled at multiple levels by transcriptional, post-transcriptional, and post-translational mechanisms under physiological and pathological conditions [119]. Deacetylation activity of SIRT1 can be modulated by multiple regulators. AROS (Active regulator of SIRT1) and DBC1 (deleted in breast cancer 1) are positive and negative regulators of SIRT1, respectively [120, 121].

Emerging evidence indicates that miRNAs are important regulators of SIRT1 expression and activity [119]. In cancer, SIRT1 mediates miR-34a activation of apoptosis by regulating p53 activity. In addition, p53 induces expression of miR-34a which suppresses SIRT1, increasing p53 activity [122]. In CRC, dysregulation of microRNA-34a expression causes drug-resistance to 5-FU in human colon cancer cells through the downregulation of Sirt1 and E2F3 [123, 124].

miRNAs play an important role in proper function and differentiation of human and mouse stem cells. Recently, it has been demonstrated that miR-34a is required for proper differentiation of mouse embryonic stem cells, mouse neural stem cell, and mouse embryonic fibroblasts and that it function in part by targeting SIRT1 and modulating p53 activity [125–127]. Also, the miR-29b-Sirt1 axis regulates self-renewal of mouse embryonic stem cells in response to reactive oxygen species [128]. miR-34a is also a critical regulator of cancer progression by the regulation of CSC characteristics, through SIRT1 as a mediator [129–133], and mainly, through up-regulation of p53/p21 [131].

5.4. SIRT1 as regulator of circadian rhythms

Two independent studies identified SIRT1 as a critical modulator of the circadian clock machinery. Asher et al. [134] observed oscillations in SIRT1 protein levels, and Nakahata et al. [135] demonstrated that SIRT1 activity, and not its protein levels, oscillates in a circadian manner. SIRT1 modulates circadian rhythms by deacetylating histone H3 Lys9 and Lys14 at promoters of rhythmic genes, BMAL1 and PER2. The CLOCK-BMAL1 complex interacts with SIRT1 and recruits it to the promoters of rhythmic genes. While BMAL1 acetylation acts as a signal for CRY recruitment, PER2 acetylation enhances its stability [134]. These findings led to the concept that SIRT1 operates as a rheostat of the circadian machinery, modulating the amplitude of CLOCK-mediated acetylation and consequent transcription cycles [135].

Circadian oscillation of SIRT1 activity suggested that cellular NAD+ levels may also oscillate. In fact, circadian clock controls the expression of NAMPT (nicotinamide phosphoribosyltransferase), a key rate-limiting enzyme in the salvage pathway of NAD+ biosynthesis. The oscillatory expression of NAMPT is abolished in Clock/Clock mice, which results in drastically reduced levels of NAD+. These results imply the existence of an enzymatic/transcriptional feedback loop, wherein SIRT1 regulates the levels of its own cofactor [135]. These results also connect the circadian machinery to cell metabolism [134].

SIRT1 either directly or indirectly can influence the redox property of the cell [136]. In addition to reduce cellular oxidative stress burden, SIRT1 is also regulated by oxidative stress [137]. Since redox homeostasis influence circadian machinery, SIR1 could regulate circadian genes trough redox status of the cell. A recent report suggests that PRDX2 regulates the TTFL oscillation by decreasing the nuclear redox levels and increasing SIRT1 enzymatic activity, although neither a direct interaction between PRX and SIRT1 nor a modulation of SIRT1 intracellular levels by PRX was found [138].

5.5. SIRT1 regulators as new tools for cancer treatment

Recently, multiple research groups have pursued the identification and development of small molecule compounds that modulate sirtuins SIRT1 regulators as new tools for cancer treatment [139]. To date, SIRT1 inhibitors and activators have been described with different effects on cancer [140].

SIRT inhibitors require combined targeting of both SIRT1 and SIRT2 to induce p53 acetylation and cell death, like sirtinol and salermide [139]. Trichostatin A (TSA) and sirtinol induce p38MAPK- and AMPK-mediated downregulation of survivin and its functional correlation with decreased colon cancer cell viability in vitro [141]. Other salermide-related sirtuin inhibitors show antiproliferative effects in colon cancer cells in vitro, including CSCs [142]. Vorinostat activates p53, but does not require p53 for inducing its anticancer action in CRC [143]. The SIRT1 selective inhibitor Amurensin G may be effective in eliminating colon CSCs and may be applicable to potentiate the sensitivity of colon CSCs to TNF-related apoptosis-inducing ligand (TRAIL) [144].

Studies have shown that the sirtuin activator resveratrol, a polyphenol found in wines has chemopreventive activity against various cancers. In CRC, resveratrol induce apoptosis and suppressed the PI3K/Akt signaling pathway. The combination treatment with resveratrol and 5-FU induced a synergistic enhancement of growth inhibition and apoptosis in colon cancer DLD-1 cells. Interestingly, resveratrol increased the intracellular expression level of miR-34a, which down-regulated the target gene E2F3 and its downstream Sirt1, resulting in growth inhibition [145].

Melatonin is the main secretory product of the pineal gland and plays important roles in several biological functions, including circadian rhythms, sleep, mood, reproductive physiology, and aging diseases [146]. Numerous studies based on animal and clinical data have provided evidence that melatonin reduces the incidence of experimentally induced cancers and may significantly inhibit the growth of some human tumors [147]. Recently, melatonin was confirmed as a novel inhibitor of SIRT1. Melatonin inhibits prostate cancer and osteosarcoma cell growth through SIRT1 inhibition [148, 149]. Interestingly, it was recently reported that melatonin decreases CSCs and dysplastic injuries in colon tissue [150].

6. Concluding remarks

SIRT1 expression correlated with depth of invasion, lymph node metastasis, and TNM stage in CRC. Simultaneously, SIRT1 overexpression predicted a poor overall survival in CRC patients, and SIRT1 is a candidate negative prognostic biomarker for CRC patients [151]. SIRT1 has also been implicated in chemoresistance in CRC patients with [152] or without metastasis [124]. Further investigations aimed at targeting SIRT1 alone or in combination with chemotherapy deserve further attention and may ultimately increase response rates in the treatment of CRC. In this sense, melatonin can significantly amplify the cytostatic and the cytotoxic effects triggered by other compounds or conventional drugs. We are far from having a satisfactory understanding about how and when melatonin exerts its beneficial effects. Melatonin in the nanomolar range induces down-regulation of SIRT1. This finding is of great relevance because there is intense research ongoing to identify nontoxic feasible inhibitors of SIRT1. Melatonin should be evaluated for the management of those cancers where this protein is overexpressed and is functional.

Author details

Sandra Ríos-Arrabal[1], José Antonio Muñoz-Gámez[2], Sergio Manuel Jiménez-Ruíz[2], Jorge Casado-Ruíz[2], Francisco Artacho-Cordón[1] and Josefa León-López[3*]

*Address all correspondence to: pepileon@ugr.es

1 Department of Radiology and Physical Medicine, University of Granada, Granada, Spain, Biosanitary Research Institute, Granada, Spain

2 Clinical Management Unit of Digestive Disease and Research Support Unit, San Cecilio University Hospital Granada, Spain; Biosanitary Research Institute Granada, Spain

3 Clinical Management Unit of Digestive Disease and Research Support Unit, San Cecilio University Hospital Granada, Spain; Biosanitary Research Institute Granada, Spain; Ciber of Hepatic and Digestive Diseases (CIBERehd), Madrid, Spain

References

[1] Ferlay J, Soerjomataram I, Dikshit R, Eser S, Mathers C, Rebelo M, Parkin DM, Forman D, Bray F. Cancer incidence and mortality worldwide: sources, methods and major patterns in GLOBOCAN 2012. International Journal of Cancer. 2015;136(5):E359–86. DOI: 10.1002/ijc.29210

[2] Vaiopoulos AG, Kostakis ID, Koutsilieris M, Papavassiliou AG. Colorectal cancer stem cells. Stem Cells. 2012;30(3):363–71. DOI: 10.1002/stem.1031

[3] Todaro M, Francipane MG, Medema JP, Stassi G. Colon cancer stem cells: promise of targeted therapy. Gastroenterology. 2010;138(6):2151–62. DOI: 10.1053/j.gastro.2009.12.063

[4] Kemper K, Grandela C, Medema JP. Molecular identification and targeting of colorectal cancer stem cells. Oncotarget. 2010;1(6):387–95.

[5] Nangia-Makker P, Yu Y, Majumdar AP. Role of cancer stem cells in age-related rise in colorectal cancer. World Journal of Gastrointestinal Pathophysiology. 2015;6(4):86–9. DOI: 10.4291/wjgp.v6.i4.86

[6] Li X, Lewis MT, Huang J, Gutierrez C, Osborne CK, Wu MF, Hilsenbeck SG, Pavlick A, Zhang X, Chamness GC, Wong H, Rosen J, Chang JC. Intrinsic resistance of tumorigenic breast cancer cells to chemotherapy. Journal of the National Cancer Institute. 2008;100(9):672–9. DOI: 10.1093/jnci/djn123

[7] Ogawa K, Yoshioka Y, Isohashi F, Seo Y, Yoshida K, Yamazaki H. Radiotherapy targeting cancer stem cells: current views and future perspectives. Anticancer Research. 2013;33(3):747–54.

[8] Meirelles K, Benedict LA, Dombkowski D, Pepin D, Preffer FI, Teixeira J, Tanwar PS, Young RH, MacLaughlin DT, Donahoe PK, Wei X. Human ovarian cancer stem/progenitor cells are stimulated by doxorubicin but inhibited by Mullerian inhibiting substance. Proceedings of the National Academy of Sciences of the United States of America. 2012;109(7):2358–63. DOI: 10.1073/pnas.1120733109

[9] Nigam A. Breast cancer stem cells, pathways and therapeutic perspectives 2011. The Indian Journal of surgery. 2013;75(3):170–80. DOI: 10.1007/s12262-012-0616-3

[10] Al-Hajj M, Wicha MS, Benito-Hernandez A, Morrison SJ, Clarke MF. Prospective identification of tumorigenic breast cancer cells. Proceedings of the National Academy of Sciences of the United States of America. 2003;100(7):3983–8. DOI: 10.1073/pnas.0530291100

[11] Dalerba P, Dylla SJ, Park IK, Liu R, Wang X, Cho RW, Hoey T, Gurney A, Huang EH, Simeone DM, Shelton AA, Parmiani G, Castelli C, Clarke MF. Phenotypic characterization of human colorectal cancer stem cells. Proceedings of the National Academy of Sciences of the United States of America. 2007;104(24):10158–63. DOI: 10.1073/pnas.0703478104

[12] Prince ME, Sivanandan R, Kaczorowski A, Wolf GT, Kaplan MJ, Dalerba P, Weissman IL, Clarke MF, Ailles LE. Identification of a subpopulation of cells with cancer stem cell properties in head and neck squamous cell carcinoma. Proceedings of the National Academy of Sciences of the United States of America. 2007;104(3):973–8. DOI: 10.1073/pnas.0610117104

[13] Ho MM, Ng AV, Lam S, Hung JY. Side population in human lung cancer cell lines and tumors is enriched with stem-like cancer cells. Cancer Research. 2007;67(10):4827–33. DOI: 10.1158/0008-5472.CAN-06-3557

[14] Li C, Lee CJ, Simeone DM. Identification of human pancreatic cancer stem cells. Methods in Molecular Biology. 2009;568:161–73. DOI: 10.1007/978-1-59745-280-9_10

[15] Singh SK, Hawkins C, Clarke ID, Squire JA, Bayani J, Hide T, Henkelman RM, Cusimano MD, Dirks PB. Identification of human brain tumour initiating cells. Nature. 2004;432(7015):396–401. DOI: 10.1038/nature03128

[16] Clarke MF, Dick JE, Dirks PB, Eaves CJ, Jamieson CH, Jones DL, Visvader J, Weissman IL, Wahl GM. Cancer stem cells--perspectives on current status and future directions: AACR Workshop on cancer stem cells. Cancer Research. 2006;66(19):9339–44. DOI: 10.1158/0008-5472.CAN-06-3126

[17] Rapp UR, Ceteci F, Schreck R. Oncogene-induced plasticity and cancer stem cells. Cell Cycle. 2008;7(1):45–51.

[18] Fearon ER, Vogelstein B. A genetic model for colorectal tumorigenesis. Cell. 1990;61(5): 759–67.

[19] Roy S, Majumdar AP. Cancer stem cells in colorectal cancer: genetic and epigenetic changes. Journal of Stem Cell Research & Therapy. 2012;Suppl 7(6). DOI: 31 10.4172/2157-7633.S7-006

[20] Rassouli FB, Matin MM, Saeinasab M. Cancer stem cells in human digestive tract malignancies. Tumour Biology: The Journal of the International Society for Oncodevelopmental Biology and Medicine. 2015. DOI: 10.1007/s13277-015-4155-y. [Epub ahead of print].

[21] Nautiyal J, Du J, Yu Y, Kanwar SS, Levi E, Majumdar AP. EGFR regulation of colon cancer stem-like cells during aging and in response to the colonic carcinogen dimethylhydrazine American Journal of Physiology. Gastrointestinal and Liver Physiology. 2012;302(7):G655-63. DOI: 10.1152/ajpgi.00323.2011

[22] Kanwar SS, Yu Y, Nautiyal J, Patel BB, Majumdar AP. The Wnt/beta-catenin pathway regulates growth and maintenance of colonospheres. Molecular Cancer. 2010;9:212. DOI: 10.1186/1476-4598-9-212

[23] Liu L, Wylie RC, Andrews LG, Tollefsbol TO. Aging, cancer and nutrition: the DNA methylation connection. Mechanisms of Ageing and Development. 2003;124(10–12): 989–98.

[24] Friedman RC, Farh KK, Burge CB, Bartel DP. Most mammalian mRNAs are conserved targets of microRNAs. Genome Research. 2009;19(1):92–105. DOI: 10.1101/gr. 082701.108

[25] Nam EJ, Yoon H, Kim SW, Kim H, Kim YT, Kim JH, Kim JW, Kim S. MicroRNA expression profiles in serous ovarian carcinoma. Clinical Cancer Research: An Official Journal of the American Association for Cancer Research. 2008;14(9):2690–5. DOI: 10.1158/1078-0432.CRC-07-1731

[26] Pourrajab F, Babaei Zarch M, BaghiYazdi M, Hekmatimoghaddam S, Zare-Khormizi MR. MicroRNA-based system in stem cell reprogramming; differentiation/dedifferentiation. The International Journal of Biochemistry & Cell Biology. 2014;55:318–28. DOI: 10.1016/j.biocel.2014.08.008

[27] Malek E, Jagannathan S, Driscoll JJ. Correlation of long non-coding RNA expression with metastasis, drug resistance and clinical outcome in cancer. Oncotarget. 2014;5(18): 8027–38.

[28] Rokavec M, Oner MG, Li H, Jackstadt R, Jiang L, Lodygin D, Kaller M, Horst D, Ziegler PK, Schwitalla S, Slotta-Huspenina J, Bader FG, Greten FR, Hermeking H. IL-6R/STAT3/miR-34a feedback loop promotes EMT-mediated colorectal cancer invasion and metastasis. The Journal of Clinical Investigation. 2014;124(4):1853–67. DOI: 10.1172/JCI73531

[29] Schetter AJ, Okayama H, Harris CC. The role of microRNAs in colorectal cancer. Cancer Journal. 2012;18(3):244–52. DOI: 10.1097/PPO.0b013e318258b78f

[30] Cekaite L, Eide PW, Lind GE, Skotheim RI, Lothe RA. MicroRNAs as growth regulators, their function and biomarker status in colorectal cancer. Oncotarget. 2015. DOI: 10.18632/oncotarget.6390. [Epub ahead of print].

[31] Meiri E, Mueller WC, Rosenwald S, Zepeniuk M, Klinke E, Edmonston TB, Werner M, Lass U, Barshack I, Feinmesser M, Huszar M, Fogt F, Ashkenazi K, Sanden M, Goren E, Dromi N, Zion O, Burnstein I, Chajut A, Spector Y, Aharonov R. A second-generation microRNA-based assay for diagnosing tumor tissue origin. The Oncologist. 2012;17(6): 801–12. DOI: 10.1634/theoncologist.2011-0466

[32] Liu X, Fu Q, Du Y, Yang Y, Cho WC. MicroRNA as regulators of cancer stem cells and chemoresistance in colorectal cancer. Current Cancer Drug Targets. 2015. [Epub ahead of print].

[33] Bitarte N, Bandres E, Boni V, Zarate R, Rodriguez J, Gonzalez-Huarriz M, Lopez I, Javier Sola J, Alonso MM, Fortes P, Garcia-Foncillas J. MicroRNA-451 is involved in the self-renewal, tumorigenicity, and chemoresistance of colorectal cancer stem cells. Stem Cells. 2011;29(11):1661–71. DOI: 10.1002/stem.741

[34] Jones MF, Hara T, Francis P, Li XL, Bilke S, Zhu Y, Pineda M, Subramanian M, Bodmer WF, Lal A. The CDX1-microRNA-215 axis regulates colorectal cancer stem cell differentiation. Proceedings of the National Academy of Sciences of the United States of America. 2015;112(13):E1550-8. DOI: 10.1073/pnas.1503370112

[35] Song B, Wang Y, Titmus MA, Botchkina G, Formentini A, Kornmann M, Ju J. Molecular mechanism of chemoresistance by miR-215 in osteosarcoma and colon cancer cells. Molecular Cancer. 2010;9:96. DOI: 10.1186/1476-4598-9-96

[36] Yu XF, Zou J, Bao ZJ, Dong J. miR-93 suppresses proliferation and colony formation of human colon cancer stem cells. World Journal of Gastroenterology. 2011;17(42):4711–7. DOI: 10.3748/wjg.v17.i42.4711

[37] Hrushesky W, Rich IN. Measuring stem cell circadian rhythm. Methods in Molecular Biology. 2015;1235:81-95. doi: 10.1007/978-1-4939-1785-3_8.

[38] Hastings MH, Herzog ED. Clock genes, oscillators, and cellular networks in the suprachiasmatic nuclei. Journal of Biological Rhythms. 2004;19(5):400–13. DOI: 10.1177/0748730404268786

[39] Mohawk JA, Green CB, Takahashi JS. Central and peripheral circadian clocks in mammals. Annual Review of Neuroscience. 2012;35:445. DOI: 10.1146/annurev-neuro-060909-153128

[40] Kohsaka A, Waki H, Cui H, Gouraud SS, Maeda M. Integration of metabolic and cardiovascular diurnal rhythms by circadian clock. Endocrine Journal. 2012;59(6):447–56. DOI: 10.1507/endocrj

[41] Chen L, Yang G. Recent advances in circadian rhythms in cardiovascular system. Frontiers in Pharmacology. 2015;6. DOI: 10.3389/fphar.2015.00071

[42] Yang G, Paschos G, Curtis AM, Musiek ES, McLoughlin SC, FitzGerald GA. Knitting up the raveled sleave of care. Science Translational Medicine. 2013;5(212):212rv3. DOI: 10.1126/scitranslmed.3007225

[43] Ukai H, Ueda HR. Systems biology of mammalian circadian clocks. Annual Review of Physiology. 2010;72:579–603. DOI: 10.1146/annurev-physiol-073109-130051

[44] Cardone L, Hirayama J, Giordano F, Tamaru T, Palvimo JJ, Sassone-Corsi P. Circadian clock control by SUMOylation of BMAL1. Science. 2005;309(5739):1390–4. DOI: 10.1126/science.1110689

[45] Liu C, Li S, Liu T, Borjigin J, Lin JD. Transcriptional coactivator PGC-1 alpha integrates the mammalian clock and energy metabolism. Nature. 2007;447(7143):477–81. DOI: 10.1038/nature05767

[46] Yang G, Jia Z, Aoyagi T, McClain D, Mortensen RM, Yang T. Systemic PPAR gamma deletion impairs circadian rhythms of behavior and metabolism. Plos One. 2012;7(8):e38117 DOI:10.1177/1534735409352083

[47] Paschos G. Circadian clocks, feeding time and metabolic homeostasis. Name: Frontiers in Pharmacology. 2015;6:112. DOI: 10.3389/fphar.2015.00112

[48] Edgar RS, Green EW, Zhao Y, van Ooijen G, Olmedo M, Qin X, Xu Y, Pan M, Valekunja UK, Feeney KA. Peroxiredoxins are conserved markers of circadian rhythms. Nature. 2012;485(7399):459–64. DOI: 10.1038/nature11088

[49] Ueda HR, Chen W, Adachi A, Wakamatsu H, Hayashi S, Takasugi T, Nagano M, Nakahama K, Suzuki Y, Sugano S. A transcription factor response element for gene expression during circadian night. Nature. 2002;418(6897):534–9. DOI: 10.1038/nature00906

[50] Storch K-F, Lipan O, Leykin I, Viswanathan N, Davis FC, Wong WH, Weitz CJ. Extensive and divergent circadian gene expression in liver and heart. Nature. 2002;417(6884):78–83. DOI: 10.1038/nature744

[51] Reddy AB, Karp NA, Maywood ES, Sage EA, Deery M, O'Neill JS, Wong GK, Chesham J, Odell M, Lilley KS. Circadian orchestration of the hepatic proteome. Current Biology. 2006;16(11):1107–15. DOI: 10.1016/j.cub.2006.04.026

[52] Robinson I, Reddy A. Molecular mechanisms of the circadian clockwork in mammals. FEBS Letters. 2014;588(15):2477–83. DOI: 10.1016/j.febslet.2014.06.005

[53] Rutter J, Reick M, Wu LC, McKnight SL. Regulation of clock and NPAS2 DNA binding by the redox state of NAD cofactors. Science. 2001;293(5529):510–4. DOI: 10.1126/science.1060698

[54] Rhee SG, Woo HA. Multiple functions of peroxiredoxins: peroxidases, sensors and regulators of the intracellular messenger H2O2, and protein chaperones. Antioxidants & Redox Signaling. 2011;15(3):781–94. DOI: 10.1089/ars.2010.3393

[55] Rhee SG, Woo HA, Kil IS, Bae SH. Peroxiredoxin functions as a peroxidase and a regulator and sensor of local peroxides. Journal of Biological Chemistry. 2012;287(7): 4403–10. DOI: 10.1074/jbc.R111.283432

[56] Hall A, Karplus PA, Poole LB. Typical 2-Cys peroxiredoxins: structures, mechanisms and functions. FEBS Journal. 2009;276(9):2469–77. DOI: 10.1111/j. 1742-4658.2009.06985.x.

[57] Hoyle NP, O'Neill JS. Oxidation-reduction cycles of peroxiredoxin proteins and nontranscriptional aspects of timekeeping. Biochemistry. 2015;54(2):184–93. DOI: 10.1021/bi5008386

[58] Avitabile D, Ranieri D, Nicolussi A, D'Inzeo S, Capriotti AL, Genovese L, Proietti S, Cucina A, Coppa A, Samperi R. Peroxiredoxin 2 nuclear levels are regulated by circadian clock synchronization in human keratinocytes. The International Journal of Biochemistry & Cell Biology. 2014;53:24–34. DOI: 10.1016/j.biocel.2014.04.024

[59] Shende VR, Kim S-M, Neuendorff N, Earnest DJ. MicroRNAs function as cis-and trans-acting modulators of peripheral circadian clocks. FEBS Letters. 2014;588(17):3015–22. DOI: 10.1016/j.febslet.2014.05.058

[60] Cheng H-YM, Papp JW, Varlamova O, Dziema H, Russell B, Curfman JP, Nakazawa T, Shimizu K, Okamura H, Impey S. microRNA modulation of circadian-clock period and entrainment. Neuron. 2007;54(5):813–29. DOI: 10.1016/j.neuron.2007.05.017

[61] Sancar A, Lindsey-Boltz LA, Gaddameedhi S, Selby CP, Ye R, Chiou Y-Y, Kemp MG, Hu J, Lee JH, Ozturk N. Circadian clock, cancer, and chemotherapy. Biochemistry. 2015;54(2):110–23. DOI: 10.1021/bi5007354

[62] Kettner NM, Katchy CA, Fu L. Circadian gene variants in cancer. Annals of Medicine. 2014;46(4):208–20. DOI: 10.3109/07853890.2014.914808

[63] Mazzoccoli G, Vinciguerra M, Papa G, Piepoli A. Circadian clock circuitry in colorectal cancer. World Journal of Gastroenterology. 2014;20(15):4197. DOI: 10.1016/jbbrc. 2006.05.094

[64] Yang X, Wood PA, Ansell C, Hrushesky WJ. Circadian time-dependent tumor suppressor function of period genes. Integrative Cancer Therapies. 2009;8(4):309–16. DOI: 10.1177/1534735409352083

[65] Wood PA, Yang X, Hrushesky WJ. Clock genes and cancer. Integrative Cancer Therapies. 2009;8(4):303–8. DOI: 10.1177/1534735409355292

[66] Alhopuro P, Björklund M, Sammalkorpi H, Turunen M, Tuupanen S, Biström M, Niittymäki I, Lehtonen HJ, Kivioja T, Launonen V. Mutations in the circadian gene

CLOCK in colorectal cancer. Molecular Cancer Research. 2010;8(7):952–60. DOI: 10.1158/1541-7786.MCR-10-0086

[67] Wang Y, Hua L, Lu C, Chen Z. Expression of circadian clock gene human Period2 (hPer2) in human colorectal carcinoma. World Journal of Surgical Oncology. 2011;9(1): 166. DOI: 10.1186/1477-7819-9-166

[68] Wang X, Yan D, Teng M, Fan J, Zhou C, Li D, Qiu G, Sun X, Li T, Xing T. Reduced expression of PER3 is associated with incidence and development of colon cancer. Annals of Surgical Oncology. 2012;19(9):3081–8. DOI: 10.1245/s10434-012-2279-5

[69] Levi F, Schibler U. Circadian rhythms: mechanisms and therapeutic implications. Annual Review of Pharmacology and Toxicology. 2007;47:593–628. DOI: 10.1146/annurev.pharmtox.47.120505.105208

[70] Asao T, Sakurai H, Harashima K, Yamaguchi S, Tsutsumi S, Nonaka T, Shioya M, Nakano T, Kuwano H. The synchronization of chemotherapy to circadian rhythms and irradiation in pre-operative chemoradiation therapy with hyperthermia for local advanced rectal cancer. Abbreviations: 5-FU 5-fluorouracil LV Leucovorin APR abdomino-perineal resection. International Journal of Hyperthermia. 2006;22(5):399–406. DOI: 10.1080/02656730600799873

[71] Janich P, Meng QJ, Benitah SA. Circadian control of tissue homeostasis and adult stem cells. Current Opinion in Cell Biology. 2014;31:8–15. DOI: 10.1016/j.ceb.2014.06.010

[72] Fujioka A, Takashima N, Shigeyoshi Y. Circadian rhythm generation in a glioma cell line. Biochemical and Biophysical Research Communications. 2006;346(1):169–74. DOI: 10.1016/jbbrc.2006.05.094

[73] Sharma VP, Anderson NT, Geusz ME. Circadian properties of cancer stem cells in glioma cell cultures and tumorspheres. Cancer Letters. 2014;345(1):65–74. DOI: 10.1016/j.canlet.2013.11.009

[74] Laerum O. Hematopoiesis occurs in rhythms. Experimental Hematology. 1995;23(11): 1145–7. DOI: 10.1111/j.1600-0609.1997.tb01680.x

[75] Bourin P, Ledain AF, Beau J, Mille D, Lévi F. In-vitro circadian rhythm of murine bone marrow progenitor production. Chronobiology International. 2002;19(1):57–67. DOI: 10.1081/CBI-120002677

[76] Lowrey PL, Takahashi JS. Genetics of circadian rhythms in mammalian model organisms. Advances in Genetics. 2011;74:175. DOI: 10.1016/B978-0-12-387690-4.00006-4

[77] Li L, Xie T. Stem cell niche: structure and function. Annual Review of Cell and Developmental Biology. 2005;21:605–31. DOI: 10.1146/annurev.cellbio.21.012704.131525

[78] McAllister SS, Weinberg RA. Tumor-host interactions: a far-reaching relationship. Journal of Clinical Oncology: Official Journal of the American Society of Clinical Oncology. 2010;28(26):4022–8. DOI: 10.1200/JCO.2010.28.4257

[79] Jung CH, Kim EM, Park JK, Hwang SG, Moon SK, Kim WJ, Um HD. Bmal1 suppresses cancer cell invasion by blocking the phosphoinositide 3-kinase-Akt-MMP-2 signaling pathway. Oncology Reports. 2013;29(6):2109–13. DOI: 10.3892/or.2013.2381

[80] Markoulli M, Papas E, Cole N, Holden BA. The diurnal variation of matrix metalloproteinase-9 and its associated factors in human tears. Investigative Ophthalmology & Visual Science. 2012;53(3):1479–84. DOI: 10.1167/iovs.11-8365

[81] Carafa V, Nebbioso A, Altucci L. Sirtuins and disease: the road ahead. Frontiers in Pharmacology. 2012;3:4. DOI: 10.3389/fphar.2012.00004

[82] Guarente L. Franklin H. Epstein lecture: sirtuins, aging, and medicine. The New England Journal of Medicine. 2011;364(23):2235–44. DOI: 10.1056/NEJMra1100831

[83] Chalkiadaki A, Guarente L. The multifaceted functions of sirtuins in cancer. Nature Reviews Cancer. 2015;15(10):608–24. DOI: 10.1038/nrc3985

[84] Yang H, Bi Y, Xue L, Wang J, Lu Y, Zhang Z, Chen X, Chu Y, Yang R, Wang R, Liu G. Multifaceted modulation of SIRT1 in cancer and inflammation. Critical Reviews in Oncogenesis. 2015;20(1–2):49–64.

[85] Fang Y, Nicholl MB. A dual role for sirtuin 1 in tumorigenesis. Current Pharmaceutical Design. 2014;20(15):2634–6.

[86] Luo J, Nikolaev AY, Imai S, Chen D, Su F, Shiloh A, Guarente L, Gu W. Negative control of p53 by Sir2alpha promotes cell survival under stress. Cell. 2001;107(2):137–48.

[87] Vaziri H, Dessain SK, Ng Eaton E, Imai SI, Frye RA, Pandita TK, Guarente L, Weinberg RA. hSIR2(SIRT1) functions as an NAD-dependent p53 deacetylase. Cell. 2001;107(2): 149–59.

[88] Dai JM, Wang ZY, Sun DC, Lin RX, Wang SQ. SIRT1 interacts with p73 and suppresses p73-dependent transcriptional activity. Journal of Cellular Physiology. 2007;210(1): 161–6. DOI: 10.1002/jcp.20831

[89] Pediconi N, Guerrieri F, Vossio S, Bruno T, Belloni L, Schinzari V, Scisciani C, Fanciulli M, Levrero M. hSirT1-dependent regulation of the PCAF-E2F1-p73 apoptotic pathway in response to DNA damage. Molecular and Cellular Biology. 2009;29(8):1989–98. DOI: 10.1128/MCB.00552-08

[90] Zhang Q, Wang SY, Fleuriel C, Leprince D, Rocheleau JV, Piston DW, Goodman RH. Metabolic regulation of SIRT1 transcription via a HIC1:CtBP corepressor complex. Proceedings of the National Academy of Sciences of the United States of America. 2007;104(3):829–33. DOI: 10.1073/pnas.0610590104

[91] Wang C, Chen L, Hou X, Li Z, Kabra N, Ma Y, Nemoto S, Finkel T, Gu W, Cress WD, Chen J. Interactions between E2F1 and SirT1 regulate apoptotic response to DNA damage. Nature Cell Biology. 2006;8(9):1025–31. DOI: 10.1038/ncb1468

[92] Wong S, Weber JD. Deacetylation of the retinoblastoma tumour suppressor protein by SIRT1. The Biochemical Journal. 2007;407(3):451–60. DOI: 10.1042/BJ20070151

[93] Ikenoue T, Inoki K, Zhao B, Guan KL. PTEN acetylation modulates its interaction with PDZ domain. Cancer Research. 2008;68(17):6908–12. DOI: 10.1158/0008-5472.CAN-08-1107

[94] Yuan H, Wang Z, Li L, Zhang H, Modi H, Horne D, Bhatia R, Chen W. Activation of stress response gene SIRT1 by BCR-ABL promotes leukemogenesis. Blood. 2012;119(8): 1904–14. DOI: 10.1182/blood-2011-06-361691

[95] Guo JY, Xia B, White E. Autophagy-mediated tumor promotion. Cell. 2013;155(6):1216–9. DOI: 10.1016/j.cell.2013.11.019

[96] Wei Y, Zou Z, Becker N, Anderson M, Sumpter R, Xiao G, Kinch L, Koduru P, Christudass CS, Veltri RW, Grishin NV, Peyton M, Minna J, Bhagat G, Levine B. EGFR-mediated Beclin 1 phosphorylation in autophagy suppression, tumor progression, and tumor chemoresistance. Cell. 2013;154(6):1269–84. DOI: 10.1016/j.cell.2013.08.015

[97] Galluzzi L, Pietrocola F, Levine B, Kroemer G. Metabolic control of autophagy. Cell. 2014;159(6):1263–76. DOI: 10.1016/j.cell.2014.11.006

[98] Lee IH, Cao L, Mostoslavsky R, Lombard DB, Liu J, Bruns NE, Tsokos M, Alt FW, Finkel T. A role for the NAD-dependent deacetylase Sirt1 in the regulation of autophagy. Proceedings of the National Academy of Sciences of the United States of America. 2008;105(9):3374–9. DOI: 10.1073/pnas.0712145105

[99] Yuan J, Minter-Dykhouse K, Lou Z. A c-Myc-SIRT1 feedback loop regulates cell growth and transformation. The Journal of Cell Biology. 2009;185(2):203–11. DOI: 10.1083/jcb.200809167

[100] Rajamohan SB, Pillai VB, Gupta M, Sundaresan NR, Birukov KG, Samant S, Hottiger MO, Gupta MP. SIRT1 promotes cell survival under stress by deacetylation-dependent deactivation of poly(ADP-ribose) polymerase 1. Molecular and Cellular Biology. 2009;29(15):4116–29. DOI: 10.1128/MCB.00121-09

[101] Ming M, Shea CR, Guo X, Li X, Soltani K, Han W, He YY. Regulation of global genome nucleotide excision repair by SIRT1 through xeroderma pigmentosum C. Proceedings of the National Academy of Sciences of the United States of America. 2010;107(52): 22623–8. DOI: 10.1073/pnas.1010377108

[102] Oberdoerffer P, Michan S, McVay M, Mostoslavsky R, Vann J, Park SK, Hartlerode A, Stegmuller J, Hafner A, Loerch P, Wright SM, Mills KD, Bonni A, Yankner BA, Scully R, Prolla TA, Alt FW, Sinclair DA. SIRT1 redistribution on chromatin promotes genomic stability but alters gene expression during aging. Cell. 2008;135(5):907–18. DOI: 10.1016/j.cell.2008.10.025

[103] Zhu X, Liu Q, Wang M, Liang M, Yang X, Xu X, Zou H, Qiu J. Activation of Sirt1 by resveratrol inhibits TNF-alpha induced inflammation in fibroblasts. PLoS One. 2011;6(11):e27081. DOI: 10.1371/journal.pone.0027081

[104] Zhang Z, Lowry SF, Guarente L, Haimovich B. Roles of SIRT1 in the acute and restorative phases following induction of inflammation. The Journal of Biological Chemistry. 2010;285(53):41391–401. DOI: 10.1074/jbc.M110.174482

[105] Yoshizaki T, Schenk S, Imamura T, Babendure JL, Sonoda N, Bae EJ, Oh DY, Lu M, Milne JC, Westphal C, Bandyopadhyay G, Olefsky JM. SIRT1 inhibits inflammatory pathways in macrophages and modulates insulin sensitivity. American Journal of Physiology: Endocrinology and Metabolism. 2010;298(3):E419-28. DOI: 10.1152/ajpendo.00417.2009

[106] Yeung F, Hoberg JE, Ramsey CS, Keller MD, Jones DR, Frye RA, Mayo MW. Modulation of NF-kappaB-dependent transcription and cell survival by the SIRT1 deacetylase. The EMBO Journal. 2004;23(12):2369–80. DOI: 10.1038/sj.emboj.7600244

[107] Nie Y, Erion DM, Yuan Z, Dietrich M, Shulman GI, Horvath TL, Gao Q. STAT3 inhibition of gluconeogenesis is downregulated by SirT1. Nature Cell Biology. 2009;11(4):492–500. DOI: 10.1038/ncb1857

[108] Zhang R, Chen HZ, Liu JJ, Jia YY, Zhang ZQ, Yang RF, Zhang Y, Xu J, Wei YS, Liu DP, Liang CC. SIRT1 suppresses activator protein-1 transcriptional activity and cyclooxygenase-2 expression in macrophages. The Journal of Biological Chemistry. 2010;285(10): 7097–110. DOI: 10.1074/jbc.M109.038604

[109] Zhang J, Lee SM, Shannon S, Gao B, Chen W, Chen A, Divekar R, McBurney MW, Braley-Mullen H, Zaghouani H, Fang D. The type III histone deacetylase Sirt1 is essential for maintenance of T cell tolerance in mice. The Journal of Clinical Investigation. 2009;119(10):3048–58. DOI: 10.1172/JCI38902

[110] Beier UH, Wang L, Bhatti TR, Liu Y, Han R, Ge G, Hancock WW. Sirtuin-1 targeting promotes Foxp3+ T-regulatory cell function and prolongs allograft survival. Molecular and Cellular Biology. 2011;31(5):1022–9. DOI: 10.1128/MCB.01206-10

[111] Chen X, Lu Y, Zhang Z, Wang J, Yang H, Liu G. Intercellular interplay between Sirt1 signalling and cell metabolism in immune cell biology. Immunology. 2015;145(4):455–67. DOI: 10.1111/imm.12473

[112] Calvanese V, Lara E, Suarez-Alvarez B, Abu Dawud R, Vazquez-Chantada M, Martinez-Chantar ML, Embade N, Lopez-Nieva P, Horrillo A, Hmadcha A, Soria B, Piazzolla D, Herranz D, Serrano M, Mato JM, Andrews PW, Lopez-Larrea C, Esteller M, Fraga MF. Sirtuin 1 regulation of developmental genes during differentiation of stem cells. Proceedings of the National Academy of Sciences of the United States of America. 2010;107(31):13736–41. DOI: 10.1073/pnas.1001399107

[113] Li L, Osdal T, Ho Y, Chun S, McDonald T, Agarwal P, Lin A, Chu S, Qi J, Hsieh YT, Dos Santos C, Yuan H, Ha TQ, Popa M, Hovland R, Bruserud O, Gjertsen BT, Kuo YH,

Chen W, Lain S, Mc Cormack E, Bhatia R. SIRT1 activation by a c-MYC oncogenic network promotes the maintenance and drug resistance of human FLT3-ITD acute myeloid leukemia stem cells. Cell Stem Cell. 2014;15(4):431–46. DOI: 10.1016/j.stem.2014.08.001

[114] Lin L, Zheng X, Qiu C, Dongol S, Lv Q, Jiang J, Kong B, Wang C. SIRT1 promotes endometrial tumor growth by targeting SREBP1 and lipogenesis. Oncology Reports. 2014;32(6):2831–5. DOI: 10.3892/or.2014.3521

[115] Lee JS, Park JR, Kwon OS, Lee TH, Nakano I, Miyoshi H, Chun KH, Park MJ, Lee HJ, Kim SU, Cha HJ. SIRT1 is required for oncogenic transformation of neural stem cells and for the survival of "cancer cells with neural stemness" in a p53-dependent manner. Neuro-oncology. 2015;17(1):95–106. DOI: 10.1093/neuonc/nou145

[116] Mao B, Hu F, Cheng J, Wang P, Xu M, Yuan F, Meng S, Wang Y, Yuan Z, Bi W. SIRT1 regulates YAP2-mediated cell proliferation and chemoresistance in hepatocellular carcinoma. Oncogene. 2014;33(11):1468–74. DOI: 10.1038/onc.2013.88

[117] Rando TA. Stem cells, ageing and the quest for immortality. Nature. 2006;441(7097): 1080–6. DOI: 10.1038/nature04958

[118] Calvanese V, Fraga MF. SirT1 brings stemness closer to cancer and aging. Aging. 2011;3(2):162–7.

[119] Choi SE, Kemper JK. Regulation of SIRT1 by microRNAs. Molecules and Cells. 2013;36(5):385–92. DOI: 10.1007/s10059-013-0297-1

[120] Kim EJ, Kho JH, Kang MR, Um SJ. Active regulator of SIRT1 cooperates with SIRT1 and facilitates suppression of p53 activity. Molecular Cell. 2007;28(2):277–90. DOI: 10.1016/j.molcel.2007.08.030

[121] Kim JE, Chen J, Lou Z. DBC1 is a negative regulator of SIRT1. Nature. 2008;451(7178): 583–6. DOI: 10.1038/nature06500

[122] Yamakuchi M, Lowenstein CJ. MiR-34, SIRT1 and p53: the feedback loop. Cell Cycle. 2009;8(5):712–5.

[123] Akao Y, Noguchi S, Iio A, Kojima K, Takagi T, Naoe T. Dysregulation of microRNA-34a expression causes drug-resistance to 5-FU in human colon cancer DLD-1 cells. Cancer Letters. 2011;300(2):197–204. DOI: 10.1016/j.canlet.2010.10.006

[124] Amirkhah R, Farazmand A, Irfan-Maqsood M, Wolkenhauer O, Schmitz U. The role of microRNAs in the resistance to colorectal cancer treatments. Cell and Molecular Biology (Noisy-le-grand). 2015;61(6):17–23.

[125] Tarantino C, Paolella G, Cozzuto L, Minopoli G, Pastore L, Parisi S, Russo T. miRNA 34a, 100, and 137 modulate differentiation of mouse embryonic stem cells. FASEB Journal: Official Publication of the Federation of American Societies for Experimental Biology. 2010;24(9):3255–63. DOI: 10.1096/fj.09-152207

[126] Aranha MM, Santos DM, Sola S, Steer CJ, Rodrigues CM. miR-34a regulates mouse neural stem cell differentiation. PLoS One. 2011;6(8):e21396. DOI: 10.1371/journal.pone.0021396

[127] Lee YL, Peng Q, Fong SW, Chen AC, Lee KF, Ng EH, Nagy A, Yeung WS. Sirtuin 1 facilitates generation of induced pluripotent stem cells from mouse embryonic fibroblasts through the miR-34a and p53 pathways. PLoS One. 2012;7(9):e45633. DOI: 10.1371/journal.pone.0045633

[128] Xu Z, Zhang L, Fei X, Yi X, Li W, Wang Q. The miR-29b-Sirt1 axis regulates self-renewal of mouse embryonic stem cells in response to reactive oxygen species. Cellular Signalling. 2014;26(7):1500–5. DOI: 10.1016/j.cellsig.2014.03.010

[129] Nalls D, Tang SN, Rodova M, Srivastava RK, Shankar S. Targeting epigenetic regulation of miR-34a for treatment of pancreatic cancer by inhibition of pancreatic cancer stem cells. PLoS One. 2011;6(8):e24099. DOI: 10.1371/journal.pone.0024099

[130] Duan K, Ge YC, Zhang XP, Wu SY, Feng JS, Chen SL, Zhang LI, Yuan ZH, Fu CH. miR-34a inhibits cell proliferation in prostate cancer by downregulation of SIRT1 expression. Oncology Letters. 2015;10(5):3223–7. DOI: 10.3892/ol.2015.3645

[131] Ye Z, Fang J, Dai S, Wang Y, Fu Z, Feng W, Wei Q, Huang P. MicroRNA-34a induces a senescence-like change via the down-regulation of SIRT1 and up-regulation of p53 protein in human esophageal squamous cancer cells with a wild-type p53 gene background. Cancer Letters. 2016;370(2):216–21. DOI: 10.1016/j.canlet.2015.10.023

[132] Ma W, Xiao GG, Mao J, Lu Y, Song B, Wang L, Fan S, Fan P, Hou Z, Li J, Yu X, Wang B, Wang H, Xu F, Li Y, Liu Q, Li L. Dysregulation of the miR-34a-SIRT1 axis inhibits breast cancer stemness. Oncotarget. 2015;6(12):10432–44. DOI: 10.18632/oncotarget.3394

[133] Wang Z, Chen CC, Chen W. CD150 Side Population Defines Leukemia Stem Cells in a BALB/c Mouse Model of CML and Is Depleted by Genetic Loss of SIRT1. Stem Cells. 2015. DOI: 10.1002/stem.2218

[134] Asher G, Gatfield D, Stratmann M, Reinke H, Dibner C, Kreppel F, Mostoslavsky R, Alt FW, Schibler U. SIRT1 regulates circadian clock gene expression through PER2 deacetylation. Cell. 2008;134(2):317–28. DOI: 10.1016/j.cell.2008.06.050

[135] Nakahata Y, Kaluzova M, Grimaldi B, Sahar S, Hirayama J, Chen D, Guarente LP, Sassone-Corsi P. The NAD+–dependent deacetylase SIRT1 modulates CLOCK-mediated chromatin remodeling and circadian control. Cell. 2008;134(2):329–40. DOI: 10.1016/j.cell.2008.07.002

[136] Chung S, Yao H, Caito S, Hwang JW, Arunachalam G, Rahman I. Regulation of SIRT1 in cellular functions: role of polyphenols. Archives of Biochemistry and Biophysics. 2010;501(1):79–90. DOI: 10.1016/j.abb.2010.05.003

[137] Volonte D, Zou H, Bartholomew JN, Liu Z, Morel PA, Galbiati F. Oxidative stress-induced inhibition of Sirt1 by caveolin-1 promotes p53-dependent premature senes-

cence and stimulates the secretion of interleukin 6 (IL-6). The Journal of Biological Chemistry. 2015;290(7):4202–14. DOI: 10.1074/jbc.M114.598268

[138] Ranieri D, Avitabile D, Shiota M, Yokomizo A, Naito S, Bizzarri M, Torrisi MR. Nuclear redox imbalance affects circadian oscillation in HaCaT keratinocytes. The International Journal of Biochemistry & Cell Biology. 2015;65:113–24. DOI: 10.1016/j.biocel.2015.05.018

[139] Villalba JM, Alcain FJ. Sirtuin activators and inhibitors. Biofactors. 2012;38(5):349–59. DOI: 10.1002/biof.1032

[140] Kozako T, Suzuki T, Yoshimitsu M, Arima N, Honda S, Soeda S. Anticancer agents targeted to sirtuins. Molecules. 2014;19(12):20295–313. DOI: 10.3390/molecules191220295

[141] Hsu YF, Sheu JR, Lin CH, Yang DS, Hsiao G, Ou G, Chiu PT, Huang YH, Kuo WH, Hsu MJ. Trichostatin A and sirtinol suppressed survivin expression through AMPK and p38MAPK in HT29 colon cancer cells. Biochimica et biophysica acta. 2012;1820(2):104–15. DOI: 10.1016/j.bbagen.2011.11.011

[142] Rotili D, Tarantino D, Nebbioso A, Paolini C, Huidobro C, Lara E, Mellini P, Lenoci A, Pezzi R, Botta G, Lahtela-Kakkonen M, Poso A, Steinkuhler C, Gallinari P, De Maria R, Fraga M, Esteller M, Altucci L, Mai A. Discovery of salermide-related sirtuin inhibitors: binding mode studies and antiproliferative effects in cancer cells including cancer stem cells. Journal of Medicinal Chemistry. 2012;55(24):10937–47. DOI: 10.1021/jm3011614

[143] Sonnemann J, Marx C, Becker S, Wittig S, Palani CD, Kramer OH, Beck JF. p53-dependent and p53-independent anticancer effects of different histone deacetylase inhibitors. British Journal of Cancer. 2014;110(3):656–67. DOI: 10.1038/bjc.2013.742

[144] Lee SH, Kim MJ, Kim DW, Kang CD, Kim SH. Amurensin G enhances the susceptibility to tumor necrosis factor-related apoptosis-inducing ligand-mediated cytotoxicity of cancer stem-like cells of HCT-15 cells. Cancer Science. 2013;104(12):1632–9. DOI: 10.1111/cas.12299

[145] Kumazaki M, Noguchi S, Yasui Y, Iwasaki J, Shinohara H, Yamada N, Akao Y. Anti-cancer effects of naturally occurring compounds through modulation of signal transduction and miRNA expression in human colon cancer cells. The Journal of Nutritional Biochemistry. 2013;24(11):1849–58. DOI: 10.1016/j.jnutbio.2013.04.006

[146] Reiter RJ, Tan DX, Galano A. Melatonin: exceeding expectations. Physiology (Bethesda). 2014;29(5):325–33. DOI: 10.1152/physiol.00011.2014

[147] Zamfir Chiru AA, Popescu CR, Gheorghe DC. Melatonin and cancer. Journal of Medicine and Life. 2014;7(3):373–4.

[148] Jung-Hynes B, Schmit TL, Reagan-Shaw SR, Siddiqui IA, Mukhtar H, Ahmad N. Melatonin, a novel Sirt1 inhibitor, imparts antiproliferative effects against prostate

cancer in vitro in culture and in vivo in TRAMP model. Journal of Pineal Research. 2011;50(2):140–9. DOI: 10.1111/j.1600-079X.2010.00823.x

[149] Cheng Y, Cai L, Jiang P, Wang J, Gao C, Feng H, Wang C, Pan H, Yang Y. SIRT1 inhibition by melatonin exerts antitumor activity in human osteosarcoma cells. European Journal of Pharmacology. 2013;715(1–3):219–29. DOI: 10.1016/j.ejphar. 2013.05.017

[150] Kannen V, Marini T, Zanette DL, Frajacomo FT, Silva GE, Silva WAJr., Garcia SB. The melatonin action on stromal stem cells within pericryptal area in colon cancer model under constant light. Biochemical and Biophysical Research Communications. 2011;405(4):593–8. DOI: 10.1016/j.bbrc.2011.01.074

[151] Zu G, Ji A, Zhou T, Che N. Clinicopathological significance of SIRT1 expression in colorectal cancer: A systematic review and meta analysis. The International Journal of Surgery. 2016;26:32–7. DOI: 10.1016/j.ijsu.2016.01.002

[152] Vellinga TT, Borovski T, de Boer VC, Fatrai S, van Schelven S, Trumpi K, Verheem A, Snoeren N, Emmink BL, Koster J, Rinkes IH, Kranenburg O. SIRT1/PGC1alpha-dependent increase in oxidative phosphorylation supports chemotherapy resistance of colon cancer. Clinical Cancer Research: An Official Journal of the American Association for Cancer Research. 2015;21(12):2870–9. DOI: 10.1158/1078-0432.CRC-14-2290

Chapter 3

Modulation of Apoptosis in Colon Cancer Cells by Bioactive Compounds

Marinela Bostan, Mirela Mihaila, Camelia Hotnog, Coralia Bleotu, Gabriela Anton, Viviana Roman and Lorelei Irina Brasoveanu

Additional information is available at the end of the chapter

http://dx.doi.org/10.5772/63382

Abstract

A big challenge for a successful colon cancer treatment is the lack of eradication of the entire tumour cell population and consequent development of chemoresistance. Control of cell number from tissues and elimination of cells predisposed to malignant transformation, having an aberrant cell cycle or presenting DNA mutations, might be performed by a cellular 'suicide' mechanism — the programmed cell death, or apoptosis. Coordinated activation and execution of multiple subprograms are needed, added by a good knowledge of the basic components of the death machinery, besides their interaction to regulate apoptosis in a coordinated manner. Triggering apoptosis in target cells is a key mechanism by which chemotherapy promotes cell killing. Many anti-cancer drugs act during physiological pathways of apoptosis, leading to tumour cell destruction. New therapeutic approaches in cancer induce tumour cells to undergo apoptosis and break the cancer cell resistance to apoptosis commands. Administrations of natural compounds that prevent induction, inhibit or delay the progression of cancer, or induce inhibition or reversal of carcinogenesis at a premalignant stage represent chemoprevention strategies. Several natural compounds have been shown to be promising based on their anti-cancer effects and low toxicity; alternative approaches might be taken into account to obtain a stronger anti-tumour response when lower concentrations of anti-cancer drugs are used, and to diminish the undesirable side-effects.

Keywords: colon cancer, apoptosis, tumour evasion, bioactive compounds, combined therapy

1. Introduction

Cancer is a disease of cells that is thought to evolve along a multi-step process: the transformation of normal cells, tumour progression and advanced metastasis, that involve a complex series of events such as genetic alterations, aberrant progression of the cell cycle, resistance to growth inhibition, proliferation without dependence on growth factors, replication without limit, evasion of apoptosis, induction of angiogenesis and modification of cell adhesion [1]. For an accurate prediction, prevention, early detection and development of anti-cancer drugs, it is essential to identify the stages of development and use basic information [2]. The lack of eradication of the entire tumour cell population and the consequent development of chemoresistance represent main obstacles to a successful treatment in many malignancies, including colon cancer [3, 4]. The control of cell number from tissues and elimination of those predisposed to malignant transformation, having an aberrant cell cycle or presenting DNA mutations, might be performed by a cellular "suicide" mechanism, the programmed cell death or apoptosis [5, 6]. Elucidating the mechanisms of programmed cell death process seems to be of great importance for carcinogenesis, tumour evasion, and to have practical implications for anti-cancer therapy since many anti-cancer drugs act during physiological pathways of apoptosis, leading to tumour cell destruction [7, 8].

Several therapeutic agents used in colon cancer treatment, e.g. fluoropyrimidines, cisplatin, oxaliplatin, irinotecan have been shown to induce resistance in cancer cell killing, and their number are rapidly increasing, possibly through the modulation of survival cell components, such as proliferative or anti-apoptotic proteins [9, 10]. Triggering apoptosis in target cells represents a key mechanism by which chemotherapy promotes cell killing. Continuing efforts are made for discovering new molecular target-based molecules [11], and new therapeutic approaches in colon cancer involve restored cellular mechanisms responsible for the induction of apoptosis in tumour cells [12–15].

A main strategy in colon cancer treatment might be the combined multi-drug chemotherapy, the reason being the potential additive or synergistic tumour cytotoxicity produced [1]. The focus on finding new therapeutic strategies has recently shifted to natural products. Various plants and their bioactive compounds have been shown to have anti-carcinogenic and anti-proliferative effects towards the colon cancer cells. Studies have also reported positive correlation between the antioxidant activity of plants and their anti-proliferative effects, suggesting the potential action of antioxidants in inhibiting cancer cell growth. For example, the flavonoids display a wide range of biological activities, including anti-inflammatory and cytoprotective activities, and several are known to act as anti-cancer reagents [16].

The administration of synthetic or natural compounds that prevent induction of cancer, inhibit or delay its progression, or reverse carcinogenesis at a premalignant stage could represent useful strategies because of their potential clinical application in combined treatments with anti-cancer drugs [17]. By combining natural compounds with anti-cancer drugs, it might be obtained an increase of cancer treatment effects, specifically in highly invasive colon cancer cells, while in non-tumour cells the use of natural compounds could reduce the cytotoxic side effects [18].

2. Biology of colon cells: normal versus carcinogenic

Colorectal cancer (CRC) is the third most common malignancy worldwide, being frequently diagnosed in advanced stages. Recent data added to the molecular explanations of growth dysregulation, metastasis formation, extension of life span, and loss of maintenance of genomic and epigenetic integrity in cancer suggest models for their causal connection. The mechanisms of growth control, senescence, and anchorage dependence are linked at the molecular level [2].

The adult colon epithelium contains three cell types that arise from a multipotent stem cell: absorptive epithelial, enteroendocrine and Goblet cells. Colonic epithelial cells are configured in deep invaginations into the wall of the colon named crypts: from stem cells located at the base of the crypt, they arise and migrate to the luminal surface of the crypt where they are shed. Stem cells divide asymmetrically: the "old" DNA is retained in the stem cell population, and the new synthesised DNA is donated to daughter cells that migrate up the crypt and are ultimately shed. Stem cells are particularly vulnerable to developing mutations that might evolve into a malignant clone. Therefore, the cells located at the base of crypts, presumably stem cells, are highly prone to apoptosis, able to counteract dangerous mutations [19]. The result of the imbalance between cell proliferation and apoptosis determines colorectal tumour growth. Relatively undifferentiated tumours with higher proliferative potential are often more aggressive than well-differentiated ones [2]. The molecular mechanisms of cell division and apoptosis are similar in normal and tumour cells, but in tumour cells, these mechanisms are aberrantly regulated. Four cellular functions are inadequate regulated in tumour cells: (1) control of cell proliferation is inefficient; (2) genetic and chromosomal structure is destabilized; (3) cellular differentiation program is frequently altered; (4) the control of apoptosis is disturbed [20].

Multiple sequential genetic changes are needed to occur in order to ensure colorectal cancer evolution. During progression of normal epithelial to carcinoma cell in colorectal cancer, TP53, KRAS, BRAF and PIK3CA gene alterations play important roles. Gene alterations cause disruption of signalling pathways in which they are involved, accompanied by increased proliferative potential and decreased apoptosis of cells [21]. Along with genetic mutations, colon carcinogenesis is accompanied by epigenetic changes that lead to altered expression of key genes. Three major epigenetic regulatory mechanisms are described: (a) DNA methylation, (b) the covalent modifications of histones and (c) non-coding RNA interference [22].

3. Programmed cell death in normal versus carcinogenic colon cells

Apoptosis represents a cellular "suicide" mechanism which allows control of the number of cells from tissues and removal of cells that present DNA mutations or have an aberrant cell cycle, predisposed to malignant transformation [5]. Thus, elucidating the mechanisms of programmed cell death process seems to be of great importance for malignant transformation, tumour evasion, and therefore for anti-cancer therapy like restoration of cellular mechanisms responsible for the induction of apoptosis in tumour cells [23, 24]. Abnormalities in apoptotic function contribute to both pathogenesis of colorectal cancer, and its resistance to chemotherapeutics and radiotherapy [19].

3.1. Apoptosis pathways

Apoptosis is an active, specialized form of cell death with distinct biochemical and genetic pathways that play a critical role in normal tissue homeostasis and development. Under stress, such as precancerous lesions, the mechanisms involved in repairing DNA damage are activated and potentially harmful cells are removed, and carcinogenesis is blocked [25]. Lack of regulation of the apoptosis pathways may promote tumorigenesis and induce resistance to treatment in cancer cells [19].

The apoptotic process displays morphological features of the cells: cellular shrinkage with nuclear chromatin condensation and nuclear fragmentation, membrane blebbing, and cell-self-fragmentation into apoptotic bodies. Apoptosis is initiated by two basic signalling pathways: **the extrinsic pathway**, initiated by external stimuli and via activation of death receptors on the cell surface, such as tumour necrosis factor-α (TNF-α), Fas (CD95/APO1) and TNF-related apoptosis-inducing ligand (TRAIL) receptors, and **the intrinsic** (or mitochondrial) **pathway,** activated by intracellular stimuli and characterized by mitochondrial outer membrane permeabilization and release of mitochondrial cytochrome *c* (cyt-c) [26]. There is an overlap between the two apoptotic pathways: the extrinsic pathway usually also activates the intrinsic pathway, and both pathways result in the recruitment and activation of cysteine-aspartic acid proteases (caspases) [27, 28]. Upon receiving specific signals instructing the cells to undergo apoptosis, the caspase family of proteins is typically activated and cleaves key cellular components required for normal cellular function, including structural proteins in the cytoskeleton and nuclear proteins such as DNA repair enzymes [29]. Caspases can directly signal apoptosis or use mitochondria as an intermediate and additional point of regulation in apoptosis signalling [30].

(a) the mitochondrial pathway (the intrinsic pathway) is activated by a wide variety of cytotoxic drugs, DNA damage, growth factor deprivation, oxidative stress, Ca^{2+} overload and oncogene activation [29, 30]. It is regulated by formation of the mitochondrial permeability transition pore (MPTP), composed by Bcl-2 family members and voltage-dependent anion channels on the outer mitochondrial membrane [31], leading to mitochondrial outer membrane permeabilization (MOMP). The drop of mitochondrial membrane potential initiates the osmotic swelling of the matrix by water influx and release of cytochrome *c* from mitochondrial intermembrane space into the cytoplasm. Cytochrome *c* then associates with apoptotic protease-activating factor 1 (APAF-1) and caspase-9 forming apoptosome complex. The activation of caspase-9 and/or caspase-8 leads to caspase-3 cleavage, endonuclease activation, and ultimately nuclear DNA fragmentation, which is the hallmark of apoptosis [31, 32]. B cell leukaemia/lymphoma 2 (Bcl-2) family proteins are central regulators of the intrinsic pathway, which either suppress or promote changes in mitochondrial membrane permeability required for the release of cyt-c and other apoptogenic proteins [33].

(b) the extrinsic pathway starts with the stimulation of specific death receptors upon binding of their ligands, like tumour necrosis factor (TNF), tumour necrosis factor-related apoptosis-inducing ligand (TRAIL) and CD95 (Fas or APO1) [34]. Death receptors are transmembrane proteins with a death domain in their cytosolic region; the ligands binding causes oligomerization of these receptors, exposing their death domains (DD) in their cytosolic tail, which rapidly bind to Fas-Associated Death Domain (FADD). Several of the DD-containing TNF-family receptors use caspase activation as a signalling mechanism, including TNFR1/CD120a, Fas/APO1/CD95, DR3/Apo2/Weasle, DR4/TrailR1, DR5/TrailR2, and DR6 [35, 36]. Binding of these receptors at the cell surface results in the recruitment of several intracellular proteins, including some procaspases, to the cytosolic domains of these receptors, forming a "death-inducing signalling complex" (DISC) that triggers caspase-8 activation [37, 38]. In the case of TNFR1, after the ligand binds to TNFR1, the cytosolic region of the receptor does not bind FADD, but TRADD adaptor, as well as several other signalling proteins, some of them being involved in the activation of NF-κB transcription factor. The initial complex is then released from the receptor, TRADD binds to FADD in the cytosol, and caspase-8 is recruited. The downstream signalling depends on additional interactions with proteins like FLICE-like inhibitory proteins (c-FLIP), forming a complex that contains heterodimers of caspase-8 and c-FLIP that will inhibit apoptosis. However, if NF-κB activity is blocked or disrupted, or c-FLIP expression is inhibited, caspase-8 is activated and cell undergoes apoptosis [30, 39]. Between the death receptor pathway and the mitochondrial pathway of apoptosis, there is an overlap. Caspase-8 has another substrate in the cell, BID, a BH3-only protein: when caspase-8 cleaves BID, the protein is translocated to the mitochondria to promote MOMP and to initiate mitochondria-dependent apoptosis [40].

3.2. Evasion mechanisms of apoptosis in colon cancer

Apoptosis is subverted during tumorigenesis through the systematic loss of regulatory control mechanisms, ultimately resulting in the generation of a malignant phenotype and resistance to chemotherapy and radiation therapy. Several potential mechanisms and factors involved were taken into account to explain the defects in apoptotic signalling and the increased activation of anti-apoptotic pathways that were observed in colon cancer cells:

(a) Disrupted balance between pro- and anti-apoptotic proteins

Many proteins exert pro- or anti-apoptotic activity in cells, and the ratio between them plays an important role in the regulation of cell death. Over- or under-expressed genes were also found to contribute to carcinogenesis by reducing apoptosis in cancer cells. Key regulatory proteins of apoptotic machinery, such as Bcl-2 (including Bcl-xl and Bax) and IAP family, undergo changes in expression during the transition from adenoma to carcinoma, and therefore, they were used as prognostic biomarkers [7]. Pro- and anti-apoptotic mediators can regulate mitochondrial outer membrane permeability and release of cytochrome *c* from the mitochondria into the cytoplasm [41] (**Figure 1**).

When there is a disruption in the balance of anti-apoptotic and pro-apoptotic members of the **Bcl-2 family**, the result is a dysregulation of apoptosis in the affected cells. This can be due to the overexpression of one or more anti-apoptotic proteins, or the underexpression of one or more pro-apoptotic proteins, or both [42, 43]. In colorectal cancer, the dysregulated expression of Bcl-2 family members may be associated with disease outcomes. Bcl-2 expression is restricted to the basal epithelial cells in normal and hyperplastic mucosa, but in dysplastic polyps and carcinomas, it is extended to the parabasal and superficial regions. Bcl-2 expression is increased in hyperplastic polyps and markedly increased in almost all adenomas, while carcinomas show weaker Bcl-2 expression, indicating the decrease of apoptosis during progression from adenoma to carcinoma [44, 45].

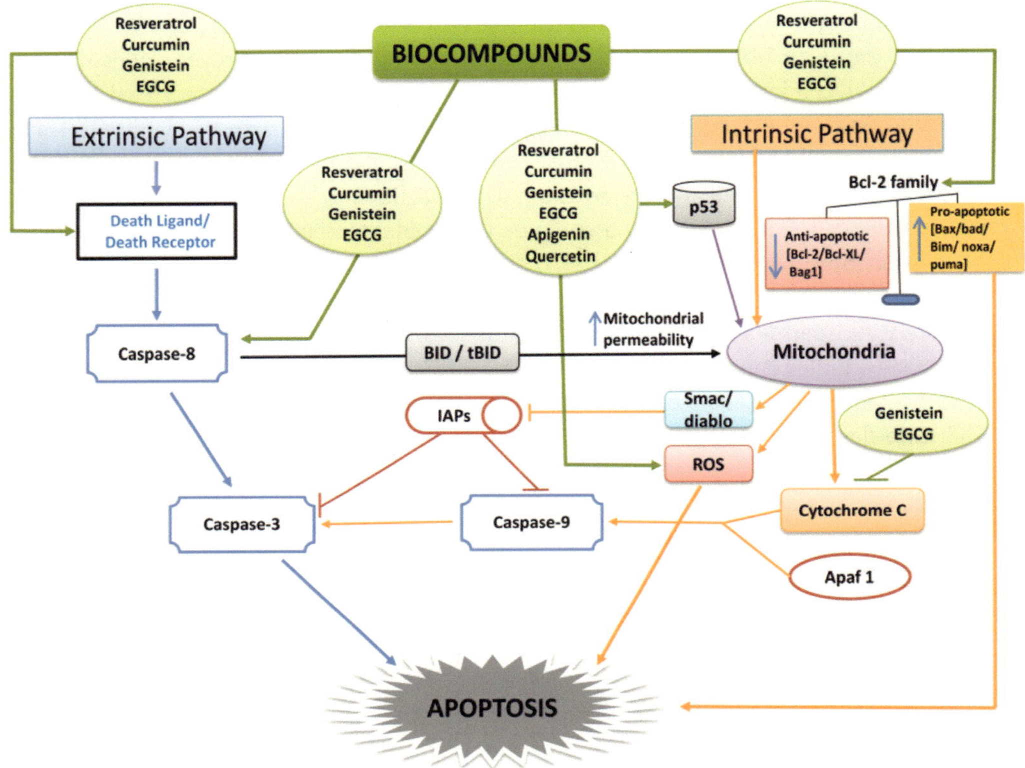

Figure 1. Role of biocompounds in modulation of intrinsic and extrinsic pathways of apoptosis.

Overexpression of the anti-apoptotic Bcl-2 family member Bcl-XL predicts poor prognosis in patients with colonic adenocarcinomas, conferring a multidrug resistance phenotype [46, 47]. Bcl-w, another anti-apoptotic Bcl-2 family protein, plays a general role in the progression from adenoma to adenocarcinoma in the colorectal epithelium; it is frequently expressed in colorectal adenocarcinomas at significant higher levels in TNM stage III tumours, positive correlated with node involvement [42]. In primary colorectal adenocarcinomas, elevated levels of expression for Bcl-xL and Bcl-w were reported to be associated with reduced expression of Bax [42]. Regarding the pro-apoptotic members of Bcl-2 family like Bcl-10, Bax, Bak, Bid, Bad, Bim, Bik, and Blk, increasing evidences suggest the involvement of Bak and Bax in the release of cytochrome *c*, based on phosphorylation of both Bak and Bax that facilitate their homo-oligomerization and subsequently the localization in mitochondria [29, 48]. Mutations in both

Bax and Bak genes confer cells the resistance to apoptosis [49, 50]. In colon cancer, Bax gene is frequently mutated in hereditary non-polyposis colorectal cancers [51] and microsatellite mutator phenotype [52, 53]. Decreased Bax expression was correlated with poor prognosis and progression towards metastasis [54].

One of the best known tumour suppressor proteins is **p53**, encoded by the tumour suppressor gene TP53 located on the short arm of chromosome 17 (17p13.1). The oncogenic property is due to a p53 mutations [55, 56], and half of all colorectal cancer cases show mutations in TP53 gene that were correlated with adenoma-to-carcinoma transitions and aggressive subsets of colorectal cancer [57, 58]. TP53 is a tumour suppressor gene in the mitochondrial apoptotic pathway, and one of the key regulators of cell-cycle control and apoptosis. Tumour cells presenting p53 mutations are defective in the induction of apoptosis. Its expression is down-regulated by survivin and Bcl-2 [59]. The molecular mechanisms that are employed by p53 to induce cell death in the context of suppressing cancer progression include the transcriptional regulation of pro-apoptotic PUMA expression, the generation of oxidative free radicals within mitochondrial components, the reduction of COX-2/PGE2 synthesis, and the induction of death receptor 5 [60, 61] (**Figure 1**).

Inhibitors of apoptosis (IAPs family) suppress apoptosis through inhibition of effector caspases [62]. The expression of inhibitor of apoptosis proteins (IAPs) is dysregulated in colorectal cancer. The anti-apoptotic regulators belonging to the IAP family, including XIAP, cIAP, and survivin, bind to caspase-3 and caspase-9 and thereby inhibit c aspase activity (**Figure 1**). Moreover, XIAP-associated factor 1 (XAF1) negatively regulates the anti-apoptotic function of XIAP. Molecules like c-FLIP, XIAP, cIAP2, and survivin have increased expression levels in colon cancer patients, and this has been correlated with disease progression and poor survival [47, 63, 64].

(b) Reduced caspase activity

During apoptosis process, the caspases implicated are either **initiator caspases** (e.g. caspase-2, caspase-8, caspase-9 and caspase-10) which are primarily responsible for the initiation of the apoptotic pathway, or **effector caspases** (caspase-3, caspase-6 and caspase-7), which are responsible in the actual cleavage of cellular components during apoptosis [65]. In the initiation and execution of apoptosis, caspases remain important players; therefore, low levels of caspases or impairment in caspase function may lead to a decrease in apoptosis and carcinogenesis [66, 67]. More than one caspase can be downregulated, contributing to colon cancer cell growth and development. Studies on differential expression by cDNA array showed a downregulation of both capase-8 and caspase-10, phenomenon that influences the pathogenesis of carcinomas [68].

(c) Impaired death receptor signalling

Several receptors and ligands that modulate the programmed cell death were described: TNF receptor superfamily, Fas/Fas-L, CD27, death receptors and ligands, receptors phosphatases. Signalling via death receptors could be impaired in human cancers via downregulation of receptor surface expression as part of an adaptive stress response. Death receptors and their ligands are key players in the extrinsic pathway of apoptosis. The extrinsic signalling pathway leading to apoptosis involves transmembrane death receptors that are members of the tumour necrosis factor (TNF) receptor gene superfamily [69]. Several abnormalities in the death signalling pathways that can lead to evasion of the extrinsic pathway of apoptosis have been identified: the downregulation of receptor expression, the impairment of its function, as well as a reduced level in the death signals, all of which contribute to impaired signalling and a reduction of apoptosis. Reduced membrane expression of death receptors and abnormal expression of decoy receptors have also been reported to play a role in the evasion of the death signalling pathways in various cancers [12, 70] (**Figure 1**).

(d) Altered redox status in apoptosis induction

The oxidative stress process is characterized by an increased generation of reactive oxygen species (ROS) accompanied by a dysfunction of the antioxidant systems which exist in every cell, dependent on the metabolic state of the cell [71, 72]. The increased metabolic activity, mitochondrial dysfunction, peroxisome activity, oncogene activity, increased activity of oxidases, cyclooxygenases, lipoxigenases could be responsible for the generation and release of reactive oxygen species in tumour cells [73–75]. Low levels of ROS may influence processes like angiogenesis, cell proliferation and survival, while intermediate levels of ROS cause transient or permanent cell-cycle arrest and induce cell differentiation. When ROS production does not irreversibly alter cell viability, they can act as primary messengers, modulating several intracellular signalling cascades that lead to cancer progression [76]. High levels of ROS induce cell apoptosis or necrosis by causing an alteration of membrane permeability, a genetic instability, oxidative modifications that lead to less active enzymes or proteins more susceptible to proteolytic degradation [77]. Furthermore, ROS plays a crucial role in regulating expression of genes associated with cancer cell proliferation, angiogenesis, invasion and metastasis by activating transcription factors such as NF-κB, activator protein-1 (AP-1) and hypoxia inducible factor-1 (HIF-1α) [78].

Excessive production of ROS in tumour cells induces apoptosis or necrosis, and acts as an important inhibitor of cancer cell proliferation. Fas ligand mediates the induction of ROS, essential for the initiation of apoptotic signalling cascade and activation of the intrinsic apoptotic machinery by disruption of mitochondrial membrane integrity [79] (**Figure 1**). The transformed cells use ROS signals to drive proliferation to tumour progression. Tumour cells present an increased basal oxidative stress, making them vulnerable to chemotherapeutic agents that further augment ROS generation or weaken antioxidant defences of the cell [80]. Human colorectal tumours have increased levels of different markers of oxidative stress, such as ROS, nitric oxide (NO), lipid peroxides, glutathione peroxidase (GPx), catalase (CAT), and decreased cytosine DNA methylation [81–83].

ROS-sensitive signalling pathways are persistently elevated in many types of cancers, including colon cancer [84]. Reactive oxygen species can act as second messengers in cellular signalling. For example, hydrogen peroxide (H_2O_2) regulates protein activity through reversible oxidation of its targets, including protein tyrosine phosphatases, protein tyrosine kinases, receptor tyrosine kinases and transcription factors [85, 86]. The mitogen-activated protein (MAP) kinase/Erk cascade, phosphoinositide-3-kinase (PI3K)/Akt-regulated signalling cascades, as well as the IκB kinase (IKK)/nuclear factor κ-B (NF-κB)-activating pathways are regulated by ROS. The extracellular signal-regulated kinase pathway (ERK) mediates signal transduction involved in cell proliferation, differentiation, and migration [87]. Activation of ERK in tumour cells by biocompounds (e.g. resveratrol, quercetin) results in anti-proliferative effects, such as apoptosis, senescence, or autophagy [88–91]. Then, ERK can activate apoptotic enzymes or phosphorylate transcription factors that regulate the expression of pro-apoptotic genes [92]. Cell death in tumour cells treated with resveratrol and quercetin was accompanied by increased ROS levels and p53 expression, decreased Bcl-2 expression, depolarization of the mitochondrial membrane, cleaved caspase-3, and DNA fragmentation [93]. Elevated levels of ROS triggered by treatment with biocompounds might inhibit dual-specificity phosphatases (DUSPs) that dephosphorylate and inactivate MAPKs, leading to ERK activation and promoting cancer cell death. Therefore, biocompounds might induce apoptosis in colon cancer cells via activation of the MEK/ERK pathway [94].

Mitochondrial release of H_2O_2 and NO upon apoptotic signals leads to the activation of c-Jun N-terminal kinases (JNKs). In response to ROS, JNKs catalyze the phosphorylation and downregulation of anti-apoptotic proteins such as Bcl-2 and Bcl-XL. JNK influences the composition of the Bax/Bcl-2 complex by increasing the expression of Bax, leading to the formation of Bax homodimers and dissipation of mitochondrial membrane integrity [95, 96]. In response to the increased generation of ROS, the MAPK family member p38MAP is also implicated in apoptotic signalling [97].

In addition, ROS play an important role in the regulation of IKK/NF-κB pathway. NF-κB is a redox-regulated sensor for oxidative stress that is activated by low doses of hydrogen peroxide. The activation of NF-κB is mediated through the NF-κB-inducing kinase (NIK) and IκB kinase (IKK) complexes. Degradation of IκB translocates NF-κB to the nucleus, where it acts as a transcription factor to induce the expression of anti-apoptotic and anti-inflammatory genes [98]. Peroxisome proliferator-activated receptor-gamma (PPARγ) has been shown to exert an inhibitory effect on cell growth in most cell types. The expression of PPARγ was significantly increased in tumour tissues from human colon cancer, and the occurrence of apoptosis induced by PPARγ ligands was sequentially accompanied by reduced levels of NF-κB and Bcl-2. PPARγ-Bcl-2 feedback loop might control the life–death continuum in colonic cells, while a deficiency in generation of PPARγ ligands could precede the development of human colon cancer [99].

4. Bioactive compounds and colon cancer

Recent studies focused on the discovery of new chemotherapeutic agents among natural products since many plants and their bioactive compounds displayed anti-carcinogenic and anti-proliferative effects towards colon cancer cells [13]. Positive correlations between antioxidant activities of plants and their anti-proliferative effects, suggesting the potential action of antioxidants in inhibiting cancer cell growth, were also reported [13]. Among them, over 5000 flavonoids were found in vegetables and fruits, wines, seeds, nuts, grains and teas, herbs, and represent a class of plant secondary metabolites, known for their antioxidant properties [100]. The position of hydroxyl groups and other features in the chemical structure of flavonoids are important for their antioxidant and free radical scavenging activities [70]. The dietary compounds could interfere with specific stages of the carcinogenic process, inhibiting cell proliferation and inducing apoptosis in different types of cancer cells [101]. In addition, they might affect the expression of several detoxifying enzymes and their ability to modulate protein-signalling cascades [102].

4.1. Dietary sources and functional features

Since the 1950s, despite extensive clinical trials, mortality from colon cancer is a major public health problem in developed countries as a result of high consumption of animal fat or red meat and low intake of fibres or vegetables [103]. Protective factors include physical activity and increased intakes of dietary fibre, fish, nuts, dairy products, fruits and vegetables, while other factors, including weight and obesity, waist circumference, smoking, alcohol consumption, and red and processed meat intakes increase the risk of colorectal cancer [104, 105]. Using simple lifestyle modifications, changing the diet might substantially reduce the risk of colorectal cancer and could complement screening, so that CRC could be preventable in 90% of cases [106]. Over the last decade, different drugs and nutritional elements have been studied in preclinical as well as clinical trials and proved to have potential benefit in the field of CRC prevention [107]. Chemoprevention, the use of drugs or other agents to inhibit the development or progression of malignant changes in cells represents an alternative approach to reduce the mortality from colorectal cancer as well as other cancers [108].

Biocompounds	Source	Mechanisms of action	Refs.
Resveratrol	Grapes and red wine, mulberries, peanuts, seeds	Caspase activation NF-κB inhibition FasL induction Activation of MEK/ERK pathway Bcl-2 downregulation Increase of ROS and p53 levels	[92–94, 111, 137, 166, 167]
Genistein	Soybeans, fava beans, lupin, coffee	NF-κB inhibition Caspase activation Inhibition of PTK Inhibition of AKT pathway mdm2 downregulation	[113, 114]
Quercetin	Vegetables (capers, radish	Bcl-2, EGFR downregulation	[91–94,

http://dx.doi.org/10.5772/63382

Biocompounds	Source	Mechanisms of action	Refs.
	leaves, dill, cilantro, fennel, red onion, radicchio, kale), fruits (cranberry, black plums, blueberry, apples), seeds, nuts, tea, red wine	Cyclin D1, survivin inhibition Inhibition of Wnt/beta-catenin signalling pathway Increase of ROS and p53 levels Activation of MEK/ERK pathway	164]
Curcumin	Turmeric, curry, mustard	NF-κB inhibition ROS induction Modulation of MAPK pathway Downregulation of survivin and IGF-1 expression	[141–143, 146, 147]
Apigenin	Parsley, celery, dandelion, coffee, chamomile tea	Modulation of survival and death effectors (PI3K, AKT, ERK, STAT3, JNK, Mcl-1)	[119, 168]
Epigallocatechin gallate (EGCG)	Green tea, white tea, black tea	Modulation of ROS production NF-κB inhibition Inhibition of growth factor-dependent signalling (EGF, VEGF, IGF-I) Inhibition of MAPK and p21 pathways Downregulation of survivin	[148, 149, 151–155, 157, 176]
Silibinin	Milk thistle seeds	Bcl-2 downregulation Bax upregulation Decrease of cyclin D1 and c-myc expression Upregulation of death receptors DR4, DR5	[17, 127, 136, 138, 139]
Naringenin	Grapefruits, oranges and tomatoes (skin)	Losses in mitochondrial membrane potential Caspase-3 activation Intracellular ROS production Sustained ERK activation	[129, 163]
Pomegranate juice	Pomegranate	Downregulation of Bcl2-XL Caspase-3 and caspase-9 activation NF-κB inhibition Suppression of AKT pathway	[131, 132, 158, 160]

Biocompounds	Source	Mechanisms of action	Refs.
Sulforaphane	Broccoli, Brussels sprouts, cabbage, cauliflower, kale, collards, kohlrabi, mustard, turnip, radish, arugula, watercress	Upregulation of Bax, p21 G_2/M cell-cycle arrest	[121, 122, 177, 178]
Ellagic acid	Strawberries, walnuts, pecans	Disruption in mitochondrial membrane potential Activation of caspase-3, caspase-8 and caspase-9 Inactivation of PI3K/Akt pathway Bax upregulation; Bcl-2 downregulation Increase of ROS production	[169, 170]
Lycopene	Tomatoes, red carrots, watermelons, papayas	Bax and FasL upregulation; Bcl-2 and Bcl-XL downregulation Downregulation of Akt, NF-κB	[171, 172]

Table 1. Biocompounds—dietary sources and mechanisms of action involved in modulation of apoptosis.

Different natural compounds display a wide range of biological activities, including anti-inflammatory and cytoprotective activities, and several are known to act as anti-cancer reagents. Curcumin from turmeric, genistein from soybean, tea polyphenols like epigallocatechin gallate from green tea, resveratrol from grapes, sulforaphane from broccoli, isothiocyanates from cruciferous vegetables, silymarin from milk thistle, diallyl sulphide from garlic, lycopene from tomato, rosmarinic acid from rosemary, apigenin from parsley, gingerol from ginger and quercetin (**Table 1**) have high antioxidant activities, and demonstrated anti-proliferative effects against various cancer cell lines [13].

Resveratrol (RSV, trans-3,4′,5-trihydroxystilbene), a naturally occurring polyphenol phytoalexin, is abundant in a wide variety of plants and their products, including grapes and red wine, mulberries, peanuts, seeds, and has anti-inflammatory, antioxidant, anti-neoplastic, anti-carcinogenic, anti-tumorigenic, cardioprotective, neuroprotective, anti-aging and antiviral effects [102, 109]. Resveratrol exhibited anti-colon cancer properties by inhibiting cell proliferation, inducing apoptosis, decreasing angiogenesis, and causing cell-cycle arrest [110, 111].

Genistein (GST, 4′,5,7-trihydroxyisoflavone) is a natural compound found in lupin, fava beans, soybeans, coffee and occurs in Asian diet, rich in soy products [112]. It is a strong topoisomerase inhibitor, similarly to etoposide and doxorubicin. It has a wide spectrum of activity, expressed in protecting cells from malignant transformation, reducing proliferation of tumour cells and stimulating apoptosis [113, 114].

Quercetin (QCT, 3,3′,4′,5,7-pentahydroxyflavone) is an important dietary flavonoid, which presents in different vegetables (e.g. capers, radish leaves, dill, cilantro, fennel, red onion, radicchio, kale), fruits (cranberry, black plums, blueberry, apples), seeds, nuts, tea and red wine. It is involved in suppression of tumour-related processes, including oxidative stress, proliferation and metastasis. QCT has also received greater attention as pro-apoptotic flavonoid with a specific and almost exclusive activity on tumour cell lines rather than normal, non-transformed cells [115]. The anti-tumour effect found in SW480 colon cancer cell line was related to the inhibition of Cyclin D (1) and survivin expression, as well as Wnt/beta-catenin signalling pathway [116].

Curcumin (CRM, 1,7-bis-(4-hydroxy-3-methoxyphenyl)-1,6-heptadiene-3,5-dione) is a diarylheptanoid and the principal curcuminoid of turmeric, extracted from *Curcuma longa*; it possesses anti-inflammatory and antioxidant properties, and has a strong inhibitory effect on cell proliferation in the HT-29 and HCT-15 human colon cancer cell lines [117, 118].

Apigenin (APG, 4′,5,7-trihydroxyflavone) is one of the most common flavonoids widely distributed in fruits and vegetables, such as parsley, celery, dandelion coffee and chamomile tea. However, apigenin only showed a modest anti-tumour activity towards cancer cells. New strategies are needed to enhance apigenin's anti-tumour efficacy [119].

Epigallocatechin 3-O-gallate (EGCG) [(2*R*,3*R*)-5,7-dihydroxy-2-(3,4,5-trihydroxyphenyl)-3,4-dihydro-2*H*-1-benzopyran-3-yl 3,4,5-trihydroxybenzoate] is the most abundant catechin in tea, a polyphenol found in high quantities in the dried leaves of white tea, green tea and, in smaller content in black tea [120]. EGCG was found to exert profound anti-inflammatory, antioxidant, anti-infective, anti-cancer, anti-angiogenic, and chemopreventive effects [120].

Sulforaphane (1-Isothiocyanato-4-methylsulfinylbutane) is found in cruciferous vegetables such as broccoli, Brussels sprouts, cabbage, cauliflower, bok choy, kale, collards, Chinese broccoli, broccoli raab, kohlrabi, mustard, turnip, radish, arugula and watercress. Young sprouts of broccoli and cauliflower are particularly rich in glucoraphanin. It is produced when the enzyme myrosinase transforms glucoraphanin, a glucosinolate, into sulforaphane upon damage to the plant which allows the two compounds to mix and react [121]. Sulforaphane (SFN) is a naturally occurring chemopreventive agent, inducing the cell-cycle arrest and apoptosis in colon cancer. However, little is known about the differential effects of SFN on colon cancer and normal cells [122].

Lycopene is a bright carotenoid pigment and phytochemical found in tomatoes, red carrots, watermelons and papayas. Although lycopene is chemically a carotene, it has no vitamin A activity. Also foods that are not red may contain lycopene, such as asparagus or parsley. Lycopene exhibited potential anti-carcinogenic activity, and the consumption of tomatoes was associated with reduced risk of several types of human cancer, including colon cancer [123, 124].

Glucobrassicin is a type of glucosinolate found in cabbages, broccoli, mustards, horseradish and woad. The main hydrolysis product after glucobrassicin is degraded by myrosinase is indole-3-carbinol, which was found to have apoptosis-inducing effects in a concentration- and time-dependent manner in human colon cancer cells [125, 126].

Silibinin is the major active constituent of **silymarin**, a standardized extract of the milk thistle seeds, that contains a mixture of flavonolignans and was shown to induce apoptosis in colon cancer cells [127, 128].

Naringenin (5,7-dihydroxy-2-(4-hydroxyphenyl)chroman-4-one) is a flavanone, considered to have a bioactive effect on human health as antioxidant, free radical scavenger, anti-inflammatory, carbohydrate metabolism promoter and immune system modulator. It can be found in grapefruits, oranges and tomatoes (skin) [129].

Pomegranate juice obtained from Punica granatum is rich in polyphenol compounds such as gallo, ellagitannin and flavonoid classes. It possesses therapeutic activity such as anti-atherogenic, anti-parasitic, anti-microbial, antioxidant, anti-carcinogenic and anti-inflammatory effects [130]; in preclinical animal studies, oral consumption of pomegranate extract inhibited the growth of lung, skin, colon and prostate tumours [131]. It was shown that pomegranate juice derivatives promote apoptosis of colon cancer cells by inducing the intrinsic pathway, but no effect was shown on the extrinsic pathway [132].

5. Bioactive compounds and their role in modulation of apoptosis in colon cancer

Results of clinical trials revealed that colon cancer can be successfully treated by chemotherapy, if the tumour selective detection can be substantial increased. In this regard, there is an increasing demand for biomarkers for risk assessment, early detection, prognosis and surrogate end points. This will be possible by the introduction of new drugs with more precise mechanisms of action, such as those acting specifically upon well-known aberrant pathways (e.g. apoptosis, cell signalling) [133]. New drugs can initiate or modulate the apoptosis cascade acting on caspases, Fas, Bax, Bid, APC or molecules which promote colon cancer cell survival (p53 mutants, Bcl-2 or COX-2) [134].

The implementation of new treatment options (and the management of metastatic colon cancer) must take into account the role of apoptosis in colon tumorigenesis with a highlight on the mechanisms leading to chemotherapeutic resistance as well as immune system evasion [69]. From this point of view, apoptosis can be considered as a potential target for cancer treatment at various stages of tumour progression, while chemoprevention as well as the apoptotic mechanisms could be utilized in the prevention and management of tumorigenesis [35, 135].

5.1. Mechanisms and targets involved

Grape seed extract that consists in a mixture of polyphenols was able to decrease cyclin D1, and c-myc expression, preventing cycle cell disruption, reduce expression of iNOS and COX-2 decreasing oxidative cellular stress [136]. On the other hand, *in vitro* studies performed on CRC cell lines showed that grape seed extract induces apoptosis via activation of caspase-3, caspase-8, and caspase-9, and also generation of ROS. It is worth mentioning that proapoptotic activity of grape seed extract has no effect in normal colonocytes [107].

Resveratrol has anti-CRC effects by inhibiting tumour initiation and progression by affecting caspase activation, NF-κB inhibition and FasL induction. Resveratrol could suppress inflammatory responses through decreasing nitric oxide levels and inhibiting the phosphorylation of the IκB enzyme complex, thus suppressing the activation of NF-κB dependent mechanisms [111, 137]. It was also described to interfere with mitochondrial functions by inhibiting mitochondrial ATP synthesis through its binding to F_1-ATPase. In addition, resveratrol can antagonize anti-apoptotic proteins that prevent the induction of apoptosis in cancer cells. Resveratrol induces p53-independent upregulation of p21, p21-triggered cell-cycle arrest and subsequently cell-cycle-dependent depletion of the anti-apoptotic protein survivin, thereby sensitizing cancer cells to TRAIL-induced apoptosis. Moreover, it suppresses expression levels of additional anti-apoptotic proteins (e.g. Bcl-x_L and MCL-1). The anti-tumour activities of resveratrol are also due to its ability to interfere with the phosphatidylinositol-3 kinase (PI-3K)/AKT and the MAPK pathways [13] (**Table 1**).

Silibinin: Studies *in vitro* and *in vivo* have shown a chemopreventive role in CRC by interfering in proliferation, signalling pathway and inflammation processes [17]. It was also found to cause decrease of cyclin D1 and c-myc expression [127]. Moreover, silibinin modulates the expression of anti-apoptotic proteins (Bcl-2, Mcl-1, X-linked inhibitor of apoptosis protein, and survivin) [136]. Silibinin can induce apoptosis by downregulation of the anti-apoptotic protein Bcl-2 and upregulation of the pro-apoptotic protein Bax, inverting the Bcl-2/Bax ratio. Sibilin also promotes apoptosis by upregulating transcription of the death receptors DR4 and DR5 [138], inhibits TNF-α activation of NF-κB, decreases expression of COX-2 and iNOS [139]. Silibinin decreased the expression of IL-1, TNF-alpha and their downstream target MMP7, all of them being upregulated during colon carcinogenesis [127, 138]. In a study evaluating silibinin pharmacodynamics, Hoh et al. [140] showed that silibinin is not toxic to normal colonic epithelium (**Table 1**).

Curcumin is effective in apoptosis triggering, inhibiting DNA mutations, cancer cell proliferation, metastasis and inflammation. Curcumin induces the production of ROS in concentration that leads to p21 protein upregulation, and consequently inhibiting cancer cell growth [141]. Moreover, curcumin interferes with the protein kinase (MAPK) pathway, which in turn decreases production of TNF-α and COX-2 as well as downregulates the expression of NF-κB and IL-6 [142, 143]. The downregulation of NF-κB levels has also effect on expression level of c-myc, cyclin D1 and Bcl-2 genes, and finally modulates the cell cycle [144]. It promotes cancer cell apoptosis by inducing expression of proapoptotic proteins (Bax, Bim, Bak, Noxa) and inhibiting expression of anti-apoptotic proteins (Bcl-2, Bcl-xl) [143]. Curcumin prevents the formation of metastases by decreasing vascular endothelial growth factor (VEGF) and matrix metalloproteinase 9 expression [144]. In recent in vitro study in CRC cells, Patel et al. [145] have shown that curcumin inhibits the receptor expression of HER2 and insulin-like growth factor 1 (IGF-1) which is well known to create resistance to 5-fluorouracil and oxaliplatin. Curcumin downregulates the expression of survivin and IGF-1 by activating the expression of p53 and reducing TNF-α levels, leading to activation of apoptotic signal [146, 147] (**Table 1**).

Epigallocatechin 3-Gallate Epigallocatechin 3-gallate (EGCG) has a strong antioxidant activity preventing ROS formation, blocking cancer cell proliferation and metastasis formation by down-regulating the expression of growth factors (epidermal growth factor, IGF-1, VEGF) [148]. EGCG blocks the cell cycle through the modulation of both MAPK and p21 pathways [149]. Furthermore, by upregulation of p53, EGCG induces apoptosis in CRC cells [150]. EGCG promotes cell growth arrest and induces apoptosis by affecting regulatory proteins of the cell cycle and inhibition of NFκB [151–153]. Some reports point out that the ROS-related effects may contribute to the anti-proliferative and pro-apoptotic activity of EGCG [154]. The effects are associated with modulation of reactive oxygen species (ROS) production. Although EGCG has a dual function of antioxidant and pro-oxidant, EGCG-mediated modulation of ROS production is reported to be responsible for its anti-cancer effects. The EGCG-mediated inhibition of NF-κB signalling is also associated with inhibition of migration, angiogenesis and cell viability [155]. Furthermore, it inhibits growth factor-dependent signalling (e.g. EGF, VEGF and IGF-I), the MAPK pathway, proteasome-dependent degradation and expression of COX-2. EGCG seems to directly interact with and modulate the character of membrane lipid rafts, which explains the ability to alter signalling processes of growth factor receptors. Furthermore, EGCG inhibits telomerase, topoisomerase II and DNA methyltransferase 1, thereby affecting the functions of chromatin [153, 156]. EGCG has a protective effect against NO-induced apoptosis in HDPC by scavenging ROS and modulating the Bcl-2 family [157] (**Table 1**).

Pomegranate may inhibit cancer cell proliferation and apoptosis through the modulation of cellular transcription factors and signalling proteins. In previous studies, pomegranate juice and its derivate inhibited proliferation and induced apoptosis in colon cancer cells, significantly suppressed TNF-α-induced COX-2 protein expression. It also reduced phosphorylation of the p65 subunit and binding to NF-κB, and abolished TNF-α induced AKT activation, playing an important role in the modulation of cell signalling in colon cancer cells [158]. The pomegranate juice exhibited a dose- and time-dependent decrease in cell proliferation, inducing cell-cycle arrest in the G_0/G_1 and G_2/M stages of the cell cycle, followed by apoptosis [159]. In the same regard, Larrosa et al. [160] have shown that induction of apoptosis was due to the downregulation of Bcl2-XL protein as well as activation of caspase-3 and caspase-9, but not caspase-8 (**Table 1**).

Citrus flavonoids: Volatile oil of *Citrus aurantifolia,* showed 78% growth inhibition of human colon cancer cells, induced the characteristic pattern of DNA fragmentation, via caspase-3 dependent pathway along with modulation of apoptosis-related protein expression [161].

Orange (*Satsuma mandarin*) juice contains a lot of flavonoids, which are potential chemoprotective compounds, with the capacity to suppress the expression of several cytokines (TNF-α, IL-1β, IL-6) as well as inflammatory enzymes (COX-2 and iNOS). In human colon cancer cell lines, the mechanism that induced the inhibition of their growth acted by blocking the cell cycle in G_0/G_1 phase and reducing levels of cyclins (A, D1 and E) [162].

Naringenin: Treatment with naringenin derivates resulted in significant apoptosis-inducing effects concomitant with losses in mitochondrial membrane potential, caspase activation, intracellular ROS production and sustained ERK activation [129]. In human colon adenocarcinomas, it induced activation of p38/MAPK, leading to the pro-apoptotic caspase-3 activation and poly (ADP-ribose) polymerase cleavage [163] (**Table 1**).

Quercetin plays a role in inhibiting tumorigenesis in colon cells through antioxidant, anti-inflammatory, anti-proliferative and pro-apoptotic mechanisms. Quercetin downregulated Bcl-2 through the inhibition of NF-κB and inhibited phosphorylation of EGFR suppressing downstream signalling in colon carcinoma cells. It augments TRAIL-induced apoptotic death and inhibits cyclin D1, survivin expression and Wnt/beta-catenin signalling pathway [91, 164] (**Table 1**).

Apigenin: Studies have shown that apigenin induces cell-cycle arrest and causes apoptosis in different cancer cells including colon cancer through modulation of various survival and death effectors, such as PI3K, AKT, ERK, STAT3, JNK and Mcl-1 [119] (**Table 1**).

Genistein inhibits the activation of NF-κB and Akt signalling pathways, both of which are known to maintain a homeostatic balance between cell survival and apoptosis; antagonizes estrogen- and androgen-mediated signalling pathways in the processes of carcinogenesis [114]. It has antioxidant properties, being a potent inhibitor of angiogenesis and metastasis. Genistein is a known inhibitor of protein-tyrosine kinase (PTK), which may attenuate the growth of cancer cells by inhibiting PTK-mediated signalling mechanisms. Genistein also inhibits topoisomerase I and II, 5α-reductase and protein histidine kinase, all of which may contribute to the anti-proliferative or pro-apoptotic effects [113]. It also down-regulates mdm2 at both transcriptional and post-translational levels [165] (**Table 1**).

5.2. Epigenetic mechanisms related to apoptosis, influenced by natural compounds

Several papers pointed the role of various natural compounds that target the **epigenetic mechanisms** in order to modulate the biologic activities, including apoptosis [173]. Epigenetic control mechanisms are reversible and natural compounds that target them may contribute to the development of new and attractive therapeutic strategies. A review of some natural compounds that target apoptosis through epigenetic mechanisms is presented below.

EGCG has a role in inhibiting histone deacetylases (HDACs) [174]. Site-specific acetylation of histones is essential to switch between permissive and repressive chromatin structures. Chromatin remodelling allows the regulation of gene expression, and it takes place under the action of enzymes responsible for acetylation (histone acetyl transferase, HAT) and deacetylation (histone deacetyl transferase, HDAC) [175]. An increased HDAC activity is characteristic to many cancers and is associated with alterations of several cellular mechanisms, including apoptosis. Therefore, by targeting HDACs, it is possible to modulate several cell processes like cell cycle, cell differentiation and apoptosis. Combined treatments of EGCG and sodium butyrate (NaB), in physiologically achievable concentrations, were shown to promote apoptosis and induce cell-cycle arrest in RKO, HCT-116 and HT-29 colon cell lines [176]. Both EGCG and NaB are epigenetic regulators, and treatment with these two compounds reduced both the expression of survivin (which has anti-apoptotic activity), as well as the expression of enzymes involved in epigenetic regulation (HDAC and DNA methyltransferase- DNMT) [176].

HDAC activity is also inhibited by **sulforaphane** (SFN) and induces an increased histone acetylation, mainly at p21 and Bax 2 promoters, events that lead to G_2/M cell-cycle arrest and apoptosis [177]. Oral administration of SFN in mice increased p21 expression via HDAC inhibition, while in APC-knock-out mice the same treatment leaded to specific increase of acetylation in H3 and H4 with decrease of intestinal polips [178]. Moreover, SFN was found to inhibit DNMTs (enzymes responsible for DNA methylation) in CaCo-2 colon cancer cell line [179]. Another epigenetic mechanism used by SFN to exert its activity is through miRNAs: in NCM460 and NCM356 normal colon epithelial cells SFN upregulated 15 miRNAs, among which several were involved in apoptosis (miR-9, miR-135b) [180].

Resveratrol activates type III HDAC inhibitors, sirtuin 1 (SIRT1) and p300 [181] which in turn negatively modulates the expression of survivin. On the other hand, in colon cancer cells, resveratrol inhibits the cell growth and induces apoptosis through miRNAs [182, 183]. Combined treatment of quercetin and resveratrol induced apoptosis in colorectal cancer cells through downregulation of miR-27a [184].

6. Combined therapy of colon cancer: current strategies and future directions

Conventional therapeutic approaches, including chemotherapy, radiotherapy and surgery, are limited for the treatment of advanced colon cancer, in prevention of the disease recurrence, and are associated with a high risk of complications, highlighting the need to develop new therapeutic strategies. The majority of CRC patients receive chemotherapy using multiple agents that are currently approved for the treatment in the appropriate setting, but many patients have tumours intrinsically resistant to them. However, it is a complex process to select the optimal chemotherapy for each patient, and the difference between theory and practice is still a problem. That's why new concepts and modern technologies are promoted by precision medicine in order to achieve a personalized treatment for cancer patients.

6.1. RTCA: useful tool for screening biocompounds and drugs

Contrast data are available on the anti-cancer effects of biocompounds in colon cancer, whether they could influence the effects of oncolytic drugs against the cell growth and apoptosis of human colon cancer cells, or which might be the proper concentrations of the compounds with cytotoxic or cytostatic potential. Real-time impedance data obtained by the xCELLigence System (ACEA Biosciences) might be used to generate compound-specific profiles which are dependent on the biological mechanisms of action of each compound used. The actual kinetic response of the cells within an assay prior or subsequent to certain manipulations provides important information regarding the biological status of the cell, such as cell growth, cell arrest, morphological changes and apoptosis [185]. Changes in a cell status, such as cell morphology, cell adhesion or cell viability lead to a change in cell index (CI), which is a quantitative measure of cell number present in a well. For example, the cytotoxicity versus proliferative capacity of genistein, resveratrol or 5-fluorouracil was assessed in LoVo colon cancer cell line in order to modulate the chemosensitivity of colon cancer cells to drug treatment, and overcome the chemo-resistance. The entire length of the assay was presented, allowing informed decisions regarding the timing of certain manipulations or treatments, choice of the proper concentrations for further end-point assays, such as flow-cytometry techniques or molecular biology approaches [186, 187].

6.2. Modulation of apoptosis by combined therapy

Many anti-cancer drugs act during physiological pathways of apoptosis, leading to tumour cell destruction. By combining natural compounds with anti-cancer drugs, an increase of the effects might be obtained, specifically in highly invasive cancer cells, while in non-tumoral cells the natural compounds could reduce the cytotoxic side effects [115] (**Figure 2**).

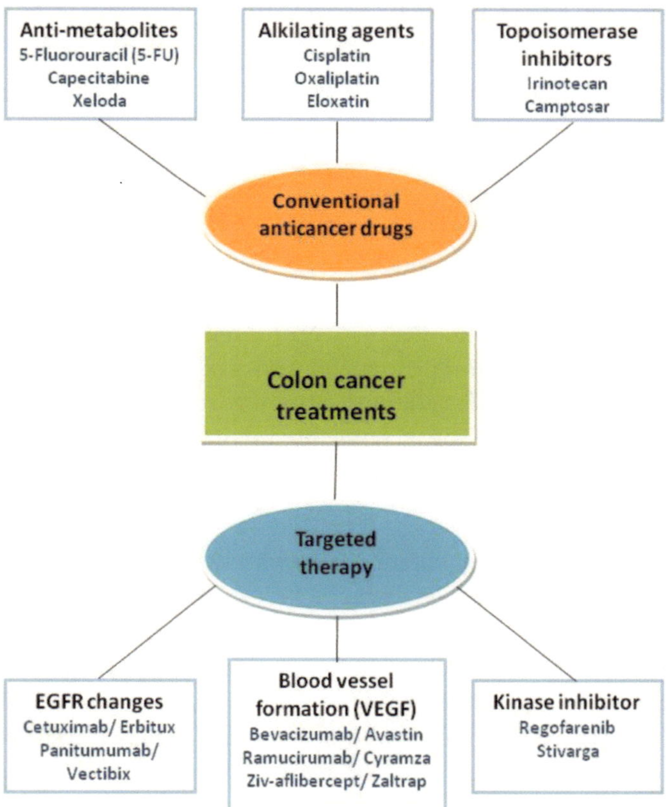

Figure 2. Available colon cancer therapeutic agents with disparate mechanisms of action.

A wide variety of currently available cancer therapeutical agents (**Figure 2**), with disparate mechanisms of actions, lead to the same mode of cell death [188]:

a. 5-Fluorouracil (5-FU) that blocks the thymidylate synthase (TS), which is essential for DNA synthesis;

b. Capecitabine that blocks thymidylate synthase (orally administered prodrug converted to 5-FU)

c. Oxaliplatin that inhibits DNA replication and transcription by forming inter- and intra-strand DNA adducts/cross-links;

d. Irinotecan that inhibits topoisomerase I, an enzyme that facilitates the uncoiling and recoiling of DNA during replication;

e. Bevacizumab, a monoclonal antibody, which binds to vascular endothelial growth factor (VEGF) ligand;

f. Cetuximab, a monoclonal antibody to epidermal growth factor receptor (EGFR) (chimeric), that blocks the ligand-binding site;

g. Panitumumab, a monoclonal antibody to EGFR (fully humanized), that blocks the ligand-binding site [188].

Several anti-cancer drugs act during physiological pathways of apoptosis, leading to tumour cell destruction [23, 189]. The pattern and extent of the cell damage induced by chemotherapeutics, like fluoropyrimidines, in human cancer cells have been suggested to depend also on the pathways downstream from drug-target interactions that once triggered will initiate programmed cell death (apoptosis) [190, 191]. 5-Fluorouracil (5-FU) is one of the widely used chemotherapeutic drugs targeting various cancers, but its chemoresistance remains as a major obstacle in clinical settings. Several groups reported the induction of apoptosis by 5-fluorouracil (5-FU) in HT29 [192] or LoVo human colon cancer cell lines [186, 187]. The long exposure of colon cells to 5-FU treatments influences both pro- and anti-apoptotic molecules like P53 and Bax, or Bcl-2 and Bcl-XL [193]. Several studies showed that 5-FU inhibits DNA proliferation in colon cancer cells by inhibiting the enzyme thymidylate synthase, leading to apoptosis, a mechanism of active cell death characterized by rapid loss of plasma membrane integrity, DNA fragmentation and altered expression of numerous genes [46, 52, 104] (**Figure 2**).

The biocompounds extracted from botanicals may be used as chemopreventive and therapeutic agents for various human cancers, inclusive colon cancer [94]. The active biocompounds might induce cancer-selective cell death by increasing production of reactive oxygen species. The cancer cells have increased levels of ROS accompanied by a highly active antioxidant defense system; therefore, the tumour cells are unable to recover from additional oxidative stress and die. It is accepted that mitochondria-derived ROS play a critical role in their pro-death and chemopreventive responses. The natural biocompounds inhibit mitochondrial electron transport chains causing ROS production, thus triggering apoptotic cell death [80]. By combining flavonoids with anti-cancer drugs, it might be obtained an increase of the desired effects, specifically in highly invasive cancer cells, while in non-tumour cells the cytotoxic side effects could be reduced [186]. In vitro, studies showed that LoVo colon cancer cells were markedly sensitized to apoptosis by both 5-FU and genistein compared to the 5-FU treatment alone. When time of incubation was increased, treatments with GST and/or 5-FU had much stronger effects on the induction of apoptosis in LoVo cells, evaluated by using annexin-V/FITC and PI double staining, followed by flow-cytometry analysis [186]. Similar studies demonstrated the additive effect of GST to anti-cancer drug treatment, and in reversing the multi-drug resistance [13, 14].

Experimental assays showed that resveratrol (RSV) induced higher levels of early and late apoptosis compared to untreated or 5-FU-treated LoVo cells. When treatments were prolonged to 72 h, stronger effects were observed both for RSV alone and combined treatments with 5-FU [187]. Flow-cytometry analyses showed that treatments with 25 μM 5-FU or 50 μM RSV slightly increased the expression of the pro-apoptotic molecules p53 and Bax. The combined treatments of 50 μM RSV and 25 μM 5-FU induced a higher increase of p53 expression compared to the non-treated cells. Also the increase of Bax expression was much higher for the combined treatments compared to non-treated cells or treated cells with 5-FU alone. Both RSV and 5-FU treatments seemed to decrease Bcl-2 expression, but the effect was stronger for the combined treatments. Combined treatments induced a higher increase of pro-apoptotic antigen expression, both for P53 and Bax, compared to 5-FU treatment [187].

Therefore, addition of flavonoids and other natural compounds might be an alternative approach in order to obtain the same or a stronger anti-tumour response, enhance the chemosensitivity of tumours to anti-cancer drugs, or diminish the undesirable side effects by using lower concentrations [194, 195].

7. Conclusions

A big challenge for a successful treatment of colon cancer is the lack of eradication of the entire tumour cell population and the consequent development of chemoresistance. Since many anti-cancer drugs act during physiological pathways of apoptosis, leading to tumour cell destruction, elucidation of the mechanisms that govern the programmed cell death process seems to be of great importance for carcinogenesis, tumour evasion, and to have practical implications for anti-cancer therapy. Many therapeutic drugs used in cancer treatment proved to induce resistance in cancer cell killing, and their number are rapidly increasing, possibly through the modulation of survival cell components such as proliferative or anti-apoptotic proteins. Contrast data are available on the anti-cancer effects of natural compounds in colon cancer, whether they could influence the effects of oncolytic drugs against the growth and apoptosis of human colon cancer cells, or which might be the proper concentrations of compounds with cytotoxic or cytostatic potential. From a large number of natural compounds investigated, several have been shown to be promising, based on their anti-cancer effects related to apoptosis. A newly arising field involves therapeutic approaches in cancer in order to induce tumour cells to undergo apoptosis and break the cancer cell resistance to apoptosis commands. Therefore, manipulation of the mechanisms of programmed cell death process could be of outstanding importance for malignant transformation, and alternative approaches might be used to obtain a stronger anti-tumour response, and/or diminish the undesirable side effects by using lower concentrations of anti-cancer drugs. Thus, new concepts and modern technologies are promoted by precision medicine in order to achieve a personalized treatment for cancer patients.

Author details

Marinela Bostan[1], Mirela Mihaila[1], Camelia Hotnog[1], Coralia Bleotu[2], Gabriela Anton[3], Viviana Roman[1] and Lorelei Irina Brasoveanu[1*]

*Address all correspondence to: luli_brasoveanu@yahoo.com

1 Center of Immunology Dept., "Stefan S. Nicolau" Institute of Virology, Bucharest, Romania

2 Cellular and Molecular Pathology Dept., "Stefan S. Nicolau" Institute of Virology, Bucharest, Romania

3 Molecular Virology Dept., "Stefan S. Nicolau" Institute of Virology, Bucharest, Romania

References

[1] Jemal, A., R. Siegel, E. Ward, Y. Hao, J. Xu, T. Murray (2008) Cancer statistics. *CA Cancer J Clin*. 58:71–96.

[2] Weber, G.F. Molecular mechanisms of cancer. Dordrecht, The Netherlands: Springer; 2007. 645 p. (p. 39, 45–54, 93–99).

[3] Desoize, B., J. Jardillier (2000) Multicellular resistance: a paradigm for clinical resistance? *Crit Rev Oncol Hematol*. 36(2–3):193–207.

[4] Gottesman, M.M. (2002) Mechanisms of cancer drug resistance. *Annu Rev Med*. 53:615–627.

[5] Zimmermann, K.C., C. Bonzon, D.R. Green (2001) The machinery of programmed cell death. *Pharmacol Ther*. 92:57–70.

[6] Townson, J.L., G.N. Naumov, A.F. Chambers (2003) The role of apoptosis in tumor progression and metastasis. *Curr Mol Med.* 3:631–42.

[7] Miura, K., W. Fujibuchi, K. Ishida, T. Naitoh, H. Ogawa, T. Ando, N. Yazaki, K. Watanabe, S. Haneda, C. Shibata, I. Sasaki (2011) Inhibitor of apoptosis protein family as diagnostic markers and therapeutic targets of colorectal cancer. *Surg Today*. 41:175–182.

[8] Meadows, G.G. (2012) Diet, nutrients, phytochemicals, and cancer metastasis suppressor genes. *Cancer Metastasis Rev*. 31(3–4):441–454.

[9] Mattern, J. (2003) Drug resistance in cancer: a multifactorial problem. *Anticancer Res.* 23(2C):1769–1772.

[10] De Angelis, P.M., D.H. Svendsrud, K.L. Kravik, T. Stokke (2006) Cellular response to 5-fluorouracil (5-FU) in 5-FU-resistant colon cancer cell lines during treatment and recovery. *Mol Cancer.* 5:20–45.

[11] Gerhauser, C. (2013) Cancer chemoprevention and nutri-epigenetics: state of the art and future challenges. *Top Curr Chem.* 329:73–132.

[12] Fulda, S. (2010) Evasion of apoptosis as a cellular stress response in cancer. *Int J Cell Biol.* 2010; 2010:370835–370841.

[13] Fulda, S. (2010) Modulation of apoptosis by natural products for cancer therapy. *Planta Med.* 76:1075–1079.

[14] Shu, L., K.L. Cheung, T.O. Khor, C. Chen, A.N. Kong (2010) Phytochemicals: cancer chemoprevention and suppression of tumor onset and metastasis. *Cancer Metastasis Rev.* 29:483–502.

[15] Thornthwaite, J.T., H.R. Shah, P. Shah, W.C. Peeples, H. Respess (2013) The formulation for cancer prevention & therapy. *Adv Biol Chem.* 3:356–387.

[16] Russo, M., C. Spagnuolo, I. Tedesco, G.L. Russo (2010) Phytochemicals in cancer prevention and therapy: truth or dare? *Toxins.* 2:517–551.

[17] Rajamanickam, S., R. Agarwal (2008) Natural products and colon cancer: current status and future prospects. *Drug Dev Res.* 69(7):460–471.

[18] Fox, J.T., S. Sakamuru, R. Huang, N. Teneva, S.O. Simmons, M. Xia, R.R. Tice, C.P. Austin, K. Myung (2012) High-throughput genotoxicity assay identifies antioxidants as inducers of DNA damage response and cell death. *Proc Natl Acad Sci. USA* 109(14): 5423–5428.

[19] Watson, A.J.M. (2004) Apoptosis and colorectal cancer. *Gut.* 53:1701–1709.

[20] Pritchard, C.C., W.M. Grady (2011) Colorectal cancer molecular biology moves into clinical practice. *Gut.* 60(1):116–29.

[21] Tejpar, S., M. Bertagnolli, F. Bosman, H.J. Lenz, L. Garraway, F. Waldman, R. Warren, A. Bild, D. Collins-Brennan, H. Hahn, D.P. Harkin, R. Kennedy, M. Ilyas, H. Morreau, V. Proutski, C. Swanton, I. Tomlinson, M. Delorenzi, R. Fiocca, E. Van Cutsem, A. Roth (2010) Prognostic and predictive biomarkers in resected colon cancer: current status and future perspectives for integrating genomics into biomarker discovery. *Oncologist.* 15(4):390–404.

[22] Samowitz, W.S. (2008) Genetic and epigenetic changes in colon cancer. *Exp Mol Pathol.* 85(1):64–67.

[23] Kim, R., K. Tanabe, Y. Uchida, M. Emi, H. Inoue, T. Toge (2002) Current status of the molecular mechanisms of anticancer drug-induced apoptosis. The contribution of molecular-level analysis to cancer chemotherapy. *Cancer Chemother Pharmacol.* 50:343–352.

[24] Kaufmann, S.H., D.L. Vaux (2003) Alterations in the apoptotic machinery and their potential role in anticancer drug resistance. *Oncogene*. 22(47):7414–7430.

[25] Negrini, S., V.G. Gorgoulis, T.D. Halazonetis (2010) Genomic instability an evolving hallmark of cancer. *Nat Rev Mol Cell Biol*. 11(3):220–228.

[26] Su, Z., Z. Yang, Y. Xu, Y. Chen, X. Yu (2015) Apoptosis, autophagy, necroptosis, and cancer metastasis. *Mol Cancer*. 14:48.

[27] Elmore, S. (2007) Apoptosis: a review of programmed cell death. *Toxicol Pathol*. 35(4): 495–516.

[28] Taylor, R.C., S.P. Cullen, S.J. Martin (2008) Apoptosis: controlled demolition at the cellular level. *Nat Rev Mol Cell Biol*. 9(3):231–241.

[29] Hassan, M., O. Feyen, E. Grinstein (2009) Fas-induced apoptosis of renal cell carcinoma is mediated by apoptosis signal-regulating kinase 1 via mitochondrial damage-dependent caspase-8 activation. *Cell Oncol*. 31(6):437–456.

[30] Mendelsohn J., P.M. Howley, M.A. Israel, J.W. Gray, C.B. Thompson, editors. The Molecular Basis of Cancer. 4th ed. Philadelphia (PA): Elsevier; 2015. 863 p.

[31] Yang, S.Y., K.M. Sales, B. Fuller, A.M. Seifalian, M.C. Winslet (2009) Apoptosis and colorectal cancer: implications for therapy. *Trends Mol Med*. 15:225–233.

[32] Giansanti, V., A. Torriglia, A.I. Scovassi (2011) Conversation between apoptosis and autophagy: is it your turn or mine? *Apoptosis*. 16(4):321–333.

[33] Danial, N.N., S.J. Korsmeyer (2004) Cell death: critical control points. *Cell*. 116:205–219.

[34] Locksley, R.M., N. Killeen, M.J. Lenardo (2001) The TNF and TNF receptor superfamilies: integrating mammalian biology. *Cell*. 104(4):487–501.

[35] Ashkenazi, A., V.M. Dixit (1998) Death receptors: signaling and modulation. *Science*. 281(5381):1305–1308.

[36] Walczak, H., P.H. Krammer (2000) The CD95 (APO-1/Fas) and the TRAIL (APO-2L) apoptosis systems. *Exp Cell Res*. 256(1):58–66.

[37] Kuwana, T., L. Bouchier-Hayes, J.E. Chipuk (2005) BH3 domains of BH3-only proteins differentially regulate Bax-mediated mitochondrial membrane permeabilization both directly and indirectly. *Mol Cell*. 2005;17(4):525–535.

[38] Hassan, M., H. Watari, A. AbuAlmaaty, Y. Ohba, N. Sakuragi (2014) Apoptosis and Molecular Targeting Therapy in Cancer. *BioMed Res Int* (2014) Article ID 150845, 23 p., http://dx.doi.org/10.1155/2014/150845: 150845.

[39] Lavrik, I., A. Golks, P.H. Krammer (2005) Death receptor signaling. *J Cell Sci*. 118(2): 265–267.

[40] Su, M., Y. Mei, S. Sinha (2013) Role of the Crosstalk Between Autophagy and Apoptosis in Cancer. *J Oncology* (2013) Article ID 102735, 14 p., http://dx.doi.org/10.1155/2013/102735.

[41] Igney, F.H., P.H. Krammer (2002) Death and anti-death: tumour resistance to apoptosis. *Nat Rev Cancer*. 2(4):277–288.

[42] Wilson, J.W., M.C. Nostro, M. Balzi, P. Faraoni, F. Cianchi, A. Becciolini, C.S. Potten (2000) Bcl-w expression in colorectal adenocarcinoma. *Br J Cancer*. 82(1):178–85.

[43] Certo, M., V. Del Gaizo Moore, M. Nishino (2006) Mitochondria primed by death signals determine cellular addiction to antiapoptotic BCL-2 family members. *Cancer Cell*. 9:351–365.

[44] Kikuchi, Y., W.N. Dinjens, F.T. Bosman (1997) Proliferation and apoptosis in proliferative lesions of the colon and rectum. *Virchows Arch*. 431(2):111–7.

[45] Ilyas, M., X.P. Hao, K. Wilkinson, I.P. Tomlinson, A.M. Abbasi, A. Forbes, W.F. Bodmer, I.C. Talbot (1998) Loss of Bcl-2 expression correlates with tumour recurrence in colorectal cancer. *Gut*. 43:383–387.

[46] Zhang, Y.L., L.Q. Pang, Y. Wu, X.Y. Wang, C.Q. Wang, Y. Fan (2008) Significance of Bcl-xL in human colon carcinoma. *World J Gastroenterol*. 14(19):3069–3073.

[47] Huang, C.Y., L. Chia-Hui Yu (2015) Pathophysiological mechanisms of death resistance in colorectal carcinoma. *World J Gastroenterol*. 21(41):11777–11792.

[48] Wei, M.C., W.X. Zong, E.H. Cheng, T. Lindsten, V. Panoutsakopoulou, A.J. Ross, K.A. Roth, G.R. MacGregor, C.B. Thompson, S.J. Korsmeyer (2001) Proapoptotic BAX and BAK: a requisite gateway to mitochondrial dysfunction and death. *Science*. 292(5517): 727–730.

[49] Kondo, S., Y. Shinomura, Y. Miyazak, T. Kiyohara, S. Tsutsui, S. Kitamura, Y. Nagasawa, M. Nakahara, S. Kanayama, Y. Matsuzawa (2000) Mutations of the bak gene in human gastric and colorectal cancers. *Cancer Res*. 60:4328–4330.

[50] Ionov, Y., H. Yamamoto, S. Krajewski, J.C. Reed, M. Perucho (2000) Mutational inactivation of the proapoptotic gene BAX confers selective advantage during tumor clonal evolution. *Proc Natl Acad Sci USA*. 97:10872–10877.

[51] Yagi, O.K., Y. Akiyama, T. Nomizu, T. Iwama, M. Endo, Y. Yuasa (1998) Proapoptotic gene BAX is frequently mutated in hereditary nonpolyposis colorectal cancers but not in adenomas. *Gastroenterology*. 114:268–274.

[52] De Angelis, P.M., T. Stokke, L. Thorstensen, R.A. Lothe, O.P. Clausenn (1998) Apoptosis and expression of Bax, Bcl-x, and Bcl-2 apoptotic regulatory proteins in colorectal carcinomas, and association with p53 genotype/phenotype. *Mol Pathol*. 51:254–261.

[53] Rampino, N., H. Yamamoto, Y. Ionov, Y. Li, H. Sawai, J.C. Reed, M. Perucho (1997) Somatic frameshift mutations in the BAX gene in colon cancers of the microsatellite mutator phenotype. *Science.* 275:967–969.

[54] Jansson, A., X.F. Sun (2002) Bax expression decreases significantly from primary tumor to metastasis in colorectal cancer. *J Clin Oncol.* 20:811–816.

[55] Bai, L., W.G. Zhu (2006) p53: structure, function and therapeutic applications. *J Cancer Mol.* 2(4):141–153.

[56] Vikhanskaya, F., M.K. Lee, M. Mazzoletti, M. Broggini, K. Sabapathy (2007) Cancer-derived p53 mutants suppress p53-target gene expression—potential mechanism for gain of function of mutant p53. *Nucl Acids Res.* 35(6):2093–2104.

[57] Russo, A., V. Bazan, B. Iacopetta, D. Kerr, T. Soussi, N. Gebbia (2005) The TP53 colorectal cancer international collaborative study on the prognostic and predictive significance of p53 mutation: influence of tumor site, type of mutation, and adjuvant treatment. *J Clin Oncol.* 23:7518–7528.

[58] Katkoori, V.R., C. Shanmugam, X. Jia, S.P. Vitta, M. Sthanam, T. Callens, L. Messiaen, D. Chen, B. Zhang, H.L. Bumpers, T. Samuel, U. Manne (2012) Prognostic significance and gene expression profiles of p53 mutations in microsatellite-stable stage III colorectal adenocarcinomas. *Plos One.* 7:e30020.

[59] Huerta, S., E.J. Goulet, E.H. Livingston (2006) Colon cancer and apoptosis. *Am J Surg.* 191:517–526.

[60] Nyiraneza, C., A. Jouret-Mourin, A. Kartheuser, P. Camby, O. Plomteux, R. Detry, K. Dahan, C. Sempoux (2011) Distinctive patterns of p53 protein expression and microsatellite instability in human colorectal cancer. *Hum Pathol.* 42(12):1897–910.

[61] Edagawa, M., J. Kawauchi, M. Hirata, H. Goshima, M. Inoue, T. Okamoto, A. Murakami, Y. Maehara, S. Kitajima (2014) Role of activating transcription factor 3 (ATF3) in endoplasmic reticulum (ER) stress-induced sensitization of p53-deficient human colon cancer cells to tumor necrosis factor (TNF)-related apoptosis inducing ligand (TRAIL)-mediated apoptosis through upregulation of death receptor 5 (DR5) by zerumbone and celecoxib. *J Biol Chem.* 289:21544–21561.

[62] Wu, W.K., X.J. Wang, A.S. Cheng, M.X. Luo, S.S. Ng, K.F. To, F.K. Chan, C.H. Cho, J.J. Sung, J. Yu (2013) Dysregulation and crosstalk of cellular signaling pathways in colon carcinogenesis. *Crit Rev Oncol Hematol.* 86(3):251–277.

[63] Mita, A.C., M.M. Mita, S.T. Nawrocki, F.J. Giles (2008) Survivin: key regulator of mitosis and apoptosis and novel target for cancer therapeutics. *Clin Cancer Res.* 14(16):5000–5005.

[64] Olsson, M., B. Zhivotovsky (2011) Caspases and cancer. *Cell Death Differ.* 18:1441–1449.

[65] Fink, S.L., B.T. Cookson (2005) Apoptosis, pyroptosis, and necrosis: mechanistic description of dead and dying eukaryotic cells. *Infect Immun.* 73(4):1907–1916.

[66] Devarajan, E., A.A. Sahin, J.S. Chen, R.R. Krishnamurthy, N. Aggarwal, A.M. Brun, A. Sapino, F. Zhang, D. Sharma, X.H. Yang, A.D. Tora, K. Mehta (2002) Downregulation of caspase 3 in breast cancer: a possible mechanism for chemoresistance. *Oncogene.* 21(57):8843–8851.

[67] Shen, X.G., C. Wang, Y. Li, L. Wang, B. Zhou, B. Xu, X. Jiang, Z.G. Zhou, X.F. Sun (2010) Downregulation of caspase-9 is a frequent event in patients with stage II colorectal cancer and correlates with poor clinical outcome. *Colorectal Dis.* 12(12):1213–1218.

[68] Fong, P.C., W.C. Xue, H.Y.S. Ngan, P.M. Chiu, K.Y.K. Chan, G.S.W. Tsao, A.N.Y. Cheung (2006) Caspase activity is downregulated in choriocarcinoma: a cDNA array differential expression study. *J Clin Pathol.* 59(2):179–183.

[69] Fulda, S., K.M. Debatin (2006) Extrinsic versus intrinsic apoptosis pathways in anticancer chemotherapy. *Oncogene.* 25:4798–4811.

[70] Fulda, S., L. Galluzzi, G. Kroemer (2010) Targeting mitochondria for cancer therapy. *Nat Rev Drug Dis.* 9(6):447–464.

[71] Acharya, A., I. Das, D. Chandhok, T. Saha (2010) Redox regulation in cancer: a double-edged sword with therapeutic potential. *Oxid Med Cell Longev.* 3:23–34.

[72] Circu, M.L., T.Y. Aw (2010) Reactive oxygen species, cellular redox systems, and apoptosis. *Free Radic Biol Med.* 48:749–762.

[73] Storz, P. (2005) Reactive oxygen species in tumor progression. *Front Biosci.* 10:1881–96.

[74] Afanas'ev, I. (2011) Reactive oxygen species signaling in cancer: comparison with aging. *Aging Dis.* 2(3):219–30.

[75] Dickinson, B.C., C.J. Chang (2011) Chemistry and biology of reactive oxygen species in signaling or stress responses. *Nat Chem Biol.* 7(8):504–11.

[76] Liou, G.Y., P. Storz (2010) Reactive oxygen species in cancer. *Free Radic Res.* 44(5):1–31.

[77] Waris, G, H. Ahsan (2006) Reactive oxygen species: role in the development of cancer and various chronic conditions. *J Carcinog.* 5:14.

[78] Gupta, R.A., R.N. DuBois, M.C. Wallace (2002) New avenues for the prevention of colorectal cancer: targeting cyclo-oxygenase-2 activity. *Best Pract Res Clin Gastroenterol.* 16:945–56.

[79] Martindale, J.L., N.J. Holbrook (2002) Cellular response to oxidative stress: signaling for suicide and survival. *J Cell Physiol.* 192(1):1–15.

[80] Trachootham, D., J. Alexandre, P. Huang (2009) Targeting cancer cells by ROSmediated mechanisms: a radical therapeutic approach? *Natl Rev Drug Dis.* 8:579–591.

[81] Oberreuther-Moschner, D.L., G. Rechkemmer, B.L. PoolZobel (2005) Basal colon crypt cells are more sensitive than surface cells toward hydrogen peroxide, a factor of oxidative stress. *Toxicol Lett.* 159(3):212–218.

[82] Rainis, T., I. Maor, A. Lanir, S. Shnizer, A. Lavy (2007) Enhanced oxidative stress and leucocyte activation in neoplastic tissues of the colon. *Dig Dis Sci.* 52(2):526–530.

[83] Slattery, M.L., A. Lundgreen, B. Welbourn, R.K. Wolff, C. Corcoran (2012) Oxidative balance and colon and rectal cancer: interaction of lifestyle factors and genes. *Mutat Res.* 734(1–2):30–40.

[84] Colin, D.J., E. Limagne, K. Ragot, G. Lizard, F. Ghiringhelli, É. Solary, B. Chauffert, N. Latruffe, D. Delmas (2014) The role of reactive oxygen species and subsequent DNA-damage response in the emergence of resistance towards resveratrol in colon cancer models. *Cell Death Dis.* 5:1533–1546.

[85] Chiarugi, P, T. Fiaschi (2007) Redox signalling in anchorage-dependent cell growth. *Cell Signal.* 19(4):672–82.

[86] Guo, Z., S. Kozlov, M.F. Lavin, M.D. Person, T.T. Paull (2010) ATM activation by oxidative stress. *Science.* 330:517–521.

[87] Dhillon, A.S., S. Hagan, O. Rath, W. Kolch (2007) MAP kinase signalling pathways in cancer. *Oncogene.* 26(22):3279–3290.

[88] She, Q.B., A.M. Bode, W.Y. Ma, N.Y. Chen, Z.G. Dong (2001) Resveratrol-induced activation of p53 and apoptosis is mediated by extracellular-signal-regulated protein kinases and p38 kinase. *Cancer Res.* 61:1604–1610.

[89] Shih, A., F.B. Davis, H.Y. Lin, P.J. Davis (2002) Resveratrol induces apoptosis in thyroid cancer cell lines via a MAPK- and p53-dependent mechanism. *J Clin Endocrinol Metab.* 87:1223–1232.

[90] Aggarwal, B.B., S. Shishodia (2006) Molecular targets of dietary agents for prevention and therapy of cancer. *Biochem Pharmacol.* 71:1397–1421.

[91] Kim, Y.H., D.H. Lee, J.H. Jeong, Z.S. Guo, Y.J. Lee (2008) Quercetin augments TRAIL induced apoptotic death: involvement of the ERK signal transduction pathway. *Biochem Pharmacol.* 75:1946–1958.

[92] Cagnol, S., J.C. Chambard (2010) ERK and cell death: mechanisms of ERK-induced cell death—apoptosis, autophagy and senescence. *FEBS J.* 277:2–21.

[93] Kong, E.H., Y.J. Kim, H.J. Cho, S.N. Yu, K.Y. Kim, J.H. Chang, S.C. Ahn (2008) Piplartine induces caspase-mediated apoptosis in PC-3 human prostate cancer cells. *Oncol Rep.* 20:785–792.

[94] Raj, L., T. Ide, A.U. Gurkar, M. Foley, M. Schenone, X. Li, N.J. Tolliday, T.R. Golub, S.A. Carr, A.F. Shamji, A.M. Stern, A. Mandinova, S.L. Schreiber, S.W. Lee (2011) Selective

killing of cancer cells by a small molecule targeting the stress response to ROS. *Nature.* 475:231–234.

[95] Cadenas, E. (2004) Mitochondrial free radical production and cell signaling. *Mol Aspects Med.* 25(1–2):17–26.

[96] Storz, P. (2007) Mitochondrial ROS—radical detoxification, mediated by protein kinase D. *Trends Cell Biol.* 17(1):13–8.

[97] You, H., K. Yamamoto, T.W. Mak (2006) Regulation of transactivation-independent proapoptotic activity of p53 by FOXO3a. *Proc Natl Acad Sci USA.* 103(24):9051–6.

[98] Janssen-Heininger, Y.M., M.E. Poynter, P.A. Baeuerle (2000) Recent advances towards understanding redox mechanisms in the activation of nuclear factor kappaB. *Free Radic Biol Med.* 28(9):1317–27.

[99] Chen, G.G., J.F.Y. Lee, S.H. Wang, U.P.F. Chan, C Ip Ping, W.Y. Lau (2002) Apoptosis induced by activation of peroxisome-proliferator activated receptor-gamma is associated with Bcl-2 and Nf-κB in human colon cancer. *Life Sci.* 70(22):2631–2646.

[100] Santandreu, F.M., A. Valle, J. Oliver, P. Roca (2011) Resveratrol potentiates the cytotoxic oxidative stress induced by chemotherapy in human colon cancer cells. *Cell Physiol Biochem.* 28(2):219–28.

[101] Radhakrishnan, S., L. Reddivari, R. Sclafani, U.N. Das, J. Vanamala (2011) Resveratrol potentiates grape seed extract induced human colon cancer cell apoptosis. *Front Biosci.* 3:1509–1523.

[102] Zhang, C., G. Lin, W. Wan, X. Li, B. Zeng, B. Yang, C. Huang (2012) Resveratrol, a polyphenol phytoalexin, protects cardiomyocytes against anoxia/reoxygenation injury via the TLR4/NF-κB signaling pathway. *Int J Mol Med.* 29(4):557–563.

[103] Connors, T.A., R. Duncan, R.J. Knox (1995) The chemotherapy of colon cancer. *Eur J Cancer.* 31(7–8):1373–1378.

[104] Chan, A.T., E.L. Giovannucci (2010) Primary prevention of colorectal cancer. *Gastroenterology.* 138(6):2029–2043.

[105] Datsis, A., A. Tsoga, V. Langouretos (2010) The role of functional foods in the prevention of colorectal cancer. *Hell J Surg.* 82(4):224–232.

[106] Boursi, B., N. Arber (2007) Current and future clinical strategies in colon cancer prevention and the emerging role of chemoprevention. *Curr Pharm Des.* 13(22):2274–2282.

[107] Derry, M.M., R. Komal, A. Chapla, A. Rajesh (2013) Identifying molecular targets of lifestyle modifications in colon cancer prevention. *Front Oncol.* 3:119.

[108] Farlex Partner Medical Dictionary. (2012) Retrieved January 26, 2016 from http://medicaldictionary.thefreedictionary.com/chemoprevention

[109] Castillo-Pichardo, L., S.F. Dharmawardhane (2012) Grape polyphenols inhibit Akt/mammalian target of rapamycin signaling and potentiate the effects of gefitinib in breast cancer. *Nutr Cancer.* 64(7):1058–1069.

[110] Mahyar-Roemer, M., H. Köhler, K. Roemer (2002) Role of Bax in resveratrol-induced apoptosis of colorectal carcinoma cells. *BMC Cancer.* 2:27.

[111] Cal, C., H. Garban, A. Jazirehi, C. Yeh, Y. Mizutani, B. Bonavida (2003) Resveratrol and cancer: chemoprevention, apoptosis, and chemoimmunosensitizing activities. *Curr Med Chem Anti-Cancer Agents.* 3:77–93.

[112] Nicastro, H.L., E.B. Trujillo, J.A. Milner (2012) Nutrigenomics and cancer prevention. *Curr Nutr Rep.* 1(1):37–43.

[113] Banerjee, S., Y. Li, Z. Wang, F.H. Sarkar (2008) Multi-targeted therapy of cancer by genistein. *Cancer Lett.* 269(2):226–242.

[114] Nakamura, Y., S. Yogosawa, Y. Izutani, H. Watanabe, E. Otsuji, T. Sakai (2009) A combination of indole-3-carbinol and genistein synergistically induces apoptosis in human colon cancer HT-29 cells by inhibiting AKT phosphorylation and progression of autophagy. *Mol Cancer.* 8:100–115.

[115] Sanchez-Gonzalez, P.D., F. Lopez-Hernandez, F.P. Barriocanal, A.I. Morales, J.M.L. Novoa (2011) Quercetin reduces cisplatin nephrotoxicity in rats without compromising its anti-tumour activity. *Nephrol Dial Transplant.* 26:3484–3495.

[116] Shan, B.E., M.X. Wang, R.Q. Li (2009) Quercetin inhibit human SW480 colon cancer growth in association with inhibition of cyclin D1 and survivin expression through Wnt/beta-catenin signaling pathway. *Cancer Investig.* 27(6):604–12.

[117] Kawamori, T., R. Lubet, V.E. Steele, G.J. Kelloff, R.B. Kaskey, C.V. Rao, B.S. Reddy (1999) Chemopreventive effect of curcumin, a naturally occurring anti-inflammatory agent, during the promotion/progression stages of colon cancer. *Cancer Res.* 59:597–601.

[118] Johnson, I.T., E.K. Lund (2007) Nutrition, obesity and colorectal cancer. *Aliment Pharmacol Ther.* 26(2):161–181.

[119] Shao, H., K. Jing, E. Mahmoud, H. Huang, X. Fang, C. Yu (2013) Apigenin sensitizes colon cancer cells to antitumor activity of ABT-263. *Mol Cancer Ther.* 12(12):2640–50.

[120] Singh, B.N., S. Shankar, R.K. Srivastava (2011) Green tea catechin, epigallocatechin-3-gallate (EGCG): mechanisms, perspectives and clinical applications. *Biochem Pharmacol.* 82(12):1807–1821.

[121] Grabacka, M.M., M. Gawin, M. Pierzchalska (2014) Phytochemical modulators of mitochondria: the search for chemopreventive agents and supportive therapeutics. *Pharmaceuticals (Basel).* 7(9):913–42.

[122] Zeng, H., O.N. Trujillo, M.P. Moyer, J.H. Botnen (2011) Prolonged sulforaphane treatment activates survival signaling in nontumorigenic NCM460 colon cells but apoptotic signaling in tumorigenic HCT116 colon cells. *Nutr Cancer.* 63(2):248–55.

[123] Tang, F.Y., C.J. Shih, L.H. Cheng, H.J. Ho, H.J. Chen (2008) Lycopene inhibits growth of human colon cancer cells via suppression of the Akt signaling pathway. *Mol Nutr Food Res.* 52(6):646–54.

[124] Lin, M.C., F.Y. Wang, Y.H. Kuo, F.Y. Tang (2011) Cancer chemopreventive effects of lycopene: suppression of MMP-7 expression and cell invasion in human colon cancer cells. *J Agric Food Chem.* 59(20):11304–18.

[125] Bonnesen, C., I.M. Eggleston, J.D. Hayes (2001) Dietary indoles and isothiocyanates that are generated from cruciferous vegetables can both stimulate apoptosis and confer protection against DNA damage in human colon cell lines. *Cancer Res.* 61(16):6120–30.

[126] Zheng, Q., Y. Hirose, N. Yoshimi, A. Murakami, K. Koshimizu, H. Ohigashi, K. Sakata, Y. Matsumoto, Y. Sayama, H. Mori (2002) Further investigation of the modifying effect of various chemopreventive agents on apoptosis and cell proliferation in human colon cancer cells. *J Cancer Res Clin Oncol.* 128(10):539–46.

[127] Kaur, M., B. Velmurugan, A. Tyagi, C. Agarwal, R.P. Singh, R. Agarwal (2010) Silibinin suppresses growth of human colorectal carcinoma SW480 cells in culture and xenograft through down-regulation of beta-catenin-dependent signaling. *Neoplasia.* 12(5):415–424.

[128] Kauntz, H., S. Bousserouel, F. Gosse, J. Marescaux, F. Raul (2012) Silibinin, a natural flavonoid, modulates the early expression of chemoprevention biomarkers in a preclinical model of colon carcinogenesis. *Int J Oncol.* 41(3):849–54.

[129] Lee, E.R., Y.J. Kang, H.J. Kim, H.Y. Choi, G.H. Kang, J.H. Kim, B.W. Kim, H.S. Jeong, Y.S. Park, S.G. Cho (2008) Regulation of apoptosis by modified naringenin derivatives in human colorectal carcinoma RKO cells. *J Cell Biochem.* 104(1):259–73.

[130] Akpinar-Bayizit, A., T. Ozcan, L. Yilmaz-Ersan (2012) The therapeutic potential of pomegranate and its products for prevention of cancer. In "*Cancer Prevention—From Mechanisms to Translational Benefits*", 331–373, InTech, Croatia, *Alexandros Georgakilas Ed.*, ISBN 978-953-51-0547-3.

[131] Adhami, V.M., N. Khan, H. Mukhtar (2009) Cancer chemoprevention by pomegranate: laboratory and clinical evidence. *Nutr Cancer.* 61(6):811–815.

[132] Jaganathan, S.K., M.V. Vellayappan, G. Narasimhan, E. Supriyanto (2014) Role of pomegranate and citrus fruit juices in colon cancer prevention. *World J Gastroenterol.* 20(16):4618–4625.

[133] Temraz, S., D. Mukherji, A. Shamseddine (2013) Potential targets for colorectal cancer prevention. *Int J Mol Sci.* 14:17279–17303.

[134] Rupnarain, C., Z. Dlamini, S. Naicker, K. Bhoola (2005) Colon cancer: genomics and apoptotic events. *Biol Chem.* 385(6):449–464.

[135] Galluzzi, L., O. Kepp, C. Trojel-Hansen, G. Kroemer (2012) Non-apoptotic functions of apoptosis-regulatory proteins. *EMBO Rep.* 13:322–330.

[136] Velmurugan, B., S.C. Gangar, M. Kaur, A. Tyagi, G. Deep, R. Agarwal (2010) Silibinin exerts sustained growth suppressive effect against human colon carcinoma SW480 xenograft by targeting multiple signaling molecules. *Pharm Res.* 27(10):2085–2097.

[137] Panaro, M.A., V. Carofiglio, A. Acquafredda, P. Cavallo, A. Cianciulli (2012) Anti-inflammatory effects of resveratrol occur via inhibition of lipopolysaccharide-induced NF-κB activation in Caco-2 and SW480 human colon cancer cells. *Br J Nutr.* 108:1623–1632.

[138] Kauntz, H., S. Bousserouel, F. Gosse, F. Raul (2012) The flavonolignan silibinin potentiates TRAIL-induced apoptosis in human colon adenocarcinoma and in derived TRAIL-resistant metastatic cells. *Apoptosis.* 17(8):797–809.

[139] Raina, K., C. Agarwal, R. Agarwal (2013) Effect of silibinin in human colorectal cancer cells: targeting the activation of NF-κB signaling. *Mol Carcinog.* 52:195–206.

[140] Hoh, C., D. Boocock, T. Marczylo, R. Singh, D.P. Berry, A.R. Dennison, A.J. Gescher (2006) Pilot study of oral silibinin, a putative chemopreventive agent, in colorectal cancer patients: Silibinin levels in plasma, colorectum, and liver and their pharmacodynamic consequences. *Clin Cancer Res.* 12(9):2944–2950.

[141] Yogosawa, S., Y. Yamada, S. Yasuda, Q. Sun, K. Takizawa, T. Sakai (2012) Dehydrozingerone, a structural analogue of curcumin, induces cell-cycle arrest at the G2/M phase and accumulates intracellular ROS in HT-29 human colon cancer cells. *J Nat Prod.* 75(12):2088–2093.

[142] Tu, S.P., H. Jin, J.D. Shi, L.M. Zhu, Y. Suo, G. Lu, A. Liu, T.C. Wang, C.S. Yang (2012) Curcumin induces the differentiation of myeloid-derived suppressor cells and inhibits their interaction with cancer cells and related tumor growth. *Cancer Prev Res.* 5(2):205–215.

[143] Camacho-Barquero, L., I. Villegas, J.M. Sánchez-Calvo, E. Talero, S. Sánchez-Fidalgo, V. Motilva, C. Alarcón de la Lastra (2007) Curcumin, a Curcuma longa constituent, acts on MAPK p38 pathway modulating COX-2 and iNOS expression in chronic experimental colitis. *Int Immunopharmacol.* 7(3):333–342.

[144] Chen, C., Y. Liu, Y. Chen, J. Xu (2011) C086, a novel analog of curcumin, induces growth inhibition and down-regulation of NFκB in colon cancer cells and xenograft tumors. C086, a novel analog of curcumin, induces growth inhibition and down-regulation of NFκB in colon cancer cells and xenograft tumors. *Cancer Biol Ther.* 12(9):797–807.

[145] Patel, B.B., D. Gupta, A.A. Elliott, V. Sengupta, Y. Yu, A.P.N. Majumdar (2010) Curcumin targets FOLFOX-surviving colon cancer cells via inhibition of EGFRs and IGF-1R. *Anticancer Res.* 30(2):319–325.

[146] He, Z.Y., C.B. Shi, H. Wen, F.L. Li, B.L. Wang, J. Wang (2011) Upregulation of p53 expression in patients with colorectal cancer by administration of curcumin. *Cancer Investig.* 29:208–213.

[147] Li, Y.H., Y.B. Niu, Y. Sun, F. Zhang, C.X. Liu, L. Fan, Q.B. Mei (2015) Role of phytochemicals in colorectal cancer prevention. *World J Gastroenterol.* 21(31):9262–9272.

[148] Khan, N., H. Mukhtar (2008) Multitargeted therapy of cancer by green tea polyphenols. *Cancer Lett.* 269(2):269–280.

[149] Larsen, C.A., R.H. Dashwood (2010) (-)-Epigallocatechin-3-gallate inhibits Met signaling, proliferation, and invasiveness in human colon cancer cells. *Arch Biochem Biophys.* 501(1):52–57.

[150] Thakur, V.S., A.R. Ruhul Amin, R.K. Paul, K. Gupta, K. Hastak, M.K. Agarwal, M.W. Jackson, D.N. Wald, H. Mukhtar, M.L. Agarwal (2010) P53-Dependent p21-mediated growth arrest pre-empts and protects HCT116 cells from PUMA-mediated apoptosis induced by EGCG. *Cancer Lett.* 296(2):225–232.

[151] Steinmann, J., J. Buer, T. Pietschmann, E. Steinmann (2013) Anti-infective properties of epigallocatechin-3-gallate (EGCG), a component of green tea. *Br J Pharmacol.* 168(5): 1059–1073.

[152] Yang, C.S., H. Wang, G.X. Li, Z. Yang, F. Guan, H. Jin (2011) Cancer prevention by tea: evidence from laboratory studies. *Pharmacol Res.* 64(2):113–122.

[153] Yang, H., K. Landis-Piwowar, T.H. Chan, Q.P. Dou (2011) Green tea polyphenols as proteasome inhibitors: implication in chemoprevention. *Curr Cancer Drug Targets.* 11(3):296–306.

[154] Carrasco-Pozo, C., M.L. Mizgier, H. Speisky, M. Gotteland (2012) Differential protective effects of quercetin, resveratrol, rutin and epigallocatechin gallate against mitochondrial dysfunction induced by indomethacin in Caco-2 cells. *Chemico-Biol. Interact.* 195:199–205.

[155] Min, K., T.K. Kwon (2014) Anticancer effects and molecular mechanisms of epigallocatechin-3-gallate. *Integr Med Res.* 3(1):16–24.

[156] Adachi, S., T. Nagao, H.I. Ingolfsson F.R. Maxfield, O.S. Andersen, L. Kopelovich, I.B. Weinstein (2007) The inhibitory effect of (-)-epigallocatechin gallate on activation of the epidermal growth factor receptor is associated with altered lipid order in HT29 colon cancer cells. *Cancer Res.* 67(13):6493–6501.

[157] Park, S.Y., Y.J. Jeong, S.H. Kim, J.Y. Jung, W.J. Kim (2013) Epigallocatechin gallate protects against nitric oxide-induced apoptosis via scavenging ROS and modulating the Bcl-2 family in human dental pulp cells. *J Toxicol Sci.* 38(3):371–8.

[158] Adams, L.S., N.P. Seeram, B.B. Aggarwal, Y. Takada, D. Sand, D. Heber (2006) Pomegranate juice, total pomegranate ellagitannins, and punicalagin suppress inflammatory cell signaling in colon cancer cells. *J Agric Food.* 54(3):980–985.

[159] Kasimsetty, S.G., D. Blalonska, M.K. Reddy, G. Ma, S.I. Khan, D. Ferreira (2010) Colon cancer chemopreventive activities of pomegranate ellagitannins and urolithins. *J Agric Food Chem.* 58:2180–2187.

[160] Larrosa, M., F.A. Tomás-Barberán, J.C. Espín (2006) The dietary hydrolysable tannin punicalagin releases ellagic acid that induces apoptosis in human colon adenocarcinoma Caco-2 cells by using the mitochondrial pathway. *J Nutr Biochem.* 17:611–625.

[161] Patil, J.R., G.K. Jayaprakasha, K.N. Chidambara Murthy, S.E. Tichy, M.B. Chetti, B.S. Patil (2009) Apoptosis-mediated proliferation inhibition of human colon cancer cells by volatile principles of Citrus aurantifolia. *Food Chem.* 114(4):1351–1358.

[162] Pan, M.H., W.J. Chen, S.Y. Lin-Shiau, C.T. Ho, J.K. Lin (2002) Tangeretin induces cell-cycle G1 arrest through inhibiting cyclin-dependent kinases 2 and 4 activities as well as elevating Cdk inhibitors p21 and p27 in human colorectal carcinoma cells. *Carcinogenesis.* 23:1677–1684.

[163] Totta, P., F. Acconcia, S. Leone, I. Cardillo, M. Marino (2004) Mechanisms of naringenin-induced apoptotic cascade in cancer cells: involvement of estrogen receptor alpha and beta signalling. *IUBMB Life.* 56(8):491–9.

[164] Fridrich, D., N. Teller, M. Esselen, G. Pahlke, D. Marko (2008) Comparison of delphinidin, quercetin and (-)-epigallocatechin-3-gallate as inhibitors of the EGFR and the ErbB2 receptor phosphorylation. *Mol Nutr Food Res.* 52:815–822.

[165] Li, M., Z. Zhang, D.L. Hill, X. Chen, H. Wang, R. Zhang (2005) Genistein, a dietary isoflavone, down-regulates the mdm2 oncogene at both transcriptional and posttranslational levels. *Cancer Res.* 65(18):8200–8.

[166] Liu, B., Z. Zhou, W. Zhou, J. Liu, Q. Zhang, J. Xia, J. Liu, N. Chen, M. Li, R. Zhu (2014) Resveratrol inhibits proliferation in human colorectal carcinoma cells by inducing G1/S-phase cell cycle arrest and apoptosis through caspase/cyclin-CDK pathways. *Mol Med Rep.* 10:1697–1702.

[167] Fouad, M.A., A.M. Agha, M.M. Merzabani, S.A. Shouman (2013) Resveratrol inhibits proliferation, angiogenesis and induces apoptosis in colon cancer cells: calorie restriction is the force to the cytotoxicity. *Hum Exp Toxicol.* 32:1067–1080.

[168] Turktekin, M., E. Konac, H.I. Onen, E. Alp, A. Yilmaz, S. Menevse (2011) Evaluation of the effects of the flavonoid apigenin on apoptotic pathway gene expression on the colon cancer cell line (HT29). *J Med Food.* 14(10):1107–17.

[169] Cho, H., H. Jung, H. Lee, H.C. Yi, H.K. Kwak, K.T. Hwang (2015) Chemopreventive activity of ellagitannins and their derivatives from black raspberry seeds on HT-29 colon cancer cells. *Food Funct.* 6(5):1675–83.

[170] Umesalma, S., P. Nagendraprabhu, G. Sudhandiran (2015) Ellagic acid inhibits proliferation and induced apoptosis via the Akt signaling pathway in HCT-15 colon adenocarcinoma cells. *Mol Cell Biochem.* 399(1–2):303–13.

[171] Huang, R.F., Y.J. Wei, B.S. Inbaraj, B.H. Chen (2015) Inhibition of colon cancer cell growth by nanoemulsion carrying gold nanoparticles and lycopene. *Int J Nanomed.* 10:2823–46.

[172] Trejo-Solís, C., J. Pedraza-Chaverrí, M. Torres-Ramos, D. Jiménez-Farfán, A. Cruz Salgado, N. Serrano-García, L. Osorio-Rico, J. Sotelo (2013) Multiple molecular and cellular mechanisms of action of lycopene in cancer inhibition. *Evid Based Complementary and Alternative Medicine* (2013) Article ID 705121, 17 p., http://dx.doi.org/10.1155/2013/705121.

[173] Stefanska, B., H. Karlic, F. Varga, K. Fabianowska-Majewska, A.G. Haslberger (2012) Epigenetic mechanisms in anti-cancer actions of bioactive food components—the implications in cancer prevention. *Br J Pharmacol.* 167:279–297.

[174] Choi, K., M.G. Jung, Y.H. Lee, J.C. Yoon, S.H. Kwon, H.B. Kang, M.J. Kim, J.H. Cha, Y.J. Kim, W.J. Jun, J.M. Lee, H.G. Yoon (2009) Epigallocatechin-3-gallate, a histone acetyltransferase inhibitor, inhibits EBV-induced B lymphocyte transformation via suppression of RelA acetylation. *Cancer Res.* 69(2):583–92.

[175] Eberhart, C.E., R.J. Coffey, A. Radhika, F.M. Giardiello, S. Ferrenbach, R.N. DuBois (1994) Up-regulation of cyclooxygenase-2 gene-expression in human colorectal adenomas and adenocarcinomas. *Gastroenterology.* 107:1183–8.

[176] Saldanha, S.N., R. Kala, T.O. Tollefsbol (2014) Molecular mechanisms for inhibition of colon cancer cells by combined epigenetic-modulating epigallocatechin gallate and sodium butyrate. *Exp Cell Res.* 324(1):40–53.

[177] Ho, E., J.D. Clarke, R.H. Dashwood (2009) Dietary sulforaphane, a histone deacetylase inhibitor for cancer prevention. *J Nutr.* 139:2393–2396.

[178] Myzak, M.C., W.M. Dashwood, G.A. Orner, E. Ho, R.H. Dashwood (2006) Sulforaphane inhibits histone deacetylase in vivo and suppresses tumorigenesis in Apc-minus mice. *FASEB J.* 20(3):506–508.

[179] Traka, M., A. Gasper, J. Smith, C. Hawkey, Y. Bao, R. Mithen (2005) Transcriptome analysis of human colon Caco-2 cells exposed to sulforaphane. *J Nutr.* 135:1865–1872.

[180] Slaby, O., M. Sachlova, V. Brezkova, R. Hezova, A. Kovarikova, S. Bischofová, S. Sevcikova, J. Bienertova-Vasku, A. Vasku, M. Svoboda, R. Vyzula (2013) Identification of microRNAs regulated by isothiocyanates and association of polymorphisms inside their target sites with risk of sporadic colorectal cancer. *Nutr Cancer.* 65:247–254.

[181] Kaeberlein, M., T. McDonagh, B. Heltweg, J. Hixon, E.A. Westman, S.D. Caldwell, A. Napper, R. Curtis, P.S. DiStefano, S. Fields, A. Bedalov, B.K. Kennedy (2005) Substrate-specific activation of sirtuins by resveratrol. *J Biol Chem.* 280(17):17038–45.

[182] Tili, E, J.J. Michaille, H. Alder, S. Volinia, D. Delmas, N. Latruffe, C.M. Croce (2010) Resveratrol modulates the levels of microRNAs targeting genes encoding tumor-suppressors and effectors of TGF-beta signaling pathway in sw480 cells. *Biochem Pharmacol.* 80:2057–2065.

[183] Kumazaki, M., S. Noguchi, Y. Yasui, J. Iwasaki, H. Shinohara, N. Yamada, et al. (2013) Anti-cancer effects of naturally occurring compounds through modulation of signal transduction and miRNA expression in human colon cancer cells. *J Nutr Biochem.* 24:1849–1858.

[184] Del Follo-Martinez, A., N. Banerjee, X. Li, S. Safe, S. Mertens-Talcott (2013) Resveratrol and quercetin in combination have anticancer activity in colon cancer cells and repress oncogenic microRNA-27a. *Nutr Cancer.* 65:494–504.

[185] Knop, C., J. Putnik, M. Scheuermann, M. Schmitz (2010) Cutting Edge Technologies: Cell Analysis/2010, B. Ziebolz, ed., Springer Medizin, Springer Verlag, Heidelberg, Germany, 4–13, 58–68, 137–141.

[186] Hotnog, D., M. Mihaila, A. Botezatu, G.G. Matei, C. Hotnog, G. Anton, M. Bostan, L.I. Brasoveanu (2013) Genistein potentiates the apoptotic effect of 5-fluorouracyl in colon cancer cell lines. *Rom Biotechnol Lett.* 18(6):8751–8760.

[187] Hotnog, D., M. Mihaila, I.V. Iancu, G.G. Matei, C. Hotnog, G. Anton, M. Bostan, L.I. Brasoveanu (2013) Resveratrol modulates apoptosis in 5-fluorouracyl treated colon cancer cell lines. *Roum Arch Microbiol Immunol.* 72(4):255–264.

[188] Ivanov, K., N. Kolev, I. Shterev, A. Tonev, V. Ignatov, V. Bojkov, T. Kirilova (2014) Adjuvant treatment in colorectal cancer. *"Colorectal Cancer—Surgery, Diagnostics and Treatment"*, 305–328, InTech, Croatia, *Jim S. Khan Ed.*, ISBN 978-953-51-1231-0.

[189] Nita, M.E., H. Nagawa, O. Tominaga, N. Tsuno, S. Fujii, S. Sasaki, C.G. Fu, T. Takenoue, T. Tsuruo, T. Muto (1998) 5-fluorouracil induces apoptosis in human colon cancer cell lines with modulation of Bcl-2 family proteins. *Br J Cancer.* 78(8):986–992.

[190] Wolmark, N., H. Rockette, B. Fisher, D.L. Wickerham, C. Redmond, E.R. Fisher, J. Jones, E.P. Mamounas, L. Ore, N.J. Petrelli, et al. (1993) The benefit of leucovorin-modulated fluorouracil as postoperative adjuvant therapy for primary colon cancer: results from National Surgical Adjuvant Breast and Bowel Project protocol C-03. *J Clin Oncol.* 11(10): 1879–87.

[191] Lowe, S.W., H.E. Ruley, T. Jacks, D.E. Housman (1993) p53-dependent apoptosis modulates the cytotoxicity of anticancer agents. *Cell.* 74(6):957–67.

[192] Piazza, G.A., A.K. Rahm, T.S. Finn, B.H. Fryer, H. Li, A.L. Stoumen, R. Pamukcu, D.J. Ahnen (1997) Apoptosis primarily accounts for the growth-inhibitory properties of

sulindac metabolites and involves a mechanism that is independent of cyclooxygenase inhibition, cell cycle arrest, and p53 induction. *Cancer Res.* 57:2452–59.

[193] Violette, S., L. Poulain, E. Dussaulx, D. Pepin, A.M. Faussat, J. Chambaz, J.M. Lacorte, C. Staedel, T. Lesuffleur (2002) Resistance of colon cancer cells to long-term 5-fluorouracil exposure is correlated to the relative level of Bcl-2 and Bcl-XL in addition to Bax and p53 status. *Int J Cancer.* 98(4):498–504.

[194] Zhang, N., Y. Yin, S.J. Xu, W.S. Chen (2008) 5-Fluorouracil: mechanisms of resistance and reversal strategies. *Molecules.* 13(8):1551–1569.

[195] Tomé-Carneiro, J., M. Larrosa, A. González-Sarrías, F.A. Tomás-Barberán, M.T. García-Conesa, J.C. Espín (2013) Resveratrol and clinical trials: the crossroad from in vitro studies to human evidence. *Curr Pharm Des.* 19(34):6064–6093.

Chapter 4

BRAF Mutation in Colorectal Cancer

Louisa Lo, Timothy Price, Joanne Young and
Amanda Townsend

Additional information is available at the end of the chapter

http://dx.doi.org/10.5772/62226

Abstract

The *BRAF* mutant colorectal cancer subgroup is a small population with unique clinicopathological and molecular features. This subgroup has been associated with particularly poor prognosis and advanced disease. The poor response of these patients to available treatments has driven much of the effort in trialling combination targeted treatments involving *BRAF* and *MEK* inhibitors. Most recently, an observed survival benefit with intensive triplet chemotherapy agents would encourage its use as first-line treatment in suitable candidates given that few of these patients proceed to second- or third-line treatments.

Keywords: BRAF, colorectal cancer, dabrafenib, trametenib, FOLFOXIRI

1. Introduction

The *BRAF* mutant (MT) colorectal cancer (CRC) population is a small and unique subgroup noted for its association with poor prognosis and survival. *BRAF* mutation occurs in approximately 10% (range, 5–22%) [1, 2] of the unselected CRC population and consistently has inferior median survival outcomes ranging from 8 to 14 months [3, 4]. Failure to achieve good survival outcomes through standard doublet chemotherapy agents in this population has ignited efforts to combine multiple target therapies, aiming for breakthroughs. In this chapter, the *BRAF* gene and its signalling pathway are explored in detail. *BRAF* gene mutation frequency and its impact on clinical presentation as well as its prognostic and predictive significance are also discussed. Updates on the current and latest management strategies as well as novel investigational treatments in this subgroup are also presented.

2. BRAF and the RAS/RAF/MEK/ERK signalling pathway

V-raf murine sarcoma viral oncogene homologue (RAF) is one of the most intensively researched mammalian effectors of RAS in the RAS/RAF/MEK/ERK signalling pathway (**Figure 1**) [5, 6]. The RAF protein itself is made up of three conserved regions: CR1, CR2, and CR3. CR1 and CR2 are situated in the N terminus. CR1 acts as the main binding domain for RAS. CR2 is the regulatory domain. CR3 is situated at the C terminus and functions as the catalytic kinase domain [7].

When GTP bound, RAS recruits RAF protein to the cell membrane and binds to it. This binding process activates RAF kinase by the phosphorylation of two amino acids (T599 and S602 of BRAF) situated in the activation segment of the kinase domain. RAF then phosphorylates its downstream effectors MEK1, MEK2, ERK1, and ERK2, leading to the activation of cellular proliferation, differentiation, and transcriptional regulation (**Figure 1**) [7].

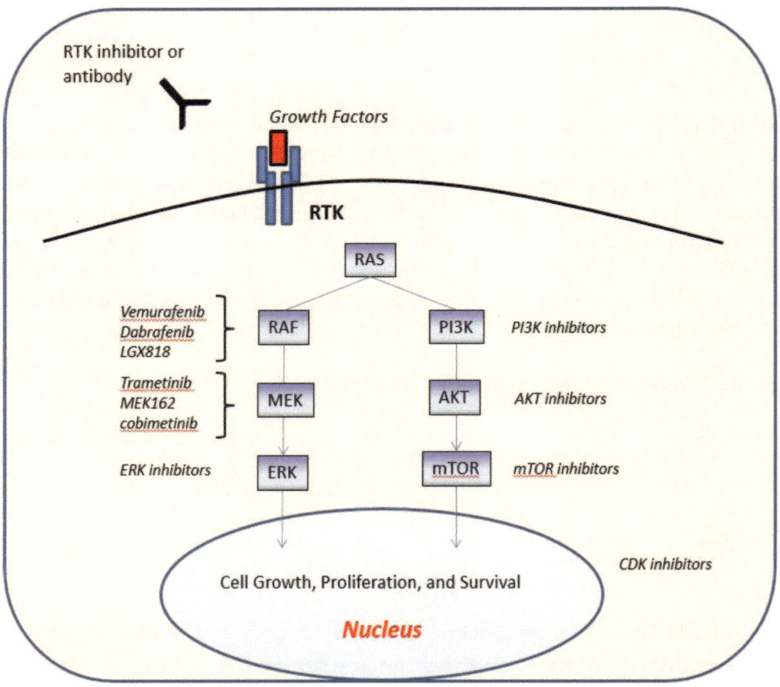

Figure 1. RAS and PIK3CA signalling pathways.

B-RAF (*BRAF*) together with A-RAF and C-RAF are the members of the RAF kinase family [8]. These three RAF isoforms are homologous in sequence and substrate specificity but do differ in their biological functions and regulations. Of these, BRAF remains the most potent activator of MEK [9].

The *BRAF* gene is a proto-oncogene located on chromosome arm 7q34, composed of 18 exons. There are more than 30 different *BRAF* mutations [10]. The most common activating mutation,

BRAF V600E (p.Val600Glu/c.1799T>A), accounts for 90% of all activating *BRAF* mutations and is found in exon 15 at nucleotide position 1799 [11]. The thymine-to-adenine transversion within codon 600 leads to the substitution of valine by glutamate at the amino acid level. This mutation occurs in the activating segment of the kinase domain, resulting in increased basal kinase activity. Compared to wild-type (WT) *BRAF*, *BRAF* V600E demonstrates an almost 500-fold increase in endogenous kinase activity [10, 12].

In solid tumours, the highest incidence of *BRAF* mutations is in malignant melanoma (27–70%), CRC (5–22%), and serous ovarian cancer (~30%) and less (1–3%) in non-small cell lung carcinoma (NSCLC) [13–15]. In colonic cell lines, the oncogenic effects of *BRAF* V600E include cell proliferation and inhibition of apoptosis [16]. Although dependent on continued BRAF activity for tumourigenic growth, *BRAF* MT cells did not require an upstream RAS function for proliferation [17].

2.1. *BRAF* mutation detection methods

CRC *BRAF* mutations can be identified using first- and second-generation direct sequencing, immunohistochemistry (IHC), and, potentially, circulating tumour cells (CTC).

Sanger sequencing is the earliest form of first-generation direct sequencing. Sanger sequencing was developed in 1975 and relies on the chain-termination sequencing of amplified DNA by polymerase chain reaction (PCR) and detection through electrophoresis. It requires approximately 18 to 19 h to process and is also 10 times less sensitive than pyrosequencing. Sanger sequencing method also cannot detect the changes in chromosomal copy number and translocations [18].

Next-generation sequencing (NGS) differs in technology using a specific reagent wash of nucleotide triphosphates with synchronised optical detection and includes pyrosequencing, allele-specific (AS) PCR, mass spectrometry, and real-time qPCR with melt-curve analysis [19]. NGS is the new gold standard test in *BRAF* mutation detection given its superior detection and speed.

Pyrosequencing is referred to as sequencing by synthesis and relies on the release of pyrophosphate (PPi) by DNA polymerase. The test detects light emitted when nucleotides are added to the target DNA template by DNA polymerase releasing PPi via a chemiluminescence reaction. It is a more rapid and sensitive test in detecting *BRAF* V600E mutations in addition to other variants such as V600D, V600K, V600R, and K601E. It can provide the percentage of DNA that harbours the *BRAF* V600E mutations. However, this method is limited by the length of DNA template and is prone to error readings in homopolymer sequences (TTTTTTTT) [18].

AS-PCR enriches known mutations in samples to increase the sensitivity of detection and is particularly useful in tissue with low tumour content. Mass spectrometry-based sequencing relies on the analysis of matrix-assisted laser desorption/ionisation time-of-flight (MALDI-TOF). This process is facilitated by the addition of mass-modified bases A, C, T, and G to the primed and amplified mutational hotspots. It is this flight time difference of the generated mass-modified complex that is measured by the mass spectrometer. Mass spectrometry-based sequencing is an even more sensitive test compared to pyrosequencing, with a detection ratio of 1:10 and 1:8, respectively [18].

Melt-curve analysis involves detecting the melting temperature for WT *BRAF* at 61°C and the V600E MT melting at 53°C. PCR methods, on the contrary, can perform as well and has advantages in terms of reduced labour (1.25 vs 16 min), faster turnaround (4 min vs 10 h), and lower cost ($2.6 vs $10.4). The sensitivity and specificity of real-time qPCR is reported to be 100% [19]. **Table 1** details the comparisons among some of the available NGS techniques.

Method	Sensitivity	Accuracy	Time	Cost/1 mill bases (USD)	Advantages/ disadvantages
Chain termination (Sanger)	Low	99.9%	20 min–3 h	2400	Requires the time-consuming step of PCR of plasmid cloning; impractical for larger sequencing projects
Pyrosequencing (454)	Medium	99.9%	24 h	10	Homopolymer errors
Sequencing by synthesis (Illumina)	High	99.9%	1–11 days	0.05–0.15	Expensive equipment; requires high DNA concentrations
Sequencing by ligation	High	99.9%	1–2 weeks	0.13	Slower; issues sequencing palindromic sequences
Ion semi conductor	High	98%	2 h	1	Homopolymer errors
Single-molecule real-time sequencing	High	87%	30 min–4 h	0.13–0.60	Expensive equipment; moderate throughput

Table 1. Available NGS techniques in detecting BRAF V600E mutation [20, 21].

The IHC detection of *BRAF* V600E with a mutation-specific antibody (clone VE1) was first described in metastatic melanoma and papillary thyroid carcinoma and is currently commercially available [22]. The advantage of IHC lies in the minimal amount of tissue needed and the availability of this technique in most pathological laboratories. Most studies have reported high sensitivities and specificities (98.8–100%) compared to PCR-based methods or sequencing [23–25]. However, there is one study that has reported sensitivity and specificity of only 71% and 74%, respectively [26]. The choice of positive control tissue and the amplification protocol is regarded to be crucial in the successful detection of *BRAF* mutation by IHC [27].

Recently, examination of CTC in peripheral blood has been explored as a new non-invasive means for detecting *BRAF* mutation in CRC [28]. Blood collected from 44 patients was enriched for CTC using a size-based microsieve technology. By incorporating the high-resolution melt-curve analysis technique, the concordance rates between CTC and tumour mutations were observed to be 90.9% (p=0.174) for *BRAF* mutation genotype status and 84.1% (p=0.000129) for KRAS mutation genotype status.

2.2. *BRAF* mutation and its frequency in CRC

A meta-analysis of 10 studies reported *BRAF* mutations in 4.8% to 20.8% of CRC [74]. **Table 2** further details the *BRAF* mutation rates and the corresponding detection methods in some notable metastatic CRC (mCRC) trials.

CRC trials	BRAF MT frequency	Method
PRIME [29, 30]	8%	Bidirectional Sanger sequencing
FIRE-3 [31]	10.5%	pyrosequencing
CRYSTAL [4]	6%	PCR clamping/melt-curve analysis
MAX [3]	10.6%	High-resolution melting point/PCR
PICCOLO [32]	14.8%	PCR/pyrosequencing
NORDIC-VII [33]	12%	Wobble enhanced ARMS*/real-time PCR
AGITG/NCIC CO.17 [59]	3.2% (overall) and 4.8% (KRAS WT)	PCR/sequencing
COIN [34]	8%	MALDI-TOF (Sequenom)/Sanger sequencing
TRIBE [35]	7.5%	Pyrosequencing

Table 2. BRAF mutation detection methods and reported frequencies in notable CRC trials.

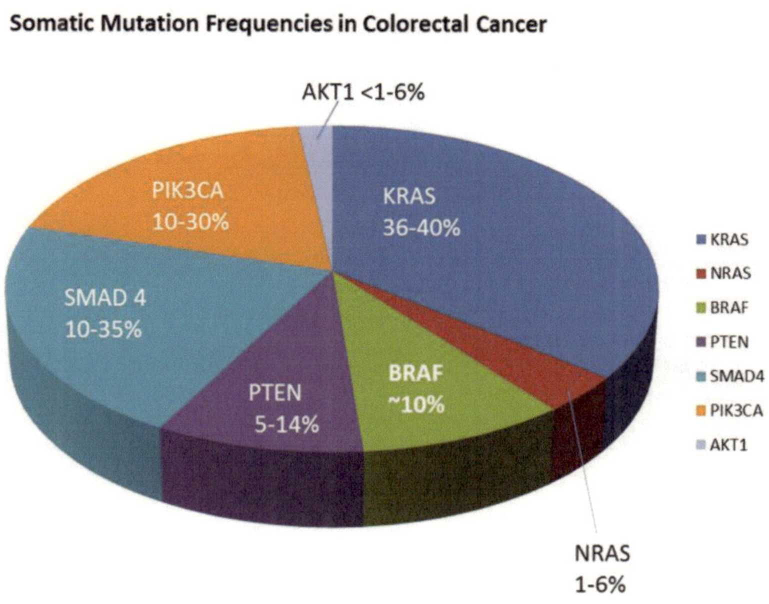

Figure 2. Somatic mutation frequencies in CRC.

Importantly, *BRAF* MT CRC is reported to be mutually exclusive to *KRAS* mutation [36]. *BRAF* mutation coexists with *PIK3CA* mutations in 13% and *PTEN* mutations in 22% of CRC [37]. **Figure 2** depicts the frequency of the different somatic mutations discovered in CRC patients.Chan, E. My Cancer Genome. Molecular Profiling of Colorectal Cancer [Internet]. January 26, 2016 [Updated:January 26, 2016]. Available from: https://www.mycancergenome.org/content/disease/colorectal-cancer/ [Accessed: January 26, 2016].

3. *BRAF* mutation and its clinical significance in CRC

3.1. CRC tumourigenesis pathways

The two main separate pathways observed in CRC development and progression are the chromosomal instability pathway (CIN), which accounts for 75% of the cases, and the microsatellite instability (MSI) pathway in 25% of the cases. Two processes are observed to contribute towards the MSI pathway: (1) germ-line mutations from Lynch syndrome and (2) sporadic MLH1 methylation from the serrated methylated pathway (**Figure 3**) [38] [100].

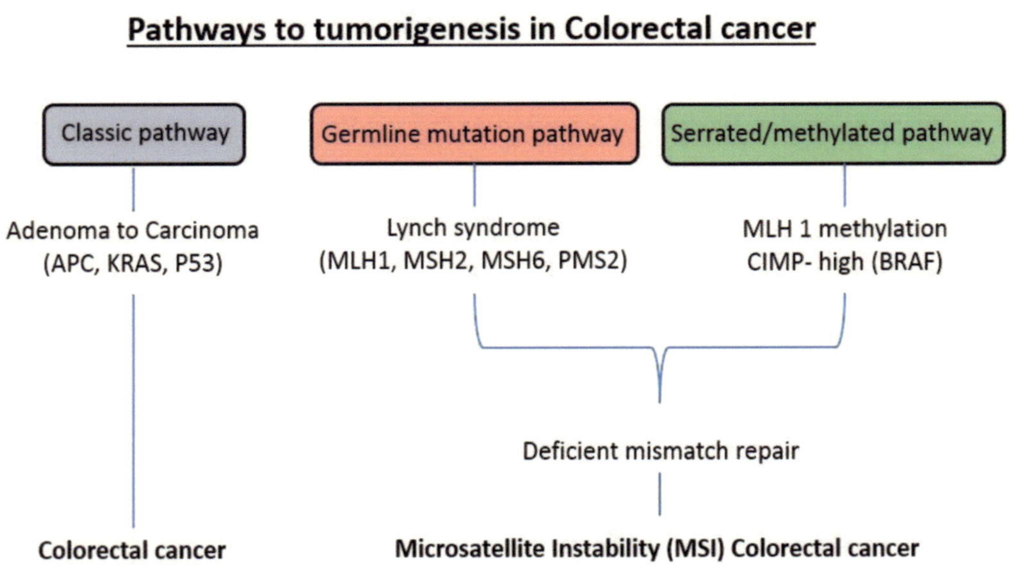

Figure 3. CRC tumourigenesis pathways.

The CIN pathway involves a defect in replication, mitosis, or DNA repair leading to genetic abnormalities, both structural and numeric, which are acquired sequentially. As a result, oncogenes are activated or tumour suppressor gene function is lost, which contributes towards malignant growth. This pathway is also often associated with aneuploidy by karyotyping. The genetic changes found in CRC arising via the CIN pathway include APC mutations (90%),

KRAS mutation (50%), TP53 mutations (70%), and allelic loss of 18q (80%) [39]. The CIN pathway has been traditionally associated with CRC arising in adenomatous polyps.

The MSI pathway is a result of defective mismatch repair (MMR) and occurs in a subset of CRC that arise from either adenomas or serrated polyps. It contributes towards tumour progression via the accumulation of tiny insertions and deletions in the repetitive sequences of microsatellites in coding genes, thereby retaining a near-diploid karyotype. This mechanism of tumourigenesis is readily recognized through a test for MSI, which categorises each tumour as MSI-high (MSI-H), MSI-low (MSI-L), or microsatellite stable (MSS), based on the proportion of microsatellites mutated. MSI-H cases usually imply an acquired or inherited defect in DNA repair.

In inherited cases of MSI-H CRC, germ-line mutation in one of the four genes that encode proteins responsible for MMR (MLH1, MSH2, PMS2, and MSH6) is responsible for a familial predisposition to cancer. This familial predisposition to CRC is known as Lynch syndrome [40], and the CRC that arise in this condition develop in adenomas.

In sporadic cases of MSI-H CRC, the serrated methylated pathway is increasingly implicated. Serrated polyps, not driven by CIN but by *BRAF* mutations, are observed to replace adenomas as precursor lesions in CRC. MSI-H CRC occur due to the epigenetic inactivation of *MLH1* by promoter methylation, which prevents MLH1 protein expression, resulting in defective MMR and producing MSI. This pathway is also closely associated with the widespread methylation of CpG islands, causing the transcriptional silencing of tumour suppressor genes, known as the CpG island methylator phenotype (CIMP) [38, 39].

3.2. *BRAF* testing to distinguish between sporadic versus germ-line MSI-H cases (Lynch syndrome)

Approximately 12% of MSI-H cases are sporadic in nature and *BRAF* mutation is implicated in nearly all (91%) of these cases [41, 42]. The methylation of *MLH1* is found only in 1.6% of germ-line Lynch syndrome cases [43], whereas it is typically found in sporadic tumour lacking MLH1 expression [44]. Hence, *BRAF* mutation testing is recommended in MSI-H CRC as a triage for Lynch syndrome. Only those lacking the *BRAF* mutation proceed with further workup for Lynch syndrome, as CRC harbouring the *BRAF* mutation are, with few exceptions, unlikely to have this condition.

MLH1 methylation testing is an alternative assay to distinguish sporadic from familial cases of CRC. However, given that methylation testing is more technically challenging than *BRAF* mutation testing, most would advocate *BRAF* testing as the more cost-effective assay to distinguish sporadic from familial MSI-H CRC [44].

3.3. Clinicopathological and molecular features of *BRAF* MT CRC

BRAF mutation has been reported in multiple studies to be associated with several clinicopathological parameters in CRC patients. *BRAF* V600E mutation is reported to increase from 10% in unselected patients to 37% in females ages >70 years [45]. *BRAF* mutations in the Western population tend to be more common in females and to have a more proximal location in the colorectum [27, 46–52]. *BRAF* mutations are rarely found in the left-sided colon (4%) and rectal cancers (2%) compared to the right-sided colon (22%; p<0.0001) [53]. *BRAF* mutation also varies by pathology. Approximately 60% of *BRAF* MT tumours are poorly differentiated and only up to 36% of them are well to moderately differentiated. Mucinous cancers tend to have a higher rate of *BRAF* mutation (22–67%) compared to non-mucinous cancers (6–21%) [39, 54, 55].

The relationship between *BRAF* mutation and these clinicopathological features was confirmed in a meta-analysis reported in 2014 [36]. Twenty-five studies of 11,955 CRC patients were included in this analysis. The mutation rate was seen to vary with the highest reported at 21.8% [2], the lowest being 5.0% [1], and the overall rate being 10.8%. Nine of the 25 studies have shown that *BRAF* mutation was associated with advanced tumor-node-metastasis (TNM) stage at diagnosis [11.6% in stage III/IV CRC vs 8.0% in stage I/II CRC; odds ratio (OR)=1.59; 95% confidence interval (CI)=1.16–2.17]. Thirteen of these studies showed that *BRAF* MT CRC was more prevalent in poorly differentiated tumours than well to moderately differentiated tumours. Of 766 patients with poorly differentiated tumours, 25.6% were *BRAF* MT, whereas only 8% of 4257 patients with well to moderately differentiated tumours were *BRAF* MT (OR=3.89; 95% CI=2.94–5.17). Six studies have also shown that more *BRAF* MT were detected in the mucinous subgroup than in the non-mucinous subgroup (19.4% vs 8.1%; OR=2.99; 95% CI=2.20–4.07). Twenty studies have also significantly demonstrated that proximal cancers (21.6%) harbour more *BRAF* mutations than distal cancers (4.8%; OR=4.85; 95% CI=3.59–6.56) [36].

Another study [56] reported a significantly increased rate of peritoneal (46% vs 24%; p<0.001) and distant lymph node metastases (53% vs 38%; p=0.001) and a lower rate of lung metastases (35% vs 49%; p=0.049) in *BRAF* MT CRC compared to *BRAF* WT tumours that might help to explain their poor prognosis.

Clinicopathological features of BRAF V600E MT CRC patients	Molecular features of BRAF V600E MT CRC
1. Age >70 years	1. More prevalent in MSI-H>MSS CRC
2. Female patients	2. More CIMP
3. Proximal right-sided tumours	3. More *MLH-1* methylation
4. High-grade and poorly differentiated	4. Mutually exclusive to KRAS mutation
5. Mucinous>non-mucinous	
6. More peritoneal and lymph node metastases	
7. Less lung metastases	

Table 3. Clinicopathological and molecular characteristics of BRAF V600E MT CRC

Relationships between *BRAF* MT and some molecular characteristics were also reported [36]. *BRAF* MT were significantly more prevalent in MSI-H CRC (38.9%) than MSS CRC (9.3%; OR=8.18; 95% CI=5.08–13.17). As mentioned above, CIMP characterized by widespread aberrant DNA methylation at select CpG islands was implicated in a minority of CRC tumourigenecity cases. Two studies were analysed for CIMP status and demonstrated a positive relationship with *BRAF* MT CRC: 45.9% (CIMP) vs 9.1% (non-CIMP; (OR=16.44; 95% CI=6.72–40.21). The methylation of the *MLH1* promoter region is an underlying cause of sporadic non-Lynch cases of MSI-H CRC. Three studies reported a relationship between *BRAF* MT and *MLH1* methylation status; 62.5% of *MLH1* methylated CRC had *BRAF* mutations compared to 9.2% of non-methylated CRC (OR=13.84; 95% CI=1.75–109.24). *BRAF* MT and *KRAS* MT were found to be mutually exclusive in this meta-analysis.

Table 3 summarises the clinicopathological and molecular characteristics of *BRAF* MT CRC.

4. *BRAF* mutation and its prognostic and predictive significance

4.1. Prognostic role and nature of progression

Multiple studies have reported poorer median overall survival (OS) in the *BRAF* MT mCRC subgroup. Regardless of treatment modality, median survival is generally reported to be between 10 and 16 months shorter than the overall population. For instance, the COIN trial, which studied 1630 patients for the effect of cetuximab and doublet chemotherapy FOLFOX in mCRC patients, had reported a median OS of 8.8 months in *BRAF* MT patients versus 20.1 months in patients with (*BRAF* and *RAS*) WT [34]. The PRIME study had reported a median OS of 10.5 months in the *BRAF* MT/RAS WT subgroup, contrasting to a median OS of 25.8 months in RAS WT group and 15.5 months in the RAS MT group. In this study, both (BRAF and RAS) WT patients also had the longest median OS of 28.3 months [29]. The pooled analysis of CRYSTAL and OPUS had also reported lower median OS in the *BRAF* MT group compared to the *BRAF* WT group (9.9 vs 21.1 months in the chemotherapy arm and 14.1 vs 24.8 months in the chemotherapy in combination with cetuximab arms) [57]. In 2013, the PLoS ONE meta-analysis analysed 21 mCRC trials of 5229 patients treated with monoclonal antibodies [58]. Fourteen of these trials were retrospective; two trials were prospective and five trials were randomised-controlled trials (RCTs). *BRAF* mutation was detected in 7.4%. Patients with *BRAF* WT showed decreased risks of progression and death with an improved progression-free survival [PFS; hazard ratio (HR)=0.38; 95% CI=0.29–0.51] and an improved OS (HR=0.35; 95% CI=0.29–0.42) compared to *BRAF* MT. Compared to *BRAF* WT patients, the updated prognostic analyses from the TRIBE study in 2014, which compared standard doublet chemotherapy to triplet chemotherapy, also reported significantly shorter PFS and OS, in the *BRAF* MT group in unresectable mCRC patients, independent of the treatment received [35]. **Table 4** summarises the reported median OS in the *BRAF* MT CRC subgroup reported from various phase III trials. It is also noted here that the *BRAF* mutation rates decrease with lines of therapy, signifying the reducing likelihood of *BRAF* MT patients surviving long enough to receive further lines of treatment.

Study	No. of patients	Treatment line/arm	BRAF MT rate	BRAF MT median PFS (months)	BRAF MT median OS (months)	KRAS WT median PFS (months)	KRAS WT median OS (months)
CRYSTAL (2011) [4]	1198	First line: FOLFIRI vs cetuximab+ FOLFIRI	6%	5.6 vs 8.0 (HR=0.93; p=0.87)	10.3 vs 14.1 (HR=0.91; p=0.74)	8.8 vs 10.9 (HR=0.67; p=0.001)	21.6 vs 25.1 (HR=0.83; p=0.055)
PRIME (2013) [29, 30]	1183	First line: FOLFOX vs panitumumab+ FOLFOX	8%	5.4 vs 6.1 (HR=0.58; p=0.12)	9.2 vs 10.5 (HR=0.90; p=0.76)	RAS/BRAF WT 9.2 vs 10.8 (HR=0.68; p<0.01)	RAS/BRAF WT 20.9 vs 28.3 (HR=0.74; p=0.02)
FIRE-3 (2013) [31]	400	First line: Avastin +FOLFIRI vs cetuximab+FOLFIRI	10.5%	6 vs 4.9 (HR=0.87; p=0.65)	13.7 vs 12.3 (HR=0.87; p=0.65)	RAS WT 10.2 vs 10.4 (HR=0.93; p=0.54)	RAS WT 25.6 vs 33.1 (HR=0.70; p=0.011)
COIN (2011) [34]	1630	First line: FOLFOX/ XELOX vs cetuximab +FOLFOX/XELOX	8%	5.6 vs 9.0 (RAS/BRAF WT) p<0.0001	8.8 vs 14.4 (KRAS MT) p<0.001	8.6 vs 8.6 (HR=0.96; p=0.60)	17.9 vs 17.0 (HR=1.04; p=0.67)
NORDIC-VII (2012) [33]	566	First line: NORDIC FLOX+cetuximab vs FLOX alone vs intermittent FLOX +cetuximab	12%	5.1 vs 8.3 (BRAF WT) p<0.001	9.5 vs 22 (BRAF WT) p<0.001	8.7 vs 7.9 vs 7.5 (HR=1.07; p=0.66)	22.0 vs 20.1 vs 21.4 (HR=1.08–1.14; p=0.77–0.80)
CO.17 (2013) [59]	572	Chemorefractory: cetuximab vs BSC	3.2%	Median PFS not reported (HR=0.76; p=0.69)	1.77 vs 2.97 (HR=0.84; p=0.81)	Favours cetuximab (HR=0.4; p<0.001)	9.7 vs 5.0 (HR=0.52; p<0.0001)
MAX (2011) [3]	471	First line: capecitabine (C) vs capecitabine/ bevacizumab (CB) or capecitabine/ bevacizumab/ mitomycin (CBM)	10.6%	2.5 vs 5.5 (HR=0.86; p=0.71)	6.3 vs 9.2 (HR=0.67; p=0.34)	5.9 vs 8.8 (HR=0.66; p=0.006)	20 vs 19.8 (HR=0.86; p=0.38)
PICCOLO (2013) [32]	460	Second line: irinotecan vs irinotecan/ panitumumab (IrPan)	14.8%	Favours irinotecan (HR=1.40; p=0.018)	Favours irinotecan (HR=1.84; p=0.029)	Favours IrPan (~6M) (HR=0.78; p=0.015)	10.5 vs 10.4 (HR=1.01; p=0.91)
181 Peeters M, Oliner KS, Price TJ, Cervantes A, Sobrero AF, Ducreux M, et al.	1015	Second line: FOLFIRI vs panitumumab/ FOLFIRI	4.4%	RAS WT 1.8 vs 2.5 (HR=0.69; p=0.34)	RAS WT 5.7 vs 4.7 (HR=0.64; p=0.20)	RAS WT 5.5 vs 6.9 (HR=0.68; p=0.006)	RAS WT 15.4 vs 18.7 (HR=0.83; p=0.15)

Study	No. of patients	Treatment line/arm	BRAF MT rate	BRAF MT median PFS (months)	BRAF MT median OS (months)	KRAS WT median PFS (months)	KRAS WT median OS (months)
Updated analysis of KRAS/NRAS and BRAF mutations in study 20050181 of panitumumab (pmab) + FOLFIRI for 2nd-line treatment (tx) of metastatic colorectal cancer (mCRC). J Clin Oncol 2014;32(Suppl.). Abstract 3568.							
TRIBE (2015) [35]	508	First line: Avastin/ FOLFIRI vs Avastin/ FOLFOXIRI	7.5%	5.5 vs 7.5 (HR=0.56)	10.8 vs 19.1 (HR=0.55)	RAS WT 11.3 vs 13.3 (HR=0.77)	RAS WT 34.4 vs 41.7 (HR=0.84)

Table 4. Poorer survival in BRAF MT CRC and mutation frequencies in subsequent lines of treatment

The *BRAF* MT CRC patients of Eastern populations were also reported to share the same fate as those in Western populations. A retrospective study [60] reported a *BRAF* mutation rate of 4.2% in 212 Chinese CRC patients. This study, which did not specifically examine the lines of treatment administered, showed that *BRAF* MT was associated with advanced TNM ($p<0.001$), more distant metastases ($p=0.025$), and worse OS (3-year OS: 16.7% in the *BRAF* MT subgroup vs 73.2% in the *BRAF* WT subgroup; $p<0.001$). The *BRAF* mutation rate of 4.2% in the Chinese population was found similar to the rates (1–7%) reported for Taiwanese and Japanese populations [61–64].

BRAF MT is also associated with poor prognosis in other stages of CRC. A review in 2013 [65] on seven studies that included stages I to IV CRC patients has concluded that *BRAF* mutation served as an independent prognostic factor for reduced OS, disease-free survival (DFS), and cancer-specific survival, especially in MSS CRC. One of the studies that included 911 stage II to IV CRC patients demonstrated *BRAF* mutation to be associated with a poor 5-year OS (*BRAF* MT vs WT, 47.5% vs 60.7%; $p<0.01$) [66]. Another study [47] looked at 1307 patients with stage II to III CRC and reported reduced OS in *BRAF* MT group (HR=2.2; 95% CI=1.4–3.4; $p=0.0003$).

To further analyse the impact of MSI status in the *BRAF* MT CRC patients, Samowitz et al. [66] have shown that survival differs for stages II to IV CRC *BRAF* MT tumours with MSI compared to MSS tumours. Poor prognosis was only demonstrated in MSS tumours (5YS: *BRAF* MT vs WT, 16.7% vs 60.0%; log-rank $p<0.01$) from a multivariate analysis adjusted for age, stage, and tumour sites. MSI tumours were reported to have good prognosis regardless of *BRAF* MT status, with 5YS 76.2% (with *BRAF* mutation) vs 75.0% (without *BRAF* mutation). Interestingly, a recent retrospective Japanese study also studied the role of *BRAF* MT in MSI tumours [67]. They examined KRAS, BRAF, and MSI status in 813 patients with curatively resected, stage I to III CRC. After adjusting for relevant variables, including MSI status, they reported that *BRAF* MT were poor prognostic factors for DFS (HR=2.20; 95% CI=1.19–4.06) and OS (HR=2.30; 95% CI=1.15–4.71) independent of MSI status. This small study, which excludes stage IV patients, suggests that MSI-H tumours without *BRAF* mutation may have the best prognosis compared to MSI-H tumours with *BRAF* mutation. MSS tumours with *BRAF* mutation would have the worst prognosis.

In accordance with their aggressive nature, *BRAF* MT cancers have also been reported to have poor PFS with sequential systemic treatments. A retrospective study on 1567 patients detected a *BRAF* mutation rate of 8%. These *BRAF* MT patients had received a median of two later lines of chemotherapy, with the median PFS for the first three lines of chemotherapy being 6.3, 2.5, and 2.6 months, respectively [68]. Another smaller study had reported even shorter median PFS (4.3 months) after first-line treatment in *BRAF* MT [69]. This observation highlights the importance of considering early intensified treatment given the propensity for these patients to not survive long enough for second- or third-line treatments.

Recently, other rare (<1%) subtypes of *BRAF* MT, which harbour mutations in codon 594 or 596, were reported to have markedly longer OS compared to *BRAF* V600E MT (median OS=62.0 vs 12.6 months; HR=0.36; 95% CI=0.20–0.64; p=0.002). These subtypes are noted to be MSS and also differ in other molecular and clinical characteristics, being more frequently rectal in origin, non-mucinous, and with no peritoneal spread [70].

4.2. Predictive role

Given that *RAS* MT are negative predictors of anti-epidermal growth factor receptor (EGFR) therapies, the predictive role of *BRAF* MT for anti-EGFR agents has been of interest given the relationship with RAS in the EGFR/RAS/RAF/MEK/ERK pathway. *BRAF* MT and its associated resistance to anti-EGFR agents have been suggested by several retrospective analyses [71–73].

To date, the predictive role of *BRAF* MT on anti-EGFR agents remains unclear, in light of differing conclusions from two separate meta-analyses [74, 75]. Pietrantonio et al. concluded that *BRAF* MT might be a negative predictor for anti-EGFR agents, supporting the meta-analysis by Yuan et al. [58]. This study included a pooled analysis of nine phase III trials and one phase II trial and shown that cetuximab- or panitumumab-based therapy did not increase the benefit of standard treatment versus best supportive care in RAS-WT/*BRAF*-MT CRC patients. Overall, the addition of cetuximab or panitumumab did not significantly improve the PFS (HR=0.88; p=0.33), OS (HR=0.91; p=0.63), and overall response rate [ORR; relative risk (RR)=1.31; p=0.25] in this subgroup population [74]. However, another recent meta-analysis reviewed seven RCTs for OS and eight RCTs for PFS and concluded on insufficient evidence to justify the exclusion of anti-EGFR agents in the *BRAF* MT population [75]. Nevertheless, these latest findings have supported the need for *BRAF* mutation assessment before the initiation of treatment to study and tailor the most effective strategies to the *BRAF* MT population.

5. Treatment strategies

5.1. Triplet chemotherapy effect

BRAF MT has not been known to be a predictor of benefit from chemotherapy or anti-vascular endothelial growth factor (VEGF) agents. The Italian TRIBE study [35] compared anti-VEGF therapy, bevacizumab added to intensified triplet chemotherapy, fluorouracil, oxaliplatin, and irinotecan (FOLFOXIRI), to standard first-line doublet chemotherapy with fluorouracil and irinotecan (FOLFIRI) plus bevacizumab in 508 unresectable mCRC patients. The study reported a higher response rate of 65% vs 53% with the triplet FOLFOXIRI and bevacizumab arm. Reassuringly, there was no increase in fatal or serious adverse events.

The updated analyses of the same study reported a BRAF mutation rate of 7.5%. In the *BRAF* MT group, there was a significant trend for better survival in the triplet arm compared to the doublet arm (19.1 vs 10.8 months; HR=0.55). Significantly, this is the only regimen to have resulted in a median OS of more than 15 months in the *BRAF* MT group compared to the more often reported median of 4.4 to 14 months in most studies [29, 57]. It was proposed that intensified triplet chemotherapy (FOLFOXIRI+bevaczicumab) is considered first line in the BRAF MT group, who usually have aggressive cancers with limited ability to undergo a more sequential approach to treat metastatic disease.

5.2. Maintenance treatment

A recent meta-analysis on five RCTs had failed to demonstrate a statistically significant OS benefit (HR=0.93; 95% CI=0.85–1.02; p=0.12; I^2=5%) with administering maintenance chemotherapy versus complete treatment interruption after first-line therapy in unselected CRC [76]. The chemotherapy free interval in the group not using maintenance treatment was 3.9 months (3.6–4.3 months). Nevertheless, the author had emphasized the importance of predictive markers to guide the selection of patients who would benefit from the maintenance strategy. Although not formally tested in the *BRAF* MT subgroup population, the maintenance strategy might prove more favourable than the intermittent strategy given its known aggressive nature. This is especially relevant given that the median reported PFS in BRAF MT as indicated previously ranged from 4.3 to 6.3 months after first-line treatment [68, 69].

In terms of the choice for maintenance treatment, there is no current recommended standard. However, practice trends could perhaps be extrapolated from the AIO KRK 0207 trial, which confirmed the prognostic impact of mutation status [77]. In all patients (irrespective of BRAF or RAS status), at a median follow-up of 27 months, the authors reported a time to failure of strategy of 3.6, 6.2, and 4.6 months among all patients receiving no treatment, fluoropyrimidine plus bevacizumab, or bevacizumab alone, respectively (p<0.001). However, in RAS/BRAF WT patients, bevacizumab monotherapy was as effective as combination treatment (fluoropyramidine/bevacizumab) for maintenance. In contrast, in the RAS or BRAF MT subgroup, the combination treatment was favoured, as single-agent bevacizumab was equivalent to no maintenance at all.

6. Investigated treatments targeting EGFR/RAF/MEK

6.1. BRAF/MEK inhibitors

As mentioned above, RAS proteins normally activate BRAF along with A-RAF and C-RAF [78]. BRAF mutations lead to the constitutive activation of BRAF kinase activity, resulting in phosphorylation and activation of the MEK kinases (MEK1 and MEK2). Once activated, MEK kinases phosphorylate and activate ERK kinases, which phosphorylate a multitude of cellular substrates involved in cell proliferation and survival (**Figure 1**).

RAF inhibitors, such as vemurafenib and dabrafenib, have produced response rates of 50 to 80% in melanomas that harbour the BRAF V600 mutations [79, 80]. This is disappointingly contrasting to the response rate of only 5%, and median PFS of 2.1 months achieved in *BRAF* MT CRC [81]. Previous observations have proposed that RAF inhibitor insensitivity in BRAF MT CRC was driven by the feedback reactivation of the RAS/RAF/MEK/ERK signalling cascade. In many BRAF MT CRC cell lines, EGFR-mediated activation of RAS and C-RAF was observed to be the culprit [82, 83]. Solit et al. had also demonstrated the critical dependency of *BRAF* MT colorectal cell lines and xenografts on MEK-ERK signalling, which renders them highly sensitive to pharmacological MEK inhibition. Pharmacological MEK inhibition completely abrogated tumour growth in BRAF MT xenografts, whereas *RAS* MT tumours were only partially inhibited [84].

Many RAF inhibitor combinations were hence evaluated in clinical trials in recent years and have shown promising results. A phase I to II clinical trial of combined RAF/MEK inhibition with dabrafenib (150 mg BD) and trametenib (2 mg OD) in 43 *BRAF* MT CRC resistant to anti-EGFR therapy produced partial responses in 12% and complete response in 2%. One patient achieved a durable complete response exceeding 36 months. Additionally, 56% achieved stable disease as the best confirmed response [85].

6.2. Dual and triplet targeting EGFR/BRAF/MEK inhibitors

The observations above have also led to a number of studies assessing the combined blockade at other sites in the EGFR pathway in addition to RAF/MEK inhibition. It was observed that the dual inhibition of anti-EGFR therapy in combination with RAF inhibition in resistant cell lines might still produce a lower degree of mitogen-activated protein kinase (MAPK) pathway inhibition in BRAF MT CRC compared to single-agent RAF inhibitors in *BRAF* MT melanoma patients. Dabrafenib and panitumumab doublet was trialled with a response rate of (partial and complete response) 2/20 (10%) and stabilised disease in 16/20 (80%) as the best overall response [86]. Another study examined the combination of vemurafenib (BRAF-inhibitor) and panitumumab in 15 patients. Two (13%) patients reported partial responses lasting 40 and 24 weeks, respectively. Eight (53%) patients stable disease lasting more than 6 months [87]. A phase II study studied dual inhibition with encorafenib (BRAF inhibitor) and cetuximab with 26 patients. Encorafenib and cetuximab doublet was reported to produce an overall RR (complete and partial) of 23.1% with a median PFS of 3.7 months. The most common treatment-related grade 3/4 adverse events associated with this doublet regimen were fatigue and hypophosphatemia (8% each) [88].

Encouragingly, the triplet combination of EGFR/RAF/MEK inhibition in *BRAF* MT CRC reported an improved response rate (26% complete and partial) in 35 patients compared to the doublet inhibition. The triplet regimen had also stabilised disease in 57%. The most common adverse events reported were diarrhoea (60% grade 1/2 and 9% grade 3) and dermatitis acneiform (47% grade 1/2 and 9% grade 3) [86].

6.3. Acquired resistance to EGFR/RAF/MEK targeted therapies

Although trials have demonstrated early efficacies of combination targeted therapies in these *BRAF* MT patients, attention was brought towards their eventual treatment resistance and disease progression. A group in Harvard recently compared pretreatment and postprogression *BRAF* MT CRC tumour biopsies by whole exome sequencing (WES) to examine the related changes that could explain treatment resistance in these cases [89]. They have identified four possible acquired molecular mechanisms that could lead to resistance to combination treatments with RAF/MEK and RAF/EGFR. These four mechanisms include (1) *KRAS* exon 2 mutation (G12D and G13D), (2) *KRAS* WT amplification [confirmed by fluorescence *in situ* hybridisation (FISH) to be ~25-fold overexpression], (3) *BRAF* MT allele amplification, and (4) *MEK1* mutation. These alterations converge on the MAPK pathway reactivation and promote resistance.

Interestingly, the group also discovered an ERK inhibitor that retained the ability to suppress MAPK signalling and overcome each of these mechanisms identified [89]. In conjunction with these findings, early-phase clinical trials are currently incorporating ERK inhibitors as potential future treatment strategies for *BRAF* MT CRC.

6.4. Other possible EGFR/RAF targeted combination treatments

6.4.1. Vemurafenib/irinotecan/cetuximab combination

The phase I vemurafenib/irinotecan/cetuximab triplet study reported a RR of 35% (partial response) in 18 mCRC patients with a median PFS of 7.7 months. The most common adverse effects were fatigue (94%), diarrhoea (89%), nausea (83%), and rash (78%). Following this, a U.S. cooperative group randomised phase II trial (NCT01787500) of irinotecan and cetuximab ±vemurafenib in BRAF-mutated mCRC (SWOG 1406) is now ongoing [90].

7. Alternative target signalling pathways

Although our increasing understanding of the complexity of the EGFR/RAF pathway has led to some advances in our understanding of possible mechanisms of resistance to BRAF inhibition, additional complex interactions with related pathways are likely to be involved, including the phosphatidylinositol 3-kinase (PI3K)/AKT pathway, mammalian target of rapamycin (mTOR), and Wnt signalling.

7.1. PI3K/AKT and mTOR pathway

The PI3K/AKT pathway is an alternative resistance mechanism to BRAF inhibition in *BRAF* MT CRC. Approximately 40% of CRC have been shown to have alterations in one of eight PI3K pathway genes. These mutations are almost always mutually exclusive to each other [91]. In addition, *BRAF* mutation co-exists with *PIK3CA* mutations in 13% and *PTEN* mutations in 22% of CRC [37]. Compared to *BRAF* MT melanoma cell lines, *BRAF* MT CRC cell lines seemed to also display a higher rate of PI3K/AKT pathway activation. These cell lines were reported to be less sensitive to the BRAF inhibitor, vemurafenib [92].

Based on the above observations, the combination triplet inhibition treatment was studied with encorafenib (BRAF inhibitor), cetuximab, and PI3K inhibitor (alpelisib) in 28 patients and reported an overall RR of 32.1% with a median PFS of 4.3 months. The most common grade 3/4 adverse events reported were hyperglycemia (11%) and increased lipase (7%) [88].

Sustained PI3K/mTOR activity was demonstrated also by Corcoran et al. [82] in BRAF MT CRC cell lines upon BRAF inhibition. Pleasingly, a potent growth-inhibitory effect was recently observed in xenografts of BRAF MT CRC with the combined BRAF/PI3K/mTOR inhibition [93].

7.2. Wnt/β-catenin pathway

A study by Lemieux et al. demonstrated the Wnt/β-catenin pathway (**Figure 3**) as a potential novel target in MEK/ERK signalling involved in CRC tumourigenesis [94]. The Wnt/β-catenin pathway is activated via the binding of Wnt1 protein to the G-protein coupled receptor, Frizzled. After the activation by Wnt1, Dishevelled protein (Dsh) induces the dissociation of the destruction complex that usually degrades β-catenin. Without the destruction complex, β-catenin is accumulated in the cytoplasm and transported to the nucleus to act as a transcriptional coactivator of transcription factors as shown in **Figure 4**. The aforementioned destruction complex comprises Axin (A), adenomatous polyposis coli (APC), and glycogen synthase kinase 3 (GSK3β). In the absence of Wnt1 activation, the destruction complex phosphorylates the downstream ubiquinating process. Here, the β-transducin repeat containing protein (βTrCP) binds β-catenin, ubiquinating it and marks it for degradation by the proteasome. Although there is conflicting literature with regards to the role of MAPK signalling in activating Wnt/β-catenin pathway, this group found Wnt signalling induction in high-grade *BRAF* MT tumours. Their data also show that the oncogenic activation of KRAS/BRAF/MEK signalling stimulates the canonical Wnt/β-catenin pathway, which in turn promotes intestinal tumour growth and invasion. This has in turn sparked trial designs to incorporate Wnt signalling as a treatment strategy.

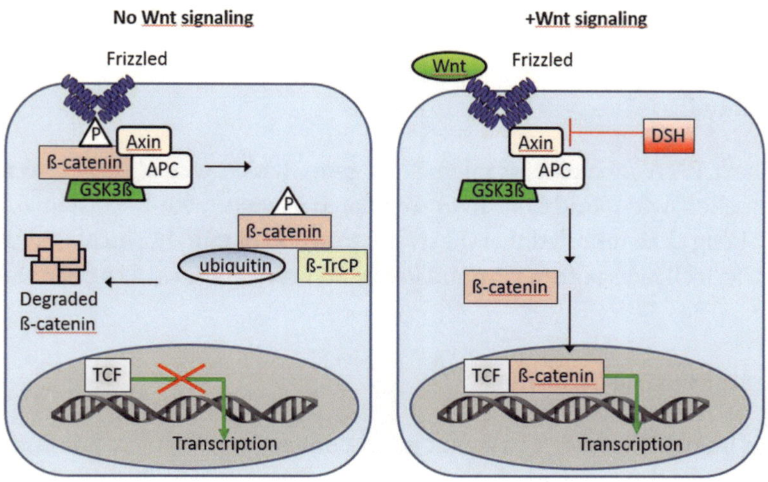

Figure 4. Wnt/β-catenin pathway.

8. Other possible therapeutic mechanisms

Recently, a number of other early studies have reported additional potential mechanisms of targeted treatment, which had shown promise in *BRAF* MT CRC xenografts or cell line studies.

8.1. Multi-targeted angiokinase inhibitor (dovitinib)

Dovitinib is a multi-target angiokinase inhibitor with activity against fibroblast growth factor receptors (FGFRs), platelet-derived growth factor receptors (PDGFRs), and VEGF receptors, which participate in tumour growth, survival, angiogenesis, and vascular development. Although not effective *in vitro*, *in vivo* studies have shown the inhibition of *BRAF* MT xenografts tumours with dovitinib. Lee et al. proposed that this observation is secondary to its angiogenesis-suppressing effect and could be a novel approach to improve the outcome of CRC patients in whom FGFR is overexpressed or amplified [95].

8.2. Proteasome inhibitor (carfilzomib)

A novel use of proteasome inhibitors (carfilzomib, bortezomib), known more for utility in haematological malignancy, has shown promising preclinical results in *BRAF* MT CRC [96]. Zecchin et al. have observed increased sensitivity of *BRAF* MT CRC to carfilzomib, whereas WT cells were significantly less affected ($p<0.05$). This response seemed to be independent of the phosphatase and tensin homologue (PTEN) or retinoblastoma protein (RB1) expression status in CRC. The mechanism of this activity was explained by the higher accumulation rate of ubiquitinated proteins in MT cells with respect to WT. It was speculated that this is secondary to the non-oncogenic addiction of *BRAF* MT cells to the protein degradation function of proteasome to counterbalance the proteotoxic stress induced by the MT protein. Interestingly, carfilzomib was also found to have antagonistic effects with the RAF inhibitor, vemurafenib, and was proposed as a possible alternative treatment to BRAF/MEK inhibition.

8.3. microRNA (miR-145)

miR-145, a short RNA molecule of microRNA gene, which was observed to have tumour suppressor function, was found to be down-regulated in vemurafenib-resistant *BRAF* MT CRC cell lines [97]. Peng et al. reported that the overexpression of miR-145 increased the sensitivity of *BRAF* MT CRC cell lines both *in vitro* and *in vivo* and could be used as a potential therapeutic target.

8.4. *In situ* cancer vaccine (Allostim)

AlloStim is an innovative design based on immunotherapy principles. It is derived from the blood of normal blood donors and is intentionally mismatched to the recipient. $CD4^+$ T cells are initially separated from the blood and differentiated and expanded for 9 days in culture to make an intermediary called T-Stim. AlloStim is made by incubating T-Stim cells for 4 h with antibody-coated microbeads. The cells with the beads still attached are suspended in infusion media and loaded into syringes. The syringes are shipped refrigerated to the point-of-care. A phase I study was completed in May 2011 and a phase II/III study is due to recruit in 2016. It involves an *in situ* (in the body) cancer vaccine step that combines killing a single metastatic tumour (usually liver metastasis) lesion by the use of cryoablation to cause the release of tumour-specific markers to the immune system and then injecting bioengineered allogeneic immune cells (AlloStim) into the lesion as an adjuvant to modulate the immune response and educate the immune system to kill other tumour cells wherever they reside in the body [98].

8.5. Apoptosis regulator (BCL-2/BCL-XL) inhibitor (Navitoclax)

Apoptosis regulator (BCL-2/BCL-XL) inhibitor (Navitoclax) was explored as a novel approach in sensitising *BRAF* MT CRC to mTOR inhibition. The results showed that this combination strategy leads to efficient apoptosis in specifically *KRAS* and *BRAF* MT but not WT CRC cells [99]. These data showed promising results with the combination strategy of apoptosis regulator inhibitors with mTOR inhibitors in *BRAF* MT CRC.

9. Ongoing trials for BRAF MT CRC

Many phase I/II trials are currently ongoing for *BRAF* MT mCRC. Most of them focus on the RAS/RAF/MEK/ERK signalling pathway, trialling combination targeted treatments. **Table 5** lists these available trials.

http://dx.doi.org/10.5772/62226

Trial name/Reg	Phase	Trialed agents	Status
NCT01543698	I/II	RAF inhibitor (dabrafenib)+MEK inhibitor (trametenib)+CDK4/6 inhibitor (LEE011)	Recruiting
NCT 01719380	IB/II	RAF inhibitor (LGX818)+cetuximab+PI3K inhibitor (BYL-719) vs LGX818+ BYL-719	Recruiting
NCT01902173	I/II	Dabrafenib+trametenib: in stage IIIC+IV CRC	Recruiting
NCT02034110	II	Dabrafenib+trametenib: BRAF MT rare cancers	Recruiting
NCT00265824	III	Avastin±erlotinib: maintenance treatment in unresectable CRC	Closed; awaiting for results
NCT02175654 (PREVIUM)	II	Regorafenib: single-agent second-line post-FOLFOXIRI+Avastin	Recruiting
NCT01750918	I/II	Dabrafenib+trametenib+panitumumab	Recruiting
NCT01787500	I	Vemurafenib+cetuximab+irinotecan	Recruiting
S1406	II	Cetuximab+irinotecan±vemurafenib	Recruiting
NCT01596140	I	Vemurafenib+mTOR inhibitor (everolimus/temsirolimus)	Recruiting
NCT02041481	I	MEK inhibitor+FOLFOX: CRC failing standard treatment	Recruiting
NCT02380443	IIB	Allostim (*in situ* cancer vaccine): third-line treatment in KRAS/BRAF MT CRC	Pending
NCT02278133	IB/II	Wnt ligand inhibitor (WNT974), RAF inhibitor and cetuximab	Recruiting
NCT01351103	I	Wnt ligand inhibitor (LGK974)	Recruiting

Table 5. Ongoing trials in BRAF MT CRC

10. Conclusion

The *BRAF* V600E MT CRC typically presents with right-sided proximal high-grade mucinous tumours in older women and may arise from serrated polyps. Molecularly, they are associated with more *MLH1* methylation, MSI, and CIMP. This small subset of CRC, which generally affects approximately 10% of CRC patients, remains a challenging group with poor response to both anti-EGFR and standard doublet chemotherapy. This CRC subgroup is typically aggressive, has short median PFS between sequential lines of treatments, and emphasises the need to use effective treatments early. New evidence suggests that triplet chemotherapy with FOLFOXIRI could be considered in suitable patients with or without bevacizumab as first-line treatment. Many trials are currently studying the effective combinations of targeted treatments involving BRAF and MEK inhibitors in this subgroup and ways to overcome resistance.

Author details

Louisa Lo[1], Timothy Price[1,2], Joanne Young[1,2] and Amanda Townsend[1,2*]

*Address all correspondence to: amanda.townsend@health.sa.gov.au

1 Medical Oncology Department, Queen Elizabeth Hospital, Birmingham, England

2 University of Adelaide, Adelaide, Australia

References

[1] Rozek LS, Herron CM, Greenson JK, Moreno V, Capella G, Rennert G, et al. Smoking, gender, and ethnicity predict somatic BRAF mutations in colorectal cancer. Cancer Epidemiol Biomarkers Prev. 2010;19(3):838–43. DOI: 10.1158/1055-9965.EPI-09-1112

[2] Shaukat A, Arain M, Thaygarajan B, Bond JH, Sawhney M. Is BRAF mutation associated with interval colorectal cancers? Dig Dis Sci. 2010;55(8):2352–6. DOI: 10.1007/s10620-010-1182-9

[3] Price TJ, Hardingham JE, Lee CK, Weickhardt A, Townsend AR, Wrin JW, et al. Impact of KRAS and BRAF gene mutation status on outcomes from the phase III AGITG MAX trial of capecitabine alone or in combination with bevacizumab and mitomycin in advanced colorectal cancer. J Clin Oncol. 2011;29(19):2675–82. DOI: 10.1200/JCO.2010.34.5520

[4] Van Cutsem E, Köhne CH, Láng I, Folprecht G, Nowacki MP, Cascinu S, et al. Cetuximab plus irinotecan, fluorouracil, and leucovorin as first-line treatment for metastatic colorectal cancer: updated analysis of overall survival according to tumor KRAS and BRAF mutation status. J Clin Oncol. 2011;29(15):2011–9. DOI: 10.1200/JCO.2010.33.5091

[5] Jansen HW, Lurz R, Bister K, Bonner TI, Mark GE, Rapp UR. Homologous cell-derived oncogenes in avian carcinoma virus MH2 and murine sarcoma virus 3611. Nature. 1984;307(5948):281–4.

[6] Sutrave P, Bonner TI, Rapp UR, Jansen HW, Patschinsky T, Bister K. Nucleotide sequence of avian retroviral oncogene v-mil: homologue of murine retroviral oncogene v-raf. Nature. 1984;309(5963):85–8.

[7] Michaloglou C, Vredeveld LC, Mooi WJ, Peeper DS. BRAF(E600) in benign and malignant human tumours. Oncogene. 2008;27(7):877–95.

[8] Chong H, Vikis HG, Guan KL. Mechanisms of regulating the Raf kinase family. Cell Signal. 2003;15(5):463–9.

[9] Schreck R, Rapp UR. Raf kinases: oncogenesis and drug discovery. Int J Cancer. 2006;119(10):2261–71.

[10] Bamford S, Dawson E, Forbes S, Clements J, Pettett R, Dogan A, et al. The COSMIC (Catalogue of Somatic Mutations in Cancer) database and website. Br J Cancer. 2004;91(2):355–8.

[11] Wan PT, Garnett MJ, Roe SM, Lee S, Niculescu-Duvaz D, Good VM, et al. Mechanism of activation of the RAF-ERK signaling pathway by oncogenic mutations of B-RAF. Cell. 2004;116(6):855–67.

[12] Stover D. BRAF c.1799T>A (V600E) Mutation in Colorectal Cancer. My Cancer Genome [Internet]. March 6, 2015 [Updated: March 6, 2015]. Available from: http://www.mycancergenome.org/content/disease/colorectal-cancer/braf/54/ [Accessed: December 23, 2015].

[13] Garnett MJ, Marais R. Guilty as charged: B-RAF is a human oncogene. Cancer Cell. 2004;6(4):313–9.

[14] Marchetti A, Felicioni L, Malatesta S, Grazia Sciarrotta M, Guetti L, Chella A, et al. Clinical features and outcome of patients with non-small-cell lung cancer harboring BRAF mutations. J Clin Oncol. 2011;29(26):3574–9. DOI: 10.1200/JCO.2011.35.9638

[15] Cardarella S, Ogino A, Nishino M, Butaney M, Shen J, Lydon C, et al. Clinical, pathologic, and biologic features associated with BRAF mutations in non-small cell lung cancer. Clin Cancer Res. 2013;19(16):4532–40. DOI: 10.1158/1078-0432.CCR-13-0657

[16] Preto A, Figueiredo J, Velho S, Ribeiro AS, Soares P, Oliveira C, et al. BRAF provides proliferation and survival signals in MSI colorectal carcinoma cells displaying BRAF(V600E) but not KRAS mutations. J Pathol. 2008;214(3):320–7.

[17] Davies H, Bignell GR, Cox C, Stephens P, Edkins S, Clegg S, et al. Mutations of the BRAF gene in human cancer. Nature. 2002;417(6892):949–54.

[18] Curry JL, Torres-Cabala CA, Tetzlaff MT, Bowman C, Prieto VG. Molecular platforms utilized to detect BRAF V600E mutation in melanoma. Semin Cutan Med Surg. 2012;31(4):267–73. DOI: 10.1016/j.sder.2012.07.007

[19] Benlloch S, PayáA, Alenda C, Bessa X, Andreu M, Jover R, et al. Detection of BRAF V600E mutation in colorectal cancer: comparison of automatic sequencing and real-time chemistry methodology. J Mol Diagn. 2006;8(5):540–3.

[20] Quail MA, Smith M, Coupland P, Otto TD, Harris SR, Connor TR, et al. A tale of three next generation sequencing platforms: comparison of Ion Torrent, Pacific Biosciences and Illumina Mi Seq sequencers. BMC Genomics. 2012;13:341. DOI: 10.1186/1471-2164-13-341

[21] Liu L, Li Y, Li S, Hu N, He Y, Pong R, et al. Comparison of next-generation sequencing systems. J Biomed Biotechnol. 2012;2012:1–11. DOI: 10.1155/2012/251364

[22] Capper D, Preusser M, Habel A, Sahm F, Ackermann U, Schindler G, et al. Assessment of BRAF V600E mutation status by immunohistochemistry with a mutation-specific monoclonal antibody. Acta Neuropathol. 2011;122(1):11–9. DOI: 10.1007/s00401-011-0841-z

[23] Capper D, Voigt A, Bozukova G, Ahadova A, Kickingereder P, von Deimling A, et al. BRAF V600E-specific immunohistochemistry for the exclusion of Lynch syndrome in MSI-H colorectal cancer. Int J Cancer. 2013;133(7):1624–30. DOI: 10.1002/ijc.28183

[24] Affolter K, Samowitz W, Tripp S, Bronner MP, Affolter K, Samowitz W, Tripp S, et al. BRAF V600E mutation detection by immunohistochemistry in colorectal carcinoma. Genes Chromosomes Cancer. 2013;52(8):748–52. DOI: 10.1002/gcc.22070

[25] Sinicrope FA, Smyrk TC, Tougeron D, Thibodeau SN, Singh S, Muranyi A, et al. Mutation-specific antibody detects mutant BRAF protein expression in human colon carcinomas. Cancer. 2013;119(15):2765–70. DOI: 10.1002/cncr.28133

[26] Adackapara CA, Sholl LM, Barletta JA, Hornick JL. Immunohistochemistry using the BRAF V600E mutation-specific monoclonal antibody VE1 is not a useful surrogate for genotyping in colorectal adenocarcinoma. Histopathology. 2013;63(2):187–93. DOI: 10.1111/his.12154

[27] Thiel A, Heinonen M, Kantonen J, Gylling A, Lahtinen L, Korhonen M, et al. BRAF mutation in sporadic colorectal cancer and Lynch syndrome. Virchows Arch. 2013;463(5):613–21. DOI: 10.1007/s00428-013-1470-9

[28] Mohamed Suhaimi NA, Foong YM, Lee DY, Phyo WM, Cima I, Lee EX, et al. Non-invasive sensitive detection of KRAS and BRAF mutation in circulating tumor cells of colorectal cancer patients. Mol Oncol. 2015;9(4):850–60. DOI: 10.1016/j.molonc.2014.12.011

[29] Douillard JY, Siena S, Cassidy J, Tabernero J, Burkes R, Barugel M, et al. Final results from PRIME: randomized phase III study of panitumumab with FOLFOX4 for first-line treatment of metastatic colorectal cancer. Ann Oncol. 2014;25(7):1346–55. DOI: 10.1093/annonc/mdu141

[30] Douillard JY, Oliner KS, Siena S, Tabernero J, Burkes R, Barugel M, et al. Panitumumab-FOLFOX4 treatment and RAS mutations in colorectal cancer. N Engl J Med. 2013;369(11):1023–34. DOI: 10.1056/NEJMoa1305275

[31] Heinemann V, Von Weikersthal LF, Decker T, Kiani A, Vehling-Kaiser U, Al-Batran S-E, et al. Randomized comparison of FOLFIRI plus cetuximab versus FOLFIRI plus bevacizumab as first-line treatment of KRAS wild-type metastatic colorectal cancer: German AIO study KRK-0306 (FIRE-3). J Clin Oncol. 2013;31(suppl):abstr LBA3506.

[32] Seymour MT, Brown SR, Middleton G, Maughan T, Richman S, Gwyther S, et al. Panitumumab and irinotecan versus irinotecan alone for patients with KRAS wild-type, fluorouracil-resistant advanced colorectal cancer (PICCOLO): a prospectively

stratified randomised trial. Lancet Oncol. 2013;14(8):749–59. DOI: 10.1016/S1470-2045(13)70163-3

[33] Tveit KM, Guren T, Glimelius B, Pfeiffer P, Sorbye H, Pyrhonen S, et al. Phase III trial of cetuximab with continuous or intermittent fluorouracil, leucovorin, and oxaliplatin (Nordic FLOX) versus FLOX alone in first-line treatment of metastatic colorectal cancer: the NORDIC-VII study. J Clin Oncol. 2012;30(15):1755–62. DOI: 10.1200/JCO.2011.38.0915

[34] Maughan TS, Adams RA, Smith CG, Meade AM, Seymour MT, Wilson RH, et al. Addition of cetuximab to oxaliplatin-based first-line combination chemotherapy for treatment of advanced colorectal cancer: results of the randomised phase 3 MRC COIN trial. Lancet. 2011;377(9783):2103–14. DOI: 10.1016/S0140-6736(11)60613-2

[35] Cremolini C, Loupakis F, Antoniotti C, Lupi C, Sensi E, Lonardi S, et al. FOLFOXIRI plus bevacizumab versus FOLFIRI plus bevacizumab as first-line treatment of patients with metastatic colorectal cancer: updated overall survival and molecular subgroup analyses of the open-label, phase 3 TRIBE study. Lancet Oncol. 2015;16(13):1306–15. DOI: 10.1016/S1470-2045(15)00122-9

[36] Chen D, Huang JF, Liu K, Zhang LQ, Yang Z, Chuai ZR, et al. BRAFV600E mutation and its association with clinicopathological features of colorectal cancer: a systematic review and meta-analysis. PLo S One. 2014;9(3):e90607. DOI: 10.1371/journal.pone.0090607

[37] Ogino S, Nosho K, Kirkner GJ, Shima K, Irahara N, Kure S, et al. PIK3CA mutation is associated with poor prognosis among patients with curatively resected colon cancer. J Clin Oncol. 2009;27(9):1477–84. DOI: 10.1200/JCO.2008.18.6544

[38] Clarke CN, Kopetz ES. BRAF mutant colorectal cancer as a distinct subset of colorectal cancer: clinical characteristics, clinical behaviour, and response to targeted therapies. J Gastrointest Oncol. 2015;6(6):660–7.

[39] Kambara T, Simms LA, Whitehall VL, Spring KJ, Wynter CV, Walsh MD, et al. BRAF mutation is associated with DNA methylation in serrated polyps and cancers of the colorectum. Gut. 2004;53(8):1137–44.

[40] The International Agency for Research on Cancer. WHO Classification of Tumours of the Digestive System (IARC WHO Classification of Tumours). 4th ed. World Health Organization; 2010. 418 pp.

[41] Imai K, Yamamoto H. Carcinogenesis and microsatellite instability: the interrelationship between genetics and epigenetics. Carcinogenesis. 2008;29(4):673–80.

[42] Jensen LH, Lindebjerg J, Byriel L, Kolvraa S, Crüger DG. Strategy in clinical practice for classification of unselected colorectal tumours based on mismatch repair deficiency. Colorectal Dis. 2008;10(5):490–7.

[43] Rahner N, Friedrichs N, Steinke V, Aretz S, Friedl W, Buettner R, et al. Coexisting somatic promoter hypermethylation and pathogenic MLH1 germline mutation in Lynch syndrome. J Pathol. 2008;214(1):10–6.

[44] Domingo E, Laiho P, Ollikainen M, Pinto M, Wang L, French AJ, et al. BRAF screening as a low-cost effective strategy for simplifying HNPCC genetic testing. J Med Genet. 2004;41(9):664–8.

[45] Tie J, Desai J. Targeting BRAF mutant metastatic colorectal cancer: clinical implications and emerging therapeutic strategies. Target Oncol. 2015;10(2):179–88. DOI: 10.1007/s11523-014-0330-0

[46] Zlobec I, Bihl MP, Schwarb H, Terracciano L, Lugli A. Clinicopathological and protein characterization of BRAF- and K-RAS-mutated colorectal cancer and implications for prognosis. Int J Cancer. 2010;127(2):367–80. DOI: 10.1002/ijc.25042

[47] Roth AD, Tejpar S, Delorenzi M, Yan P, Fiocca R, Klingbiel D, et al. Prognostic role of KRAS and BRAF in stage II and III resected colon cancer: results of the translational study on the PETACC-3, EORTC 40993, SAKK 60-00 trial. J Clin Oncol. 2010;28(3):466–74. DOI: 10.1200/JCO.2009.23.3452

[48] Fariña-Sarasqueta A, van Lijnschoten G, Moerland E, Creemers GJ, Lemmens VE, Rutten HJ, et al. The BRAF V600E mutation is an independent prognostic factor for survival in stage II and stage III colon cancer patients. Ann Oncol. 2010;21(12):2396–402. DOI: 10.1093/annonc/mdq258

[49] Ogino S, Shima K, Meyerhardt JA, Mc Cleary NJ, Ng K, Hollis D, et al. Predictive and prognostic roles of BRAF mutation in stage III colon cancer: results from intergroup trial CALGB 89803. Clin Cancer Res. 2012;18(3):890–900. DOI: 10.1158/1078-0432.CCR-11-2246

[50] Pai RK, Jayachandran P, Koong AC, Chang DT, Kwok S, Ma L, et al. BRAF-mutated, microsatellite-stable adenocarcinoma of the proximal colon: an aggressive adenocarcinoma with poor survival, mucinous differentiation, and adverse morphologic features. Am J Surg Pathol. 2012;36(5):744–52. DOI: 10.1097/PAS.0b013e31824430d7

[51] Kalady MF, Dejulius KL, Sanchez JA, Jarrar A, Liu X, Manilich E, et al. BRAF mutations in colorectal cancer are associated with distinct clinical characteristics and worse prognosis. Dis Colon Rectum. 2012;55(2):128–33. DOI: 10.1097/DCR.0b013e31823c08b3

[52] Eklöf V, Wikberg ML, Edin S, Dahlin AM, Jonsson BA, ÖbergÅ, et al. The prognostic role of KRAS, BRAF, PIK3CA and PTEN in colorectal cancer. Br J Cancer. 2013;108(10):2153–63. DOI: 10.1038/bjc.2013.212

[53] Tie J, Gibbs P, Lipton L, Christie M, Jorissen RN, Burgess AW, et al. Optimizing targeted therapeutic development: analysis of a colorectal cancer patient population with the BRAF(V600E) mutation. Int J Cancer. 2011;128(9):2075–84. DOI: 10.1002/ijc.25555

[54] Li WQ, Kawakami K, Ruszkiewicz A, Bennett G, Moore J, Iacopetta B. BRAF mutations are associated with distinctive clinical, pathological and molecular features of colorectal cancer independently of microsatellite instability status. Mol Cancer. 2006;5:2.

[55] Ogino S, Brahmandam M, Cantor M, Namgyal C, Kawasaki T, Kirkner G. Distinct molecular features of colorectal carcinoma with signet ring cell component and colorectal carcinoma with mucinous component. Mod Pathol. 2006;19(1):59–68.

[56] Tran B, Kopetz S, Tie J, Gibbs P, Jiang ZQ, Lieu CH, et al. Impact of BRAF mutation and microsatellite instability on the pattern of metastatic spread and prognosis in metastatic colorectal cancer. Cancer. 2011;117(20):4623–32. DOI: 10.1002/cncr.26086

[57] Bokemeyer C, Van Cutsem E, Rougier P, Ciardiello F, Heeger S, Schlichting M, et al. Addition of cetuximab to chemotherapy as first-line treatment for KRAS wild-type metastatic colorectal cancer: pooled analysis of the CRYSTAL and OPUS randomised clinical trials. Eur J Cancer. 2012;48(10):1466–75. DOI: 10.1016/j.ejca.2012.02.057

[58] Yuan ZX, Wang XY, Qin QY, Chen DF, Zhong QH, Wang L, et al. The prognostic role of BRAF mutation in metastatic colorectal cancer receiving anti-EGFR monoclonal antibodies: a meta-analysis. PLoS One. 2013;8(6):e65995. DOI: 10.1371/journal.pone.0065995

[59] Karapetis CS, Jonker D, Daneshmand M, Hanson JE, O'Callaghan CJ, Marginean C, et al. PIK3CA, BRAF, and PTEN status and benefit from cetuximab in the treatment of advanced colorectal cancer—results from NCIC CTG/AGITG CO.17. Clin Cancer Res. 2014;20(3):744–53. DOI: 10.1158/1078-0432.CCR-13-0606

[60] Chen J, Guo F, Shi X, Zhang L, Zhang A, Jin H, et al. BRAF V600E mutation and KRAS codon 13 mutations predict poor survival in Chinese colorectal cancer patients. BMC Cancer. 2014;14:802. DOI: 10.1186/1471-2407-14-802

[61] Yokota T, Ura T, Shibata N, Takahari D, Shitara K, Nomura M, et al. BRAF mutation is a powerful prognostic factor in advanced and recurrent colorectal cancer. Br J Cancer. 2011;104(5):856–62. DOI: 10.1038/bjc.2011.19

[62] Li HT, Lu YY, An YX, Wang X, Zhao QC. KRAS, BRAF and PIK3CA mutations in human colorectal cancer: relationship with metastatic colorectal cancer. Oncol Rep. 2011;25(6): 1691–7. DOI: 10.3892/or.2011.1217

[63] Hsieh LL, Er TK, Chen CC, Hsieh JS, Chang JG, Liu TC. Characteristics and prevalence of KRAS, BRAF, and PIK3CA mutations in colorectal cancer by high-resolution melting analysis in Taiwanese population. Clin Chim Acta. 2012;413(19–20):1605–11. DOI: 10.1016/j.cca.2012.04.029

[64] Shen Y, Wang J, Han X, Yang H, Wang S, Lin D, et al. Effectors of epidermal growth factor receptor pathway: the genetic profiling of KRAS, BRAF, PIK3CA, NRAS mutations in colorectal cancer characteristics and personalized medicine. PLo S One. 2013;8(12):e81628. DOI: 10.1371/journal.pone.0081628

[65] Thiel A, Ristimäki A. Toward a molecular classification of colorectal cancer: the role of BRAF. Front Oncol. 2013;3:281. DOI: 10.3389/fonc.2013.00281

[66] Samowitz WS, Sweeney C, Herrick J, Albertsen H, Levin TR, Murtaugh MA, et al. Poor survival associated with the BRAF V600E mutation in microsatellite-stable colon cancers. Cancer Res. 2005;65(14):6063–9.

[67] Kadowaki S, Kakuta M, Takahashi S, Takahashi A, Arai Y, Nishimura Y, et al. Prognostic value of KRAS and BRAF mutations in curatively resected colorectal cancer. World J Gastroenterol. 2015;21(4):1275–83. DOI: 10.3748/wjg.v21.i4.1275

[68] Morris V, Overman MJ, Jiang ZQ, Garrett C, Agarwal S, Eng C, et al. Progression-free survival remains poor over sequential lines of systemic therapy in patients with BRAF-mutated colorectal cancer. Clin Colorectal Cancer. 2014;13(3):164–71. DOI:10.1016/j.clcc.2014.06.001

[69] Souglakos J, Philips J, Wang R, Marwah S, Silver M, Tzardi M, et al. Prognostic and predictive value of common mutations for treatment response and survival in patients with metastatic colorectal cancer. Br J Cancer. 2009;101(3):465–72. DOI: 10.1038/sj.bjc.660516

[70] Cremolini C, Di Bartolomeo M, Amatu A, Antoniotti C, Moretto R, Berenato R, et al. BRAF codons 594 and 596 mutations identify a new molecular subtype of metastatic colorectal cancer at favorable prognosis. Ann Oncol. 2015;26(10):2092–7. DOI: 10.1093/annonc/mdv290

[71] Di Nicolantonio F, Martini M, Molinari F, Sartore-Bianchi A, Arena S, Saletti P, et al. Wild-type BRAF is required for response to panitumumab or cetuximab in metastatic colorectal cancer. J Clin Oncol. 2008;26(35):5705–12. DOI: 10.1200/JCO.2008.18.0786

[72] Loupakis F, Ruzzo A, Cremolini C, Vincenzi B, Salvatore L, Santini D, et al. KRAS codon 61, 146 and BRAF mutations predict resistance to cetuximab plus irinotecan in KRAS codon 12 and 13 wild-type metastatic colorectal cancer. Br J Cancer. 2009;101(4):715–21. DOI: 10.1038/sj.bjc.6605177

[73] De Roock W, Claes B, Bernasconi D, De Schutter J, Biesmans B, Fountzilas G, et al. Effects of KRAS, BRAF, NRAS, and PIK3CA mutations on the efficacy of cetuximab plus chemotherapy in chemotherapy-refractory metastatic colorectal cancer: a retrospective consortium analysis. Lancet Oncol. 2010;11(8):753–62. DOI: 10.1016/S1470-2045(10)70130-3

[74] Pietrantonio F, Petrelli F, Coinu A, Di Bartolomeo M, Borgonovo K, Maggi C, et al. Predictive role of BRAF mutations in patients with advanced colorectal cancer receiving cetuximab and panitumumab: a meta-analysis. Eur J Cancer. 2015;51(5): 587–94. DOI: 10.1016/j.ejca.2015.01.054

[75] Rowland A, Dias MM, Wiese MD, Kichenadasse G, Mc Kinnon RA, Karapetis CS, et al. Meta-analysis of BRAF mutation as a predictive biomarker of benefit from anti-EGFR

monoclonal antibody therapy for RAS wild-type metastatic colorectal cancer. Br J Cancer. 2015;112(12):1888–94. DOI: 10.1038/bjc.2015.173

[76] Pereira AA, Rego JF, Munhoz RR, Hoff PM, Sasse AD, Riechelmann RP, et al. The impact of complete chemotherapy stop on the overall survival of patients with advanced colorectal cancer in first-line setting: a meta-analysis of randomized trials. Acta Oncol. 2015;54(10):1737–46. DOI: 10.3109/0284186X.2015.1044022

[77] Hegewisch-Becker S, Graeven U, Lerchenmüller C, Killing B, Depenbusch R, Steffens C, et al. Maintenance strategy with fluoropyrimidines (FP) plus bevacizumab (BEV), BEV alone or no treatment, following a 24-week first-line induction with FP, oxaliplatin (OX) and BEV for patients with metastatic colorectal cancer: mature data and subgroup analysis of the AIO KRK 0207 phase III study. In: ESMO; 27.09.2014; Madrid. Ann Oncol: Oxford University Press; 2014. p. 25 (suppl 4): iv167. DOI: 10.1093/annonc/mdu333.2

[78] Montagut C, Settleman J. Targeting the RAF-MEK-ERK pathway in cancer therapy. Cancer Lett. 2009;283(2):125–34. DOI: 10.1016/j.canlet.2009.01.02

[79] Flaherty KT, Puzanov I, Kim KB, Ribas A, Mc Arthur GA, Sosman JA, et al. Inhibition of mutated, activated BRAF in metastatic melanoma. N Engl J Med. 2010;363(9):809–19. DOI: 10.1056/NEJMoa1002011

[80] Long GV, Stroyakovskiy D, Gogas H, Levchenko E, de Braud F, Larkin J, et al. Combined BRAF and MEK inhibition versus BRAF inhibition alone in melanoma. N Engl J Med. 2014;371(20):1877–88. DOI: 10.1056/NEJMoa1406037

[81] Kopetz S, Desai J, Chan E, Hecht JR, O'Dwyer PJ, Lee RJ, et al. PLX4032 in metastatic colorectal cancer patients with mutant BRAF tumors. J Clin Oncol. 2010;28(15s):abstr 3534.

[82] Corcoran RB, Ebi H, Turke AB, Coffee EM, Nishino M, Cogdill AP, et al. EGFR-mediated re-activation of MAPK signaling contributes to insensitivity of BRAF mutant colorectal cancers to RAF inhibition with vemurafenib. Cancer Discov. 2012;2(3):227–35. DOI: 10.1158/2159-8290.CD-11-0341

[83] Prahallad A, Sun C, Huang S, Di Nicolantonio F, Salazar R, Zecchin D, et al. Unresponsiveness of colon cancer to BRAF(V600E) inhibition through feedback activation of EGFR. Nature. 2012;483(7387):100–3. DOI: 10.1038/nature10868

[84] Solit DB, Garraway LA, Pratilas CA, Sawai A, Getz G, Basso A, et al. BRAF mutation predicts sensitivity to MEK inhibition. Nature. 2006;439(7074):358–62.

[85] Corcoran RB, Atreya CE, Falchook GS, Kwak EL, Ryan DP, Bendell JC. Combined BRAF and MEK inhibition with dabrafenib and trametinib in BRAF V600-mutant colorectal cancer. J Clin Oncol. 2015;33(34):4023–31. DOI: 10.1200/JCO.2015.63.2471

[86] Atreya CE, Van Cutsem E, Bendell JC, Andre T, Schellens JHM, Gordon MS, et al. Updated efficacy of the MEK inhibitor trametinib (T), BRAF inhibitor dabrafenib (D),

and anti-EGFR antibody panitumumab (P) in patients (pts) with BRAF V600E mutated (BRAFm) metastatic colorectal cancer (mCRC). J Clin Oncol. 2015;33:abstr 103.

[87] Yaeger RD, Cercek A, O'Reilly EM, Reidy DL, Kemeny NE, Wolinsky T, et al. Pilot study of vemurafenib and panitumumab combination therapy in patients with BRAF V600E mutated metastatic colorectal cancer. J Clin Oncol. 2015;33(suppl 3):abstr 611.

[88] Elez E, Schellens J, Van Geel R, Bendell JC, Spreafico A, Schuler M, et al. Results of a phase 1b study of the selective BRAF V600 inhibitor encorafenib in combination with cetuximab alone or cetuximab + alpelisib for treatment of patients with advanced BRAF-mutant metastatic colorectal cancer. Ann Oncol. 2015;26(suppl 4):117–22. DOI: 10.1093/annonc/mdv262.08

[89] Ahronian LG, Sennott EM, Van Allen EM, Wagle N, Kwak EL, Faris JE, et al. Clinical acquired resistance to RAF inhibitor combinations in BRAF-mutant colorectal cancer through MAPK pathway alterations. Cancer Discov. 2015;5(4):358–67. DOI: 10.1158/2159-8290.CD-14-1518

[90] Hong DS, Morris VK, El Osta BE, Fu S, Overman MJ, Piha-Paul SA, et al. Phase Ib study of vemurafenib in combination with irinotecan and cetuximab in patients with BRAF-mutated metastatic colorectal cancer and advanced cancers. J Clin Oncol. 2015;33(suppl 15):abstr 3511.

[91] Parsons DW, Wang TL, Samuels Y, Bardelli A, Cummins JM, De Long L, et al. Colorectal cancer: mutations in a signalling pathway. Nature. 2005;436(7052):792.

[92] Mao M, Tian F, Mariadason JM, Tsao CC, Lemos RJr, Dayyani F, et al. Resistance to BRAF inhibition in BRAF-mutant colon cancer can be overcome with PI3K inhibition or demethylating agents. Clin Cancer Res. 2013;19(3):657–67. DOI: 10.1158/1078-0432.CCR-11-1446

[93] Coffee EM, Faber AC, Roper J, Sinnamon MJ, Goel G, Keung L, et al. Concomitant BRAF and PI3K/m TOR blockade is required for effective treatment of BRAF(V600E) colorectal cancer. Clin Cancer Res. 2013;19(10):2688–98. DOI: 10.1158/1078-0432.CCR-12-2556

[94] Lemieux E, Cagnol S, Beaudry K, Carrier J, Rivard N. Oncogenic KRAS signalling promotes the Wnt/β-catenin pathway through LRP6 in colorectal cancer. Oncogene. 2015;34(38):4914–27. DOI: 10.1038/onc.2014.416

[95] Lee CK, Lee ME, Lee WS, Kim JM, Park KH, Kim TS, et al. Dovitinib (TKI258), a multi-target angiokinase inhibitor, is effective regardless of KRAS or BRAF mutation status in colorectal cancer. Am J Cancer Res. 2014;5(1):72–86.

[96] Zecchin D, Boscaro V, Medico E, Barault L, Martini M, Arena S, et al. BRAF V600E is a determinant of sensitivity to proteasome inhibitors. Mol Cancer Ther. 2013;12(12):2950–61. DOI: 10.1158/1535-7163.MCT-13-0243

[97] Peng W, Hu J, Zhu XD, Liu X, Wang CC, Li WH, et al. Overexpression of mi R-145 increases the sensitivity of vemurafenib in drug-resistant colo205 cell line. Tumour Biol. 2014;35(4):2983–8. DOI: 10.1007/s13277-013-1383-x

[98] Immunovative Therapies Ltd. Increased Frequency of Allo Stim(TM) Dosing in Combination With Cryoablation in Metastatic Colorectal Cancer [Internet]. March 2, 2015 [Updated: December 7, 2015]. Available from: https://clinicaltrials.gov/ct2/show/record/NCT02380443 [Accessed: December 28, 2015].

[99] Faber AC, Coffee EM, Costa C, Dastur A, Ebi H, Hata AN, et al. m TOR inhibition specifically sensitizes colorectal cancers with KRAS or BRAF mutations to BCL-2/BCL-XL inhibition by suppressing MCL-1. Cancer Discov. 2014;4(1):42–52. DOI: 10.1158/2159-8290.CD-13-0315

[100] Worthley DL, Whitehall VL, Spring KJ, Leggett BA. Colorectal carcinogenesis: road maps to cancer. World J Gastroenterol. 2007;13(28):3784–91.

Section 2

Diagnosis

Chapter 5

Colorectal Cancer Prevention and Risk Counseling

Serife Koc, Melek Nihal Esin and Aysun Ardic

Additional information is available at the end of the chapter

http://dx.doi.org/10.5772/63206

Abstract

Colorectal cancer (CRC) is one of the leading causes of cancer death in the world. Many risk factors have been identified in the development of colorectal cancer. It is necessary to carry out activities related to risk factors in order to implement effective CRC early diagnosis and screening programs and achieve positive outcomes. International screening guidelines have been created and these are being implemented by individual countries according to their own health policies. Colorectal cancer prevention and early training in terms of disease identification, counseling against negative disease perceptions, and changing false beliefs will reduce the fear of CRC and ensure the development of positive health behaviors and acceptance of screening. Among recent developments in cancer prevention, "cancer risk counseling" has become quite prominent. Individual-specific colorectal cancer risk counseling programs are developed through the assessment of individual risk factors by focusing on a genetic assessment and the development of a risk management plan. This chapter will examine and define colorectal cancer prevention and risk counseling strategies in relation with the relative literature.

Keywords: Colorectal cancer, prevention, cancer risk counseling, screening, clinical guidelines

1. Introduction

Colorectal cancer (CRC) is one of the leading causes of cancer death in the world. Colorectal cancer is a significant public health problem in many countries considering its incidence, mortality rate, and treatment costs [1]. Among all cancer deaths, mortality due to CRC ranks second in the world and accounts for 9–10% of all cancers deaths [2–4]. Colorectal cancer is the second most common cancer worldwide [5]. The incidence of CRC in North America and highly industrialized areas such as northwestern Europe and Australia is high, but is low in less developed regions such as Asia, Africa, and South America [2, 5, 6]. Lifetime risk of developing CRC varies between 2.4 and 6%. Risk factors possessed by individuals may increase this rate [2, 3]. It is necessary to carry out activities related to risk factors in order to implement effective CRC early diagnosis and screening programs and achieve positive outcomes. Moreover, implementing cost-effective screening programs decreases costs and increases the effectiveness of CRC screening [7, 8]. Many people do not know the risk factors for CRC; it is reported that those who do know them should be encouraged and supported by professionals to apply safeguard measures and effective interventions. More than half of CRC incidents can be prevented by implementing protection strategies in accordance with risk factors [9, 10]. However, to achieve this, negative behaviors must be changed to positive, and individuals should be directed toward early diagnosis in accordance with their risk conditions and monitored [11, 12]. In the realization of primary and secondary prevention strategies, bespoke colon cancer risk counseling is important for reducing morbidity and mortality [11–13].

2. Colorectal cancer prevention and risk counseling

2.1. Colorectal cancer prevention

2.1.1. Colorectal cancer risk factors

Advancing age, familial and genetic factors, environmental factors, and lifestyle/behavioral factors affect the development of CRC [2, 6–8]. Colorectal cancer risk factors are divided into two groups, those that can be changed and those that cannot [1, 6, 10].

Nonchangeable risk factors: These factors cannot be taken under control by the individual. These include age, sex, genetics (personal or family history of CRC), chronic colon diseases such as ulcerative colitis, inflammatory bowel disease or Crohn's disease, and a history of adenomatous polyps [6, 8, 10, 13].

Changeable risk factors: These are behavioral factors that can be altered or managed to help reduce the risk of CRC. It is reported that more than half of all cancers are linked to risky health behaviors. Changeable factors include but are not limited to smoking, moderate-to-heavy levels of alcohol consumption, being overweight and obesity, unbalanced diet, excessive consumption of red meat and/or processed meat products, physical inactivity, and/or sedentary lifestyle [3, 4, 6, 8–10, 13–19]. Risk factors and their relative risk for CRC are shown in **Table 1**. Colorectal cancer risk with relative risk above 1 indicates high risk, and less than 1 indicates low risk [10].

2.1.2. Colorectal cancer prevention strategies

The aim is to prevent cancer, precancerous lesions, and reduce the incidence of cancer-related morbidity and mortality and cancer spread, or at least diagnose it at earlier stages. Cancer prevention research, and the reduction of cancer morbidity and mortality, requires a three-dimensional approach: primary, secondary, and tertiary prevention [4, 6, 11, 20].

http://dx.doi.org/10.5772/63206

Factors increasing the risk	Relative risk
Family history and genetics	
One first-degree relative	2.2
More than one relative	4.0
Relative diagnosed before 45	3.9
Individual history	
Crohn's disease	2.6
Ulcerative colitis	2.8
Colon	1.9
Rectum	
Diabetes	1.2
Behavioral risk factors	
Excessive alcohol consumption	1.6
Obesity	1,.2
Red meat consumption	1.2
Processed meat consumption	1.2
Smoking cigarette	1.2
Risk reducing factors	
Physical activity (colon)	0.7
Consumption of dairy products	0.8
Fruit consumption	0.9
Vegetable consumption	0.9
Total dietary fiber consumption (10 g/day)	0.9

Table 1. Colorectal cancer risk factors and relative risk.

2.1.2.1. Primary prevention strategies

Primary prevention includes reducing the effects of carcinogens by using chemopreventive agents or removing environmental carcinogens. The goal of primary prevention is to prevent cancer from starting by reducing individual risk. Primary prevention focuses on lifestyle changes and risk factors related to chemoprevention. Primary prevention measures focus on two areas: making lifestyle changes toward changing primary risk factors and chemoprevention (chemical protection) strategies [20, 21].

2.1.2.1.1. Lifestyle changes

Healthy body weight: Being overweight obesity increases the risk of CRC, independent of physical activity. It is noted that abdominal obesity as measured by waist diameter is a more important risk factor than general obesity for both women and men [8, 10]. Patient education about ways to gain and maintain a healthy body weight is an important health professional task. Most people know its importance but there is a need for the encouragement and support of health professionals to implement effective interventions for individuals. Excess body fat can be reduced by reducing caloric intake and increasing physical activity. Reducing daily calorie intake by 50–100 calories can prevent gradual weight gain in adults, 500 calories/day or more weight loss program is the first joint reduction target. Research has shown that up to 60 minutes a day of moderate to vigorous physical activity may be necessary to prevent weight gain. For overweight people, daily physical activity up to 90 minutes of moderate intensity can help in losing weight [21].

Healthy nutrition and diet: Positive dietary factors that reduce the risk of cancer include low-fat diet (less than 24% of dietary fat content), high in fiber, high in omega 3, high fruits and vegetables, citrus fruits, cruciferous vegetables, carotene and lycopene-rich foods, plant-based diet, calcium, selenium, vitamin D, folic acid, omega 3 nutritional factors, and fatty acids. Dietary factors that increase the risk of cancer include animal fat, saturated fat, red meat, burnt/charred meat, trans fatty acids, and excessive alcohol consumption. Animal fats and consumption of excessive red meat and processed meat products increase the risk of high-calorie diet and consumptionless fiber-rich foods [2, 6, 8, 15, 16]. An oil-poor fiber-rich diet, 20–35 g of fiber daily for adults, and reducing total daily calories from fat by about 30%, with limited consumption of red meat is said to help reduce the risk of CRC. Also, regular consumption of fruits, vegetables, and calcium are recommended to reduce the risk for CRC for women and men. Nutritional advice for cancer prevention includes plant-derived diet containing at least five servings of fruits and vegetables every day, choosing whole grains instead of refined carbohydrates, eating saturated fat, and restricting alcohol and excessive calorie intake [11, 17, 19, 21].

Physical activity: Physical inactivity is one of the behavioral risk factors most often associated with CRC. Risk of CRC is lower for physically active people. Risk of CRC for very physically active people is 25% lower than in most physically inactive people [10]. Being physically active during both work and leisure time also reduces the risk. The American Cancer Society recommends a minimum of 150 minutes of moderate intensity every week, and preferably spread over the week, or 75 minutes of vigorous physical activity (or combination thereof) [10].

Avoidance of tobacco and alcohol: Smoking is more related to lung cancer but it also has quite harmful effects on the colon and rectum. Cigarette smoking increases the risk of colorectal adenoma [2, 6, 10, 17] and long-term use is associated with large polyps in the colon/rectum. The numbers of polyps have been reported to increase in patients even after they quit smoking 10 years previously [8, 17]. It is stated that the relative risk of CRC development is 1.64 in current smokers relative to nonsmokers [2], and 12% of all CRC deaths are related to tobacco use [8, 17]. Age of smoking initiation, duration of smoking, and the amount of cigarettes consumed per day increase the risk of CRC [18]. The difference in life risk of developing CRC in individuals who consume —two to four alcoholic beverages per day is greater than 23% compared with those who consume less than one alcoholic beverage per day. Alcohol consumption as a factor that plays a role in CRC is seen at an earlier age. The relative risk is 1.08 for alcohol intake of 25 g/day. Smoking together with alcohol consumption doubles the risk of CRC [10, 17, 19].

2.1.2.1.2. Chemopreventive measures

The administration of drugs or natural compounds to prevent the development of CRC is called chemoprevention. Colorectal cancer chemoprevention can be considered for advanced adenomas greater than 1 cm with villous histology, and more than two adenomas independent of the size of the adenoma and histology. Also, patients with a family history of cancer or cancer in first-degree relatives benefit from chemoprevention. Some 10% of all CRC groups can benefit from chemoprevention [22]. Research into chemoprevention of CRC is very active and chemical measures are recommended to more people in the high-risk group [6, 18, 21, 22]. Results of studies on chemical measures vary. Nonsteroidal anti-inflammatory drugs (NSAIDs) and aspirin have been determined to inhibit the enzyme cyclo-oxygenase (COX-1 and COX-2), which is involved in development of CRC. Regular aspirin or other NSAID use in humans reduces CRC development by 30–50%. In the recent past, these agents were not recommended for the general population (average risk), but today aspirin and other NSAIDs are recommended for the average-risk group. However, aspirin and other NSAIDs have adverse effects such as gastrointestinal bleeding and stroke, thus the benefit/risk balance of these drugs has restricted their use. In addition, calcium, vitamin D, folic acid, hormone replacement therapy, and the protection provided by statins need to be evaluated in further studies [6, 18, 21, 22].

2.1.2.2. Secondary prevention strategies

Secondary prevention, which enables slow-growing lesions to be diagnosed at early stages, includes early diagnosis and screening methods. Screening achieves better results because it avoids the onset of new cases and enables treatment of tumors at an early stage, which provides a better prognosis. Screening methods such as colonoscopy can identify abnormal cancerous changes so cancer can be prevented from fully developing. Secondary prevention is often associated with the removal of precancerous lesions or intraepithelial neoplasia (e.g., ductal carcinoma in situ, adenoma, or hyperplasia). In this way, disease is caught at an early stage, and the incidence of patients with advanced stage disease and mortality decreases [20, 23]. Polyps, especially adenomatous-type polyps, are known to be the precursor of CRC. The estimated 5-year survival rate of localized tumor (limited to the bowel wall) is 90%, it is 68% when the regional lymph node is involved, and 10% in the presence of distant metastases. CRC screening is recommended for the entire population; some people have a higher risk of developing CRC than others. The most important step is to assess the correct risk of developing CRC, screening is most effective test for individuals [6, 21, 23–27].

Colorectal cancer screening tests are divided into two groups:

- Stool tests: guaiac-based fecal occult blood test (gFOBT), fecal immunochemical test, stool DNA test.
- Structural analysis: flexible sigmoidoscopy (FS), colonoscopy, double barium contrast radiography, computed tomographic (CT) colonography, virtual colonoscopy, capsule endoscopy.

Each test has different advantages and disadvantages and can be used alone or in combination according to the request and the status of the individual [6]. Secondary prevention measures "Who should be screened and how?" The answer to the questions of who and which test brings clarity to the issue of how and how much will be applied at intervals, which is why CRC screening recommendations/guidelines have been established in many countries [6, 11, 21].

2.1.2.3. Clinical guidelines on colorectal cancer prevention

The aim of screening is to detect a precancer condition in the healthy population, as well as very early-stage malignancies that can be treated with a clearly curative intervention. In this context, international clinical guidelines have been created by the following organizations:

- American Cancer Society (ACS), The US Multi-Society Task Force on Colorectal Cancer (USMSTF), and American College of Radiology
- U.S. Preventive Services Task Force (USPSTF)
- National Comprehensive Cancer Network (NCCN)
- European Society for Medical Oncology (ESMO)

Screening tests and follow-up intervals are implemented and updated frequently by these organizations, depending on study results and technical improvements. The recommendations are not applied in the same way for the whole population; there are variations between countries and appropriate tests are recommended based on individual risk situations [6, 11, 16, 21, 24–28]. Although all guidelines recommend starting routine screening for CRC and adenomatous polyps in asymptomatic adults at age 50, there is less agreement as to the screening method, frequency of screening, and at which age screening may be safely discontinued. The recommendations differ for the method, frequency, and age of screening commencement in high-risk patients.

American Cancer Society, the US Multi-Society Task Force on Colorectal Cancer, and American College of Radiology (ACR) guidelines were published in 2008 [6, 21, 24]. These guidelines recommend starting screening in asymptomatic men and women at age 50 years. Any test that can detect adenomatous polyps can be used for screening adults at average risk. **Table 2** lists the tests and their recommended frequency of use. Individuals with family history of CRC, polyps, or one of the hereditary CRC syndromes, or a personal history of CRC or chronic inflammatory bowel disease are recommended to undergo colonoscopy at younger ages and more frequently than individuals at average risk (**Tables 3** and **4**) [24, 28].

Test	Interval recommendations	Training issues to facilitate decision-making advantage/disadvantage
Flexible sigmoidoscopy	Every 5 years[1,2] Every 10 years[3] The optimal interval should not be <10 years and may even be extended to 20 years[3]	• Full or partial bowel preparation is required • Sedation is not generally used, so there may be some difficulties during the process • The protective effect is limited to the examined column section • If results are positive, people are generally directed to colonoscopy • Low risk of bleeding, infection, and perforation
Colonoscopy	Every 10 years[1,2,3] The optimal interval should not be <10 years and may even be extended up to 20 years[3]	• Full bowel preparation is required • Awareness under sedation used in most centers • A business day may be needed for resting before the preparation and after the process • Transportation (car cannot be used after sedation) and travel companion is required • Biopsy can be taken during the procedure, polyps can be removed • Rare but potentially serious risk of perforation and hemorrhage; risk increases with polypectomy
Double-contrast colonography	Every 5 years[1,2] Uncertain[3]	• Full bowel preparation is required • The biopsy cannot be done during the procedure • If one or more polyps >6 mm, colonoscopy will be recommended; follow-up colonoscopy will require full bowel preparation • Sedation is generally not used, so there may be some difficulties during the process • Low-risk, rare perforations have been reported
Virtual colonoscopy/ CT colonography	Every 5 years[1] Uncertain[2,3]	• Full bowel preparation is required • If one or more polyps > 6 mm, colonoscopy will be recommended; if colonoscopy is not possible on the same day, full bowel preparation is needed before the colonoscopy • Sedation is not used, so there may be some difficulties during the process

Test	Interval recommendations	Training issues to facilitate decision-making advantage/disadvantage
		• Low-risk, rare perforations have been reported • Extracolonic abnormalities can be identified and require further evaluation

[1]American Cancer Society, USMSTF, American College of Radiology screening guide.
[2]National Comprehensive Cancer Network (NCCN).
[3]ESMO guidelines and European guidelines for quality assurance in colorectal cancer screening and diagnosis [6, 13, 21, 24–27].

Table 2. Average risk for colorectal cancer, tips for individuals in the group, follow-up frequency, and advantages and disadvantages.

Test	Recommendations interval	Training issues to facilitate decision-making advantage/disadvantage
Guiac-based FOBT	Annually[1], [2] Annually[3] The test interval should not exceed 2 years[3]	• Depending on the manufacturer's recommendation, 2–3 stool samples collected at home are required to complete the test; stool sample collected during a single examination at the clinic, touching stool test is not acceptable and should not be used • No risk of perforation of the intestine • Can be done at home, increase the protection of privacy • It is relatively cheap compared with other tests • If results are positive, further evaluation with colonoscopy is needed • Avoid consumption aspirin, NSAIDs, vitamin C, red meat, poultry, fish, and raw vegetables for 48 hours before the test
Fecal immuno-chemical test	Annually[1] Uncertain[2] The test interval should not exceed 3 years[3]	• If results are positive, further evaluation with colonoscopy I needed • Single tests are often ineffective • The transportation of the material to the laboratory requires specific instructions and appropriate protective material • No risk of perforation • Protection of privacy as can be done at home
Stool DNA test	Uncertain[1],[2],[3]	• A test sample should be sufficient and should be packaged in suitable preservative for transportation to the laboratory • More expensive than other stool tests • If the test result is positive, further evaluation with colonoscopy is needed. If the test is negative, it is not clear, the test should be

Test	Recommendations interval	Training issues to facilitate decision-making advantage/disadvantage
		repeated at appropriate intervals • No dietary restrictions • Protection of privacy increased as can be done at home • No risk of perforation

[1]American Cancer Society, USMSTF, American College of Radiology screening guide.
[2]National Comprehensive Cancer Network (NCCN).
[3]ESMO guidelines and European guidelines for quality assurance in colorectal cancer screening and diagnosis [6, 13, 21, 24–27].

Table 2. Moderate risk for colorectal cancer, tips for individuals in the group, follow-up frequency, advantages and disadvantages (continued).

Risk category	Starting year	Recommendations/interval	Comment
CRC or adenomatous polyps in the first 60 years of first-degree relative or two or more first-degree relatives at any age	40 years, or 10 years younger than the age of the CRC diagnosis in the youngest relative CRC diagnosis[1,2] 40 years, or 5 years younger than the age of cancer onset in first-degree relatives[3]	Colonoscopy[1,2] FOBT and colonoscopy[3] Every 5 years[1,2,3]	
Two adenomatous/CRC polyps in first- or second-degree relatives aged over 60 years	40 years[1,2] or 5 years younger than the age of disease onset in first-degree relatives[3]	Screening frequency and recommendations for moderate risk individuals are applied[1,2] Screening/follow-up procedure will be determined by clinical follow-up of patients[3]	Individuals can now scan any screening test but should begin at an early age

[1]American Cancer Society, USMSTF, American College of Radiology screening guide.
[2]National Comprehensive Cancer Network (NCCN).
[3]ESMO guidelines and European guidelines for quality assurance in colorectal cancer screening and diagnosis [6, 13, 21, 24–27].

Table 3. Recommendations and colorectal cancer screening tests for individuals in the increased-risk group.

Risk category	Starting year	Recommendations/interval	Comment
Genetically diagnosed with FAP or without evidence of	10 or 12 years old[1,2] Starting at age 12–14 years and continued lifelong in mutation carriers[3]	Individual genetic anomaly that carries genetic tests to determine the annual FSA and consulting requirements[1,2] Sigmoidoscopy every 2 years[3]	If genetic testing is positive, colectomy should be considered Screening and monitoring procedures following clinical cases will be determined[3]

Risk category	Starting year	Recommendations/interval	Comment
genetic testing and those suspected in FAP			Once adenomas are detected, annual colonoscopy should be carried out until colectomy is planned[3]
For AFAP	Starting at age 18–20 years and continued lifelong in mutation carriers. [3]	Colonoscopy every 2 years[3]	After adenomas are detected, colonoscopy should be carried out annually[3]
Genetically or clinically diagnosed with HNPCC individuals, or high-risk individuals for HNPCC	20–25 years of age or their immediate family members or 10 years younger than the age of the CRC diagnosis in the youngest relative[1],[2] Starting at age 20–25 or 5 years before the youngest case in the family[3]	Colonoscopy every 1–2 years and counseling on whether the genetic testing is necessary[1],[2]Colonoscopy every 1–2 years.[3] Upper limit is not established.[3]	First-degree relatives of people with known hereditary MMR gene mutations should be offered genetic testing for HNPCC. Family mutation as yet unknown, but also those having one of the first three criteria of modified Bethesda should be recommended Screening and monitoring procedures following clinical cases will be determined[3]

[1]American Cancer Society, USMSTF, American College of Radiology screening guide.
[2]National Comprehensive Cancer Network (NCCN).
[3]ESMO guidelines and European guidelines for quality assurance in colorectal cancer screening and diagnosis [6, 13, 21, 24–27].

Table 4. Recommendations and colorectal cancer screening tests for individuals in the high-risk group.

US Preventive Services Task Force (USPSTF):

The US Preventive Services Task Force (USPSTF) recommends using high-sensitivity fecal occult blood testing, sigmoidoscopy, or colonoscopy from the age 50 years and to continue until the age of 75 years [28]. Higher risk individuals should begin screening at a younger age, and likely more frequently. Whether individuals need to be screened beyond the age of 75 years must be decided on an individual basis. Recommended screening tests and intervals are as follows:

- High-sensitivity fecal occult blood test (FOBT)—annual
- Flexible sigmoidoscopy—5 yearly (every 3 years with FOBT)
- Colonoscopy—every 10 years

Colonoscopy can be used for screening or as a follow-up diagnostic tool in symptomatic patients, or when the results of another CRC screening test are unclear or abnormal [28].

The National Comprehensive Cancer Network (NCCN):

The National Comprehensive Cancer Network (NCCN) has released separate guidelines for average- (**Table 2**), increased- (**Table 3**), and high-risk individuals (**Table 4**). For average individuals, the NNCN's guidance is almost identical to that of the ACS, USMSTF, and ACR. These guidelines make recommendations for each risk factor for individuals at high risk [27, 28].

European Society for Medical Oncology (ESMO):

According to all international guidelines, screening tests are stratified according to the personal risk of disease. The CRC screening guidelines of ESMO are in parallel with the guiding principles of the European guidelines. The ESMO recommendations for average-, increased-, and high-risk individuals are shown in **Tables 2–4**, respectively. Guaiac (g) FOBT reduced CRC mortality in average-risk populations by 15% in different age groups. To date, only FOBT has been recommended for men and women aged 50–74 years. Fecal immunochemical testing appears to be superior to gFOBT with respect to detection rates and positive predictive values for adenomas and cancer. Flexible sigmoidoscopy has been demonstrated to reduce CRC and mortality rates when conducted in organized screening programs. FS screening should be discontinued in patients of average risk aged more than 74 years because of the increased number of comorbidities in this population. There is no current evidence to support adding in a one-off sigmoidoscopy to FOBT screening. There is limited efficacy of colonoscopy in reducing CRC incidence and mortality. The optimal age for a single colonoscopy is circa 55 years but the age range for this test is 50–74 years. Newer screening techniques such as computed tomography colonography, stool DNA testing, and capsule endoscopy are still under evaluation and as such should not yet be relied upon to screen the average-risk population [29, 30].

Colorectal cancer screening remains a subject of debate regarding to whom, with which method, and at what frequency; however, its cost-effectiveness has been demonstrated and this is key in influencing the decision to implement CRC screening programs [7, 31]. Policy-makers and health professionals who decide on which CRC screening strategy to recommend or implement must be well informed. It is vital that resources are used efficiently when planning or implementing nationwide CRC screening programs, and that a cost-effective option for CRC screening is selected. According to the results of recent review studies, there is a complexity which screening test is the most cost-effective and which screening test should be chosen [7, 31].

Individuals are divided into categories according to their risk of CRC, and the type and frequency of screening methods varies depending on the risk category [6, 21, 23–27]. The risk of developing CRC for an individual is classified into three categories: moderate risk, increased risk, and high risk; screening is recommended in accordance with the risk group of individuals [6, 13]. Persons with known gene mutation or those with suspected gene mutations have a very high risk of contracting the disease [6, 13, 21, 24–27].

2.1.2.3.1. Moderate/average-risk group

Everyone is under the lowest risk for CRC [21]. Personal and family history of colorectal polyps or ulcerative colitis without CRC, chronic inflammatory bowel disease such as Crohn's disease without CRC, and all individuals aged 50 years and over are at average risk [6, 21, 24–27].

Individuals at average risk are recommended for screening; the frequency of follow-up is shown in **Table 2**.

2.1.2.3.2. Increased risk group

In this group, risk of CRC is growing twice according to the individuals in average risk. Individuals with a history of adenomatous polyps are at significantly higher risk. A family history of CRC or adenoma increases a person's risk of developing CRC. If there is a family history CRC or adenomas including first-degree relatives (mother, father, sibling, or child) before the age of 60, the risk of developing CRC at any age (—three to four times the average risk) significantly increases. Screening recommendations for high-risk individuals are shown in **Table 3**.

2.1.2.3.3. High-risk group

The risk of CRC in individuals with a known genetic mutation is high. The most common hereditary CRC syndrome, HNPCC, also known as Lynch syndrome, is an autosomal dominant syndrome and accounts for 3–5% of all CRCs. Familial adenomatous polyposis, which is characterized by multiple adenomatous colonic polyps, is an autosomal dominant syndrome comprising 1% of all CRC cases. For the FAP, the average age of cancer diagnosed is 39 years for FAP, but in the individuals with FAP 75% of adenomas occurred in 20 years. Recommended screening and surveillance programs for high-risk individuals are shown in **Table 4** [6, 21, 24, 30].

2.1.2.4. Tertiary prevention strategies

Tertiary prevention is used in the treatment of specified diseases or prevention of complications associated with the disease, is often used to treat one type of cancer and metastasis, or involves treating patients at risk for development of a secondary primary cancer [20]. The target of tertiary prevention in cancer patients is to reduce morbidity and mortality with the optimal treatment. Primary and secondary prevention practices are recommended in developing or less developed countries due to the fact that greater economic burden of tertiary prevention [20].

2.2. Colon cancer risk counseling

Today, although advances in treatment and screening standards established successful tests for CRC, it is not perceived as a curable and preventable disease. Many people do not know that even simple measures can prevent CRC. Cancer can be prevented in some individual cases, and it is very important to develop the perception in the community and belief that cancer can be prevented and is curable. Determining the level of risk and interpretation, encouraging preventive behaviors, and improving the early diagnosis and screening behaviors are important parts of early detection and screening programs. Prevention of colon cancer will be successful with the health efforts of professionals to increase awareness of the disease, risk assessments, counseling programs with appropriate recommendations, and diagnose the patients in an early stage [32, 33]. In studies conducted in recent years in the prevention of cancer, "cancer risk counseling" concept stands out [32, 34]. Physicians and nurses who work in primary healthcare services and oncology units have an important role and responsibilities in implementing programs and changing behavior that encourages early screening and diagnosis of cancer. Cancer risk counseling focuses on genetic assessment, assessment of individual risk factors, and the development of a risk management plan [35]. At this point, health professionals trained in CRC counseling can take control of their risk by reaching the individuals at an early stage [11, 12, 32, 36, 37]. Cancer risk counseling should be done in a second step in primary care with asymptomatic individuals at moderate risk and members of the increased-risk and high-risk groups. For example, risk counseling to individuals who have registered in family medicine and family health centers in the moderate-risk group is given by public health nurses. Family of individuals with hereditary CRC and of patients are counseled by doctors and nurses in clinical oncology for as long as treatment continues, or by clinical staff of family cancer clinics/genetic private surveillance programs or outpatient clinics, for those with chronic bowel disease if they are under follow-up [32, 36–38]. To conduct CRC risk counseling, physicians and nurses must have the authority and knowledge on this subject.

This risk counseling process encompasses a comprehensive cancer risk assessment, and determining genetic predisposition, information, guidance training and screening, genetic counseling, and creation of a risk management plan that includes the monitoring and evaluation plan. To achieve effective results in risk counseling, giving individual-specific messages, making an assessment of risk status together with the individual, and supporting the individual in the decision-making process is essential. In addition, it is aimed to follow-up screening participation of the individuals, and guide individuals who receive abnormal test results. Thus, CRC risk counseling aims to reduce morbidity and mortality with an increase in screening rates and to detect disease at an early stage [33, 35, 38].

Risk advisor staff who conduct risk counseling and risk assessments must have certain characteristics. CRC staff have to have adequate current information about hardware, communication techniques, good training, and counseling skills. Also, a counseling room should have adequate ventilation and lighting systems suitable for training and counseling. Colorectal cancer risk counseling identifies risk factors for an individual that can and cannot be changed (hazard identification/risk assessment); screening for risk factors proposition includes monitoring of behavior change initiatives and behavioral changes [38].

2.2.1. Stages of colorectal cancer risk counseling

Colorectal cancer risk counseling includes individual education and counseling and is implemented in three stages [32, 38]:

Stage 1: Application phase

Stage 2: Follow-up phase

Stage 3: Evaluation phase

2.2.1.1. *Application phase*

The creation of awareness through risk assessment and transfer of disease-specific information/education consist of three parts. Before making giving detailed information, disease awareness should be created for the individual, the individual's attention should be directed toward the subject and they should be allowed to ask questions [38]. At this stage, awareness about factors that increase the risk of disease must be created, and behavioral changes must be implemented in order to ensure appropriate counseling skills and evidence-based interventions [14]. A wide range of communication media have been used in studies aiming to increase awareness of CRC screening ranging from personal letters to TV advertisements. While facilitating effective participation in CRC screening initiatives, such as reminders, mass media and the media, group training, personal training, and assessments, are taken by reducing structural barriers to healthcare professionals and include initiatives such as feedback. The effectiveness of personal reminders, personal training, and counseling in improving CRC screening has been proven [10, 25, 39–44].

Sections	Initiatives/methods	Tools
Application phase		
Creating awareness	**Initiative:** CRC risk factors, prevention, information about early diagnosis **Method:** Face-to-face interviews, telephone interviews, video/slide show, introduce role models, motivational interviewing, send letters	Banners, posters, models, TV and newspaper advertisements, letters, mail/invitation via e-mail, phone messages, calendars, giveaway/inducers such as promotion, promotional stands
Risk assessment	**Initiative:** Determine the risk rating of the individual **Method:** Face-to-face interviews, computer-aided risk assessment models	Risk assessment tables, pedigree charts, graphs, histograms, electronic health records
Disease-specific information	**Initiative:** Provide adequate and appropriate information about the disease **Method:** Face to face interviews	Slides, posters, pamphlets, educational videos, health beliefs scales, written materials
Follow-up phase		
	Initiative: Maintain awareness, support positive behavior, follow-up/surveillance of screening behavior **Method:** Interview	Phone calls, text messages, e-mail, reminders, call center awards
Evaluation phase		
	Initiative: Preventive screening behavior and participation in evaluation, assessment test results **Method:** Face-to-face interviews	Automated phone calls Web-based assessment

Table 5. Colorectal cancer risk counseling can be applied in all stages of evidence-based initiatives.

Creating awareness: Various implications may be used in order to create awareness in the individuals about the importance of their protective behaviors in the prevention of CRC and their health. Evidence-based interventions recommended in the recent relevant studies are shown in **Table 5** [10, 25, 39–44]. Due to purpose of encouraging individuals take action to protective behaviors, it is important to give positive messages in materials (e.g., posters, banners) that it is possible to protect against CRC [11, 36, 37]. Risk assessment is required for each individual in order to determine the screening interval and proper test [21, 33].

Risk assessment: It is important to be able to receive adequate health history. The scope of individual members in the counseling process assessment includes the following:

- demographic, socioeconomic, cultural characteristics, and medical history (previous/ existing diseases, especially chronic bowel disease, polyps),
- a detailed family history (especially first- and second-degree relatives),
- cognitive and psychosocial (cognitive capacity, CRC knowledge, risk perception, CRC-related health beliefs and attitudes, perceptions, motivation, concerns, barriers, CRC relevant experience, anxiety and fears, coping mechanisms and social support status, decision-making and decision support systems),
- lifestyle behaviors (habits that increase the risk of CRC, dietary behaviors, physical activity status, smoking and alcohol use, stress level, given the importance of such a negative attitude and a healthy lifestyle),
- do not collect data on exposure to environmental risk factors and other characteristics.

Risk assessment tools for practical risk assessment (risk calculation tool, pedigram) can be made using electronic health records [10, 25, 33, 35, 39, 45]. According to the data obtained, a risk rating of the risk assessment is performed. The risk rating is how to determine whether an individual is at risk and making orientation relative to the risk. The degree of risk of cancer is important in guiding the individual screening tests [6, 11, 21]. In this regard, national/ international guidelines should be considered. Risk assessment, web-based tools, and mathematical models of interpretation of risk may make it easier to use directed individual protection proposals. Graphical presentation of risk status (bar, pie, histogram) makes it easier to explain and to understand the risk [6, 21, 33, 45]. Health behavior models have been developed for people to understand why there are different health behaviors or practices they are going to implement. While counseling individuals, health behavior models act as a "black box" to determine factors that affect preventive behaviors and to change negative behaviors to positive. These models are Health Belief Model, Transtheoretic Model, Health Promotion, and Preventive Health Model [11, 12, 14, 38, 39].

The risk status of the individual is described in a way that can be understood. Words, tone of voice, body images, and facial expressions of health personnel can affect the understanding individual risk information. The level of education of the individual, age, cultural, and linguistic differences should be taken into account. In addition, the cost of diagnosis and treatment, transportation requirements, communication, and cultural characteristics are important for the care of the patient's decision. Particular circumstances of the individual (e.g., affected my social and personal values, and economic and environmental conditions) should be considered. Individuals are given information regarding their assessment and risk diagnostics; when interpreting cancer risks, results that will disrupt the motivation for the individual's protection behavior or descriptions that will cause anxiety/fear should be avoided [33, 45].

Sufficient disease-specific information: The aim is to address the lack of knowledge about the disease and the individual CRC screening tests (fecal occult blood test, colonoscopy, double-contrast bowel X-ray, sigmoidoscopy). Patients training sessions should include information on colon and rectal anatomy of the digestive system, CRC generation, CRC signs and symptoms, risk factors, the importance of disease prevention, prevention, healthy lifestyle behaviors, early diagnosis and screening tests, the advantages and disadvantages of each test, and information about CRC protection behavior information [11, 21, 32, 35, 38, 39, 45]. Taking appropriate initiatives to scan an individual's risk rating should be provided and monitored (see **Table 5**). Encouragement of positive behavior aimed at reducing CRC risk and altering health beliefs associated with the disease are very important. Therefore, the individual's health beliefs during counseling, motivation, and barriers to education in this direction may be determined by a variety of scales [11, 21, 38]. Video display and printed materials in the education department, presentations, and motivational interviewing techniques such as active listening are available. There are no studies on the use of individual incentives that promote screening (a small amount of money, coupons, gift certificates); therefore, there is insufficient evidence to support this initiative alone. After the training, short appropriate tests should be conducted in order to evaluate the effectiveness of the training; individuals who then wish to undergo screening should be referred to the relevant departments and clinics [38].

2.2.1.2. Follow-up phase

Maintainance of awareness of the individual is intended to support the CRC protection behavior. It will increase the importance of the disease and practical initiatives to ensure the consistency of behavior covered in the training. The next follow-up face-to-face meeting in the implementation phase can be done through methods such as e-mail or telephone (**Table 5**). During these initiatives, any information that was given during training that was not clear can be questioned. For example, healthy lifestyle behaviors and screening recommendations for prevention of CRC can be repeated/reviewed, and information can be discussed about where to go in the event of receiving negative test results. At this stage, the behavior of individuals regarding disease protection is expected to show increased enthusiasm. All associated individuals (family, friends, healthcare professionals) are encouraged to support positive and protective behavior [11, 12, 21, 25, 35, 38].

2.2.1.3. Evaluation phase

At this stage, CRC protection behavior exhibited by the individual is evaluated. Changing an individual's behavior is not a goal that can be realized in a short time, it requires long-term follow-up. In order to ensure continuity, to maintain positive behaviors and enable behavior changes to occur, regular implementation of risk counseling (e.g., 3, 6, 12, 24 months) should be carried out [34, 35, 39]. The evaluation phase, which allows for obtaining feedback from individuals, is usually advised to be face to face. Reasons for an individual wishing to end the

http://dx.doi.org/10.5772/63206

program should be taken to identify obstacles and need to reschedule procedures overcome these barriers [11, 12, 21, 32, 35, 38, 41, 45].

3. Conclusions

Primary and secondary prevention practices in the management of CRC are to be carried out together. Applying primary measures alone will not be enough, only having screening tests will not prevent the disease occurrence. Primary healthcare physicians and nurses have an important role in the implementation of risk counseling. Colorectal cancer risk counsellers are required to have special knowledge and skills. Therefore, the staff who undertake counseling are required to have received appropriate training. Colorectal cancer risk counseling is a process that applies to all stages of implementation, including monitoring, evaluation stages, and health services. Many initiatives and recommended methods for each stage of the process have been demonstrated in research. Adequate training in CRC risk counseling practice of health professionals, all relevant employees in surgery, oncology, and public health has been estimated to reduce the incidence of CRC.

Author details

Serife Koc[1*], Melek Nihal Esin[2] and Aysun Ardic[2]

*Address all correspondence to: serife.koc@istanbul.edu.tr

1 Karamanoglu Mehmetbey University, Karaman School of Health, Karaman, Turkey

2 Istanbul University, Florence Nightingale Faculty of Nursing, Istanbul, Turkey

References

[1] Chan AD, Giovannucci ED. Primary prevention of colorectal cancer. Gastroenterology. 2010; 138: 2029–2043.

[2] Wilkes GM. Colon, rectal, and anal cancers. In: Yarbro CH, Wujcik D, Gobel BH, editors. Cancer Nursing Principles and Practice. 7th ed. Sudbury, MA: Jones and Barlett Publishers; 2011. pp. 1205–1257.

[3] Johnson CM, Wei C, Ensor JE, Smolenski DJ, Amos CI, Levin B. et al. Meta-analyses of colorectal cancer risk factors. Cancer Causes Control. 2013; 24: 1207–1222.

[4] Tarraga LPJ, Albero JS, Rodriguez-Montes JA. Primary and secondary prevention of colorectal cancer. Clinical Medicine Insights: Gastroenterology. 2014; 7: 33–46.

[5] Ferlay J, Soerjomataram I, Ervik M, Dikshit R, Eser S, Mathers C, Rebelo M, Parkin DM, Forman D, Bray F. GLOBOCAN 2012 v1.0, Cancer Incidence and Mortality Worldwide: IARC CancerBase No. 11 [Internet]. Lyon, France: International Agency for Research on Cancer; 2013. Available from: http://globocan.iarc.fr [Accesssed: 2014/08/30].

[6] Erturk S. Colorectal cancers: Epidemiology, factors that play a role in the etiology, screening and chemoprevention. In: Baykan A, Zorluoglu A, Gecim E, Terzi C, editors. Colon and Rectum Cancers. Istanbul: Turkish Society of Colon and Rectal Surgery, Secil Offset Printing and Packaging Industry Co.Ltd.; 2010. pp. 15-30. [in Turkish]

[7] Patel SS, Kilgore ML. Cost effectiveness of colorectal cancer screening strategies. Cancer Control: Journal of the Moffitt Cancer Center. 2015; 22(2): 248–258.

[8] Oxentenko AS, Wei EK, Limburg PJ, Giovanucci E. Risk factors and prevention. In: Couric K, editor. American Cancer Society's Complete Guide to Colorectal Cancer. Atlanta: American Cancer Society; 2006. pp. 11–34.

[9] Glasper A. Can nurses help to promote earlier diagnosis of bowel cancer? British Journal of Nursing. 2012; 21(1): 50–51.

[10] American Cancer Society (ACS). Colorectal Cancer Facts and Figures 2014-2016. Atlanta: American Cancer Society, Inc.; 2014. Available from: http://www.cancer.org/acs/groups/content/documents/document/acspc-042280.pdf [Accesssed: 2015/10/30].

[11] Price AS. Primary and secondary prevention of colorectal cancer. Gastroenterology Nursing. 2003; 26(2): 73–81.

[12] Myers ER. Decision counseling in cancer prevention and control. Health Psychology. 2005; 24(4): 71–77.

[13] Cavdar I. Colon Rectum and Anal Cancers. In: Can G, editor. Oncology Nursing. Istanbul: Nobel Medical Publishers; 2015. pp. 707–717. [in Turkish]

[14] Simons VA, Flynn SP, Flocke SA. Practical behavior change counseling in primary care. Primary Care: Clinics in Office Practice. 2007; 34(3): 611–622.

[15] Thomson CA, Chen Z. The role of diet, physical activity and body composition in cancer prevention. In: Alberts DS, Hess LM, editors. Fundamentals of Cancer Prevention. 2nd ed. Tucson: Springer; 2010. pp. 31–78. DOI: 10.1007/978-3-540-68986-7.

[16] James, WPT. The role of nutrition in cancer prevention. In: Miller AB, editor. Epidemiologic studies in cancer prevention and screening. New York: Springer; 2013; pp. 121–140.

[17] Bazensky I, Shoobridge-Moran C, Yoder LH. Colorectal cancer: an overview of the epidemiology, risk factors, symptoms, and screening guidelines. Medsurg Nursing. 2007; 16(1): 46–51.

[18] Kahler CJ, Rex D, Imperiale TF. Screening for Colorectal Cancer, Social Follow-up and Primary Prevention: An Overview of Current Literature. Gastroenterology Turkish pressure. 2008; 3 (4): 193–217. [in Turkish]

[19] Keith JN, Jackson SC. Environmental factors and colorectal cancer. In: Kim KE, editor. Early Detection and Prevention of Colorectal Cancer. New Jersey: Slack Incorporated; 2009. pp. 49–71.

[20] Alberts DS, Hess LM. Introduction to cancer prevention. In: Alberts DS, Hess LM, editors. Fundamentals of Cancer Prevention. 2nd ed. Tucson: Springer; 2010. pp. 1–12. DOI: 10.1007/978-3-540-68986-7.

[21] Mahon SM. Prevention and screening of gastrointestinal cancers. Seminars in Oncology Nursing. 2009; 25(1): 15–31.

[22] Lance P. Chemical prevention for colorectal cancer: There is a long way to go although some progress. Gastroenterology Turkish pressure. 2008; 3(2): 98–106. [in Turkish]

[23] Patel SG, Ahnen DJ. Screening for colon polyps and cancer. In: Miller AB, editor. Epidemiologic Studies in Cancer Prevention and Screening. New York: Springer; 2013; pp. 169–182.

[24] Levin B, Lieberman BA, McFarland B, Andrews KS, Brooks D, Bond J. et al. Screening and surveillance for the early detection of colorectal cancer and adenomatous polyps, 2008: a joint guideline from the American Cancer Society, the US Multi-Society Task Force on Colorectal Cancer, and the American College of Radiology. Gastroenterology. 2008; 134(5): 1570–1595.

[25] European Commission. European guidelines for quality assurance in colorectal cancer screening and diagnosis. [Internet]. First ed., Luxemburg: Publication Office of the European Union; 2010. DOI: 10.2772/15379. Available from: http://www.kolorektum.cz/file/guidelines [Accessed: 2016/01/03].

[26] Lionis C, Petelos E. Early detection of colorectal cancer and population screening tests. In: Ettarh R, editor. Colorectal Cancer—From Prevention to Patient Care. Rijeka: InTech; 2012. pp. 45–66. Available from: http://www.intechopen.com/books/colorectal-cancer-from-prevention-to-patientcare/early-detection-of-colorectal-cancer-and-population-screening-tests [Accessed: 2015/12/30].

[27] NCCN Guidelines Version 2.2014, Colorectal Cancer Screening. Available from: http://www.nccn.org [Accessed: 2015/10/04].

[28] Cabebe EC. Colorectal cancer guidelines: colorectal cancer screening. In: Espat NJ, editor. [Internet]. 2015. Available from: http://emedicine.medscape.com/article/2500006-overview#a1 [Accessed: 2016/02/25].

[29] Labianca R, Nordlinger B, Beretta GD, Mosconi S, Mandalà M, Cervantes A, Arnold D. Early colon cancer: ESMO clinical practice guidelines for diagnosis, treatment and follow up. Annals of Oncology. 2013; 24(6): 64–72.

[30] Balmaña J, Balaguer F, Cervantes A, Arnold D. Familial risk-colorectal cancer: ESMO Clinical Practice Guidelines. Annals of Oncology. 2013; 24(6): 73–80.

[31] Lansdorp-Vogelaar I, Knudsen AB, Brenner H. Cost-effectiveness of colorectal cancer screening. Epidemiologic Reviews. 2011; 33(1): 88–100.

[32] Koc S, Esin MN. Screening behaviors, health beliefs, and related factors of first-degree relatives of colorectal cancer patients with ongoing treatment in Turkey. Cancer Nursing. 2014; 37(6): E51–60.

[33] Mahon SM. Screening and detection for asymptomatic individuals. In: Yarbro CH, Wujcik D, Gobel BH, editors. Cancer Nursing Principles and Practice. 7th ed. Sudbury, MA: Jones and Barlett Publishers; 2011. pp. 115–134.

[34] Glanz K, Steffen AD, Taglialatela LA. Effects of colon cancer risk counseling for first degree relatives. Cancer Epidemiology, Biomarkers and Prevention. 2007; 16(7): 1485–1491.

[35] MacDonald DJ. The oncology nurse's role in cancer risk assessment and counseling. Seminars in Oncology Nursing. 1997; 13(2): 123–128.

[36] Greenwald B. Health fairs: an avenue for colon health promotion in the community. Gastroenterology Nursing. 2003; 26(5): 191–194.

[37] Greenwald B. How to market colorectal cancer screening awareness and colonoscopy services. Gastroenterology Nursing. 2005; 28(5): 435–437.

[38] Koc S. The effect of colorectal cancer risk counseling on the promoting of primary and secondary preventive behaviors of the individuals at risk. [thesis] Istanbul: Istanbul University; 2014. [in Turkish]

[39] Gimeno Garcia AZ, Hernandez Alvarez Buylla N, Nicolas-Perez D, Quintero E. Public awareness of colorectal cancer screening: knowledge, attitudes, and interventions for increasing screening uptake. ISRN Oncology. 2014; 2014: 1–19.

[40] Rawl SM, Menon U, Burness A, Breslau ES. Interventions to promote colorectal cancer 26 screening: an integrative review. Nursing Outlook. 2012; 60(4): 172–181.

[41] Sabatino SA, Lawrence B, Elder R, Mercer SL, Wilson KM, DeVinney B, et al. Effectiveness of interventions to increase screening for breast, cervical, and colorectal cancers: nine updated systematic reviews for the guide to community preventive services. American Journal of Preventive Medicine. 2012; 43(1): 97–118.

[42] Brouwers CM, Vito C, Bahirathan L, Carol A, Carroll JC, Cotterchio M, et al. Effective interventions to facilitate the uptake of breast, cervical and colorectal cancer screening: an implementation guideline. Implementation Science. 2011a; 6(112): 1–8.

[43] Brouwers CM, Vito C, Bahirathan L, Carol A, Carroll JC, Cotterchio M, et al. What implementation interventions increase cancer screening rates? A systematic review. Implementation Science. 2011b; 6(111): 1–17.

[44] Holden DJ, Jonas DE, Porterfield DS, Reuland D, Harris R. Systematic review: enhancing the use and quality of colorectal cancer screening. Annals of Internal Medicine. 2010; 152(10): 668–676.

[45] National Cancer Institute. Cancer Genetics Risk Assessment and Counseling-for health professionals. [Internet]. Bethesda, MD: National Cancer Institute; 2015. Available from: http://www.cancer.gov/about-cancer/causes-prevention/genetics/risk-assessment-pdq#link/_323_toc [Accessed: 2015/12/30].

Chapter 6

Imaging of Colonic and Rectal Cancer

Radu I Badea, Cosmin N Caraiani and Diana I Florian

Additional information is available at the end of the chapter

http://dx.doi.org/10.5772/62307

Abstract

Colorectal cancer is one of the most common cancers worldwide. Thus, its early detection through screening and diagnostic techniques is the key in managing this condition. For this to be possible, it is necessary to know the risk factors and to choose the appropriate screening and diagnostic techniques for each case. Imaging also plays a key role in treatment planning by assessing both local and distance extension of the disease.

The aim of this chapter is to make an overview of the currently available imaging techniques for diagnosis of colorectal cancer (ultrasound, computed tomography—CT, magnetic resonance imaging—MRI, and positron emission tomography—PET/CT), focusing on specific and technical elements, benefits, costs, and limitations of each technique.

Keywords: colon, rectum, imaging, ultrasonography, CT, MRI

1. General

1.1. Epidemiology

Colorectal cancer (CRC) is a major human health issue. Globally, it ranks third in incidence after lung and breast cancers. In developed areas such as North America, Australia, New Zealand and Western Europe, it appears even more frequently, being ranked the second [1, 2]. In terms of etiology, it is divided into two categories: genetic and non-genetic. The non-genetic ("sporadic") category is the most common one (~70–80%), its known cause being the malignant transformation of the adenomatous polyps. This phenomenon occurs over years, related to an unstable lifestyle. An improper diet (low in fruit and vegetables and high in red meat and saturated fat), consumption of toxic products (alcohol and tobacco), obesity, sedentarism, as well as the presence of inflammatory bowel diseases (ulcerative colitis and Crohn's disease) are all considered as being predisposing factors [3, 4]. In recent years, a decrease in the mortality from colorectal neoplasia and an increase in the survival by up to 5 years has been reported. These are due to the evolution of early detection techniques through screening, as well as to the improved therapeutic procedures. Even if in this disease the prognosis is better than in other cancers, the main concern regards its management which should be directed toward prevention and early diagnosis.

1.2. Techniques used for early detection

Screening methods used are in full development. They are classified into biological assays (for the detection of occult stool blood, DNA, RNA, and feces protein) and colorectal exploration techniques. Among the biological assays, the one used for the detection of occult blood in the stool is the most widely used because of its accessibility, low-cost, and proven effectiveness in reducing the CRC incidence and mortality (by ~15–33%) [4]. The assay for the detection of DNA, RNA, and some proteins in plasma and feces represents another biological category. Due to the variability of literature data related to their diagnosis value as well as their high cost, their usefulness on a large scale is still reduced [4]. The genetic syndromes with increased risk of CRC (the familial adenomatous polyposis and the hereditary non-polyposis colorectal cancer—Lynch syndrome) can be diagnosed through different genetic assays.

In the category of the colorectal exploration tests, optical colonoscopy is the method of choice. This technique is used as a screening assay at different time intervals depending on the probability of disease occurrence. One of its major advantages is the possibility of polyps biopsy/resection (in spite of the high cost and low acceptance by the population!) [4].

Other colorectal exploration assays include imaging methods. The techniques used are the double-contrast irrigoscopy and the CT virtual colonoscopy (CT colonography). It is currently recommended to replace the double-contrast irrigoscopy with the CT virtual colonoscopy because of a lower discomfort and a better tolerance, as well as its increasing affordability [5, 6]. There are studies that are showing an increased sensitivity (96%) of the CT virtual colonoscopy, similar to the optical colonoscopy, but the values vary depending on the lesion size [6].

1.3. Criteria to be included in the screening programs

The population at an average risk of developing CRC is represented by subjects older than 50 years old, without other associated risk factors. They can be followed up annually for the detection of occult stool blood, as well as by flexible sigmoidoscopy (only for the left colon, technique that does not require special preparation). The combination of the two assays may be carried out every 5 years. Other availabilities are double-contrast irrigoscopy and virtual colonoscopy done every 5 years, or optical colonoscopy, every 10 years [5–7].

The population with increased risk of developing CRC is represented by subjects with personal or familial history of CRC or adenomatous polyps, those with genetic syndromes, or patients with chronic inflammatory diseases. Each of them can benefit from a customized screening program. The screening program must begin at the age of 40, or 10 years earlier than the age of the youngest relative affected by the disease. The American College of Physicians recommends the use of the optical colonoscopy as a screening method for the high risk population group, noting that the choice of the tests must be carried out according to the risk/benefit ratio, affordability, and the patient's preferences. In addition, it is recommended to cease the screening in patients over 75 years old or those with a life expectancy of less than 10 years [7].

2. Imaging in colorectal cancer

This category contains a series of diagnostic procedures, the main purpose being that of providing information in the form of images. Every method has specific physical principles, technology, benefits, costs, and limitations. For this reason, each method should be discussed separately.

2.1. Transabdominal ultrasonography (ultrasound)

The ultrasound examination of the digestive tract is a challenge for the performing physician. This is because of the sinuosity of the bowel loops that makes it difficult to perform a full examination using a transducer with a small surface, as well as because of the high air content of the digestive tract, source of sonographic artifacts. It should also be kept in mind that the ultrasound appearance of the digestive structures varies from one time of the examination to another because of the intestinal peristalsis. The ultrasound examination of the digestive tract highly depends on the experience and patience of the examiner, to a much higher extent than the exploration of parenchymal organs. Ultrasonography is the imaging technique with the best space and time resolution in the assessment of the digestive wall, higher than computer-assisted tomography or magnetic resonance imaging. Depending on the frequency of the transducer, we can identify three layers of the wall (when using the convex probe) or five layers (when using the linear probe). Thus, the difficulties of examining the whole digestive tract are offset by a more accurate appreciation of the details.

Ultrasonography is, on many occasions, the first method of choice for patients with abdominal pain, bowel movements impairments, or other symptoms in the abdominal area [8]. It is a very accessible method, non-irradiating and painless, easily accepted by the patient, and widely available. Also, in many cases, it provides very useful information for patient diagnosis, allowing the exclusion of other diseases with similar symptoms to the CRC. The examining physician must be familiar with the ultrasound appearance of the colon cancer, which is that of a parietal hypoechoic thickening with loss of normal stratification [9]. The extent of the affected colonic wall is variable. Also, the tumor formation can be eccentric, circumferential, or semicircumferential. The colonic lumen can be stenosed [**Figure 1**]. At palpation with the transducer, the modified region may show an increased stiffness. The pericolic fat has, if invaded by tumor, an "infiltrated" (hyperechogenic) appearance. Peritumoral adenopathies can also be highlighted, with malignant aspect—being hypoechogenic and round [9]. The anorectal administration of contrast fluid (water enema) known as hydrosonography will increase the performance of ultrasonography in diagnosing colon cancer [10] [**Figure 2**]. A study on 145 patients showed a sensitivity of 79.06% and a specificity of 92.15% for ultrasound in the diagnosis of colon cancer [11], performances which can be improved by the use of hydrosonography. Studies demonstrate that using water enema, the accuracy of the ultrasound in the T staging of the colon cancer increases to 88% and the tumoral infiltration of the lymph nodes can be predicted in approximately 70% of cases.

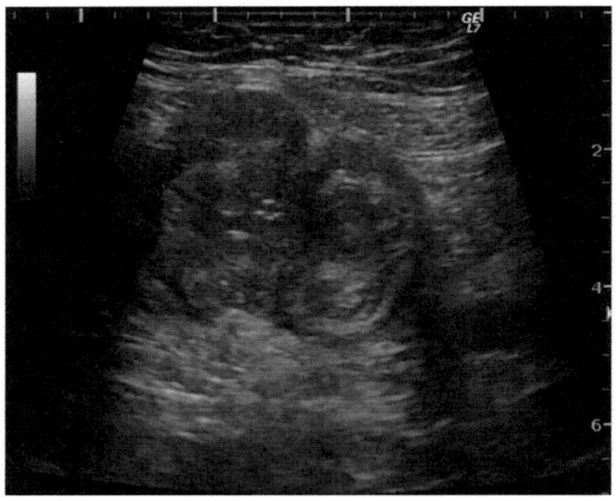

Figure 1. Transabdominal ultrasonography. Appearance of colon cancer.

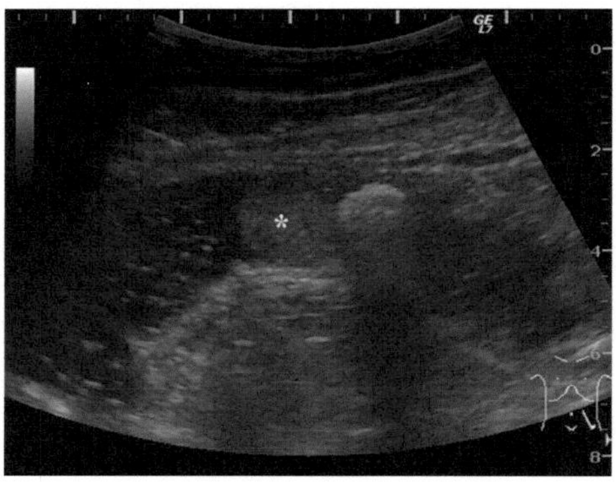

Figure 2. Transabdominal ultrasonography. Appearance of polypoid tumor. The ultrasonographic image is optimized by hydrosonography (anorectal administration of water).

Asserting the existence of a colonic tumor does not represent a complete diagnosis. We also need to know if the pathological process in the colon is a candidate for a treatment with curative purpose or the disease is in an advanced stage and the patient can only receive palliative treatment. The main reason for which we consider incurable a colon tumor process is the presence of distant metastases. Most often, colon cancer leads to liver metastases [12]. Even if the imaging method recommended for the staging of the colon cancer is computed tomography, ultrasound still plays an important role because it is the first imaging technique currently used. Ultrasound examination improved by the intravenous administration of contrast agents has a complementary role to computed tomography in the characterization of small, hypo-

http://dx.doi.org/10.5772/62307

vascular liver lesions, difficult to be characterized by the means of computed tomography. The ultrasound appearance of the hepatic metastases from colorectal tumors is variable. They are most commonly hypoechoic, but they can also be iso- or hyperechoic [**Figure 3**]. They are, in most of the cases, surrounded by a hypoechoic halo. The presence of the halo around a focal liver lesion makes it very likely that the lesion is malignant [13]. Sensitivity of ultrasound in the diagnosis of liver metastases is, according to various studies, between 53 and 72%. It is much improved, reaching values of 80–90%, after the administration of an intravenous contrast agent [14, 15]. After the administration of ultrasound contrast media, most of CRC liver metastases will have a hypovascular appearance. In the arterial phase of the examination, they will show peripheral enhancement like a "halo". Later, during portal/venous phases, this peripheral enhancement will wash out, remaining hypoechoic compared to the liver parenchyma. The portal and especially the late phase will be very important in liver metastases diagnosis; in these phases, they appear like "black spots" on the hyperechoic and shiny background of the normal surrounding parenchyma that captured avidly the contrast agent [**Figure 4**].

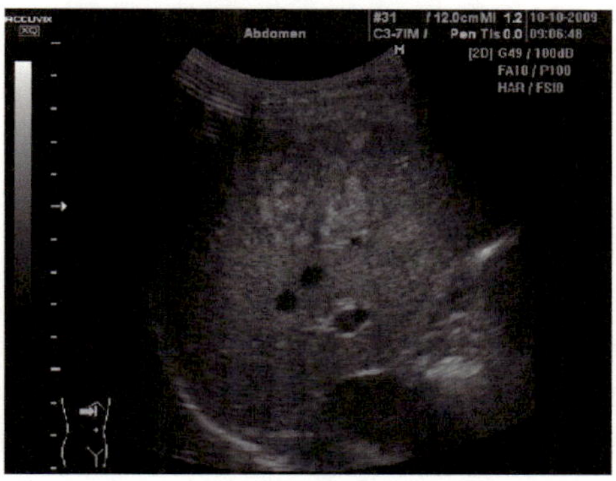

Figure 3. Transabdominal ultrasonography (gray scale). Appearance of liver metastases.

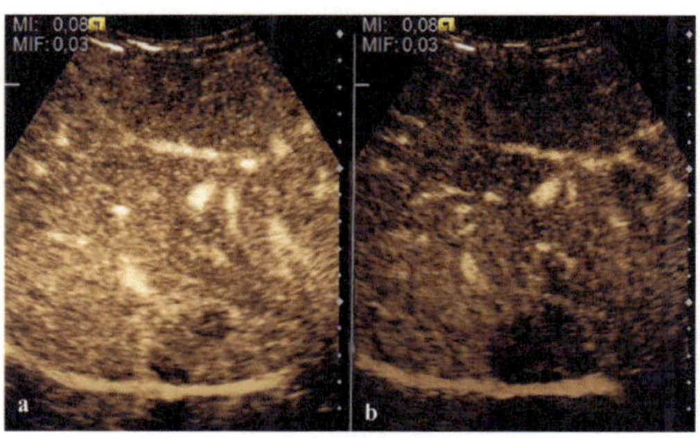

Figure 4. Transabdominal ultrasonography with i.v. contrast agent (CEUS). Liver metastases. Peripheral enhancement after contrast administration in the arterial phase (a) and wash-out in the late phase (b).

During abdominal ultrasound in patients with colon tumors, the retroperitoneum must also be assessed. The area between the inferior vena cava and the aorta is the location of metastases in 1–2% of patients with colon cancer. The assessment of this area can be difficult in overweight patients and those with overlap of gas-distended bowel loops. The presence of ascites in a patient with colon tumor raises the suspicion of peritoneal carcinomatosis. The carcinomatosis nodules will be sought mainly in the interhepatophrenic area, at the level of peritoneal recesses, and in the rectovesical space. Searching small-sized carcinoma nodules also requires the assessment of the anterior peritoneum using the high-frequency linear probe [16] [**Figure 5**].

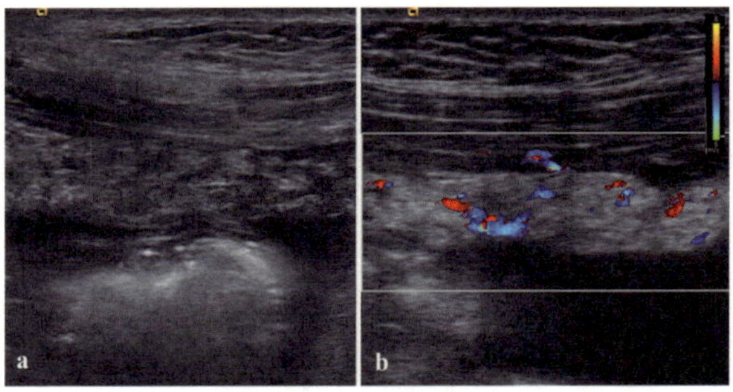

Figure 5. Peritoneal carcinomatosis. Examination was performed with high frequency probe. (a) gray scale ultrasonography and (b) color Doppler ultrasonography).

2.2. Transrectal ultrasonography

This is strictly a staging procedure. The rectal ultrasound exploration is only possible through endocavitary approach. The transperineal approach may be used in case of stenosing or prolapsing low rectal tumors in the anal canal, or if the patient shows intolerance to endocavitary procedure. In women, the rectum exploration can be achieved also by endovaginal examination [17]. The preferred ultrasound approach is transrectal, because of the visualization of the five parietal layers and the surrounding organs in the pelvis. From a technical standpoint, the ultrasound device must be equipped with a mechanic and rotating transducer with the frequency between 5–10 MHz. Attached to it there is a rubber bag filled with water (~30–60 ml) (dedicated transducer). In this way, the region to be assessed can be explored more accurately, the ultrasound beam being perpendicular to the rectal wall [18]. Alternatively, the endocavitary transducer for general use can be utilised (adapted equipment). In this case, the ultrasound waves are emitted at an angle of 135 degrees to the plane of the rod, and the obtained information is indicative. However, because of the multidirectional orientation of the examination plan, this equipment can be used to explore larger rectal tumors and even those located in the upper rectum.

There are several ultrasound procedures useful in the diagnosis of rectal tumors. Among them, the ultrasound in "gray scale" allows the analysis of morphological features (the affected parietal layers) [**Figure 6**]. Doppler ultrasonography and contrast-enhanced ultrasonography (CEUS) provide information about tumor microcirculation by analyzing specific parameters

[19–21] [**Figure 7**]. 3D ultrasound assesses the position of the tumor mass, and it provides the performance of measurements in the three space dimensions using a special transducer [22] [**Figure 8**]. Sonoelastography is a newly emerging technique and its principle is based on the analysis of the target tissue response (in our case, the tumor tissue) when compressed. Thus, this technique provides information about the degree of the tumor stiffness and surrounding tumoral adenopathies [**Figure 9, Figure 10**].

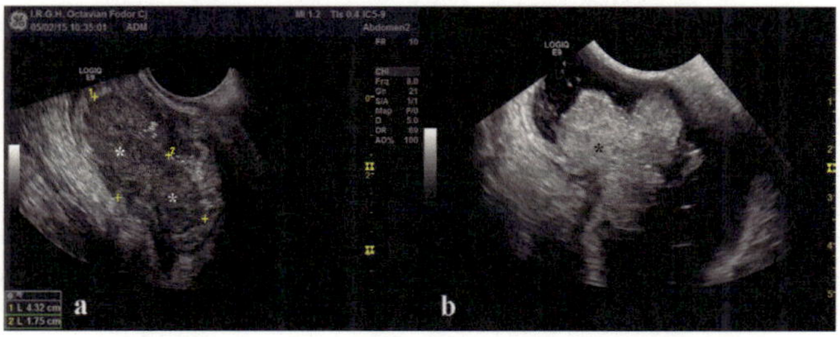

Figure 6. Rectal tumor (a and b). Endorectal gray scale appearance (asterisk).

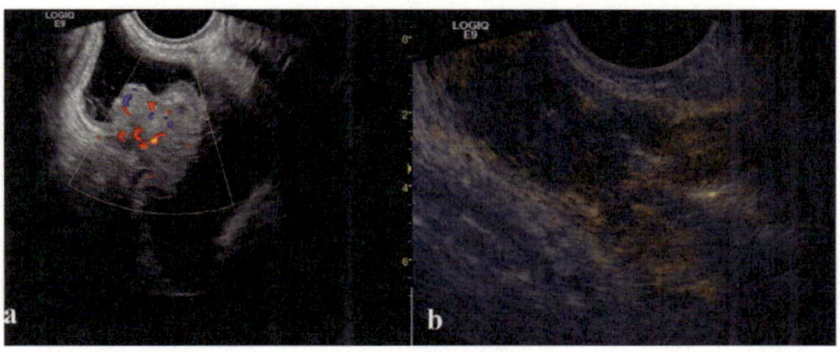

Figure 7. Rectal tumor investigated with Doppler ultrasound (a) and with CEUS (b). The contrast examination is performed after radiotherapy. Note the partial response to the treatment.

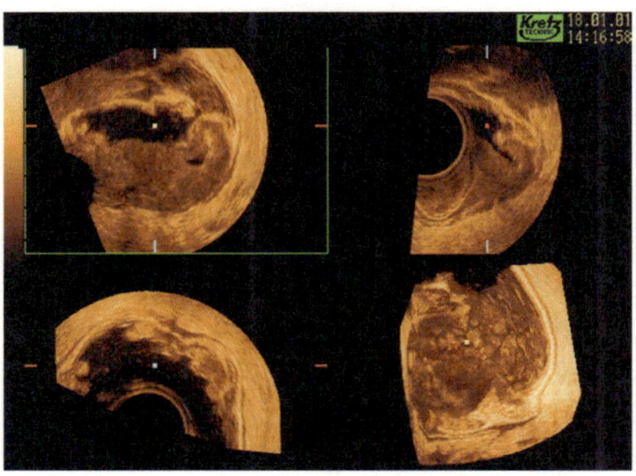

Figure 8. Rectal tumor—multidirectional tridimensional appearance.

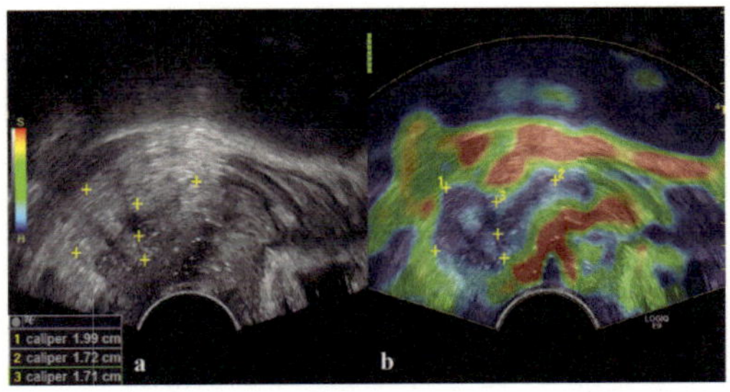

Figure 9. Rectal tumor. Gray scale ultrasound (a) and sonoelastographic examination (b). To be noticed the perirectal fat invasion.

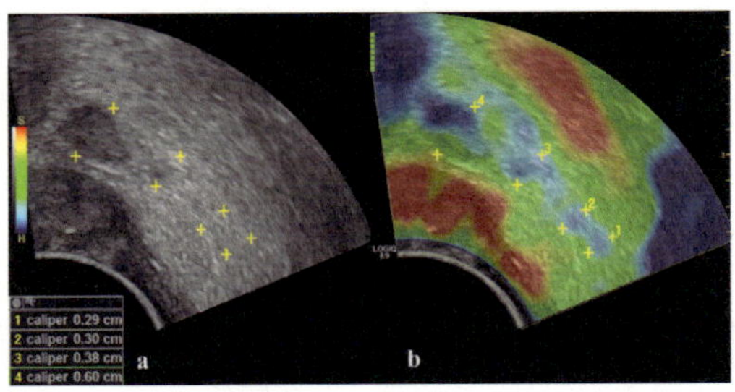

Figure 10. Neoplastic perirectal lymphadenopathies (a and b). Sonoelastographic appearance (real-time elastography, color, contact elastography). The marked rigidity of perirectal adenopathies, characteristic of malignancy, is noticed.

The examination takes place after a previous preparation of the patient by an evacuation enema. The patient is positioned in the left lateral decubitus, and the transducer is inserted into the rectum. To optimize the ultrasound image, water can be introduced previously, intrarectally (200–300 ml), but this applies only to patients with sphincter continence and to the compliant ones [22]. Transrectal ultrasound enables the visualization, tracking and assessment of tumor extension to the rectal wall and adjacent organs. The ultrasonographic appearance of rectal infiltrative tumors consists in the presence of circumferential or focal parietal thickening, along with the loss of parietal stratification. Proliferative tumors appear as endoluminal hypoechogenic masses. At the Doppler investigation, they have a disorganized vascularization. At the sonoelastography examination, the tumors are rigid. The staging of rectal cancer through transrectal ultrasound can only be performed locally (T and N stage) because of the reduced field of view of the method. The assessment of tumor invasion in the rectal wall is possible by ultrasound, with an overall diagnosis accuracy of approximately 80–95% [23]. However, the diagnostic performance of the method varies depending on the T stage, being higher for the diagnosis of the rectal tumors in early stages (T1 and T2). This is mainly because of the increased spatial resolution, enabling the differentiation of the rectal wall layers [24]. For the diagnosis of advanced stages, the MRI is preferred because it allows a better visualization of the mesorectum fascia, the peritoneum, and the surrounding organs [25]. Because of the reduced field of view of the transrectal ultrasound, the assessment of the tumoral attaint of the mesorectal fascia is difficult [23]. The tumoral invasion within lymph nodes is another decisive element in determining the therapeutic protocol in patients with rectal cancer. The dimensional and morphological criteria are not sufficient to establish lymph node malignancy. The latest studies show that transrectal ultrasound sensitivity is similar to that of MRI (75.8% versus 77%) for lymph nodes assessment [24, 26].

Among the technical limitations of endocavitary ultrasound is the presence of a tumoral stenosis, which does not allow the transducer to pass the obstacle, thus the tumor cannot be properly assessed. Other limitations are related to post-surgery and post-radiation changes of the rectal wall. The use of the universal endocavitary transducer and the transperineal or transvaginal approach may represent alternative techniques that can provide additional information. Another drawback is differentiating the post-surgery/radiation appearance from a possible tumor residue, or a relapse, and the differentiation of stage T2 from stage T3 can be difficult in some cases because of local inflammatory or fibrotic changes.

2.3. Computer tomography

Abdominal CT (including CT virtual colonoscopy) is one of the imaging options in the diagnosis of colon tumors, allowing their detection, characterization, and staging. Discovering a colon tumor under CT can be accidental or in the context of some complications (intestinal obstruction, invagination, perforation, or fistulization) [27]. In terms of the examining technique, it is recommended to perform a luminal distension, with oral contrast, water or air, along with the intravenous administration of the iodinated contrast agent. Currently, it is preferred to replace the oral contrast agent with water, allowing a better individualization of bleeding and tumor iodophilia [27]. A typical CT appearance of a colorectal tumor is that of a polypoid mass [**Figure 11**] with possible areas of necrosis and air inclusions. Another presentation of CRC is that of an irregular focal or circumferential parietal thickening, associated with endoluminal narrowing or colon stenosis [**Figure 12**]. The local extracolonic invasion is assessed by the infiltration of the pericolonic fat [**Figure 13**]. After the administration of the iodinated contrast agent, both the adenomatous polyps and the adenocarcinomas show iodophilia. In the case of a tumoral occlusion, the colon appears dilated upstream of the stenosis and the transition zone is easily viewed using multiplanar reconstructions. The tumoral perforation is more common in the cecum area, and it is detected by the presence of pneumoperitoneum and the infiltration of pericolonic fat [27]. Local staging (stage "T") of the CRC via

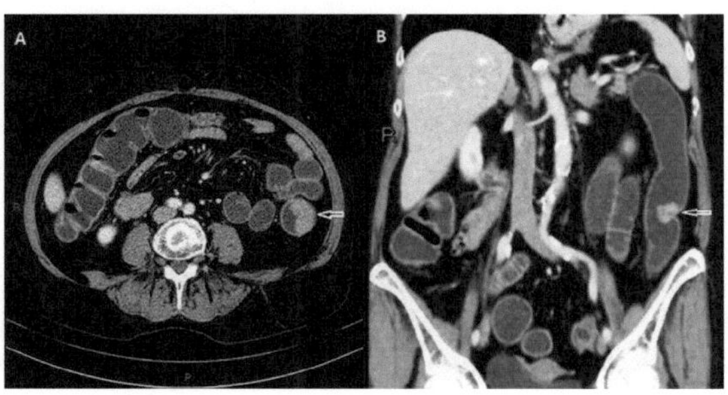

Figure 11. Water enema CT performed to a 50-year-old female patient with suspicion of adenomatous polyps. (a) Axial and (b) coronal images show a polypoid T2 lesion, located on the lateral wall of the descending colon.

CT is difficult because of the impossibility of differentiating its early stages. Erasing the (fatty) cleavage plane between the colon and the surrounding structures (retroperitoneum, anterior abdominal wall, liver, spleen, pancreas, or stomach) suggests their tumoral invasion and it grades the tumor in stage T4 [28].

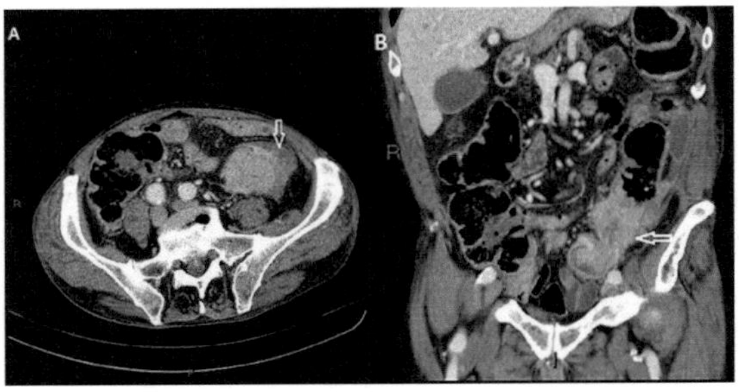

Figure 12. Contrast enhanced abdominal CT performed for suspicion of intestinal occlusion. (a) Axial image (portal phase) shows a voluminous iodophilic sigmoid tumor that obstructs the lumen and seems to invade the peritoneum, associated with a thin layer of perilesional fluid. (b) Coronal image shows perilesional fat stranding and the tendency to invagination.

The value of the method for tumoral staging is centered by its ability to identify the local invasion, the lymph nodes, and parenchymal metastases, firstly in the liver, but also peritoneal, in the lungs and within bones. The size of the lymph nodes is not a good indicator of malignancy because tumor foci may exist in the case of small ones too. However, the alteration of lymph nodes may be suspected in CT when there are associated morphological signs. Thus, the presence of an irregular border, a central necrosis, as well as calcifications or a tendency to conglomerate, may all be suggestive of tumoral lymph node invasion [29]. On the other hand, primary tumor location is closely related to the impairment of certain lymph node stations [27].

The most commonly affected organ by distal dissemination of CRC is the liver. The CT appearance of CRC liver metastases is that of hypodense and hypovascular liver masses as compared with the adjacent healthy liver parenchyma [**Figure 13**]. Sometimes the hepatic metastases reveal the peripheral ring iodophilia during the arterial phase. They may also have a cystic or calcified character; this being often seen in the mucinous colon cancer [27, 29]. CT examination cannot differentiate small liver metastases from benign focal liver lesions. The association of the hepatic steatosis (often seen after chemotherapy) also hinders the diagnosis of liver metastases [30]. However, the abdominal CT with intravenous iodinated contrast, during portal phase, represents the imaging technique of choice for the detection of liver metastases, with high diagnostic accuracy (95%) [5]. The distal dissemination of the (lower) rectal cancer can take place only in the lungs without affecting the liver because of the venous drainage of the rectum (in the inferior vena cava). The chest CT can detect lung metastases that have a unique nodular appearance, sometimes cavitary or calcified. Lymphangitic carcinomatosis associated with pleural effusion is another form of pulmonary metastasis [29, 30]. Peritoneal dissemination is identifiable by the presence of peritoneal thickening and of the tumoral deposits in the omentum, associated with intra-abdominal fluid collections. Bone metastases are rare, and they have a lytic or mixed appearance (lytic and sclerotic) [30]. Brain metastases from colorectal cancer do not have a specific CT appearance, and they cannot be distinguished in imaging from those with other origin [30].

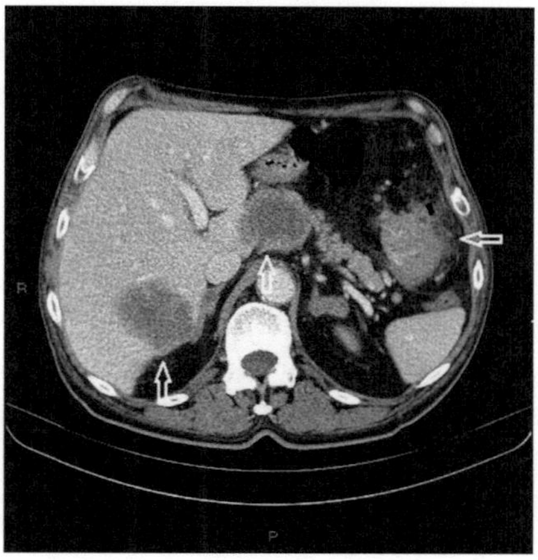

Figure 13. Abdominal CT scan of a 60-year-old male with colon cancer. Axial image (portal phase) shows a tumoral thickening of the colonic wall associated with pericolonic fat stranding, some extra-luminal gas bubbles (tumor perforation) and liver metastases (in segments I and VI).

2.3.1. *CT virtual colonoscopy*

CT virtual colonoscopy is a minimally invasive imaging technique that allows the assessment of both colon and rectum, and also of the extracolonic organs. Its use as a screening method in CRC is much discussed in the literature. Studies about the sensitivity and specificity of this method are varied but the highest values of sensitivity were obtained for the detection of polyps with sizes over 10 mm (95%) [5, 6]. Despite some controversy, CT virtual colonoscopy is useful in elderly subjects with comorbidities, in case of an incomplete optical colonoscopy or if the patient refuses it [5, 6]. Another indication is the evaluation of the entire colon for the exclusion of a synchronous cancer. In addition, a balance of the disease extension can be performed if the examination is made using intravenous contrast agent [5, 31]. The most important contraindications are the acute colic disease (diverticulitis, inflammatory bowel disease in acute stages), presence of intestinal perforation, recent post-polypectomy or immediately after surgery [31, 32]. It is necessary to prepare the colon 24 hours before the examination. This is possible through a diet low in fiber and administration of sodium phosphate, magnesium citrate, or polyethylene glycol. The administration of oral barium or iodine contrast agents allows the "tagging" of the residual stool deposits and the differentiation from colonic polyps. Another method of preparation consists of the use of an oral hyperosmolar contrast agent, thereby achieving an increase in patient compliance [33, 34]. The next step in performing a virtual colonoscopy is the luminal distension by air or by carbon dioxide, under pressure control through a rectal tube. In practice, the carbon dioxide is preferred because of an increased tolerance of the patient and its absorption in the colon mucosa [31, 34]. The acquired images are analyzed in at least two positions (supination and pronation, sometimes lateral decubitus), which allows the differentiation of the colon polyps from residual stool deposits [34]. The interpretation is done by analyzing the 2D and 3D images, along with virtual endoluminal navigation. There is also a software (Computer Aided Detection—CAD) that automatically detects the lesions in the colon. This facilitates lesion detection but it should not exclude the primary analysis of 2D and 3D images [34]. Lesion characterization and classification is possible using the reporting system according to the model "CT Colonography Reporting and Data System (C-RADS)" [35]. This system allows the location, the morphological (sessile, flat, or pedicle tumor), and dimensional analysis of the detected lesion. C0 suggests an inadequate examination and C1 represents the normal appearance of the colon. C2 lesions represent their indeterminate character and they refer to identification of less than three polyps with the diameter between 6 and 9 mm. C3 lesions are represented by either a polyp over 10 mm, or more than three polyps ranging in size from 6 to 9 mm. C4 lesions describe the presence of a colonic tumor mass, with luminal narrowing or the invasion of adjacent organs [32, 35]. The main disadvantages of this method are irradiation (currently decreasing!) and the impossibility to perform biopsy or to treat the detected lesions. There is also a great variability among examiners in image interpretation because of different levels of experience [33].

2.3.2. Water enema CT

Water enema CT is applicable in the case of an inconclusive or impossible optical colonoscopy [36]. The method involves luminal distension of the colon by water enema for about 3 minutes. Water is introduced through an endorectal tube connected to a bag with a volume of approximately 2 L. Initially, images are acquired without the intravenous administration of contrast agent, followed by a post-contrast acquisition. At the end of the examination, the colonic content is discharged by simply lowering the enema bag. Image interpretation is possible in the axial plane with the reconstruction in all three space dimensions [28]. Luminal distension of the colon with water provides a good contrast between the colonic wall and its luminal content. The tumor-free colonic wall is thin, regular, with a thickness below 3 mm and an enhancement in portal phase [28, 36]. A colorectal tumor may appear as an endoluminal polypoid lesion or as a semi- or circumferential irregular parietal thickening, with heterogeneous iodophilia [28]. Some studies show a high accuracy of the method in differentiating the T1-2 tumors from the T3-4 ones. A study performed on a group of 53 patients reveals that the deep parietal invasion (T3-T4) is suggested by the irregular appearance of the outer (peritoneal) tumor margin associated with an angular transition area to the healthy colon [37]. Besides the loco-regional staging (T), the water enema CT allows the overall assessment of the distal colorectal tumor dissemination, with the simultaneous detection of the liver metastases and peritoneal carcinomatosis [37]. Finally, water enema CT is an imaging technique useful in the CRC diagnosis, staging, and characterization because it is cheap, accessible, and easy to perform. In addition, it is easily accepted by patients and it requires no previous colon preparation [28, 37].

http://dx.doi.org/10.5772/62307

2.4. Colon imaging through magnetic resonance

The situation in which we may incidentally detect a colon tumor upon acquiring MRI scans of the abdomen for other purposes is rare. The MRI appearance of the colic tumor is non-specific. Generally, there is a thickening of the colonic wall, with loss of stratification and a slight hypersignal on T2 sequence with fat suppression. The pericolic fat infiltration and the presence of perilesional adenopathies are important additional signs, which may direct the diagnosis toward a colonic tumoral pathology. From a practical standpoint, however, the radiologist must refer toward gastroenterology and colonscopy every patient without known enteral pathology, with suspect thickening of the colon wall. The preferred imaging technique for the staging of colon tumors is computed tomography. Computed tomography has the advantage that allows, on a single imaging examination, to assess both the abdominal and thoracic cavities, including bones and lungs. However, there are situations where the physician can request abdominal MRI for staging an initial colon cancer.

2.5. MRI imaging of the rectum

Because of the critically important information it offers, pelvic MRI examination is mandatory in staging rectal tumors. The sequences to be achieved primarily are the high resolution (HR) T2 weighted images, in all three planes. The examination shall be completed with diffusion sequences. The injection of the intravenous contrast agent is not needed in the local staging of rectal cancer. On the HR T2 sequences, a rectal tumor will appear slightly in hypersignal reported to parietal muscles, and respectively in hyposignal reported to perirectal fat. Because of the existing contrast between the tumor, on the one hand, and the perirectal fat, on the other hand, we do not recommend using the fat suppression. Fat suppression will lead to the underestimation of the perirectal extension of the tumoral process. Most of the times the rectal lumen will also have a content in hypersignal in the plane of the tumor because of mucin secretion. In tumoral stages T1 and T2, tumor growth is limited to the rectal wall [**Figure 14**]. In tumoral stage T1, the tumoral growth does not exceed the submucosa, and in stage T2 it

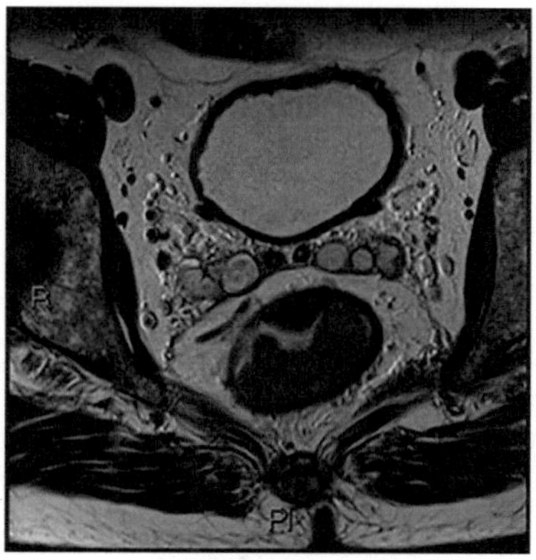

Figure 14. Pelvis MRI, T2 weighted images, axial section. Rectal tumor prominent in rectal lumen. Note that the tumor does not surpass the thin line in hyposignal representing the muscular layer and the perirectal fat is homogeneous. The appearance suggests a T2 stage tumor.

does not exceed the muscularis layer. The MRI examination is not accurate in differentiating tumor stages T1 and T2, but it is very good in determining the existence or absence of the tumoral invasion of the perirectal fat (it can thus differentiate tumors limited to the rectal wall, stages T1 and T2, from the ones extending outside the wall). MRI has a great accuracy in determining the depth of the perirectal invasion [38]. Most of rectal tumors (approximately 80%) will be in T3 stage when imaging diagnosis is performed [**Figure 15**]. Because the depth of the perirectal invasion is an important independent prognostic factor for the survival and chances of curing a rectal tumor, the layering of T3 stage according to the depth of the invasion was necessary (**Table 1**). Thus it is considered that a depth of the perirectal invasion higher than 5mm will lead to a decrease in the survival expectancy at 5 years, from 85 to 54% [39]. The invasion of adjacent organs or structures (bladder, prostate, or seminal vesicles, uterus or ovaries, vagina, peritoneum recesses, the levator ani muscles or the pelvic wall) is considered T4 stage [**Figure 16**]. Apart from a correct local staging, the MRI examination must provide information related to the relationship between the tumor and certain surrounding structures. One of these structures is the mesorectal fascia. A mesorectal fascia without tumoral invasion will allow the total excision of the mesorectum, as this surgical procedure leads to the smallest chance of tumor recurrence. To consider mesorectal fascia as invaded, it is necessary that the tumor exceed it,or that tumoral tissue exists less than 1 mm away from the fascia (the tumoral tissue can be represented either by a direct extension of the tumoral mass, by tumoral deposits within the mesorectum, or by the presence of metastatic lymph nodes). Establishing the invasion or the relationship the tumor has with the mesorectal fascia is one of the advantages of magnetic resonance imaging as compared with transrectal ultrasound. The peritoneum recess is reflected on the upper side of the urinary bladder and on the anterior wall of the upper rectum to form the rectovesical recess. Its invasion is difficult to reveal and it requires knowledge of the normal anatomy. Tumors that will invade the peritoneum will be staged as T4a. Also, MRI examination is superior to transrectal ultrasound in establishing the existence of peritoneal invasion. Furthermore, the existence of invasion of the anal sphincter should be established before surgery because it has great significance in the preoperative planning. It is considered that in the cases of tumoral extension to the rear side of the pubis-rectal muscles,

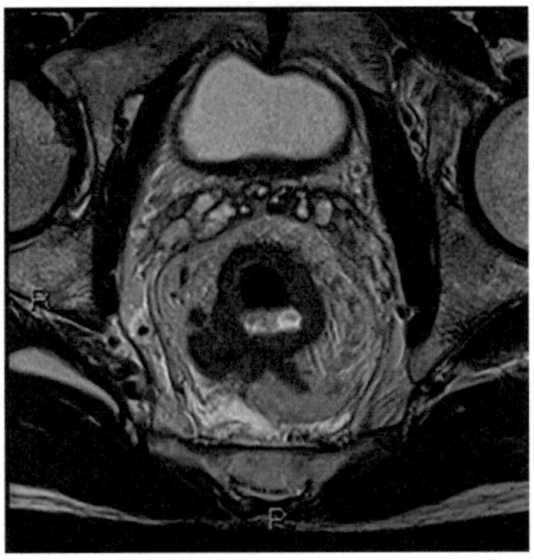

Figure 15. Pelvis MRI, T2 weighted images, axial section. Circumferential rectal tumor, extending into all wall layers and invading the perirectal fat, in right lateral and posterior area.

http://dx.doi.org/10.5772/62307

the surgery with the preservation of the anal sphincter is not feasible. In the case of tumors with sphincter infiltration its extension and the interested structures should be carefully specified on the imaging report because, according to this extension, we will be able to determine whether it is possible or not to perform recto-anal reconstruction procedures or if the patient will be a candidate for the rectum amputation.

Tumoral mass	
Tx	Determination of tumor extension cannot be assessed on the performed examination
T1	Tumor has not spread deeper than the submucosa
T2	Tumor invades muscularis propria, but does not extend into the perirectal fat
T3	Tumor grows through the muscularis propria in mesorectum
T3a	Tumor extends to a depth less than 5 mm beyond the muscularis propria
T3b	Tumor extends 5–10 mm from muscularis propria
T3c	Tumor extends more than 10 mm from muscularis propria
T4a	Tumor invades visceral peritoneum
T4b	Tumor invades organs and structures near the rectum
Adenopathies	
Nx	Lymph node staging cannot be assessed on the performed examination
N0	No obvious metastatic adenopathies
N1a	Tumor invades one lymph node
N1b	Tumor invades two or three lymph nodes
N1c	Tumoral deposits in the subserosa, mesentery, non-peritonealized pericolic, or perirectal tissues without lymph node metastasis
N2a	Metastasis in four up to 6 lymph nodes
N2b	Metastasis in seven or more lymph nodes
M0	No distant metastasis (other than in regional lymph nodes)
M1a	Distant metastasis confined to one organ
M1b	Distant metastasis in more organs or peritoneal carcinomatosis

Table 1. TNM classification adapted from American Joint Committee on Cancer. AJCC Cancer Staging Manual. 7th edition. New York, NY: Springer, 2010.

Lymph nodes that must be assessed during the staging of a rectal tumor belong to the following groups: mesorectum, superior rectal, inferior mesenteric, internal and external iliac, retroperitoneal, and inguinal areas. The most commonly affected lymph nodes are the ones located at mesorectal level, inside the mesorectal fascia. However, it is also important to mention if we consider that lymph nodes located outside the mesorectal fascia are affected by tumoral metastases—they will have to be surgically excised to avoid relapse, or the preoperative radiation therapy should be done on a broader field. If transrectal ultrasound is considered to have roughly similar performances to MRI in revealing the existence of mesorectal lymph nodes, MRI will certainly be better in diagnosing the presence of lymph nodes located outside the mesorectal fascia. MRI is still limited in revealing the malignant or benign character of the detected lymph nodes. Thus, if we use the classic criterion linked to the size of the lymph nodes, using a limit of 5 mm to differentiate the benign lymph nodes from the malignant ones, we will have a sensitivity of 68% and a specificity of 78% for the diagnosis of malignancy [40]. The accuracy of this criterion in the differential diagnosis of benign/malignant perirectal adenopathies is more limited as, between 30 and 50% of the metastatic adenopathies have diameters of less than 5 mm [41]. An irregular outline of lymph nodes, associated with non-homogeneity of the signal inside them, would be considered as being a key indicator of malignancy [40].

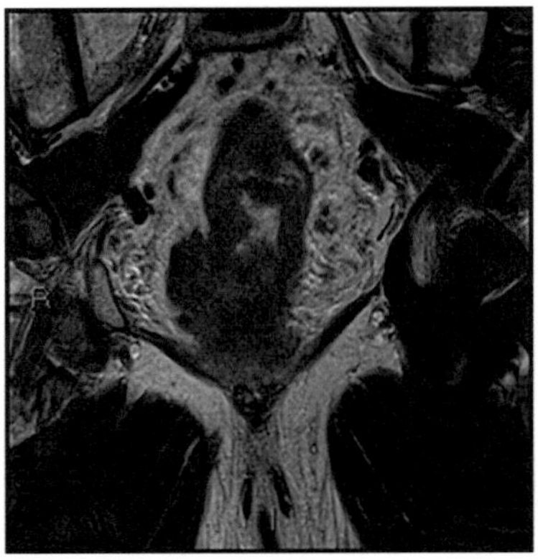

Figure 16. Pelvis MRI, T2 weighted images, coronal section. Rectal tumor with invasion of the perirectal space. Inferior and on the right side the tumor determines the invasion of the levator ani muscles.

2.6. Positron emission tomography (PET-CT)

It is considered that PET-CT does not bring additional information compared with thoraco-abdomino-pelvic CT in the initial staging of colon cancer [42, 43]. There are two situations where PET-CT is recommended in patients with colorectal tumors: (a) patients in which the values of the carcinoembryonic antigen are growing during oncological monitoring and the conventional imaging cannot detect the location of the tumoral recurrence and (b) patients with single liver metastasis, candidates for liver resections. It is considered that, in these patients, performing PET-CT before surgery leads to a decrease in the number of useless laparotomies [44, 45]. It is believed that chemotherapy decreases the sensitivity of PET-CT for diagnosing the colorectal cancer metastases. For this reason, in patients which are potential candidates for liver metastasectomy, we prefer to perform the PET-CT examination before starting chemotherapy to detect other possible tumoral locations.

3. Protocols for the imaging examination of the patient with colon cancer

Most of the times colon tumors are identified through colonoscopy, and imaging helps staging these tumors. If the tumor is located in the colon, the initial staging will be done through abdominal ultrasound and thoraco-abdomino-pelvic CT. In most cases, this will be sufficient for an accurate staging and the images will be later used as reference for the post-treatment examinations. In case lesions detected are considered as being indeterminate, with non-specific computer-tomographic and ultrasound appearance, it will be necessary to complete with other imaging examinations or sampling via an intraoperative biopsy or percutaneous punctures. The imaging techniques that can be used in this situation are contrast enhanced ultrasound (CEUS), magnetic resonance imaging (MRI) or PET-CT. The rectal tumors will benefit from the high-resolution pelvic MRI or transrectal ultrasound for their initial staging. There are situations in which we will find colon tumor formations incidentally in the course of imaging explorations performed for other purposes or for non-specific symptoms. In these cases, we should be advised first of all on the imaging appearance of such tumors. Then, we shall refer to colonoscopy for the confirmation of the existence of a tumoral process.

The staging of the tumor will be made in the same manner as in the case of the tumors diagnosed through colonoscopy. The imaging monitoring of the patients treated for colonic tumors is made through computerized tomography every 6 months. Because of the difficulties in the detection and diagnosis of small liver metastases through computed tomography, our work team recommends to complete the investigations with a liver ultrasound. The images will be permanently correlated with those obtained prior to the treatment, and the lesions with undetermined appearance will benefit from additional diagnostic investigations, similar to those described in the initial staging of the colon tumors. In the patients with tumors found in a later stage, which cannot benefit from curative treatments, it is recommended that the monitoring by thoraco-abdomino-pelvic computer-tomography be made even more often (every 3 months) to evaluate the efficiency of the administered chemotherapy. If, after a series of examinations, the disease evolution is clear, an early change of the chemotherapy scheme can lead to an increased life expectancy.

The patients with operated rectal tumors, especially those who have received neoadjuvant radiotherapy, may receive the recommendation to undergo the pelvic MRI periodically, complementary to the thoraco-abdomino-pelvic computed tomography. This is because MRI is more accurate, compared with the computed tomography, in the differentiation of the tumoral relapses in the pelvic area from the post-irradiation fibrosis.

Author details

Radu I Badea[1], Cosmin N Caraiani[2] and Diana I Florian[2*]

*Address all correspondence to: florian.diana2@yahoo.com

1 Department of Ultrasonography, 3rd Medical Clinic, "Octavian Fodor" Gastroenterology and Hepatology Institute and Imaging Department, "Iuliu Hatieganu" University of Medicine and Pharmacy, Cluj-Napoca, Romania

2 Department of Radiology and Imaging, Hiperdia Clinic and "Octavian Fodor" Gastroenterology and Hepatology Institute, Cluj-Napoca, Romania

References

[1] Carroll MR, Seaman HE, Halloran SP. Tests and investigations for colorectal cancer screening. Clin Biochem 2014;47(10–11):921–939.

[2] Tamas K, Walenkamp AM, de Vries EG, et al. Rectal and colon cancer: Not just a different anatomic site. Cancer Treat Rev 2015;41(8):671–679.

[3] Ferlay J, Steliarova-Foucher E, Lortet-Tieulent J, et al. Cancer incidence and mortality patterns in Europe: Estimates for 40 countries in 2012. Eur J Cancer 2013;49(6):1374–1403.

[4] Binefa G, Rodríguez-Moranta F, Teule A, et al. Colorectal cancer: From prevention to personalized medicine. World J Gastroenterol 2014;20(22):6786–6808.

[5] van de Velde CJ, Boelens PG, Borras JM, et al. EURECCA colorectal: Multidisciplinary management: European consensus conference colon & rectum. Eur J Cancer 2014;50(1): 1–34.

[6] Tudyka V, Blomqvist L, Beets-Tan RG, et al. EURECCA consensus conference highlights about colon &rectal cancer multidisciplinary management: The radiology experts review. Eur J Surg Oncol 2014;40(4):469–475.

[7] Qaseem A, Denberg TD, Hopkins RH, et al. Screening for colorectal cancer: A guidance Statement From the American College of Physicians. Ann Intern Med 2012;156:378–386.

[8] O'Malley M, Wilson S. US of gastrointestinal tract abnormalities with CT correlation. Radiographics 2003;23:59–72.

[9] Chung HW, Chung JB, Park SW, et al. Comparison of hydrocolonic sonography accuracy in preoperative staging between colon and rectal cancer. World J Gastroenterol 2004;10(8):1157–1161.

[10] Liao D, Frokjaer JB, Yang J, et al. Three-dimensional surface model analysis in the gastrointestinal tract. World J Gastroenterol 2006;12:2870–2875.

[11] Martínez-Ares D, Martín-Granizo Barrenechea I, Souto-Ruzo J, et al. The value of abdominal ultrasound in the diagnosis of colon cancer. Rev Esp Enferm Dig 2005;97:877–886.

[12] Glover C, Douse P, Kane P, et al. Accuracy of investigations for asymptomatic colorectal liver metastases. Dis Colon Rectum 2002;45:476–484.

[13] Robinson PJ. Imaging liver metastases: current limitations and future prospects. Br J Radiol 2000;73:234–241.

[14] Dietrich CF, Kratzer W, Strobe D, et al. Assessment of metastatic liver disease in patients with primary extrahepatic tumors by contrast-enhanced sonography versus CT and MRI. World J Gastroenterol 2006;12:1699–1705.

[15] Claudon M, Cosgrove D, Albrecht T, et al. Guidelines and good clinical practice recommendations for contrast enhanced ultrasound (CEUS) – update 2008. Ultraschall Med 2008;29:28–44.

[16] Hanbidge AE, Lynch D, Wilson SR. US of the peritoneum. Radio Graphics 2003;23:663–684.

[17] Badea R, Badea Gh, Philippi W, et al. The value and limits of endorectal sonography in the preoperative stage classification of rectal cancer. Ultraschall Med 1988;9(6): 265 – 269.

[18] Santoro GA, D'Elia A, Battistella G, et al. The use of a dedicated rectosigmoidoscope for ultrasound staging of tumours of the upper and middle third of the rectum. Colorectal Dis 2006;9: 61 – 66.

[19] Neciu C, Badea R, Chiorean L, et al. Oral and IV Contrast Enhanced Ultrasonography of the digestive tract – a useful completion of the B-mode examination: A literature review and an exhaustive illustration through images. Med Ultrason 2015;17(1):62–73.

[20] Lu M, Yan B, Song J, et al. Double-contrast-enhanced sonography for diagnosis of rectal lesions with pathologic correlation. J Ultrasound Med 2014;33:575–583.

[21] Waage JE, Havre RF, Odegaard S, et al. Endorectal elastography in the evaluation of rectal tumours. Colorectal Dis 2011;13:1130–1137.

[22] Badea R, Vasile T, Seiceanu A. Romanian three dimensional ultrasonography of the lower gastrointestinal tract – A new ultrasound examination technique or an alternative to endoscopy? J Gastroenterol 2001;10(3):251 –257.

[23] Kim MJ. Transrectal ultrasonography of anorectal diseases: advantages and disadvantages. Ultrasonography 2015;34(1):19–31.

[24] Puli SR, Reddy JB, Bechtold ML, et al. Accuracy of endoscopic ultrasound to diagnose nodal invasion by rectal cancers: A meta-analysis and systematic review. Ann Surg Oncol 2009;16:1255–1265.

[25] Wang Y, Zhou CW, Hao YZ, et al. Improvement in T-staging of rectal carcinoma: Using a novel endorectal ultrasonography technique with sterile coupling gel filling the rectum. Ultrasound Med Biol 2012;38:574–579.

[26] Al-Sukhni E, Milot L, Fruitman M, et al. Diagnostic accuracy of MRI for assessment of T category, lymph node metastases, and circumferential resection margin involvement in patients with rectal cancer: a systematic review and meta-analysis. Ann Surg Oncol 2012;19:2212–2223.

[27] Horton KM, Abrams RA, Fishman EK. Spiral CT of colon cancer: Imaging features and role in management. Radiographics 2000;20(2):419–430.

[28] Ridereau-Zins C. Imaging in colonic cancer. Diagn Interv Imaging 2014;95(5):475–483.

[29] Kijima S, Sasaki T, Nagata K, et al. Preoperative evaluation of colorectal cancer using CT colonography, MRI, and PET/CT. World J Gastroenterol 2014;20(45):16964–16975.

[30] Tirumani SH, Kim KW, Nishino M, et al. Update on the role of imaging in management of metastatic colorectal cancer. Radiographics 2014;34(7):1908–1928.

[31] Laghi A. Computed tomography colonography in 2014: An update on technique and indications. World J Gastroenterol 2014;20(45):16858–16867.

[32] American College of Radiology. ACR practice guideline for the performance of computed tomography (CT) colonography in adults: Reston VA. ACR Practice Guideline: American College of Radiology 2009;36:1–10.

[33] Levine MS, Yee J. History, evolution, and current status of radiologic imaging tests for colorectal cancer screening. Radiology 2014;273(2):S160-S180.

[34] Gandon Y. Screening for colorectal cancer: The role of CT colonography. Diagn Interv Imaging 2014;95(5):467–474.

[35] Zalis ME, Barish MA, Choi JR, et al. CT colonography reporting and data system: A consensus proposal. Radiology 2005;236(1):3–9.

[36] Ridereau-Zins C, AubéC, Luet D, et al. Assessment of water enema computed tomography: An effective imaging technique for the diagnosis of colon cancer: Colon cancer: Computed tomography using a water enema. Abdom Imaging 2010;35(4):407–413.

[37] Sibileau E, Ridereau-Zins C, Vanel D, et al. Accuracy of water-enema multidetector computed tomography (WE-MDCT) in colon cancer staging: A prospective study. Abdom Imaging 2014;39(5):941–948.

[38] MERCURY Study Group. Extramural depth of tumor invasion at thin-section MR in patients with rectal cancer: Results of the MERCURY study. Radiology 2007;243(1):132–139.

[39] Merkel S, Mansmann U, Siassi M, et al. The prognostic inhomogeneity in p T3 rectal carcinomas. Int J Colorectal Dis 2001;16(5):298–304.

[40] Brown G, Richards CJ, Bourne MW, et al. Morphologic predictors of lymph node status in rectal cancer with use of high-spatial-resolution MR imaging with histopathologic comparison. Radiology 2003;227(2):371–377.

[41] Kotanagi H, Fukuoka T, Shibata Y, et al. The size of regional lymph nodes does not correlate with the presence or absence of metastasis in lymph nodes in rectal cancer. J Surg Oncol 1993;54(4):252–254.

[42] Furukawa H, Ikuma H, Seki A, et al. Positron emission tomography scanning is not superior to whole body multidetector helical computed tomography in the preoperative staging of colorectal cancer. Gut 2006; 55:1007-1011.

[43] Nahas CS, Akhurst T, Yeung H, et al. Positron emission tomography detection of distant metastatic or synchronous disease in patients with locally advanced rectal cancer receiving preoperative chemoradiation. Ann Surg Oncol 2008;15:704-711.

[44] Whiteford MH, Whiteford HM, Yee LF, et al. Usefulness of FDG-PET scan in the assessment of suspected metastatic or recurrent adenocarcinoma of the colon and rectum. Dis Colon Rectum 2000;43:759-767.

[45] Flamen P, Hoekstra OS, Homans F, et al. Unexplained rising carcinoembryonic antigen (CEA) in the postoperative surveillance of colorectal cancer: the utility of positron emission tomography (PET). Eur J Cancer 2001;37:862-869.

Chapter 7

Endoscopic Submucosal Dissection for Early Colon Cancer

Valentin Ignatov, Anton Tonev, Nikola Kolev,
Aleksandar Zlatarov, Shteryu Shterev,
Tanya Kirilova and Krasimir Ivanov

Additional information is available at the end of the chapter

http://dx.doi.org/10.5772/63441

Abstract

Endoscopic submucosal dissection (ESD) was first implemented in early gastric cancer allowing for en-bloc resection of the lesions. With the experience came the expertise to introduce ESD for early colon cancer (ECC). ESD demonstrates several advantages in comparison with the endoscopic mucosa resection. It allows accurate histological assessment of the depth of invasion, minimizes the risk of local recurrence and helps in the determination of additional therapy. Indications for ESD are placed only after adequate endoscopic morphological classification of the lesions excluding higher risk of nodal metastases. This chapter provides an overview of the application of ESD techniques in ESD for ECC and provides assessment on its technical aspects and complications. In order to decrease the rate of complications a standard protocol for the ESD should be adopted. The protocol includes recommendations for patient selection, bowel and patient preparation, appropriate equipment (knives, endoscopes, and power devices). The chapter will review the current ESD techniques and oncological results. ESD could have great impact on the treatment of early colon cancer. Its role is already proven in rectal localizations and despite the challenges it should be adopted for the colon. Safe strategy for ESD is the cornerstone in decreasing complications, which includes suitable resection of specialized ESD devices.

Keywords: Early colon cancer, endoscopic submucosal dissection, minimally invasive treatment

1. Introduction

The endoscopic treatment method for gastrointestinal neoplastic lesion has developed in recent years. Another modality to the existing techniques is the endoscopic submucosal dissection which is a novel method which broadens the possibilities for endoscopic treatment of neoplastic lesion. First introduced in Japan for early gastric cancer, now the method has advanced and is also applied for early colon cancer. After gaining initial experience the ESD can be used safely on condition that the indications are strictly followed and the technical issues and associated complications are recognized. The chapter will review the current ESD techniques and oncological results. ESD could have great impact on the treatment of early colon cancer. Its role is already proven in rectal localizations and despite the challenges it should be adopted for the colon. Safe strategy for ESD is the cornerstone in decreasing complications, which includes suitable resection of specialized ESD devices.

2. Indications for colonic ESD

The indications for ESD are object of debate. The Colon ESD standardization Implementation Working Group has proposed a draft of "Criteria of Indications for Colorectal ESD). They include large-sized (more than 20 mm in diameter) lesion, which are unsuitable for snare endoscopic mucosal resection, non-granular types of laterally spreading tumours, lesion with type VI pit pattern, cancer with less than 1000 μm submucosal infiltration, large depressed-type lesions, large elevated lesion, suspected of cancer [1]. Additional indications for ESD include sporadic tumours in IBD, local residual carcinoma after endoscopic piecemeal resection, mucosal lesion with fibrosis, adenoma with non-lifting sign.

The diagnostic process includes chromo-endoscopy, magnified endoscopy, NBI-enhanced magnified endoscopy or EUS. The histological confirmation of diagnosis is not required because the adequate chromo-endoscopic evaluation is confirmed to be sufficient. Biopsy is not always required. The occurring submucosal fibrosis may increases the difficulty of the procedure and the associated risk [2].

3. Muscle retracting sign

Other useful criteria which may help the selection of patients suitable for ESD is the muscle retracting (MR) sign. The MR sign is described as retraction of muscularis propria with submucosal fibrosis. ESD of lesions with positive MR sign is more difficult, which poses as a threat for a safe procedure [2]. Usually in such cases ESD is aborted. The sign is not universally exhibited by all larger lesions with protruding areas, despite the morphological similarities. The conclusion is that MR sign may serve as indication for difficult ESD with risk of resection failure. Therefore it may indicate patients for surgical resection to avoid adverse events and complications of the ESD.

http://dx.doi.org/10.5772/63441

4. CO2 insufflation

The ESD is performed after insufflation of the colon lumen with CO 2, which has been proven to be effective [3]. It decreases the risk of pneumoperitoneum in cases of perforation and further complications, related to the ESD.

5. Treatment devices

ESD is technically dependent method and various devices have been introduced. Most of them have been developed in Japan [1, 4–21] (**Figure 1**). The devices can be divided in two more general categories: needle-knife type and grasping type.

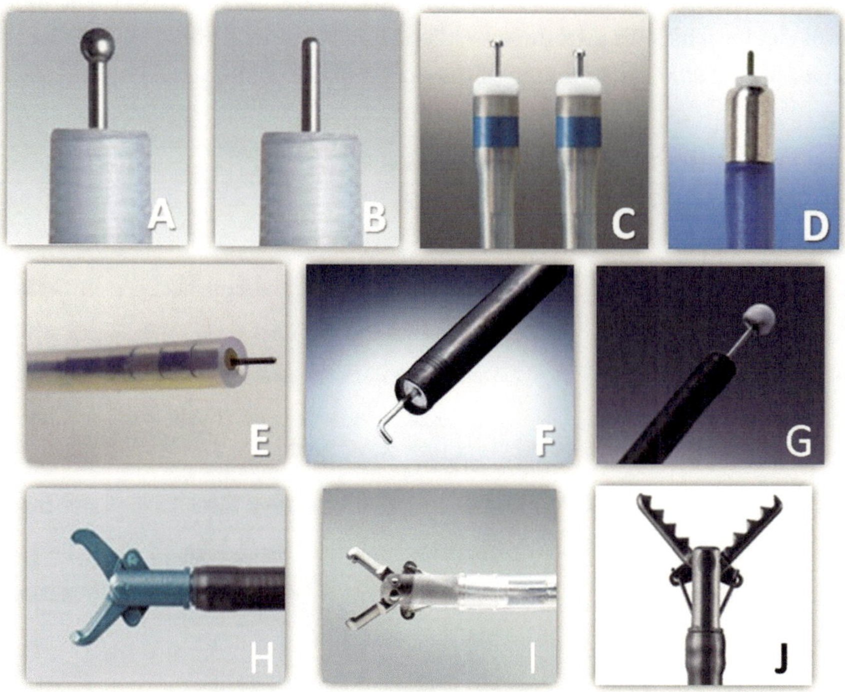

Figure 1. Devices used for colonic endoscopic submucosal dssection: A: Flush Knife (Fujifilm Medical, Tokyo, Japan); B: Flush Knife Ball Tip (Fujifilm Medical, Tokyo, Japan); C: DualKnife (Olympus Medical Systems Co., Tokyo, Japan); D: B-Knife (Zeon Medical, Tokyo, Japan); E: Splash needle (Pentax Co., Tokyo, Japan); F: Hook Knife (Olympus Medical Systems Co., Tokyo, Japan); G: IT Knife 2 (Olympus Medical Systems Co., Tokyo, Japan); H: Clutch Cutter (Fujifilm, Tokyo, Japan); I: SB knife Jr (Sumitomo Bakelite); J: Hemostat-Y forceps (PENTAX Medical, Germany).

The needle-type knife device has two modifications – uncovered and covered type. The Flush Knife (Fujifilm Medical, Tokyo, Japan), the DualKnife (OlympusMedical Systems Co., Tokyo, Japan), the B-Knife (Zeon Medical, Tokyo, Japan), and the Splash needle (Pentax Co., Tokyo, Japan) belong to the obtuse, short tipped types [22–24]. As suggested by their name, the Flush Knife and the Splash needle also have the capability to inject substances in the submucosa.

This option is very helpful, because it obviates the need to change the injection and the cutting device during the procedure [23, 25]. Having a ball-disk at the tip, the Dual Knife is able to hook the submucosa, separate it from the muscularis propria. In contrast to the monopolar devices, the BKnife is a bipolar knife and therefore it may reduce the risk of complications. The HookKnife is usually used in cases of poor submucosal elevation [26]. Because of the special tip, the submucosa can be hooked and separated from muscularis propria and be safely cut [30]. On the other hand, the DualKnife and the Flush Knife are short tipped and may cause perforation of the thin wall of the colon in the presence of folds. The Flush Knife has two modifications – with needle tip and ball tip. Another product of Olympus Medical Systems Co. is the insulated-tipped knife 2 (IT Knife 2). Its efficacy is reported to be high when used for gastric lesion [27]. The procedure time is reported to be shortened because of the faster dissection time due to the longer blade. It also enables coagulation of small vessels. However, it is difficult to manipulate with this device and the long blade may also cause long perforations. A new device was later introduced, called IT knife nano. Its blade is smaller than of the IT Knife 2 and is targeted for submucosal dissection of the colon.

Author	**Year**	**Country**	**Number of cases**	**Main device**	**Generator**
Tamegai et al.	2007	Japan	71	Hook Knife	
Hurlstone et al.	2007	UK	42	Flex knife, IT knife	–
Fujishiro et al.	2007	Japan	200	Flex knife, Hook Knife, electrosurgical knife	ICC-2(X) or VI0300D
Zhou et al.	2009	China	74	Needle-knife, IT knife, Hook Knife	ICC-200
Isomoto et al.	2009	Japan	292	Flex knife, Hash knife, Hook Knife	ICC-200 or VI0300D
Saito et al.	2009	Japan	405	Bipolar needle knife (B-knife), IT knife	–
Iizuka et al.	2009	Japan	38	Flex knife	ICC-200 or VI0300D
Hotta et al.	2010	Japan	120	Flex knife, Flush Knife, Hook Knife	ICC-200 or VI0300D
Niimi et al.	2010	Japan	310	Flex knife, Hook Knife, electrosurgical knife	ICC-200 or VI0300D
Yoshida et al.	2010	Japan	250	Flush Knife	VI0300D
Toyonaga et al.	2010	Japan	512	Flex knife, Flush Knife	–
Matsumoto et al.	2010	Japan	203	Flex knife, Hook Knife, Dual Knife	–
Uraoka et al.	2011	Japan	202	B-Knife, Dual Knife, IT knife, mucoscctome	–
Shono et al.	2011	Japan	137	Flush Knife, Hook Knife, precutting knife	–
Kim et al.	2011	Korea	108	Flex knife, Hook Knife	VI0300D
Lee et al.	2011	Korea	499	Flex knife, Hook Knife	VI0300D
Probst et al.	2012	Germany	76	Hook Knife, IT knife, triangle knife	VI0300D
Okamoto et al.	2013	Japan	30	Dual Knife, mucosectome-2	VI0300D
Nawata et al.	2014	Japan	150	SB knife Jr, IT knife nano	–

Table 1. List of most commonly used devices and generators.

The grasping type devices have two major representatives – Clutch Cutter device (Fujifilm, Tokyo, Japan) and SB knife Jr (Sumitomo Bakelite) [21, 28]. The cutting method involves use of grasping type scissor forceps. It avoids fixing the knife to the target, although their use is associated with higher risk of perforation and bleeding after unexpected bowel movement [28]. Another useful device is the Hemostat-Y forceps (H-S2518; Pentax Co., Tokyo, Japan), which is used in bipolar mode to control visible bleeding and minimize the risk of any burning effect on the muscle layer. Some authors describe the use of double-balloon colonoscope in cases of difficult lesion location or to avoid paradoxical movement [29]. The procedure requires electrosurgical device. On **Table 1** are presented the most commonly used generators.

6. Practical aspects of the ESD

The bowel preparation is essential for a successful ESD. Any feces and liquid should be cleared from the colon. If any still remains in the lumen, ESD should not be initiated. The feces do not only prevent adequate dissection, but also pose as a serious treat in case of perforation.

A single channel general lower gastrointestinal endoscope is used for the procedure. Some centres have adopted the use of upper gastrointestinal endoscope. It is slimmer and can be used in retroflexed position [4]. The tip of the endoscope can be fitted with a transparent cap (Olympus Medical Systems Co., Tokyo, Japan).

ESD starts with submucosal injection. It is crucial to maintain adequate elevation during the procedure. Different solutions have been used. Some centres use in their practice two solutions: Glyceol (10% glycerin and 5% fructose; Chugai Pharmaceutical Co., Ltd., Tokyo, Japan) mixed with a small amount of Indigo Carmine and epinephrine, and 0.4% sodium hyaluronate solution (MucoUp; Seikagaku Corp, Tokyo, Japan) [30]. First, small amount of Glyceol is injected in the submucosal layer to confirm the appropriate localization and then MucoUp is injected until proper elevation is achieved. The final step is to inject small amout of Glyceol to flush the residual MucoUp [31]. Repeated submucosal injections are required during the procedure to maintain adequate submucosal elevation [29].

7. Sedation

ESD is usually a long procedure and can continue for more than 2.5 hours. Additionally, the abdominal discomfort caused by gas insufflation causes restlessness. Restlessness due to abdominal fullness and pain occurs frequently in cases with an operation time exceeding 2.5 h. Several medicaments are used for sedation. Some authors report use of midazolam and pentazocine with monitoring by automatic blood pressure monitor. They observed restlessness in 15 out of these 22 cases (68.1%) despite conscious sedation when the procedure lasted more than 2.5 hours. When the procedure lasted less than 2.5 h, restlessness was observed in only 10 out of 83 cases (12.0%) [32]. Carbon dioxide insufflations have also been reported to be effective for the prevention of abdominal fullness [33]. Another option is the use of propofol for conscious sedation which could be used for longer procedure without restlessness and discomfort [10].

8. Technique of ESD

The process of ESD is divided in several consecutive steps which are presented on **Figure 2**. After adequate elevation of the mucosa has been achieved, the process is initiated. The first step is mucosal incision and simultaneous incision to the deep submucosa layer. The lifting solution is injected at the proximal end of the lesion and mucosal incision is made. Sometimes the insertion of the endoscopic tip into the submucosal layer may become difficult and in these cases trimming of the mucosa is performed. To clear space for dissection after the trimming the submucosal layer near the mucosa is precisely cut. One of the practices for the mucosal incision is to circumvent the tumour. In cases where partial circumferential incision is performed the proximal side of the lesion is incised after the submucosal injection. Various endocut modes are recommended for the incision, which depend on the generator used. The described techniques for incision have their advantages and disadvantages. The circumferential incision may lead to undesired leakage of lifting liquid and loss of submucosal elevation. When injected at the distal side the tumour takes perpendicular to the endoscope position, which may hamper the dissection. The remaining uncut mucosa at the distal side pulls the tumour upward and also changes the position of the tumour. These situations are observed for tumours larger than 50 mm. When the incision is partially circumferential the elevation of the mucosa is easily maintained, because the uncut residual mucosa prevents liquid leakage. On the other hand after the partial resection of the tumour, the residual mucosa may become difficult for resection. Therefore each approach has its advantages and disadvantages. The specific type of incision should be chosen according to the tumour characteristics such as size,

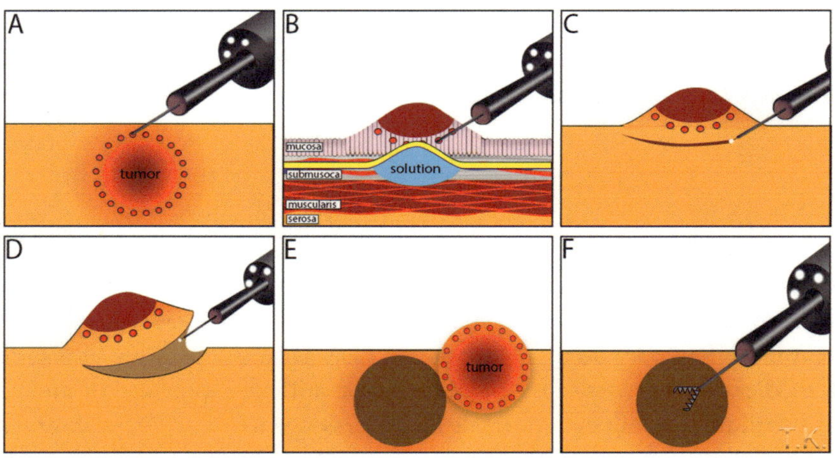

Figure 2. Steps of endoscopic submucosal dissection for early stage colon cancer: A: electrocautery marking around the lesion; B: injection of solution underneath the lesion; C: incision around the lesion; D: lifting and removal of the lesion; E: extraction of the tumor; F: meticulous hemostasis.

location, types of knives. During the submucosal dissection, the endoscopist can easily recognize the advantages of ESD. Structures such as vessels, fibrosis, etc. are clearly visible. Hemorrhage is controlled by precoagulation of the blood vessels. The thinner vessels are coagulated by cutting devices. The thicker ones can be dealt with forceps. Unlike for adenomatous lesion, in cases of early colon cancer the cutting line should be near the mucosal layer in order to achieve R0 resection. This step should be carried out with precision due to the higher perforation risk. The ESD is only finalized after careful inspection for any bleeding vessels. If any are found these are coagulated.

9. Complications

ESD in the colon is technically challenging procedure due to the anatomical characteristic of the colon. The latter is a long luminal organ with many folds, which impede the manipulation of the endoscope. The thin walls are easier to penetrate in comparison to the gastric wall. The insuflated gas during longer procedures may cause paradoxical movement of the endoscope. This situation occurs specifically in tumour, located above the sigmoid colon. It is difficult to find specific studies only on colon ESD. Therefore the presented data will cover also outcomes of colorectal ESD, bearing in mind that the rectal manipulations are easier due to the length of this segment. The rate of perforation of ESD is dramatically high when compared with that observed for endoscopic mucosal resection (EMR) [34–36] and has been reported to be 1.4–10.4%. According to several clinical studies the predicting factors for perforation are large lesions (>30 mm), fibrosis, colonic location and less experience with ESD [12, 22, 37, 38]. (**Table 2**).

The use of knife coagulation is considered the most common cause of perforation [39]. As described in the previous section, the obtuse knives such as DualKnife and the Flush Knife can easily cause perforation. In contrast the Hook Knife is able to hook up the mucosa, separate it from the submucosal layer and cut it safely. Other reasons for perforation include snare resection, coagulation by special haemostatic forceps with soft coagulation, endoscopic clipping onto coagulated submucosa [39]. The complications following ESD for colon tumour can be severe and even fatal in case of peritonitis. Alarming symptoms for perforation are abdominal tympanism, emphysema, and abdominal pain and muscle resistance. Most of the perforation cases are treated conservatively without emergency surgery. Although the closure of the mucus defect is practiced in several centres in Japan, this practice is currently considered impractical and technically challenging with the available devices, e.g. hemo-clips. Endoscopic clipping is possible for small perforation [40, 41]. The abdominal distention can be treated by decompression of the peritoneum via 20 Fr needle [10]. A new closure device which consists of clip with a loop may come in handy [42]. In some cases the perforation is not detected during endoscopy and only later on computed tomography. The possible explanation is that microperforations occur during ESD on deep injection by the needle. Those cases are not clinically significant and can be safely treated by conservative measures, such as stopping of oral intake. Another specific case of perforation is the delayed perforation. It accounts to 0.3% to 0.7% of the perforations [4, 5, 43] and is considered to be related to excessive coagulation in the muscularis propria. Usually delayed perforations are large in size and therefore require emergency surgery [4, 5, 43]. Bleeding after ESD is another common complication. The usual practice is to cut any vessel below 2 mm in diameter with a knife in coagulation mode. For vessels larger than 2 mm in diameter, a special haemostatic forceps should be used in soft coagulation mode. These forceps have the ability to gently catch the vessel and lift it upwards from muscularis propria. The surrounding mucosa around the vessel is also resected with the forceps. Removal of the coagulated vessel and the surrounding submucosa ensures safer and easier submucosal dissection. In cases when bleeding cannot be stopped by the knife the haemostatic forceps can be used as well with SOFT coagulation mode. The rate of postoperative haemorrhage in ESD is reported to be 0–12.0% (**Table 1**) [4, 5, 8–10, 22, 23, 25, 26, 44]. Most cases of postoperative haemorrhage are treated only by endoscopic clipping and withholding oral intake without emergency surgery or blood transfusion.

Author	Year	Country	Number of cases	Post-ESD perforation rate	Bleeding rate
Tamegai et al.	2007	Japan	71	–	1.4%
Hurlstone et al.	2007	UK	42	2.4%	9.5%
Fujishiro et al.	2007	Japan	200	6.0%	0.5%
Zhou et al.	2009	China	74	8.1%	1.4%
Isomoto et al.	2009	Japan	292	7.9%	0.7%
Saito et al.	2009	Japan	405	3.5%	1.0%
Iizuka et al.	2009	Japan	38	7.9%	–
Hotta et al.	2010	Japan	120	7.5%	–
Niimi et al.	2010	Japan	310	4.8%	1.6%
Yoshida et al.	2010	Japan	250	6.0%	2.4%
Toyonaga et al.	2010	Japan	512	1.8%	1.6%
Matsumoto et al.	2010	Japan	203	6.9%	–
Uraoka et al.	2011	Japan	202	2.5%	0.5%
Shono et al.	2011	Japan	137	3.6%	3.6%
Kim et al.	2011	Korea	108	20.4%	–
Lee et al.	2011	Korea	499	7.4%	–
Probst et al.	2012	Germany	76	1.3%	7.9%
Okamoto et al.	2013	Japan	30	0.0%	0.0%
Nawata et al.	2014	Japan	150	0.0%	0.0%

Table 2. Rate of complications after colorectal ESD from single center studies.

Another common effect after ESD is local inflammation to a certain degree. C-reactive protein level may rise to 5,82 ± 12.10 mg/L 2 days after the procedure in cases with perforation and

1.27 ± 2.00 mg/L in cases without perforation [45]. Fever and abdominal pain were also reported without perforation. A rare complication was acute colon obstruction after ESD of a colonic tumour located at the cecal base [46].

10. Clinical Studies on Colorectal ESD

Several large series on colorectal ESD have been published from Asian centres. However, most of the data are retrospective, and direct prospective comparative data on ESD versus EMR or surgery are not available. The Japan Society for Cancer of the Colon and Rectum conducted a multi-centre, observational study for all patients treated by conventional endoscopic resection and ESD for colorectal neoplasms exceeding 20 mm in size from October 2007 to December 2010 [9]. A total of 816 lesions were treated by ESD and the short-term outcomes were as follows. The mean lesion size was about 40 mm in diameter. *En bloc* resection was achieved in more than 90% of the cases, regardless of lesion size, with a perforation rate of 2.0% and delayed bleeding rate of 2.2%. None of the perforation cases needed emergency surgery as most

Author	Year	Country	Number of cases	En bloc resection rate	Complete en bloc resection rate
Tamegai et al.	2007	Japan	71	98.6%	95.8%
Hurlstone et al.	2007	UK	42	78.6%	73.8%
Fujishiro et al.	2007	Japan	200	91.5%	70.5%
Zhou et al.	2009	China	74	93.2%	89.2%
Isomoto et al.	2009	Japan	292	90.1%	79.8%
Saito et al.	2009	Japan	405	86.9%	–
Iizuka et al.	2009	Japan	38	60.5%	57.9%
Hotta et al.	2010	Japan	120	93.3%	51.0%
Niimi et al.	2010	Japan	310	90.3%	74.5%
Yoshida et al.	2010	Japan	250	86.8%	81.2%
Toyonaga et al.	2010	Japan	512	98.2%	
Matsumoto et al.	2010	Japan	203	–	85.7%
Uraoka et al.	2011	Japan	202	90.6%	–
Shono et al.	2011	Japan	137	89.1%	85.4%
Kim et al.	2011	Korea	108	–	78.7%
Lee et al.	2011	Korea	499	95.0%	–
Probst et al.	2012	Germany	76	81.6%	69.7%
Okamoto et al.	2013	Japan	30	100.0%	–
Nawata et al.	2014	Japan	150	98.7%	97.3%

Table 3. Rate of en-bloc resections and complete en-bloc resections after colorectal ESD from single center studies.

iatrogenic perforations is very small, and can be successfully closed with endoscopic clip placement alone followed by intravenous antibacterial therapy (nothing *per os*).

A recent systematic review reported resection rates of 90.5% (61–98.2%) for endoscopic en bloc resection and of 76.9% (58–95.6%) for histologically confirmed complete resection, with associated local recurrence rates of 1.9% (0–11%) (**Table 3**) [30]. In addition, there are several studies with >500 ESD procedures, including large single centre series [47, 48], multi-centre surveys [49, 50], and a prospective multi-centre study [51]. These series confirm the high "en bloc" resection rates (up to 88.8% histologically confirmed complete resections) and the reported complication rates (perforation 4.8–5.4%, delayed perforation 0.4–0.7%, bleeding 1.5–1.7%). It was also demonstrated that ESD is feasible not only for the resection of adenoma or superficial cancers, but is also curative for submucosal invasive cancer. Thus, submucosal invasion limited to the upper 1,000 inlinegraphic m of the submucosal layer (sm1) is sufficiently treated with local resection if the tumour has a G1/G2 differentiation and no lymphatic or vascular invasion (L0, V0) [52–55]. When compared to EMR, data on ESD consistently show a higher en bloc resection rate/lower recurrence rate. Thus, in an analysis of 26 studies on EMR, en bloc resection for relatively smaller target lesions was possible in only 42.6% (19.2–91.8%) and recurrence rates were 17% (4.8–31.4%) for lesions resected in a piecemeal fashion [9]. In addition, several retrospective case series [35, 56–58], a matched case control analysis [59], and a meta-analysis [60] were published on the comparative analysis of EMR versus ESD. All these reports show a higher efficacy of ESD for the resection of larger sessile or flat lesions, resulting in a lower recurrence rate. When analysing risk factors for adenoma recurrence after EMR, associations were reported with size and morphology of the lesions (higher risk of incomplete resection for serrated adenoma/flat adenoma), piecemeal resection, and number of fragments [61–65]. Data on complications after EMR/ESD show similar bleeding rates (EMR 0–11.1%; ESD 0.5–9.5%), but the perforation rate is higher for ESD (1.3–20%) than for EMR (0–5.8%). However, the vast majority of perforations occurring during ESD are small and easily treated during the procedure, and thus the actual need for emergency surgery does not differ for EMR versus ESD [14, 18, 49, 66–68]. ESD is technically demanding and does require long procedure times. Thus, a recent study comparing 1,029 cases of conventional EMR with 816 ESD procedures showed a significantly higher procedure time for ESD (96 min) than for EMR (18 min). Procedure times increased with the size of the lesion, although for very large lesions a comparison to laparoscopic surgery would be more appropriate [66, 67]. Comparative data are available for ESD versus surgery, but again without a formal head-to-head study. Two smaller retrospective studies found no significant difference for efficacy (including procedure time) and safety between ESD versus transanal endoscopic microsurgery (TEM) for the treatment of early rectal cancer [69, 70]. A recently published systematic review and meta-analysis of 11 ESD and 10 TEM studies showed higher en bloc resection rates and a reduced need for additional surgery for TEM, while recurrence rates were significantly lower after ESD and no difference in the overall complication rate was observed [71]. Finally, a comparative retrospective study from the National Cancer Centre Tokyo found that ESD is equally effective as laparoscopic surgery for the treatment of early colorectal cancer, with significantly lower complication rates and shorter procedure times [72]. Indeed, the accompanying editorial called for an initiative to disseminate ESD for optimal treatment of early colorectal cancer [73]. While larger studies on colorectal ESD are almost exclusively from Asia, data on colorectal ESD from Western countries is mostly limited to the distal colon [9, 19, 74–77](**Table 1**). Taken together, there are considerable advantages of ESD over EMR for the resection of larger sessile or flat lesions, in particular high enbloc resection rates and low recurrence rates. The major problem of ESD is the technical challenge and the relatively long procedure time. Compared with surgery, ESD shows similar performance as TEM for rectal lesions, while a clear advantage – both for clinical outcome and procedure time – was observed in a single comparative study for ESD versus laparoscopic surgery for the treatment of T1 colorectal carcinoma. Nevertheless, there still is a need for prospective comparative trials to better define the role of ESD in comparison to EMR or surgery.

11. Conclusion

ESD is an attractive endoscopic treatment modality for larger sessile or flat adenomas/ superficial or slightly submucosal invasive colorectal cancers. ESD is a reliable method for achieving en bloc resection of relatively large colorectal superficial neoplasms, with superior curability. Still, ESD is associated with technical difficulties and complications, including perforation. Therefore patients should be selected for ESD only according to strict criteria, including tumour characteristics. The prerequisite for ESD is proper diagnosis, established by magnifying endoscopy, endoscopic ultrasound, etc. While colorectal ESD has recently become a standard procedure in major Asian endoscopy centres, propagation of ESD in Western countries will critically depend on opportunities for specialized training and probably also on technical developments to facilitate ESD and reduce procedure times.

Author details

Valentin Ignatov, Anton Tonev*, Nikola Kolev, Aleksandar Zlatarov, Shteryu Shterev, Tanya Kirilova and Krasimir Ivanov

*Address all correspondence to: teraton@abv.bg

Department of General and Operative Surgery, Medical University Varna, Bulgaria

References

[1] Shono T, Ishikawa K, Ochiai Y, Nakao M, Togawa O, Nishimura M, et al. Feasibility of endoscopic submucosal dissection: a new technique for en bloc resection of a large superficial tumor in the colon and rectum. Int J SurgOncol. 2011;2011:948293.

[2] Toyonaga T, Tanaka S, Man-I M, East J, Ono W, Nishino E, et al. Clinical significance of the muscle-retracting sign during colorectal endoscopic submucosal dissection. EndoscInt Open. 2015 May 5;3(03):E246–251.

[3] Fujishiro M, Kodashima S, Ono S, Goto O, Yamamichi N, Yahagi N, et al. Submucosal injection of normal saline can prevent unexpected deep thermal injury of Argon plasma coagulation in the in vivo porcine stomach. Gut Liver. 2008 Sep;2(2):95–98.

[4] Fujishiro M, Yahagi N, Kakushima N, Kodashima S, Muraki Y, Ono S, et al. Outcomes of endoscopic submucosal dissection for colorectal epithelial neoplasms in 200 consecutive cases. ClinGastroenterolHepatol. 2007;5(6):678–683.

[5] Isomoto H, Nishiyama H, Yamaguchi N, Fukuda E, Ishii H, Ikeda K, et al. Clinicopathological factors associated with clinical outcomes of endoscopic submucosal dissection for colorectal epithelial neoplasms. Endoscopy. 2009 Aug;41(8):679–683.

[6] Matsumoto A, Tanaka S, Oba S, Kanao H, Oka S, Yoshihara M, et al. Outcome of endoscopic submucosal dissection for colorectal tumors accompanied by fibrosis. Scand J Gastroenterol. 2010;45(11):1329–1337.

[7] Matsui N, Akahoshi K, Nakamura K, Ihara E, Kita H. Endoscopic submucosal dissection for removal of superficial gastrointestinal neoplasms: A technical review. World J GastrointestEndosc. 2012 Apr 16;4(4):123–136.

[8] Tamegai Y, Saito Y, Masaki N, Hinohara C, Oshima T, Kogure E, et al. Endoscopic submucosal dissection: a safe technique for colorectal tumors. Endoscopy. 2007 May; 39(5):418–422.

[9] Hurlstone DP, Atkinson R, Sanders DS, Thomson M, Cross SS, Brown S. Achieving R0 resection in the colorectum using endoscopic submucosal dissection. Br J Surg. 2007 Dec;94(12):1536–1542.

[10] Zhou P-H, Yao L-Q, Qin X-Y. Endoscopic submucosal dissection for colorectal epithelial neoplasm. Surg Endosc. 2009 Jul;23(7):1546–1551.

[11] Saito Y, Sakamoto T, Fukunaga S, Nakajima T, Kiriyama S, Kuriyama S, et al. Endoscopic submucosal dissection (ESD) for colorectal tumors. Dig Endosc Off J JpnGastroenterolEndosc Soc. 2009 Jul;21Suppl 1:S7–12.

[12] Iizuka H, Okamura S, Onozato Y, Ishihara H, Kakizaki S, Mori M. Endoscopic submucosal dissection for colorectal tumors. GastroentérologieClin Biol. 2009;33(10–11):1004–11.

[13] Hotta K, Oyama T, Shinohara T, Miyata Y, Takahashi A, Kitamura Y, et al. Learning curve for endoscopic submucosal dissection of large colorectal tumors. Dig Endosc. 2010;22(4):302–306.

[14] Niimi K, Fujishiro M, Kodashima S, Goto O, Ono S, Hirano K, et al. Long-term outcomes of endoscopic submucosal dissection for colorectal epithelial neoplasms. Endoscopy. 2010 Sep;42(09):723–729.

[15] Yoshida N, Naito Y, Kugai M, Inoue K, Wakabayashi N, Yagi N, et al. Efficient hemostatic method for endoscopic submucosal dissection of colorectal tumors. World J Gastroenterol WJG. 2010 Sep 7;16(33):4180–4186.

[16] Toyonaga T, Man-i M, Chinzei R, Takada N, Iwata Y, Morita Y, et al. Endoscopic treatment for early stage colorectal tumors: the comparison between EMR with small incision, simplified ESD, and ESD using the standard flush knife and the ball tipped flush knife. ActaChirIugosl. 2010;57(3):41–46.

[17] Uraoka T, Higashi R, Kato J, Kaji E, Suzuki H, Ishikawa S, et al. Colorectal endoscopic submucosal dissection for elderly patients at least 80 years of age. SurgEndosc. 2011 Sep;25(9):3000–3007.

[18] Kim ES, Cho KB, Park KS, Lee KI, Jang BK, Chung WJ, et al. Factors predictive of perforation during endoscopic submucosal dissection for the treatment of colorectal tumors. Endoscopy. 2011 Jul;43(7):573–578.

[19] Probst A, Golger D, Anthuber M, Märkl B, Messmann H. Endoscopic submucosal dissection in large sessile lesions of the rectosigmoid: learning curve in a European center. Endoscopy. 2012 Jul;44(7):660–667.

[20] Okamoto K, Kitamura S, Muguruma N, Takaoka T, Fujino Y, Kawahara Y, et al. Mucosectom2-short blade for safe and efficient endoscopic submucosal dissection of colorectal tumors. Endoscopy. 2013 Nov;45(11):928–930.

[21] Nawata Y, Homma K, Suzuki Y. Retrospective study of technical aspects and complications of endoscopic submucosal dissection for large superficial colorectal tumors. Dig Endosc Off J JpnGastroenterolEndosc Soc. 2014 Jul;26(4):552–555.

[22] Saito Y, Uraoka T, Matsuda T, Emura F, Ikehara H, Mashimo Y, et al. Endoscopic treatment of large superficial colorectal tumors: a case series of 200 endoscopic submucosal dissections (with video). GastrointestEndosc. 2007 Nov;66(5):966–973.

[23] Toyonaga T, Man-I M, Morita Y, Sanuki T, Yoshida M, Kutsumi H, et al. The new resources of treatment for early stage colorectal tumors: EMR with small incision and simplified endoscopic submucosal dissection. Dig EndoscOff J JpnGastroenterolEndosc Soc. 2009 Jul;21Suppl 1:S31–37.

[24] Fujishiro M, Kodashima S, Goto O, Ono S, Muraki Y, Kakushima N, et al. Technical feasibility of endoscopic submucosal dissection of gastrointestinal epithelial neoplasms with a splash-needle. SurgLaparoscEndoscPercutan Tech. 2008 Dec;18(6):592–597.

[25] Takeuchi Y, Uedo N, Ishihara R, Iishi H, Kizu T, Inoue T, et al. Efficacy of an endo-knife with a water-jet function (Flushknife) for endoscopic submucosal dissection of superficial colorectal neoplasms. Am J Gastroenterol. 2010 Feb;105(2):314–322.

[26] Yoshida N, Naito Y, Sakai K, Sumida Y, Kanemasa K, Inoue K, et al. Outcome of endoscopic submucosal dissection for colorectal tumors in elderly people. Int J Colorectal Dis. 2010 Apr;25(4):455–461.

[27] Saito Y, Kawano H, Takeuchi Y, Ohata K, Oka S, Hotta K, et al. Current status of colorectal endoscopic submucosal dissection in Japan and other Asian countries: progressing towards technical standardization. Dig Endosc Off J JpnGastroenterolEndosc Soc. 2012 May;24Suppl 1:67–72.

[28] Akahoshi K, Akahane H, Murata A, Akiba H, Oya M. Endoscopic submucosal dissection using a novel grasping type scissors forceps. Endoscopy. 2007 Dec;39(12):1103–1105.

[29] Jung YS, Park DI. Submucosal injection solutions for endoscopic mucosal resection and endoscopic submucosal dissection of gastrointestinal neoplasms. GastrointestInterv. 2013;2(2):73–77.

[30] Matsuda T, Fujii T, Saito Y, Nakajima T, Uraoka T, Kobayashi N, et al. Efficacy of the invasive/non-invasive pattern by magnifying chromoendoscopy to estimate the depth of invasion of early colorectal neoplasms. Am J Gastroenterol. 2008 Nov;103(11):2700–2706.

[31] Hayashi N, Tanaka S, Hewett DG, Kaltenbach TR, Sano Y, Ponchon T, et al. Endoscopic prediction of deep submucosal invasive carcinoma: validation of the narrow-band imaging international colorectal endoscopic (NICE) classification. GastrointestEndosc. 2013 Oct;78(4):625–632.

[32] Yoshida N, Yagi N, Naito Y, Yoshikawa T. Safe procedure in endoscopic submucosal dissection for colorectal tumors focused on preventing complications. World J Gastroenterol. 2010 Apr 14;16(14):1688–1695.

[33] Saito Y, Uraoka T, Matsuda T, Emura F, Ikehara H, Mashimo Y, et al. A pilot study to assess the safety and efficacy of carbon dioxide insufflation during colorectal endoscopic submucosal dissection with the patient under conscious sedation. GastrointestEndosc. 2007;65(3):537–542.

[34] Tanaka S, Haruma K, Oka S, Takahashi R, Kunihiro M, Kitadai Y, et al. Clinicopathologic features and endoscopic treatment of superficially spreading colorectal neoplasms larger than 20 mm. GastrointestEndosc. 2001 Jul;54(1):62–66.

[35] Saito Y, Fukuzawa M, Matsuda T, Fukunaga S, Sakamoto T, Uraoka T, et al. Clinical outcome of endoscopic submucosal dissection versus endoscopic mucosal resection of large colorectal tumors as determined by curative resection. SurgEndosc. 2010 Feb; 24(2):343–352.

[36] Iishi H, Tatsuta M, Iseki K, Narahara H, Uedo N, Sakai N, et al. Endoscopic piecemeal resection with submucosal saline injection of large sessile colorectal polyps. GastrointestEndosc. 2000 Jun;51(6):697–700.

[37] Jeong G, Lee JH, Yu MK, Moon W, Rhee P-L, Paik SW, et al. Non-surgical management of microperforation induced by EMR of the stomach. Dig Liver Dis Off J Ital SocGastroenterol Ital Assoc Study Liver. 2006 Aug;38(8):605–608.

[38] Seebach L, Bauerfeind P, Gubler C. "Sparing the surgeon": clinical experience with over-the-scope clips for gastrointestinal perforation. Endoscopy. 2010 Dec;42(12):1108–1111.

[39] Yoshida N, Wakabayashi N, Kanemasa K, Sumida Y, Hasegawa D, Inoue K, et al. Endoscopic submucosal dissection for colorectal tumors: technical difficulties and rate of perforation. Endoscopy. 2009 Sep;41(09):758–761.

[40] Fujishiro M, Yahagi N, Kakushima N, Kodashima S, Muraki Y, Ono S, et al. Successful nonsurgical management of perforation complicating endoscopic submucosal dissection of gastrointestinal epithelial neoplasms. Endoscopy. 2006 Oct;38(10):1001–1006.

[41] Uraoka T, Kawahara Y, Kato J, Saito Y, Yamamoto K. Endoscopic submucosal dissection in the colorectum: present status and future prospects. Dig Endosc. 2009;21:S13–16.

[42] Sakamoto N, Beppu K, Matsumoto K, Shibuya T, Osada T, Mori H, et al. "Loop Clip", a new closure device for large mucosal defects after EMR and ESD. Endoscopy. 2008 Sep;40Suppl 2:E97–98.

[43] Toyanaga T, Man-I M, Ivanov D, Sanuki T, Morita Y, Kutsumi H, et al. The results and limitations of endoscopic submucosal dissection for colorectal tumors. ActaChirIugosl. 2008;55(3):17–23.

[44] Tanaka S, Oka S, Kaneko I, Hirata M, Mouri R, Kanao H, et al. Endoscopic submucosal dissection for colorectal neoplasia: possibility of standardization. GastrointestEndosc. 2007;66(1):100–107.

[45] Yoshida N, Kanemasa K, Sakai K. Experience of endoscopic submucosal dissection (ESD) to colorectal tumor-especially about clinical course of cases with perforation. 2008 [cited 2016 Jan 8]; Available from: http://inis.iaea.org/Search/search.aspx?orig_q=RN:39103526

[46] Park SY, Jeon SW. Acute intestinal obstruction after endoscopic submucosal dissection: report of a case. Dis Colon Rectum. 2008 Jun 7;51(8):1295–1297.

[47] Yoshida N, Yagi N, Inada Y, Kugai M, Yanagisawa A, Naito Y. Prevention and management of complications of and training for colorectal endoscopic submucosal dissection. Gastroenterol Res Pract. 2013;2013:287173.

[48] Lee E-J, Lee JB, Lee SH, Kim DS, Lee DH, Lee DS, et al. Endoscopic submucosal dissection for colorectal tumors--1,000 colorectal ESD cases: one specialized institute's experiences. SurgEndosc. 2013 Jan;27(1):31–39.

[49] Tanaka S, Terasaki M, Kanao H, Oka S, Chayama K. Current status and future perspectives of endoscopic submucosal dissection for colorectal tumors. Dig Endosc. 2012;24(s1):73–79.

[50] Tanaka S, Tamegai Y, Tsuda S, Saito Y, Yahagi N, Yamano H. Multicenter questionnaire survey on the current situation of colorectal endoscopic submucosal dissection in Japan. Dig Endosc. 2010;22(s1):S2–8.

[51] Saito Y, Uraoka T, Yamaguchi Y, Hotta K, Sakamoto N, Ikematsu H, et al. A prospective, multicenter study of 1111 colorectal endoscopic submucosal dissections (with video). GastrointestEndosc. 2010 Dec;72(6):1217–1225.

[52] Oka S, Tanaka S, Kanao H, Ishikawa H, Watanabe T, Igarashi M, et al. Mid-term prognosis after endoscopic resection for submucosal colorectal carcinoma: summary of a multicenter questionnaire survey conducted by the colorectal endoscopic resection standardization implementation working group in Japanese Society for Cancer of the Colon and Rectum. Dig Endosc Off J JpnGastroenterolEndosc Soc. 2011 Apr;23(2):190–194.

[53] S Y, M W, H H, H B, K Y, J S, et al. The risk of lymph node metastasis in T1 colorectal carcinoma. Hepatogastroenterology. 2003 Dec;51(58):998–1000.

[54] Bosch SL, Teerenstra S, de Wilt JHW, Cunningham C, Nagtegaal ID. Predicting lymph node metastasis in pT1 colorectal cancer: a systematic review of risk factors providing rationale for therapy decisions. Endoscopy. 2013 Oct;45(10):827–834.

[55] Carrara A, Mangiola D, Pertile R, Ricci A, Motter M, Ghezzi G, et al. Analysis of risk factors for lymph nodal involvement in early stages of rectal cancer: When can local excision be considered an appropriate treatment? Systematic review and meta-analysis of the literature. Int J SurgOncol. 2012 Jun 19;2012:e438450.

[56] Lee E-J, Lee JB, Lee SH, Youk EG. Endoscopic treatment of large colorectal tumors: comparison of endoscopic mucosal resection, endoscopic mucosal resection–precutting, and endoscopic submucosal dissection. SurgEndosc. 2012 Jan 26;26(8):2220–2230.

[57] Terasaki M, Tanaka S, Oka S, Nakadoi K, Takata S, Kanao H, et al. Clinical outcomes of endoscopic submucosal dissection and endoscopic mucosal resection for laterally spreading tumors larger than 20 mm. J GastroenterolHepatol. 2012 Apr;27(4):734–740.

[58] Tajika M, Niwa Y, Bhatia V, Kondo S, Tanaka T, Mizuno N, et al. Comparison of endoscopic submucosal dissection and endoscopic mucosal resection for large colorectal tumors. Eur J GastroenterolHepatol. 2011 Nov;23(11):1042–1049.

[59] Kobayashi N, Yoshitake N, Hirahara Y, Konishi J, Saito Y, Matsuda T, et al. Matched case-control study comparing endoscopic submucosal dissection and endoscopic mucosal resection for colorectal tumors. J GastroenterolHepatol. 2012 Apr;27(4):728–733.

[60] Cao Y, Liao C, Tan A, Gao Y, Mo Z, Gao F. Meta-analysis of endoscopic submucosal dissection versus endoscopic mucosal resection for tumors of the gastrointestinal tract. Endoscopy. 2009 Sep;41(09):751–757.

[61] Pohl H, Srivastava A, Bensen SP, Anderson P, Rothstein RI, Gordon SR, et al. Incomplete polyp resection during colonoscopy—Results of the complete adenoma resection (CARE) Study. Gastroenterology. 2013;144(1):74–80.e1.

[62] Woodward TA, Heckman MG, Cleveland P, De Melo S, Raimondo M, Wallace M. Predictors of Complete Endoscopic Mucosal Resection of Flat and Depressed Gastrointestinal Neoplasia of the Colon. Am J Gastroenterol. 2012;107(5):650–4.

[63] Kim HH, Kim JH, Park SJ, Park MI, Moon W. Risk factors for incomplete resection and complications in endoscopic mucosal resection for lateral spreading tumors. Dig Endosc. 2012;24(4):259–266.

[64] Mannath J, Subramanian V, Singh R, Telakis E, Ragunath K. Polyp recurrence after endoscopic mucosal resection of sessile and flat colonic adenomas. Dig Dis Sci. 2011 Feb 16;56(8):2389–2395.

[65] Sakamoto T, Matsuda T, Otake Y, Nakajima T, Saito Y. Predictive factors of local recurrence after endoscopic piecemeal mucosal resection. J Gastroenterol. 2012 Jan 6;47(6):635–640.

[66] Ohata K, Nonaka K, Minato Y, Misumi Y, Tashima T, Shozushima M, et al. Endoscopic submucosal dissection for large colorectal tumor in a Japanese general hospital. J Oncol. 2013;2013:218670.

[67] Nakajima T, Saito Y, Tanaka S, Iishi H, Kudo S, Ikematsu H, et al. Current status of endoscopic resection strategy for large, early colorectal neoplasia in Japan. SurgEndosc. 2013 Sep;27(9):3262–3270.

[68] Lee E-J, Lee JB, Choi YS, Lee SH, Lee DH, Kim DS, et al. Clinical risk factors for perforation during endoscopic submucosal dissection (ESD) for large-sized, nonpedunculated colorectal tumors. SurgEndosc. 2012 Jun;26(6):1587–1594.

[69] Kawaguti FS, Nahas CSR, Marques CFS, Martins B da C, Retes FA, Medeiros RSS, et al. Endoscopic submucosal dissection versus transanal endoscopic microsurgery for the treatment of early rectal cancer. SurgEndosc. 2014 Apr;28(4):1173–1179.

[70] Park SU, Min YW, Shin JU, Choi JH, Kim Y-H, Kim JJ, et al. Endoscopic submucosal dissection or transanal endoscopic microsurgery for nonpolypoid rectal high grade dysplasia and submucosa-invading rectal cancer. Endoscopy. 2012 Nov;44(11):1031–1036.

[71] Arezzo A, Passera R, Saito Y, Sakamoto T, Kobayashi N, Sakamoto N, et al. Systematic review and meta-analysis of endoscopic submucosal dissection versus transanal endoscopic microsurgery for large noninvasive rectal lesions. SurgEndosc. 2014 Feb; 28(2):427–438.

[72] Kiriyama S, Saito Y, Yamamoto S, Soetikno R, Matsuda T, Nakajima T, et al. Comparison of endoscopic submucosal dissection with laparoscopic-assisted colorectal surgery for early-stage colorectal cancer: a retrospective analysis. Endoscopy. 2012 Nov;44(11): 1024–1030.

[73] Swanström LL. Treatment of early colorectal cancers: too many choices? Endoscopy. 2012 Nov;44(11):991–992.

[74] Farhat S, Chaussade S, Ponchon T, Coumaros D, Charachon A, Barrioz T, et al. Endoscopic submucosal dissection in a European setting. A multi-institutional report of a technique in development. Endoscopy. 2011 Aug;43(8):664–670.

[75] Repici A, Hassan C, Pagano N, Rando G, Romeo F, Spaggiari P, et al. High efficacy of endoscopic submucosal dissection for rectal laterally spreading tumors larger than 3 cm. GastrointestEndosc. 2013 Jan;77(1):96–101.

[76] Thorlacius H, Uedo N, Toth E. Implementation of endoscopic submucosal dissection for early colorectal neoplasms in Sweden. Gastroenterol Res Pract. 2013;2013:758202.

[77] Sauer M, Hildenbrand R, Bollmann R, Sido B, Dumoulin FL. Tu1426 Endoscopic Submucosal Dissection (ESD) of large sessile and flat neoplastic lesions in the colon: a single-center series with 83 procedures from Europe. GastrointestEndosc. 2014 May; 79(5):AB536.

Section 3

Classic Treatments

Chapter 8

Colorectal Cancer and Inflammatory Bowel Disease

Paul Mitrut, Anca Oana Docea, Adina Maria Kamal,
Radu Mitrut, Daniela Calina, Eliza Gofita,
Vlad Padureanu, Corina Gruia and Liliana Streba

Additional information is available at the end of the chapter

http://dx.doi.org/10.5772/63408

Abstract

Inflammatory bowel disease (IBD) with its two entities, ulcerative colitis and Crohn's disease, is at increased risk of developing colorectal cancer (CRC). Risk factors for CRC are represented by the duration of the disease, extent of disease, the association of primary sclerosing cholangitis, family history, and early age at onset. In inflammatory bowel disease, colonic carcinogenesis appears on an inflamed colon, being determined by different genetic alterations. The main element of the process of carcinogenesis is the dysplasia, which is a neoplastic intraepithelial transformation, limited to the basal membrane surrounding the glands around which it appears. The stages of carcinogenesis process start with dysplasia of varying degrees as follows: indefinite dysplasia, low-grade dysplasia, high-grade dysplasia, and finally invasive adenocarcinoma.

Endoscopic surveillance in IBD is absolutely necessary for early detection of dysplastic lesions. The endoscopic surveillance process begins after 7–10 years of disease progression, performed every 1 or 2 years, depending on the severity of the disease.

General principles of endoscopic surveillance involve the use of modern diagnostic methods (high definition, chromoendoscopy, indigo carmine with high definition, high-definition narrow band imaging).

The current standard-of-care (colonoscopy plus randomized biopsies) to detect dysplasia in IBD patients is inadequate. Guidelines now support to use of chromoendoscopy with targeted biopsy in the detection of dysplasia and/or colorectal cancer in patients with IBD.

Chemopreventive drugs involve the administration of therapeutic agents such as 5-ASA derivatives, ursodeoxycholic acid and folic acid, and possibly statins.

As for future goals, understanding the mechanisms of colonic carcinogenesis in IBD can identify patients at high risk for developing CRC and thus chemoprevention can be initiated. The discovery of new therapeutic agents plays an important role in chemoprevention and represents a significant desideratum among researchers.

Keywords: colorectal cancer, inflammatory bowel disease, carcinogenesis, colonoscopic surveillance, chromoendoscopy, high-definition narrow band imaging

1. Introduction

Inflammatory bowel diseases with its two separate entities (ulcerative colitis and Crohn's disease) are conditions considered at high risk for developing colorectal cancer. Because inflammatory bowel diseases are relatively rare in the general population, only about 1% of colorectal cancers are attributed to them. Meta-analyzes showed that the risk is 2% at 10 years, 8% at 20 years, and 18% at 30 years after onset [1]. Absolute cumulative frequencies of colorectal cancer to Crohn's disease and ulcerative colitis are almost identical 7% for the first to 8% for the second, after 20 years of evolution [2]. Most knowledge about the pathogenesis of colorectal cancer come from studies on sporadic cancers or those associated with increased risk of hereditary disease (familial adenomatous polyposis or non-polyposis colorectal cancer), this data being then extrapolated for inflammatory bowel diseases.

Eaden et al. [3] reviewed 116 studies involving 55,000 patients with ulcerative colitis. One thousand seven hundred of these patients developed colorectal cancer, having an incidence of 2% after 10 years of evolution, and of 8% after 20 years finally increasing to 18% after 30 years.

2. Risk factors for colorectal cancer in inflammatory bowel disease

In ulcerative colitis, onset of colorectal cancer is correlated with many factors. Thus, the duration of the disease is recognized as one of the leading risk factors for developing colorectal cancer in ulcerative colitis. Neoplastic risk occurs after 8 years of evolution and increases exponentially after 20 years [1].

A systematic colonoscopy surveillance can detect early dysplastic lesions, and the systematic use of 5-ASA therapy can lower the risk of developing colorectal cancer in patients with IBD. The reduced incidence of prophylactic colectomy for dysplastic lesions determines a high risk for colorectal cancer. This information is an argument for preventive colonoscopy surveillance of patients with IBD and surgical prophylaxis in case of dysplasia [4, 5].

Younger age at onset is in the opinion of some authors, an independent risk factor for colorectal cancer. Younger patients have a potentially greater lifespan and therefore higher risks, which may reflect the longer duration of the disease [1, 4–6]. The association of PSC increases the risk of colorectal cancer. Its incidence in patients with ulcerative colitis is 2–5% [1]. In 1992, Broome et al. reported an increased risk of colorectal cancer in patients with ulcerative colitis associating PSC. Subsequent studies have shown that the cumulative risk of colorectal cancer is higher in patients with combination of cholangitis and ulcerative colitis compared with the ones only known for ulcerative colitis, that is, 9% after 10 years compared to 2, 31% after 20 years compared to 5, and 50% after 25 years to 10% [7].

The extent of the disease is also an important risk factor for the risk of developing colorectal cancer. Pancolitis presents the highest risk of malignancy [1]. The extension of inflammatory areas is an independent risk factor involved in the carcinogenesis and Crohn's disease.

A family history of colon cancer cancer is associated with an increased risk of colorectal −2 or 3 times higher, in the general population, which remains increased in patients with ulcerative colitis. A case–control study conducted on 297 patients at the Mayo Clinic found that a family history of sporadic colorectal cancer represents an independent risk factor for malignancy in patients with ulcerative colitis [7].

An interesting finding is that patients with asymptomatic disease (therapeutically controlled) have higher risks of malignancy compared with fulminant forms of ulcerative colitis that often require colectomy before the onset of dysplasia. In centers where a large number of colectomies are performed, the incidence of colorectal cancer (CRC) is significantly lower because the procedure eliminates the risk [1].

In Crohn's disease, the risk factors involved in carcinogenesis are areas of stenosis, inflammatory extension areas, younger age at onset and age >45 years at diagnosis. Risk factors specific to patients with inflammatory bowel disease [8]:

- Coexisting primary sclerosing cholangitis
- Increasing cumulative extent of colonic inflammatory lesions
- Increasing duration of inflammatory bowel disease
- Active chronic inflammation endoscopically assessed
- Active chronic inflammation histologically assessed
- Anatomical abnormalities such as:
  - Foreshortened colon
  - Strictures
  - Pseudo polyps
- Personal history of flat dysplasia.

The severity of inflammatory colonic lesion correlates with the risk of colorectal cancer in patients with IBD. There is a correlation between the degree of inflammation and the risk of dysplastic lesions and indirectly with the colorectal cancer incidence. Various studies have shown the relationship between the risk of colorectal cancer in patients with IBD and the degree of inflammation, extent of lesions and coexistence of other sites of inflammation [9]. Involved in the colonic carcinogenesis in patients with IBD are, besides inflammation areas of various degrees, also genetic and immunological factors.

3. Molecular and genetic markers

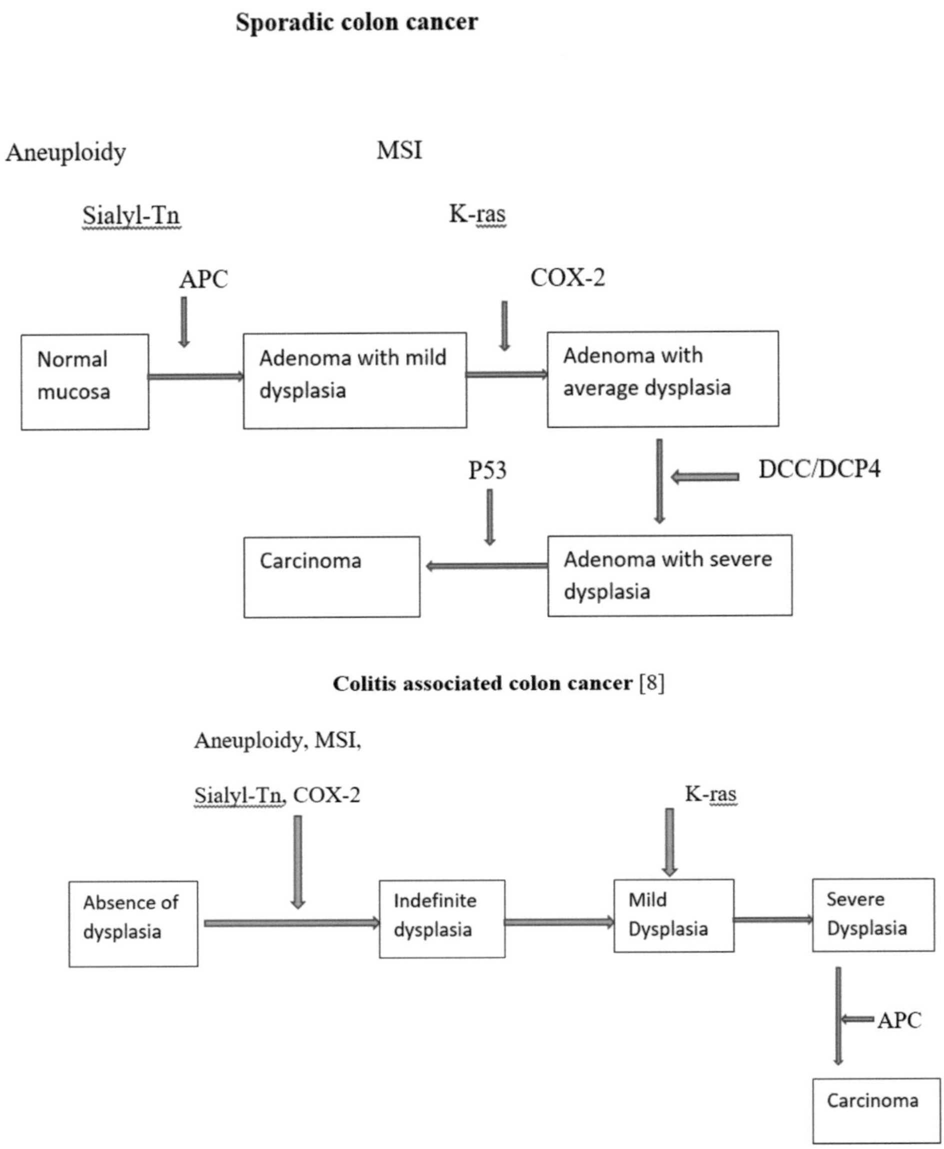

Pathogenesis of sporadic colon cancer and colitis-associated colon cancer [8].

Involved in the appearance of colorectal cancer associated with inflammatory bowel disease, are, on the one hand the chromosomal instability caused by abnormal chromosome separation (CRS) aneuploidy and loss of genetic material, and on the other hand, the microsatellite instability (MSI) mechanisms found in sporadic carcinogenesis. The trigger element for chromosomal instability is represented by impairing the function of APC associated with the induction of K-ras oncogene and inactivation of tumor suppressor gene on CRS 18q in DCC and DPC4 region. Adenoma–carcinoma transformation is a direct result of the loss of p53 gene function [1, 6, 8].

Microsatellite instability, which is absent on normal mucosa, is described as an early event in non-dysplastic mucosa in patients with ulcerative colitis.

It is important to understand what mechanisms and factors can contribute to dysplastic lesions and colorectal cancer in IBD. Inflammation and genetic mutations play a major role. The supervision and therapeutic intervention in these disorders depends on understanding of these pathological processes. Thus, some genes associated with inflammation such as cyclo-oxygenase-2, nitric oxide synthase-2, and 1–8 interferon inducible genes are increased in inflamed colonic mucosa and remain elevated in colonic neoplasms [10, 11].

Genetic changes, responsible for colorectal cancer in inflammatory bowel disease, are similar to those involved in sporadic colon cancer [8].

Oxidative stress and its role in cell destruction in inflamed tissue may also play an important role in the pathogenesis of colorectal cancer in IBD [12].

Figures 1 and **2** depict some pathology aspects of colon mucosa with inflammatory changes. The inflammatory context is suggested by an abundant lymphoplasmocitary infiltrate and polimorphonucleated within the mucosal corion.

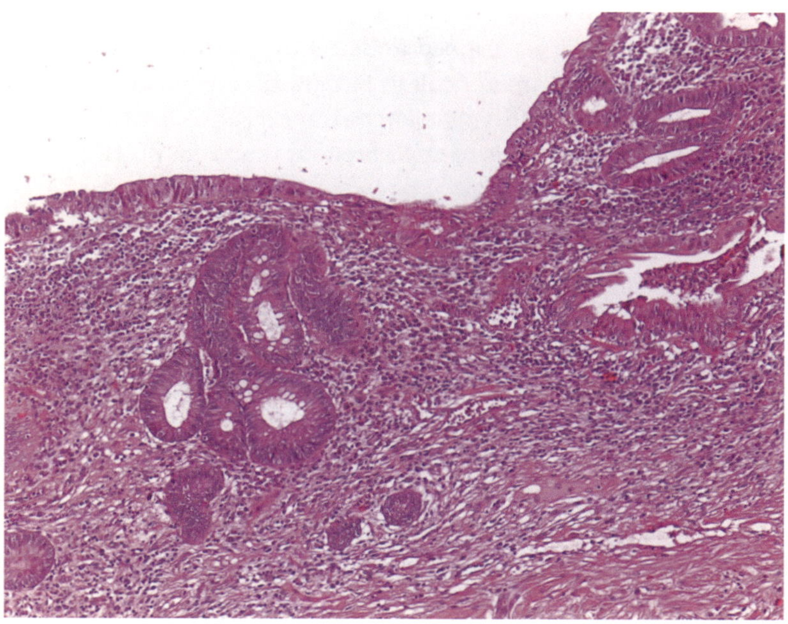

Figure 1. Inflammatory aspect of colonic mucosa. Modified cytoarchitectonics. Epithelial pseudostratification of the glandular tissue.

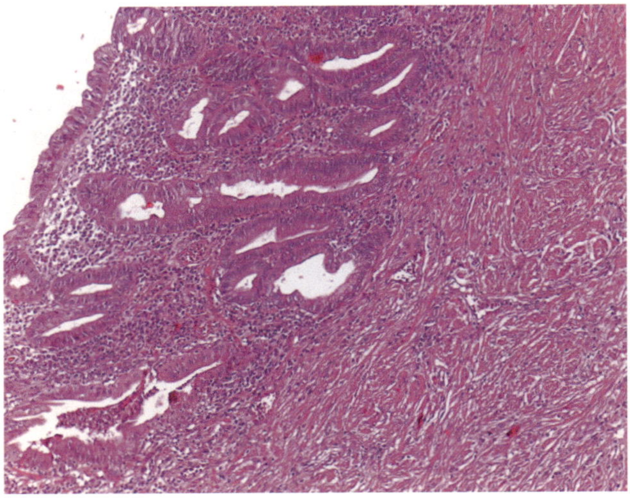

Figure 2. Inflammatory aspect of colonic mucosa. Nuclear pleomorphism. Mucus depletion, with a decreased number of secretory cells within normal glands.

4. Prevention of colorectal cancer in inflammatory bowel disease

4.1. Endoscopic surveillance in IBD

Endoscopic surveillance in IBD is designed to detect dysplastic lesions that can be treated surgically. As dysplastic lesions are difficult to recognize via endoscopic examination, their detection requires colectomy that prevents colorectal cancer (CRC). This fact is also determined by the risk of developing synchronous or metachronous cancer in IBD [13].

Colonoscopy surveillance reduces the risk of death from CRC in patients with long-term evolution of inflammatory disease. Given the cost–benefit ratio, this surveillance is especially recommended in patients with evolving active disease of over 7–10 years. The first colonoscopy screening program will be carried out in a remission period of the disease to avoid difficulties in identifying dysplasia in areas of increased inflammatory activity (**Figures 3** and **4**). The entire colonic mucosa will be examined and four biopsies will be taken from 10 to 10 cm. Any suspicious lesions will be biopsied. If the initial biopsy does not describe dysplastic foci, the colonoscopy is recommended to be repeated after 2 years or annually if the disease has more than 20 years of evolution when the risk of cancer increases exponentially. This interval is reduced to 6 months, 1-year maximum if the pathology result of the lesions comes back as indefinite dysplasia. The most controversial attitude is regarding mild dysplasia. In the case of dysplastic lesions associated with IBD, there are opinions saying that endoscopic resection can be done if the pathological examination of the fragments collected from the base of the polyp and also from the colon are negative for dysplasia [14]. The marking of the polypectomy site is recommended, and the colonoscopy should be repeated after 3–6 months. The confir-

http://dx.doi.org/10.5772/63408

mation of unifocal or multifocal dysplasia by a second expert requires that a colectomy should be performed. High-grade dysplasia is an absolute indication for colectomy.

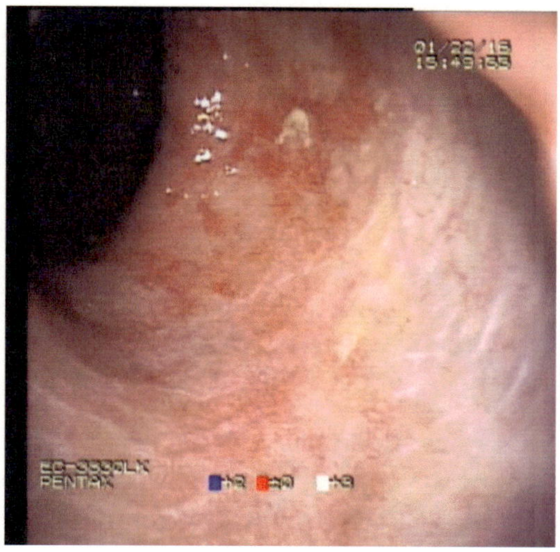

Figure 3. Ulcerative colitis with areas of low grade dysplasia.

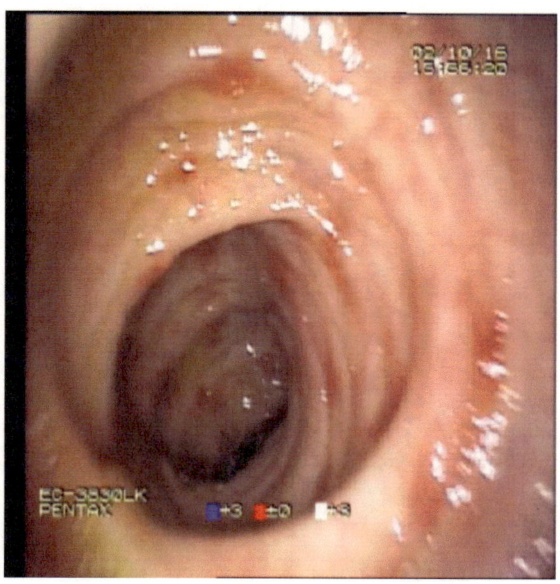

Figure 4. Ulcerative colitis with high grade dysplasia.

There is an evolution of the inflammatory lesions that either do not have dysplastic lesions or evolve from indefinite dysplasia to low-grade dysplasia, high-grade dysplasia, and finally carcinoma.

Dysplasia, detected at colonoscopic examination, represents an indication for colectomy. When low-grade dysplasia is detected, it is considered that the risk of developing colorectal cancer is nine times higher than in normal individuals and there is a 12 times higher risk of developing other advanced dysplastic lesions.

In patients with low-grade dysplasia, when colectomy is performed immediately, it was noted that 19% of the cases had high-grade dysplasia and 29–54% were at risk of developing advanced neoplasia in the following 5 years. High-grade dysplasia has a risk of 43% of combination with synchronous malignancy [14].

Dysplastic lesions are lesions that precede colorectal cancer development. Flat dysplasia can be discovered through microscopic examination of biopsy fragments, collected through random biopsies, sometimes from apparently normal mucosa. Often, flat dysplasia can be discovered with superior detection techniques such as chromoendoscopy, high-definition, and high magnification endoscopy [15–18].

Treatment for patients with dysplastic lesions and IBD depends on the degree of dysplasia. Patients presenting with multifocal flat low-grade dysplasia lesions or repetitive flat low-grade dysplasia should be advised to undertake prophylactic proctocolectomy.

Dysplasia-associated lesion or mass (DALM) is a specific endoscopic feature found in patients with ulcerative colitis. DALM is associated in a proportion of 40% with colorectal cancer; this

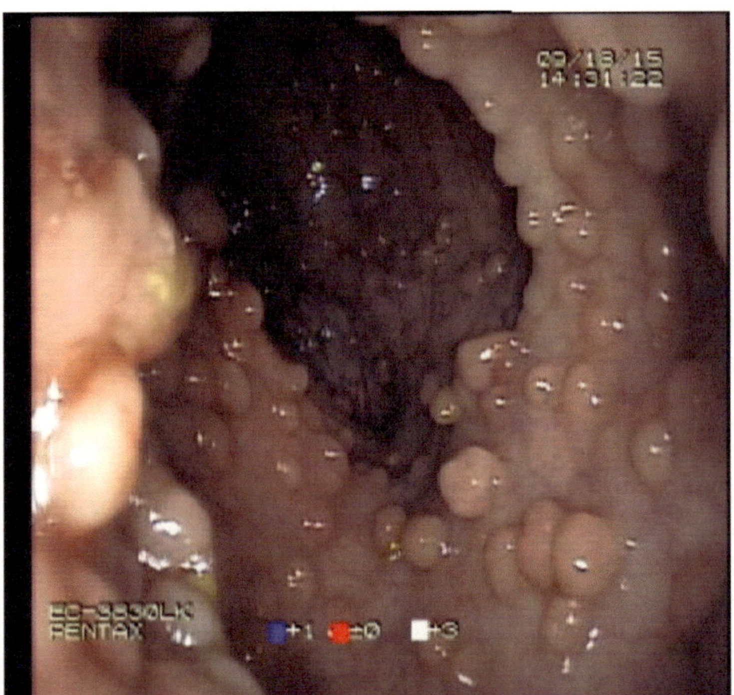

Figure 5. Polipoid lesions in a patient suffering from Crohn's disease.

http://dx.doi.org/10.5772/63408

association is enhanced by the presence of high-grade dysplasia lesions. DALM is an indication of proctocolectomy regardless of the degree of dysplasia.

Polypoid lesions identified in patients with IBD are not always malignant and can be treated with endoscopic polypectomy, especially if the polyps are adenomatous [19] (**Figure 5**).

Dysplastic lesions detected in biopsy samples from patients with IBD usually occur in areas of inflammation and can be polypoid, ulcerated lesions, or plague-like lesions (DALM). (**Figure 6** describes various instances of lesions in a patient with IBD).

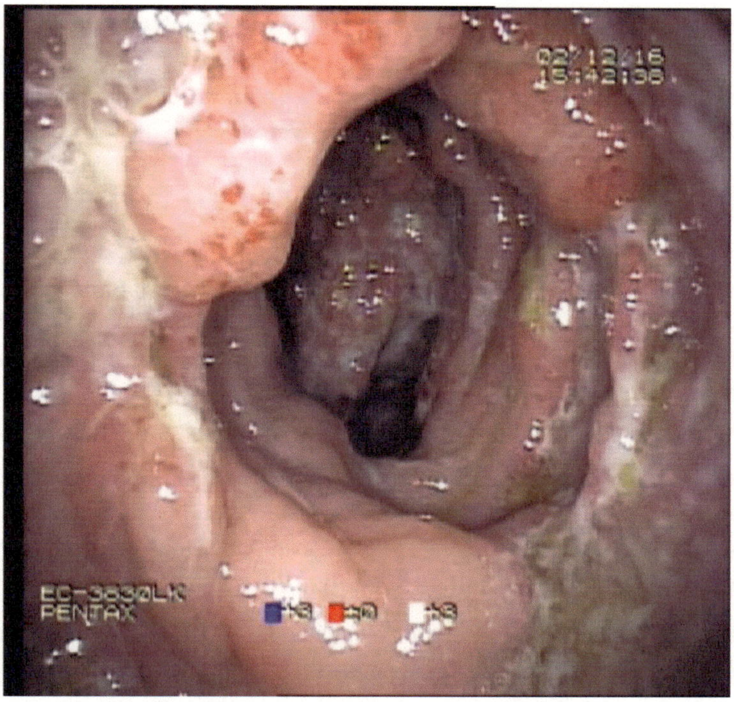

Figure 6. High grade dysplasia in a patient with Crohn's disease.

Although prophylactic proctocolectomy ensures the elimination of the risk of colon cancer (42% of cases in patients with high-grade dysplasia and 19% of cases in patients with low-grade dysplasia), there are practitioners who opt for a lifelong schedule of surveillance. They choose periodic examination at 6 months to 1 year by endoscopically investigating the entire colon, harvesting biopsy fragments and using preventive treatment with anti-inflammatory drugs and potentially chemopreventive agents. There are some major limitations to this attitude, namely the possibility of omission of malignant or dysplastic lesions during colonoscopy, especially if the number of biopsies is insufficient. Also, the lack of compliance of patients to colonoscopy surveillance programs is also an important risk factor for malignant lesions.

Guidelines from the Crohn's and Colitis Foundation of America (CCFA) and from European Crohn's and Colitis Organization (ECCO) mention the same methods for Crohn's colitis surveillance and ulcerative colitis as well due to the similar risk of developing colorectal. Colonoscopic screening is performed during remission of the disease, every 1 or 2 years, after 8–10 years of evolution. Screening interval may decrease with increasing duration of disease progression. Patients with proctosigmoiditis, who have a lower risk of malignancy compared to the general population, will be monitored using standard colorectal cancer prevention measures.

Patients with PSC, who have an increased risk of malignancy, should be monitored annually. Biopsy samples are collected from 10 to 10 cm (2–4 random biopsy specimens) and from suspect areas. In addition, in ulcerative colitis, biopsies are harvested from every 5 cm from the rectum and sigmoid, because the risk of developing colorectal cancer is higher in these regions. The degree of detection of dysplastic lesions is higher if a greater number of randomized biopsies are taken (90% if 33 and 95% if 56 random biopsies were taken) [20, 21].

4.2. New methods for early detection of dysplasia

To increase the rate of detection of dysplastic lesions, targeted biopsy represents an alternative. Guidelines now support the use of chromoendoscopy with targeted biopsy in the detection of dysplasia and/or colorectal cancer in patients with inflammatory bowel disease (IBD). Chromoendoscopy can see injuries that are not visible in the white light of standard endoscopy. Two substances are used, namely methylene blue and indigo carmine. High-magnification chromoendoscopy increases the detection of dysplastic lesions 3–4.5 times over [22–26].

Because of these arguments chromoendoscopy is used for routine surveillance of patients with IBD. With this method, the majority of dysplastic lesions can be discovered in patients with IBD during surveillance colonoscopy. Using only conventional colonoscopy is obviously insufficient in detecting dysplastic lesions [27–30].

Confocal laser endomicroscopy (CLE) is a modern technique for visualization of the histology of colonic mucosa in real time, being extremely useful for diagnosing intraepithelial neoplasia. With concomitant use of chromoendoscopic and CLE evaluation, the detection rate of dysplastic lesions was increased by 4.75 times compared to classical colonoscopy [21, 28–30].

Confocal chromoscopic endomicroscopy is superior to chromoscopy alone for the detection of intraepithelial neoplasia. Difficulties are caused by the high cost of exploration and biopsy interpretation difficulty that often requires an experienced pathologist.

The use of narrow band imaging (NBI) is not superior to conventional colonoscopy in detecting dysplastic lesions [31, 32].

Although many lesions can be identified by NBI, unfortunately equal numbers of dysplastic lesions can be missed by both conventional colonoscopy and this method. More studies are needed to clarify these issues.

We again underline that chromoendoscopy with targeted biopsy is indicated by all current guidelines for detecting dysplastic lesions in IBD.

http://dx.doi.org/10.5772/63408

4.3. Chemoprevention

Surveillance colonoscopy does not prevent colorectal cancer but allows early detection of dysplastic lesions and surgical therapeutic intervention.

Treatment of inflammatory lesions of IBD with specific anti-inflammatory therapy represents an important method of primary chemoprevention of colorectal cancer [33–36].

4.3.1. Aminosalicylates and other anti-inflammatory agents

IBD anti-inflammatory treatment in addition to relieving symptoms and improving lesions can prevent dysplastic lesions and colorectal cancer. Although studies are contradictory, most authors recommend administration of anti-inflammatory therapy for colorectal cancer prevention [37].

5-aminosalicylic acid preparations (5-ASA) are the main anti-inflammatory drugs used for the treatment of digestive tract inflammation in patients with IBD. Aminosalicylates inhibit cyclooxygenase and 5-lipoxygenase, thus inhibiting the synthesis of leukotriene B4, thromboxane A2 and prostaglandins and thus intervene in the immune response, reducing the production of antibodies and phagocytic activity. The administration of 5-ASA preparations reduces the risk of colorectal cancer, especially at higher doses of 2 g per day.

Mesalazine is effective in preventing colorectal cancer in IBD, proven experimentally on colon cancer cell lines [38].

4.3.2. Ursodeoxycholic acid

Ursodeoxycholic acid (UDCA) used for treating PSC has a preventive effect in colorectal cancer by decreasing the concentration of biliary acids in the colon and through its antioxidant properties. On the other hand, it is unclear whether ursodeoxycholic acid is effective in preventing colorectal cancer in patients with IBD without the association of primary sclerosing cholangitis. In IBD forms associated with PSC, UDCA can reduce mortality and prevent the evolution of dysplastic lesions [39].

Further studies are necessary to establish the dose of UDCA to be used for secondary chemoprevention.

4.3.3. Folic acid

There are numerous studies showing that as in sporadic CRC, folic acid supplementation would decrease the risk of CRC in patients with IBD. Although there is no consensus in this regard, given that it is a cheap drug, that offers long-term safety, folic acid is recommended in patients with IBD as chemopreventive purposes. The mechanism of action is possibly related to the process of maintenance of DNA methylation and maintenance of DNA precursors level.

4.3.4. Statins

There is little data on the protective effect of statins on the development of CRC. It seems that the protective effect is lower in sporadic colorectal cancer and more expressed in colorectal cancer associated with inflammatory bowel disease. Experimental studies on mice show the protective effect of statins in reducing colorectal Dysplasia by inhibiting DNA destruction. Also in experimental models simvastatin significantly reduced tumor development by inducing apoptosis and inhibiting angiogenesis [40, 41].

These experiments provide important arguments that statins could be a potential chemopreventive and therapeutic agent effective in CRC associated with IBD. Extensive studies over long periods of time are needed to bring new arguments and insights on these aspects.

Author details

Paul Mitrut*, Anca Oana Docea, Adina Maria Kamal, Radu Mitrut, Daniela Calina, Eliza Gofita, Vlad Padureanu, Corina Gruia and Liliana Streba

*Address all correspondence to: paulmitrut@yahoo.com

University of Medicine and Pharmacy of Craiova, Craiova, Romania

References

[1] Farraye FA, Odze RD, Eaden J, Itzkowitz SH. AGA technical review on the diagnosis and management of colorectal neoplasia in inflammatory bowel disease. Gastroenterology. 2010;138:746–774.

[2] Gillen CD, Walmsley RS, Prior B, et al. Primary sclerosing cholangitis and ulcerative colitis: evidence for increased neoplastic potential. Hepatology. 1995;22:1404–1408.

[3] Eaden JA, Abrams KR, Mayberry JF. The risk of colorectal cancer in ulcerative colitis: a metaanalysis. Gut. 2001;48:526–535.

[4] Lakatos PL, Lakatos L. Risk for colorectal cancer in ulcerative colitis: changes causes and management strategies. World J Gastroenterol. 2008;14(25):3937–3947.

[5] Ha F1, Khalil H. Crohn's disease: a clinical update. Ther Adv Gastroenterol. 2015;8(6): 352–9.

[6] Jiang D1, Zhong S2, McPeek MS. Retrospective Binary-Trait Association Test Elucidates Genetic Architecture of Crohn Disease. Am J Hum Genet. 2016;98(2):243–55.

[7] Nuako KW, Ahlquist DA, Mahoney DW, et al. Familial predisposition for colorectal cancer in chronic ulcerative colitis: a case control study. Gastroenterology. 1998;115:1079–1083.

[8] Beaugerie L, Itzkowitz SH. Cancers complicating inflammatory bowel disease. N Engl J Med. 2015;372:1441–1452.

[9] Gupta RB, Harpaz N, Itzkowitz S, Hossain S, Matula S, Kornbluth A, Bodian C, Ullman T. Histologic inflammation is a risk factor for progression to colorectal neoplasia in ulcerative colitis: a cohort study. Gastroenterology. 2007;133(4):1099–105.

[10] Cosnes J. Smoking and diet: impact on disease course? Dig Dis. 2016;34(1–2):72–77. [Epub ahead of print]

[11] Itzkowitz S. Colon carcinogenesis in inflammatory bowel disease: applying molecular genetics to clinical practice. J Clin Gastroenterol. 2003;36:S70–74.

[12] Clevers H. Colon cancer-understanding how NSAIDs work. N Engl J Med. 2006;354:761–763.

[13] Roessner A, Kuester D, Malfertheiner P, Schneider-Stock R. Oxidative stress in ulcerative colitis-associated carcinogenesis. Pathol Res Pract. 2008;204:511–524.

[14] Soetikno R, Kaltenbach T, McQuaid KR, Subramanian V, Laine L, Kumar R, Barkun AN. Paradigm shift in the surveillance and management of dysplasia in inflammatory bowel disease. Dig Endosc. 2016. doi:10.1111/den.12634. [Epub ahead of print]

[15] Wanders LK, Kuiper T, Kiesslich R, Karstensen JG, Leong RW, Dekker E, Bisschops R. Limited applicability of chromoendoscopy-guided confocal laser endomicroscopy as daily-practice surveillance strategy in Crohn's disease. Gastrointest Endosc. 2015. pii: S0016-5107(15)02834-5. doi:10.1016/j.gie.2015.09.001. [Epub ahead of print]

[16] Rubin PN, Friedman S, Harpaz N, et al. Colonosopicpolypectomy in chronic colitis: conservative management after endoscopic resection of dysplastic polyps. Gastroenterology. 1999;117:1295–300.

[17] Marion JF, Waye JD, Israel Y, Present DH, Suprun M, Bodian C, Harpaz N, Chapman M, Itzkowitz S, Abreu MT, Ullman TA, McBride RB, Aisenberg J, Mayer L. Chromoendoscopy is more effective than standard colonoscopy in detecting dysplasia during long-term surveillance of patients with colitis. Clin Gastroenterol Hepatol. 2015. pii: S1542-3565(15)01597-9. doi:10.1016/j.cgh.2015.11.011. [Epub ahead of print]

[18] Welman CJ. Crohn's disease imaging in the emergency department. J Gastroenterol Hepatol. 2016. doi:10.1111/jgh.13352. [Epub ahead of print]

[19] Aalykke C, Jensen MD, Fallingborg J, Jess T, Langholz E, Meisner S, Andersen NN, Riis LB, Thomsen OØ, Tøttrup A. Colonoscopy surveillance for dysplasia and colorectal cancer in patients with inflammatory bowel disease. Dan Med J. 2015;62(1):B4995.

[20] Triantafillidis JK, Nasivelos G, Kosmidis PA. "Colorectal cancer and inflammatory bowel disease: epidemiology, risk factors, mechanisms of carcinogenesis and prevention strategies". Auction Res. 2009;29(7):727–2737.

[21] Mattar MC, Lough D, Charabaty A. Current management of inflammatory bowel disease and colorectal cancer. Gastrointest Cancer Res. 2011;4(2):5361.

[22] Kiesslich R, Hoffman A, Neurath M-F. Colonoscopy, and inflamatory bowel disease. Tumors New Diagn Methods Endosc. 2006;38(1):5–10.

[23] Nakai Y, Isayama H, Shinoura S, IwashitaT, Samarasena J. Confocal laser endomicroscopy in gastrointestinal and pancreatobiliary diseases. Dig Endosc. 2014;26(Suppl 1): 86–94.

[24] Negrón ME1, Kaplan GG, Barkema HW, Eksteen B, Clement F, Manns BJ, Coward S, Panaccione R, Ghosh S, Heitman SJ. Colorectal cancer surveillance in patients with inflammatory bowel disease and primary sclerosing cholangitis: an economic evaluation. Inflamm Bowel Dis. 2014;20(11):2046–55.

[25] Lutgens M, van Oijen M, Mooiweer E, van der Valk M, Vleggaar F, Siersema P, Oldenburg B. A risk-profiling approach for surveillance of inflammatory bowel disease-colorectal carcinoma is more cost-effective: a comparative cost-effectiveness analysis between international guidelines. Gastrointest Endosc. 2014;80(5):842–8.

[26] Efthymiou M, Allen PB, Taylor AC, Desmond PV, Jayasakera C, De Cruz P, Kamm MA. Chromoendoscopy versus narrow band imaging for colonic surveillance in inflammatory bowel disease. Inflamm Bowel Dis. 2013;19(10):2132–8.

[27] Subramanian V, Bisschops R. Image-enhanced endoscopy is critical in the surveillance of patients with colonic IBD. Gastrointest Endosc Clin N Am. 2014;24(3):393–403.

[28] Rogler G. Chronic ulcerative colitis and colorectal cancer. Cancer Lett. 2014;345(2):235–41.

[29] Genta RM, Feagins LA. Advanced precancerous lesions in the small bowel mucosa. Best Pract Res Clin Gastroenterol. 2013;27(2):225–33.

[30] Beaugerie L, Svrcek M, Seksik P, Bouvier AM, Simon T, Allez M, Brixi H, Gornet JM, Altwegg R, Beau P, Duclos B, Bourreille A, Faivre J, Peyrin-Biroulet L, Fléjou JF, Carrat F. Risk of colorectal high-grade dysplasia and cancer in a prospective observational cohort of patients with inflammatory bowel disease. Gastroenterology. 2013;145(1): 166–175.

[31] Dekker E, van den Broek FJC, Reitsma JB, Hardwick JC, Johan Offerhaus G, van Deventer SJ, Hommes DW, Fockens P. "Narrow band imaging compared with conventional colonoscopy for the detection of dysplasia in patients with longstanding ulcerative colitis". Endoscopy. 2007;39(3):216–221.

[32] Moody GA, Jayanthi V, Probert CSJ, Mac Kay H, Mayberry JF. Long-term therapy with sulphasalazine protects against colorectal cancer in ulcerative colitis: a retrospective

study of colorectal cancer risk and compliance with treatment in Leicestershire. Eur J Gastroenterol Hepatol. 1996;8:1179–83.

[33] Qin X. Is colonic Crohn's disease more closely related to ulcerative colitis or Crohn's disease by nature? Inflamm Bowel Dis. 2016. [Epub ahead of print]

[34] Velayos FS, Loftus Jr. EV, Jess T, Scott Harmsen W, Bida J, Zinsmeister AR, Tremaine WJ, Sandborn WJ. Predictive and protective factors associated with colorectal cancer in ulcerative colitis: a case-control study. Gastroenterology. 2006;130:941–1949.

[35] Burman S, Hoedt EC, Pottenger S, Mohd-Najman NS, Ó Cuív P, Morrison M. An (anti)-inflammatory microbiota: defining the role in inflammatory bowel disease? Dig Dis. 2016;34(1–2):64–71.

[36] Herfarth HH. Methotrexate for inflammatory bowel diseases—new developments. Dig Dis. 2016;34(1–2):140–146.

[37] Megna BW, Carney PR, Kennedy GD. Intestinal inflammation and the diet: is food friend or foe? World J Gastrointest Surg. 2016;8(2):115–23.

[38] Gearry RB. IBD and environment: are there differences between east and west. Dig Dis. 2016;34(1–2):84–89.

[39] Sjooqvist U, Tribukait B, Öst A, Einarsson C, Oxelmark L, Lofberg R. Ursodeoxycholic acid treatment in IBD-patients with colorectal dysplasia and/or DNA-aneuploidy: a prospective, double-blind, randomized controlled pilot study. Anticancer Res. 2004;24(5B):3121–3127.

[40] Suzuki S, Tajima T, Sassa S, Kudo H, Okayasu I, Sakamoto S. Preventive effect of fluvastatin on ulcerative colitis-associated carcinogenesis in mice. Anticancer Res. 2006;26(6B):4223–4228.

[41] Cho S-J, Kim JS, Kim JM, Lee JY, Jung HC, Song IS. Simvastatin induces apoptosis in human colon cancer cells and in tumor xenografts, and attenuates colitis-associated colon cancer in mice. Int J Cancer. 2008;123:951–957.

Chapter 9

Laparoscopy in the Management of Colon Cancer

Valentin Ignatov, Anton Tonev, Nikola Kolev,
Aleksandar Zlatarov, Shteryu Shterev, Dilyan Petrov,
Tanya Kirilova and Krasimir Ivanov

Additional information is available at the end of the chapter

http://dx.doi.org/10.5772/64507

Abstract

The minimally invasive techniques in surgical practice have been well introduced and widely accepted for certain procedures, including surgery for colon cancer. The advantages of the laparoscopic approach in terms of early and late postoperative results and the oncological safety have been established by numerous reports, including randomized controlled trials. The application of laparoscopic colon surgery for cancer has been adopted in various institutions. This chapter reviews the available literature data regarding the use of minimally invasive surgery for colon cancer, including early and late surgical and oncological results and new trends. Retrospective and prospective trials published in the last 20 years are reviewed to address the issues. Technological advantages such as intracorproreal anastomosis, single incision, and natural orifice surgery are commented in the chapter.

Keywords: minimally invasive surgery, laparoscopy, colon cancer, hemicolectomy, colectomy, sigma resection

1. Introduction

The mainstay of treatment of colon cancer is the multidisciplinary approach. The advances of medical technology in various areas have led to improvement of cancer staging, surgical technique, medical oncology, and cancer biology. The logical consequence led to better treatment options. It was well stated in the article by Dinu et al. that a multidisciplinary team consisting of oncologists, surgeons, radiologists, physicists, and pathologists should provide the patient with a specific elaborate protocol of treatment, given the generally accepted treatment guidelines that are based on the efficacy of the multimodal treatment [1].

Reference	Procedure	Conversion to open surgery, % (number of total)		Operating time, min		Length of hospital stay, days		Postoperative morbidity, % (number of total)	
		HALS	LAC	HALS	LAC	HALS	LAC	HALS	LAC
HALS Study Group♦ [3]	All	14% (3/22)	22% (4/18)	152 ± 66	141 ± 54	7 (2–12)	6 (2–10)	5% (1/22)	22% (4/18)
Hassan♦ [6]	All	15% (16/109)	11% (17/149)	277 ± 96*	211 ± 108*	6 ± 3*	5 ± 3*	20% (18/109)	17% (11/149)
Segmental colectomy									
Targarona [10]	Left and right colectomy	7% (2/27)	7% (2/27)	140 ± 56 (70–300)	152 ± 34 (109–240)	6.5 ± 3.7	7.2 ± 3.9	26% (7/27)	22% (6/27)
Chang [14]	Sigmoidectomy/ left colectomy	0% (0/66)*	13% (11/85)*	189 ± 40 (120–290)	205 ± 60 (90–380)	5.2 ± 3.0 (3–22)	5.0 ± 2.4 (2–17)	21% (11/66)	16% (14/85)
Yano [16]	Low anterior resection	0% (0/5)	12.5% (1/8)	211 ± 48*	311 ± 78*	–	–	–	–
Lee [18]	Sigmoidectomy diverticulitis	4.8% (1/21)	14% (3/21)	171 ± 34*	197 ± 42*	6.7 ± 2.1	7.5 ± 8.2	24% (5/21)	19% (4/21)
Anderson [24]	Sigmoidectomy diverticulitis	6.1% (6/98)	23.5% (4/17)	142 ± 46.5	153 ± 40.4	5.0 ± 3.0	5.1 ± 3.3	14.6% (14/98)*	29.4% (5/17)*
Ringley♦ [26]	Left and right colectomy	–	–	120 (78–181)*	156 (74–300)*	4 (2–11)	4 (2–14)	–	–
Tjandra♦ [28]	Ultralow anterior resection	0% (0/32)	0% (0/31)	170 ± 20*	188 ± 16*	5.9 ± 0.8	5.8 ± 1.2	22% (7/32)	26% (8/31)
Total (procto)colectomy									
Nakajima [29]	Total (procto-)colectomy	0% (0/12)	9.1% (1/11)	217 ± 63*	281 ± 62*	7.6 ± 2.7	8.1 ± 2.4	33% (4/12)	45% (5/11)
Rivadeneira [30]	Proctocolectomy	10% (1/10)	0% (0/13)	265 ± 57 (210–390)*	311 ± 40 (240–400)*	6.1 ± 3.3 (3–13)	7.2 ± 3.9 (4–17)	40% (4/10)	31% (4/13)
Boushey♦ [31]	Total (procto-) colectomy	2% (1/45)*	7% (6/85)*	TAC: 240 ± 49 TPC: 297 ± 52	271 ± 60 315 ± 70	TAC: 6 (3–34) TPC: 5 (4–14)	5 (4–25) 5 (3–24)	TAC: 24% (4/17) TPC: 32% (9/28)	35% (18/52) 24% (8/33)
Polle [32]	Total restorative proctocolectomy	0% (0/30)	0% (0/35)	231 ± 60 (149–400)	297 ± 38.5 (235–375)	11.8 ± 5.7 (5–31)			

Table 1. Characteristics of HALS and LAC in several studies included in the metaanalysis on hand-assisted and laparoscopic assisted approach in colorectal surgery by Aalbers et al. [33].

Laparoscopic approach is used with increased frequency for many surgical procedures. The laparoscopic colectomy follows the principles of open oncological surgery – low ligation of the blood vessels at their origin and no-touch isolation [2]. Usually the anastomosis for right-colon tumors is performed extracorporally, and thus minimal laparotomy is required. The laparoscopic technique decreases length of hospital stay and pain and allows sooner restoration of food intake. Laparoscopy can be safely used if the following criteria are absent: severe adhesions, advanced tumor (e.g., T4),and/ or complicated colon cancer. The similarity between oncological results and the defined short-term clinical advantages of laparoscopic and open surgery for colon cancer have been proven in various multicenter studies. [14]. The patients with previous abdominal surgery (PAS) are at risk due to severe adhesions. The laparoscopic adhesiolysis is more technically challenging and time consuming. The study of Zanghi et al. reviews that matter and concludes that laparoscopic adhesiolysis increases the risk of bowel injury [7]. PAS is not universally accepted as contraindication for laparoscopic surgery, although it complicates the procedure as a whole. Law et al. reported patients with PAS who did not develop short-term postoperative complications such as ileus, prolonged hospital stay, or conversion rate after colorectal surgery [4]. In contrast, Yamamoto et al. described relatively higher rates of intraoperative intestinal injury and postoperative complications, including ileus and delayed time to diet in patients with a history of abdominal surgery [5] (**Table 1**).

2. Laparoscopy for colon cancer

2.1. Patients

In results from a single-center study from Tajima et al., patients were compared according to their age, gender, and tumor location between the hand-assisted laparoscopy (HALS) and CL groups [8] (**Table 2**). Less bleeding during surgery, faster postoperative recovery, and shorter stay are some of numerous advantages of laparoscopic resection of colon. After all, there are doubts of the radical curative effect of complete tumor resection, lymph node dissection, and puncture implantation metastasis by laparoscopic surgery. However, the most important indicator for the radical curative effect of laparoscopic surgery is the number of dissected lymph nodes. CRM is significant for the assessing of the prognosis of colorectal cancer surgery. The long-term survival rate of colorectal cancer patients undergoing laparoscopic surgery compared to open surgery procedures is also analyzed. No statistical difference in 3- or 5-year OS and 3-or 5-year DFS between the two procedures was reported ($P>0.05$) [8].

Surgical time of colorectal cancer laparoscopic surgery is longer compared to open surgery, and laparoscopic surgery requires a more skilful surgeon. The surgeons undergo rigorous training and development for a period of time, which improves the surgical procedure [9]. Also the nonneoplasm technique is important, which is the same as the open surgery is. The previously used method for the quality assessment with digital score may cause deviation.

Surgical methods	HALS, % (n)	CL, % (n)	P-value
Right hemicolectomy	26.5 (26)	24.6 (28)	0.743
Transverse colectomy	2.0 (2)	7.0 (8)	0.088
Left hemicolectomy	8.2 (8)	7.0 (8)	0.753
Anterior resection	27.6 (27)	33.3 (38)	0.363

Table 2. Comparison of stage I/II/III patients (n = 145) who underwent HALS (n = 63) or CL (n = 82).

2.2. Hand-Assisted Laparoscopic Surgery

Over the last years, minimally invasive laparoscopic surgery is being used more and more. Additional bowel resection for stage I rectal cancer, radical resection of stage II or III rectal cancer, and palliative surgery in patients with stage IV rectal cancer are among the indications of laparoscopic surgery. Traditional laparotomy for rectal cancer makes it difficult to visualize certain areas, including the pelvic floor, the ventral part of the bladder, and the posterior to apical regions of the prostate.

The traditional laparoscopic approach has been well established. In some cases a hybrid approach is required, e.g., rectal cancer surgery. The traditional laparotomy may reveal certain anatomical areas. On the other hand, the laparoscope provides magnified view of the structures and allows for safer approach. Laparoscopy-assisted colorectal surgery (LACS) is used in Japan and several drawbacks are reported – is more time consuming and requires specific experience and technical equipment, which makes it more challenging. In Europe and the United States, the so-called hybrid-hand assisted laparoscopic surgery (HALS) is more widespread, which allows for direct vision. The advantages of HALS include direct safe palpation and grasping with the hand, shorter operative time, and shorter learning-curve.

2.3. Outcomes

2.3.1. Short-term benefits of laparoscopic surgery

Laparoscopic procedures have several short-term benefits that are well described in all reports on the topic of minimally invasive procedures. Those include earlier restoration of bowel function, oral food intake, smaller incision, and less operative trauma (therefore less need for analgesia) and were proven in various randomized control trials. In the case of cancer surgery, the laparoscopic approach allows for faster recovery, which may influence the oncological results by sooner initiation of systemic therapy. The hospital stay is shorter in comparison to open surgery. In elderly and comorbid patients, the laparoscopic surgery may lead to cardiovascular and pulmonary complications, although the mortality and morbidity rates are lower than in open surgery.

2.3.2. Long-term outcomes

Oncological outcomes of LS and OS for colorectal cancer patients were similar in most randomized studies. The random trial conducted by Lacy et al. [11] showed excellent long-term oncologic outcomes following LS, when compared with OS in patients with curable colon cancer. This study had a median follow-up of 95 months, but there was only one difference between the two techniques including the higher survival rate of patients with stage III colon cancer.

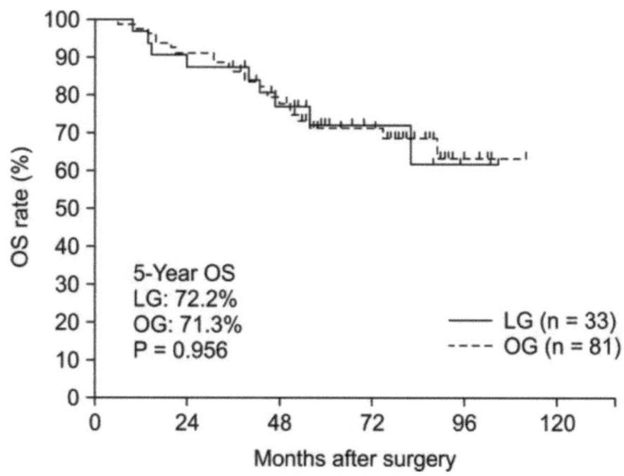

Figure 1. Overall survival (OS) of stage III colon cancer patients. LG, laparoscopic surgery group; OG, open surgery group [11].

The oncologic outcomes after performing LS instead of OS are still being analyzed when treating colorectal cancer patients. Recurrences and disease-free and overall survivals following LS compared to OS for stage III colorectal cancer patients are shown on **Figure 1** [11].

The long-term results are similar for laparoscopy and open surgery. On the contrary, a study made by Lacy et al. [11] has noted some oncological benefits for stage III colon cancer, including better local recurrence rates and higher rates of long-term and overall survival. For stage I and II, there were no significant oncological differences. Those results could be explained by patient's immunity response, dissemination of cancer cells, and earlier start of systemic treatment. The rates of local and distant metastases are found to be lower after laparoscopic surgery [12]. Despite that peritoneal carcinomatosis rates remain the same. The local recurrence rate of right colon cancer is relatively higher in compared to the left localization, although this is not confirmed by randomized studies [13].

3. New trends

3.1. SILS

The increasing patients' interest in cosmetic results has led to the more frequent use of single-incision surgery, even for colon cancer. The ultimate goal of "scarless surgery" could be achieved only when oncological results are proven to be equivalent to standard laparoscopic surgery. SILS ports are placed at the umbilicus or in case of rectal cancer at the planned site of a stoma. SILS reduces the abdominal incision trauma, provides better cosmesis, and reportedly, shorter hospital stay. SILS approach is successfully applied in laparoscopic colorectal procedures. For last few years, there are more data about this approach, which confirmed benefits of and interests in this technique. The SILS technique is administered to patients and the achieved results are promising. The development of SILS went from simple surgical procedures to the first colorectal resections in 2008. The first sigmoidectomy for benign disease was performed by Bucher et al. [17]. This approach was also used for anterior rectal resection, proctocolectomy, and total proctocolectomy. Lu C-C et al. as well as some other authors suggested that SILS could be applied both for benign and malignant cases [17, 20, 22, 23].

The operative time compared to conventional laparoscopic surgery is varying, and according to some retrospective studies the difference is not statistically significant. The operative time yet is longer, regardless of the procedure according to a study by Kwag et al [20]. The difference of operative times could be explained also by the fact that this techniques is not that widely used and the learning curve is steeper. Other criteria such as pain are reported to be more severe after SILS [20], although other authors report decrease of pain [22, 23].

4. NOTES

The first human colorectal natural orifice endoscopic surgery (NOTES) procedure was initiated with the reports of Bernhardt et al. [19] and Palanivelu et al. [25], who performed appendectomy in 2008. Performance of more complex procedures was limited by the instrumentation. In addition the colorectal procedures require restoration of continuity, which is a major limitation for NOTES. The hybrid NOTES procedures such as trans- anal total mesocolic excision (TEM) broaden the possibilities for this technique (**Figure 2**).

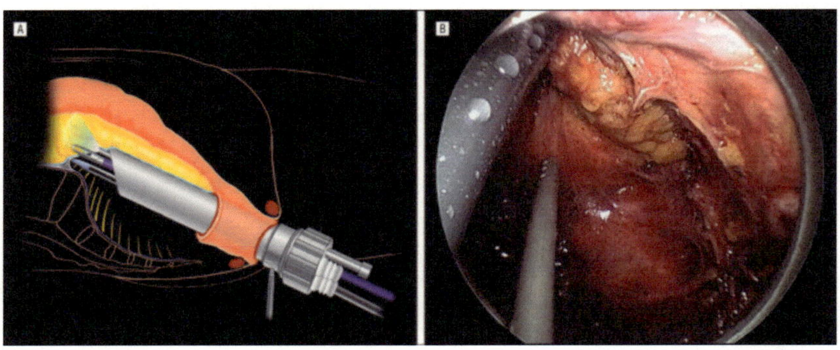

Figure 2. Schematic of retroperitoneal dissection with the transluminal transanal endoscopic operation device (A) and intraoperative view of the retroperitoneal approach at the sacral promontory (B) [24].

SILS evolved starting with cadavers and swines [25]. Sylla et al. [15] reported successful total mesorectum excision (TME) with laparoscopic assistance in a human. Two cases of laparoscopically assisted transanal TME were reported by Dumont et al. [21]. The clinical and oncological advantages are yet to be analyzed [2, 27–29].

Alternative technique is the mini-laparoscopy-assisted natural orifice surgery (MA-NOS), which includes additional laparoscopic ports less than 5mm and main port inserted in the natural orifice. The largest port is placed in the natural orifice. Lacy et al. [27] has pioneered this technique and presented a case of total colectomy. The authors suggest that the lack of dedicated NOTES instruments requires laparoscopic assistance.

5. Summary

Laparoscopic colon resection for cancer can be performed safely and accurately with many short-term benefits to the patients while resulting in at least equivalent long-term results as open surgery procedures. Other potential benefits may include better preservation of cell-mediated immune function and reduced tumor cell proliferation. The scientific confirmation of the efficacy of laparoscopic surgery is needed to implement it further in the practice and accept it as a worldwide standard. The available level 1 data support safety, patient-related benefits, and oncological similarity. Innovative approaches are being tested, including less abdominal wall trauma. Mastering the laparoscopic approach still has a steep learning curve, although the even more available laparoscopic courses will diminish that issue.

Author details

Valentin Ignatov, Anton Tonev*, Nikola Kolev, Aleksandar Zlatarov, Shteryu Shterev, Dilyan Petrov, Tanya Kirilova and Krasimir Ivanov

*Address all correspondence to: teraton@abv.bg

Department of General and Operative Surgery, Medical University of Varna, Varna, Bulgaria

References

[1] Therapeutic strategies in colonic cancer. Chir Buchar Rom 1990. 2014 Dec;109(6):741–6.

[2] García- Valdecasas JC, Delgado S, Castells A, Taurá P, Piqué JM,. Laparoscopy-assisted colectomy versus open colectomy for treatment of non-metastatic colon cancer: a randomised trial. The Lancet. 2002 Jun 29;359(9325):2224–9.

[3] HALS Study Group (2000) Hand-assisted laparoscopic surgery vs. standard laparoscopic surgery for colorectal disease: a prospective randomized trial. Surg Endosc 14:896–901 CrossRef

[4] Law WL, Lee YM, Chu KW. Previous abdominal operations do not affect the outcomes of laparoscopic colorectal surgery. Surg Endosc Interv Tech. 2005;19(3):326–30.

[5] Yamamoto M, Okuda J, Tanaka K, Kondo K, Asai K, Kayano H, . Effect of Previous Abdominal Surgery on Outcomes Following Laparoscopic Colorectal Surgery: Dis Colon Rectum. 2013 Mar;56(3):336–42.

[6] Hassan I, Nancy You Y, Cima RR, Larson DW, Dozois EJ, Barnes SA, Pemberton JH (2007) Hand-assisted versus laparoscopic-assisted colorectal surgery: practice patterns and clinical outcomes in a minimally-invasive colorectal practice. Surg Endosc Aug [Epub ahead of print]

[7] Zanghì A, Cavallaro A, Piccolo G, Fisichella R, Di Vita M, Spartà D, . Dissemination metastasis after laparoscopic colorectal surgery versus conventional open surgery for colorectal cancer: a metaanalysis. Eur Rev Med Pharmacol Sci. 2013 May;17(9):1174–84.

[8] Tajima T, Mukai M, Noguchi W, Higami S, Uda S, Yamamoto S, . Comparison of hand-assisted laparoscopic surgery and conventional laparotomy for rectal cancer: Interim results from a single center. Mol Clin Oncol [Internet]. 2015 Feb 9 [cited 2016 Feb 5]; Available from: http://www.spandidos-publications.com/10.3892/mco.2015.508

[9] Lee S. Laparoscopic Procedures for Colon and Rectal Cancer Surgery. Clin Colon Rectal Surg. 2009 Nov;22(04):218–24.

[10] Targarona EM, Gracia E, Garriga J, Martinez-Bru C, Cortes M, Boluda R, Lerma L, Trias M (2002) Prospective randomized trial comparing conventional laparoscopic colectomy with hand-assisted laparoscopic colectomy: applicability, immediate clinical outcome, inflammatory response, and cost. Surg Endosc 16:234–239 PubMed Cross Ref.

[11] Lacy AM, Delgado S, Castells A, Prins HA, Arroyo V, Ibarzabal A, . The long-term results of a randomized clinical trial of laparoscopy-assisted versus open surgery for colon cancer. Ann Surg. 2008 Jul;248(1):1–7.

[12] Baek J-H, Lee G-J, Lee W-S. Comparison of long-term oncologic outcomes of stage III colorectal cancer following laparoscopic versus open surgery. Ann Surg Treat Res. 2015;88(1):8.

[13] Guerrieri M, Campagnacci R, De Sanctis A, Lezoche G, Massucco P, Summa M, . Laparoscopic versus open colectomy for TNM stage III colon cancer: results of a prospective multicenter study in Italy. Surg Today. 2012 Nov;42(11):1071–7.

[14] Chang YJ, Marcello PW, Rusin LC, Roberts PL, Schoetz DJ (2005) Hand-assisted laparoscopic sigmoid colectomy: helping hand or hindrance? Surg Endosc 19:656–661 PubMed CrossRef.

[15] Sylla P, Bordeianou LG, Berger D, Han KS, Lauwers GY, Sahani DV, . A pilot study of natural orifice transanal endoscopic total mesorectal excision with laparoscopic assistance for rectal cancer. Surg Endosc. 2013 Sep;27(9):3396–405.

[16] Yano H, Ohnishi T, Kanoh T, Monden T (2005) Hand-assisted laparoscopic low anterior resection for rectal carcinoma. J Laparoendosc Adv Surg Tech A 15:611–614 PubMed CrossRef.

[17] Bucher P, Pugin F, Morel P. Single port access laparoscopic right hemicolectomy. Int J Colorectal Dis. 2008 Oct;23(10):1013–6.

[18] Lee SW, Yoo J, Dujovny N, Sonoda T, Milsom JW (2006) Laparoscopic vs. hand-assisted laparoscopic sigmoidectomy for diverticulitis. Dis Colon Rectum 49:464–469 PubMed CrossRef.

[19] Bernhardt J, Gerber B, Schober H-C, Kähler G, Ludwig K. NOTES--case report of a unidirectional flexible appendectomy. Int J Colorectal Dis. 2008 May;23(5):547–50.

[20] Kwag S-J, Kim J-G, Oh S-T, Kang W-K. Single incision vs conventional laparoscopic anterior resection for sigmoid colon cancer: a case-matched study. Am J Surg. 2013 Sep; 206(3):320–5.

[21] Dumont F, Goéré D, Honoré C, Elias D. Transanal endoscopic total mesorectal excision combined with single-port laparoscopy. Dis Colon Rectum. 2012 Sep;55(9):996–1001.

[22] Kim S-J, Ryu G-O, Choi B-J, Kim J-G, Lee K-J, Lee SC, . The short-term outcomes of conventional and single-port laparoscopic surgery for colorectal cancer. Ann Surg. 2011 Dec;254(6):933–40.

[23] Lu C-C, Lin S-E, Chung K-C, Rau K-M. Comparison of clinical outcome of single-incision laparoscopic surgery using a simplified access system with conventional laparoscopic surgery for malignant colorectal disease: Single-incision laparoscopic colectomy. Colorectal Dis. 2012 Apr;14(4):e171–6.

[24] Anderson J, Luchtefeld M, Dujovny N, Hoedema R, Kim D, Butcher J (2007) A comparison of laparoscopic, hand-assist and open sigmoid resection in the treatment of diverticular disease. Am J Surg 193:400–403 PubMed CrossRef.

[25] Palanivelu C, Rajan PS, Rangarajan M, Parthasarathi R, Senthilnathan P, Prasad M. Transvaginal endoscopic appendectomy in humans: a unique approach to NOTES--world's first report. Surg Endosc. 2008 May;22(5):1343–7.

[26] Ringley C, Lee YK, Iqbal A, Bocharev V, Sasson A, McBride CL, Thompson JS, Vitamvas ML, Oleynikov D (2007) Comparison of conventional laparoscopic and hand-assisted oncologic segmental colonic resection. Surg Endosc 24: Epub ahead of print.

[27] Lacy AM, Adelsdorfer C, Delgado S, Sylla P, Rattner DW. Minilaparoscopy-assisted transrectal low anterior resection (LAR): a preliminary study. Surg Endosc. 2013 Jan; 27(1):339–46.

[28] Tjandra JJ, Chan MKY, Yeh CH (2007) Laparoscopic-vs. hand-assisted ultralow anterior resection: a prospective study. Dis Colon Rectum Dec [Epub ahead of print]

[29] Nakajima K, Lee SW, Cocilovo C, Foglia C, Sonoda T, Milsom JW (2004) Laparoscopic total colectomy: hand-assisted vs. standard technique. Surg Endosc 18:582–586 PubMed CrossRef

[30] Rivadeneira DE, Marcello PW, Roberts PL, Rusin LC, Murray JJ, Coller JA, Schoetz DJ Jr (2004) Benefits of hand-assisted laparoscopic restorative proctocolectomy: a comparative study. Dis Colon Rectum 47:1371–1376 PubMed CrossRef

[31] Boushey RP, Marcello PW, Martel G, Rusin LC, Roberts PL, Schoetz DJ Jr (2007) Laparoscopic total colectomy: an evolutionary experience. Dis Colon Rectum 50: 1512–1519 PubMed CrossRef

[32] Polle SW, van Berge Henegouwen MI, Slors FM, Cuesta MA, Gouma DJ, Bemelman WA (2008) Total laparoscopic restorative proctocolectomy: are there any advantages compared with the open and hand-assisted approach? Dis Colon Rectum [Epub ahead of print]

[33] Aalbers AGJ, Biere SSAY, van Berge Henegouwen MI, Bemelman WA. Hand-assisted or laparoscopic-assisted approach in colorectal surgery: a systematic review and meta-analysis. Surg Endosc. 2008;22(8):1769–80.

Chapter 10

Current Immunotherapeutic Treatments in Colon Cancer

Zodwa Dlamini, Thandeka Khoza, Rodney Hull,
Mpho Choene and Zilungile Mkhize-Kwitshana

Additional information is available at the end of the chapter

http://dx.doi.org/10.5772/63212

Abstract

The immune system is able to act against cancer cells and consequently these cells have developed a range of responses to evade or suppress the immune systems anticancer responses. The concept of cancer immunotherapy is based on techniques developed to restore or boost the ability of the immune system to recognize and target tumor cells. It is known that colon cancer does initiate an immune response and that this type of cancer initiates pathways and responses to evade or suppress the immune system. This chapter will discuss some of the dominant therapies being developed to treat colon cancer based on the concept of cancer immunotherapy. Cancer vaccines are based on the concept of providing the immune system with antigen targets derived from tumor-specific molecules, while monoclonal antibodies involve the development of antibodies specifically targeting proteins expressed on the surface of tumor cells. Antibody-based immunotherapy has further applications in the use of bispecific antibodies (BsAb), which are synthetic antibodies designed to be able to recognize two different antigens or epitopes and in this way can increase the immunoresponse and limit immune evasion observed in mono-targeted therapy. Immune checkpoint inhibitors target proteins that are responsible for keeping immune responses in check. Tumor cells overexpress these proteins in order to evade the immune response. Blocking these proteins will lead to an increased immune response against these cells. Cytokine-based immunotherapies involve the use of the immune systems' own molecular messengers that are responsible for a robust immune response, to boost the antitumor response of the immune system. Oncolytic viral therapy is based on the use of viruses that selectively infect and replicate in cancer and associated endothelial cells and subsequently kills these cells. Adoptive immunotherapy involves the use of immune cells from the patient to be cultured and altered in the laboratory and then reintroduced to boost the immune response. This is normally performed with T cells. Immunotherapy may be the next logical step in the development of an effective therapy for colon cancer and other cancers. The combination of these therapies with traditional chemotherapy or radiotherapy has shown promise in cancer treatment.

Keywords: Cancer vaccines, Monoclonal antibodies, Bispecific antibodies, Cytokines, Immune checkpoint inhibitors, Adoptive therapy, Immunotherapy

---

1. Introduction: immunotherapy

Tumor-associated antigens (TAAs) are antigens that can elicit a specific immune response. Immune cells and immune-related components such as macrophages, neutrophils, complement components, $\gamma\delta$ T cells, natural killer (NK) cells, NKT cells, and certain cytokines (interleukin (IL)-12, interferon gamma (IFN-γ)) and cells of the adaptive immune system, including B lymphocytes, helper T cells (Th cells), and cytotoxic T lymphocytes (CTLs), are all active against cancer cells [1]. TAAs are presented to the cells of the adaptive immune system by cells such as dendritic cells (DCs) or other antigen-presenting cells (APCs). These antigens are processed and presented by major histocompatibility complex (MHC) class I and class II molecules leading to the activation of antigen-specific lymphocytes, resulting in antibody production [1].

Colon cancer evades the immune system through the shift from Th1 to Th2 immune responses [2] loss/downregulation of human leukocyte antigen (HLA) class I antigen processing and presentation [3], defective DC function [4, 5], T-cell loss of signaling molecules [6, 7], escaping death receptors, HLA G expression, alterations in transforming growth factor (TGF) beta signaling [8], Increased vascular endothelial growth factor (VEGF) expression, impaired NK activity, regulatory T-cell downregulation [9], and complement decay accelerating factor CD55 [2]. A shift is known to occur in the white blood cell composition with elevated numbers of CD8 T cells in the initial stages, but an overall reduction in the numbers of circulating immune-related cells. At the same time the levels of cytokines such as IFN-γ and tumor necrosis factor-α (TNFα) are reduced during vascular invasion [10]. Antitumor T cells can be inhibited through NO production by the enzyme arginase [11].

Immunotherapy can be divided into two main categories: passive and active immunotherapy. Passive immunotherapy makes use of *in vitro* produced immunologic effectors that are capable of influencing tumor cell growth. This includes monoclonal antibody (mAb) therapy and adaptive transfer of antigen-specific effector cells. Active immunotherapy aims at inducing or boosting immune effector cells [1].

2. Cancer vaccines

Cancer vaccines are active immunotherapeutic approaches that are intended to activate and expand tumor-specific T cells to induce an antitumor response. Conventional vaccines are preventative in nature, but current cancer vaccines activate the immune system to destroy tumors once present. A range of tumor antigens have been identified. These include T-cell epitope peptides, defined carbohydrates of glycoproteins and glycolipids, antibody-based anti-idiotype vaccines, plasmid DNA and recombinant viral vector vaccines, allogeneic or autologous whole tumor cell vaccines, DC-based vaccines, oncolysates, or autologous heat-shock protein (HSP)-peptide complex vaccines. An ideal prophylactic cancer vaccine would be affordable, stable, and safe. It would induce effective immunity rapidly and require few immunizations (ideally one) to induce protection [12]. This section aims to address advances made in developing vaccines against colon cancer. This will include vaccines that are currently in use and vaccines still undergoing clinical trials. It will report on the safety, side effects, and efficacy of these vaccines.

Colon cancers express multiple immunogenic proteins, all of which may serve as targets for the development of T-cell-mediated adaptive immune responses [10]. It is also known that colorectal cancers do activate the immune system, leading to the attenuation of metastasis and increasing the survival of patients [10]. In order to evade the immune response, colorectal cancer suppresses the immune response or displays only weak immunogenicity. Additionally, studies have shown that restoration or supplementation of the immune function toward these tumors is possible [10, 13, 14]. Peptides used to inoculate a patient suffering from colon cancer will be degraded and the resulting fragments will be endocytosed by APCs. These cells will then present the antigen to the T cells. CTLs or CD8+ T cells induce apoptosis in tumor cells through the release of granzymes and perforins and through the Fas death receptor pathway. Type 1 CD4+ T cells and T-helper cells secrete cytokines leading to the recruitment of CTLs, macrophages, and NK cells. These secrete cytokines that activate cytotoxic pathways [11] (**Figure 1**). It is also known that colorectal cancers do activate the immune system, leading to the attenuation of metastasis and an increase in the survival rate and time of patients [10]. The effectiveness of peptide vaccines can be enhanced by altering the amino acid sequence of the peptide to enhance the interaction with the T-cell receptor (TCR), to improve binding to MHC, and finally to improve biostability and reduce degradation by proteases [11].

2.1. Evasion of the immune system by altered ligand expression

One mechanism utilized by cancer cells to evade the immune system involves the expression of FasL. This ligand binds to the Fas receptor present on CTL, leading to the CTL to undergo apoptosis. The expression of FasL leads to the increased resistance to Fas-induced apoptosis. Altered peptide ligands (APLs) are analogs of immunogenic peptides which are ligands for TCRs. These altered ligands bind the TCR, but does not lead to lysis of the tumor cell [11]. Regulatory T cells can inhibit antitumor immunity by upregulating cell membrane molecules that lead to the inhibition of effector T-cell activation and function. Cancer cells have defective antigen presentation allowing them to avoid recognition by the immune system. This is accomplished by reduced expression of MHC I, antigen-processing machinery, or Tumor-associated antigens themselves [11].

2.2. Tumor-associated antigens (TAAs)

Defined TAA epitopes can be used to vaccinate cancer patients. The peptide fragments are presented by the two MHC proteins, MHC classes I and II (HLA I and II) to the TCRs. MHC class I presents the vaccine-derived peptide to naive CTLs. Primed CTLs recognize the tumor antigen on the surface of the tumor and send out a death signal to the tumor. Helper T cells are generated by MHC class II proteins [11] (**Figure 1**). However, there are not many specific peptides that can be targeted as cancer specific. In order to increase uptake and presentation of the antigens by APCs, an adjuvant is added [1]. Another strategy is to inject the DNA sequences coding for specific TAAs to be taken up. The target ill be transcribed into mRNA, translated into a protein, and processed into peptides by APCs. This can be done by using viruses engineered to express TAAs. However, the immune system may preferentially react to the viral antigens rather than the TAAs, leading to the attenuation of the antitumor immune response [1]. The earliest example of the therapeutic use of tumor antigens was in the form of crude tumor lysates being administered to patients. These lysates are still used as a means to prime DCs, facilitating peptide presentation [11]. This is because the ideal source of TAAs is all the TAAs the tumor itself expresses. By incubating DCs with dead tumor cell lysate, these antigens will all be presented by MHC class I (cross-presentation) and MHC class II pathways. This will result in a diversified immune response involving CTLs as well as CD4+ T-helper cells [1].

The use of tumor lysates has largely been superseded by the use of synthetic peptides. These have certain advantages over tumor lysates. They provide a higher amount of specific antigen and allow for modification of the target peptide. It is also easy to monitor the immune response to vaccination with a single peptide as only one CTL type requires evaluation [11]. Tumor-specific antigens (TSAs) are mutated or virus-derived epitopes and contain unique immunogenic neo-antigens that can be recognized by the immune system. These include N-RAS and p53 [1].

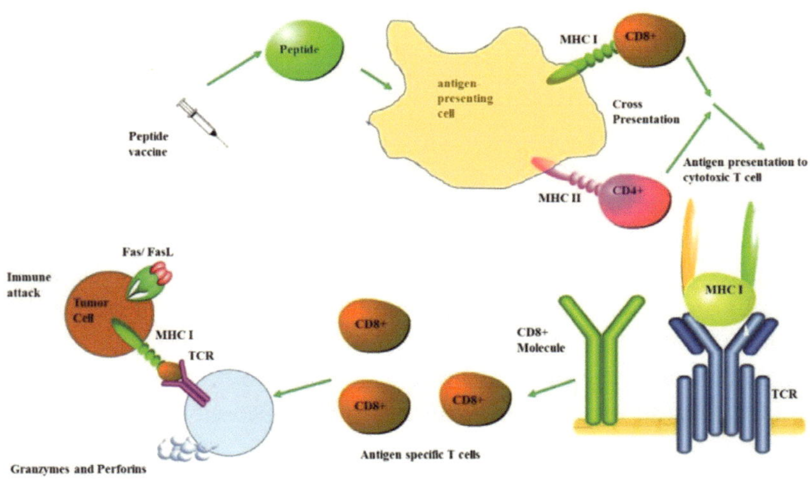

Figure 1. Antitumor effect of peptide vaccine therapy: following introduction of peptide vaccine to the bloodstream, it is processed and presented by the APC leading to the activation of CD4+ helper T cells and CD8+ cytotoxic T cells. Interaction between MHC I molecules on APC and TCR during antigen presentation facilitated by CD8 molecule leads to the generation of tumor-specific CTLs capable of lysing tumor cells.

Peptides	Mechanism	Study details	References
Tyrosine kinase receptor ephrin type-A receptor 2 (EphA2-derived peptide)	EphaA2 EphA2-specific CTL	High level of immunity against colorectal cancer in murine model	[15]
RNF43-721		Phase 1 clinical trial	[16]
ABT-737	Inhibition of antiapoptotic Bcl-2 family	Sensitized cancer cells in mouse colon cancer model	[17]
Epitopes of HER2, MVF, GMP, and n-MDP	Multiple targets	Phase 1 clinical trial	[18]
Endoglin	Inhibition of angiogenesis	Inhibition of tumor growth in mouse model	[19]
CEA CEA691	Induction of tumor-specific CTLs	Increase in survival rate in colon carcinoma mouse model	[20]
OX40L – TNF family protein		Inhibition of tumor growth in mouse model	[21]
Mucin 1: MUC1 a cell surface-associated protein		Stimulation of antigen-specific CTL, abundant secretion of IFN-γ. Tumor burden was significantly reduced in colon cancer mouse model	[22]
Heat-shock protein Gp96	Induction of tumor-specific CTLs	Two-year overall survival and disease-free survival were significantly improved	
SART3-tumor-rejection antigen	Induction of tumor-specific CTLs	Increased cellular immune responses to the tumor. No improved clinical outcome	[23, 24]
Lck-derived peptides	Induction of tumor-specific CTLs		[24]
Survivin-2B	Induction of HLA-A24-restricted cytotoxic T cells resulting in high toxicity against HLA-A24-positive survivin-2B-positive cancer in vitro	Increased proportion of peptide-specific CTL. No significantly improved clinical outcome	[25]
βHCG CTP37-DT (Avicine)		Phase II trials showed improved patient survival	[26]
CDX 1307	Fusion between βHCG and an antibody against the mannose receptor	Phase I trial. Inoculation leads to DC activation as well as cytotoxic T-cell activity against tumor cells	[27]
p53 (SLP)	p53-specific CD4+ Th cell SLP is a p53 synthetic long peptide	Antitumor response against p53-overexpressing tumors. The p53-SLP vaccine induces p53-specific T-cell responses	[10]

Peptides	Mechanism	Study details	References
EGFR2 gefitinib or erlotinib	EGFR mutations enhance tyrosine kinase activity in response to EGF, increasing the efficacy of anti-EGFR	In a phase I trial, the vaccine elicited antibody response phase II cancer	[28]
Gastrin: G17DT (gastroimmune)	Antigastrin-17 immunogen, raising antibodies that blockade gastrin-stimulated tumor growth	Phase II trials showed gastroimmune combined with irinotecan chemotherapy increased patient survival	[29]

Examples of peptide-based vaccine targets, their mechanism, as well as the current results of any trials performed using the vaccines to treat colon cancer.

Table 1. Peptide targets and mechanism of action.

Discussed below are examples of peptide-based vaccines and their targets that have been used to treat colon cancer. More examples are listed in **Table 1**. Beta human chorionic gonadotropin (βHCG) is not produced by normal colorectal cells. The increase in the expression of this antigen in colon cancer cells leads to an increase in tumor invasiveness, higher metastatic incidence and promotion of tumor growth, neovascularization, and immune system suppression. This makes it an attractive target for the development of an antibody-based vaccine [10]. Carcinoembryonic antigen (CEA) is an oncofetal antigen that can serve as a target for vaccine development. It is found overexpressed on the surface of colon cancer cells, with very low levels of expression on normal cells. Unfortunately this protein is normally expressed during fetal development and is therefore tolerated by the immune system. This led to the creation of an artificial CEA. CeaVac is based on anti-idiotypic antibodies and mimics CEA [10]. Another oncofetal protein 5T4 is a leucine-rich membrane glycoprotein. Once again it is nearly absent in normal tissues but is overexpressed in colon cancer cells and developing cells. Its presence is associated with poor survival. The drug TroVax uses 5T4 with a pox virus vector and a modified vaccinia virus. Preclinical trials in mouse models resulted in a 90% reduction of tumor burden [10].

Onyvax-105 is another anti-idiotype antibody mimicking the glycosylphosphatidylinositol-anchored protein CD55. CD55 regulates complement activation protecting cells against complement attack thereby enhancing tumor cell survival. The gastric acid–stimulating hormone gastrin is a hormone the precursors of which are overexpressed in colon cancer, where they act as growth factors. This leads to increases in angiogenesis and cell proliferation. Vaccines raised against this protein would therefore result in inhibition of cell growth, proliferation, and metastasis [10]. Onartuzumab is a mAb that targets human growth factor receptor (HGFR). It is a monovalent HGF antagonist antibody against MET Proto-Oncogene, Receptor Tyrosine Kinase that benefits patients who overexpress HGFR [30].

The FANG ™ vaccine consists of tumor cells from the patient and a plasmid expressing granulocyte-macrophage colony-stimulating factor (GM-CSF) and bifunctional short hairpin RNAfurin (bi-shRNAfurin). The growth and production of DCs are induced by GM-CSF. The enzyme furin transforms precursor proteins into active proteins and the presence of bi-shRNAi furin inhibits the production of active proteins. This particularly inhibits the production of TGF β1 and 2 (TGFβ). Overexpression of TGFβ is associated with cancer progression and immune suppression by inhibiting GM-CSF and the consequent production of dendritic and other APCs. The vaccine therefore prevents the overexpression of TGFβ and leads to immune cell activation and the inhibition of cancer cell proliferation [30]. The vaccine was manufactured using GM-CSF and IL-13 to generate DCs from monocytes. The DCs were loaded with 6HLA-A*0201-binding peptides derived, among others, from CEA, MAGE-2 (melanoma antigen overexpressed in gastrointestinal cancer), and HER2/neu [10, 30].

TroVax is an attenuated strain of vaccinia virus that encodes the 5T4 protein. This protein is an oncofetal antigen and is a transmembrane glycoprotein. It is highly expressed in colon cancers and is virtually absent in normal tissue. The receptor is thought to play a role in metastasis and the expression level increases with the advancement of the stage of the cancer. This vaccine is able to induce an effective immune response, as it results in the formation of antibodies for both the 5T4 antigen and the viral particle [31].

2.3. Heat-shock proteins (HSPs)

HSPs are widely expressed in tumors, where they promote cancer progression. HSP 72 and glucose-regulated protein 96 (gp96) are two of these proteins that are highly expressed in colon cancer [32]. These proteins are thought to play a role in cell growth and signal transduction and expression of these proteins is higher in tumors undergoing metastasis. This makes them useful as diagnostic and prognostic markers. However, this expression is not related to patient survival [32].

HSPs enhance antigen-specific tumor immunity as they play an important role in the presentation of antigens to $CD8^{+}$ T cells through the MHC I pathway. This is because of the roles HSP 70s play as chaperones and in the transport of peptides to the heterodimeric transporters associated with antigen processing [33]. Similarly gp96 is a major chaperone involved in the lumen of the endoplasmic reticulum (ER), where it facilitates the folding of the MHC Iβ-2 microglobulin-peptide complexes in the ER [34].

Vaccines based on HSPs have been tested in animal trials and been found to be highly effective in the treatment of cancers [32, 35]. The function of the HSP in transporting and presenting other peptides as surface antigens has led many researchers to propose that HSPs can be used to create a HSP target protein fusion. This booster strategy would therefore enhance the ability of the target protein to be used as an antigen by T cells [36]. Two of these proteins that can be coupled to HSPs to improve their immunogenicity and usefulness as a cancer vaccine are alpha-fetoprotein (AFP) in hepatocellular carcinoma and CD44 in colonic carcinomas [32].

3. Targeted therapy: monoclonal antibodies

Recently, a new class of targeted agents have been identified, which bind to the ligand or the extracellular domain of a receptor. This results in alteration of intracellular signal transduction pathways which will affect cell proliferation, dedifferentiation, inhibition of apoptosis, and stimulation of neoangiogenesis [37]. This section will look into VEGF-targeted drugs (e.g., ramucirumab (Cyramza®) and bevacizumab (Avastin®)), EGFR-targeted drugs (e.g., cetuximab (Erbitux®) and panitumumab (Vectibix®)), and others such as those that target kinases [37].

3.1. Bevacizumab and ramucirumab

VEGF is a potent angiogenic factor and functions by binding to one of three VEGF receptors located on endothelial cells and angioblasts. The VEGF receptor-2 is overexpressed on up to 50% of colorectal cancer cell surfaces. VEGF-A and other proangiogenic factors promote the degradation of the extracellular matrix. This enables proliferation and migration of endothelial cells [37]. The ligands of the VEGF family include VEGF-A, VEGF-B, VEGF-C, VEGF-D, and VEGF-E; and the receptors are VEGFR-1, R-2, and R-3. In colon cancer the ligand that is most abundant is VEGF-A [38]. Sustained angiogenesis is a hallmark of cancer; and targeted inhibition of blood vessel development is an established strategy for antitumor therapy [38]. Anti-VEGF therapies have been associated with a survival benefit across multiple malignancies including colon cancer [38].

Bevacizumab is a humanized mAb against VEGF and it acts by preventing ligand binding by binding to VEGF. This prevents downstream intracellular signal transduction; however, the response to bevacizumab appears to be independent of VEGF expression or high microvessel density (MVD) [37]. MVD assessment is a good predictor of metastasis, with selective antibodies, such as endoglin, distinguishing between tumor neovascularization and preexisting vessels. VEGF expression is highest in patients with metastatic tumors and the level is associated with cancer stage [38]. Bevacizumab is typically used in combination with other chemotherapeutic agents, and it is also indicated in improving the delivery of chemotherapy by changing tumor vasculature and decreasing the elevated interstitial pressure in tumors. The combination of therapies results in improved survival [38].

Ramucirumab is a fully humanized IgG1 mAb targeting the extracellular domain of VEGF receptor 2 (VEGFR2). Large-scale trials have indicated that ramucirumab shows promising antitumor effects and is well tolerated. The origin of this antibody was through the use of a large phage display library with tailored *in vitro* selection methods to identify a high-affinity antibody [39]. Measurement of VEGFA and soluble VEGFR1/2 during phase I trials of the antibody indicated that there is an increase in the expression of VEGF as well as a decrease in VEGFR1/2 levels. These changes were not dose related, which suggests that the receptor was saturated [39]. Phase I trial results were promising and phase II trials resulted in a high percentage of patients presenting with progression free survival at 6 months. Phase III trials showed an increase in overall patient survival [39]. Adverse reactions to ramucirumab included hypertension, vascular thrombotic events, and proteinuria [40].

Aflibercept is a recombinant fusion protein consisting of the second immunoglobulin (Ig) domain of VEGFR-1 and the third Ig domain of VEGFR-2, fused to human IgG1. It exhibits affinity for VEGF-A, VEGF-B, and PlGF. The antibody displayed effective activity against colon cancers with improvements in the primary endpoint of overall survival and overall response rate, as well as displaying a high degree of tolerability in patients [40]. VEGFR-1 also plays a role in colon cancer and inhibiting its signaling could also play a role in cancer treatment. An antibody developed to target this receptor named IMC-18F1 has been developed. This is a high-affinity human VEGFR-1-neutralizing antibody that specifically binds the extracellular domain of VEGFR-1. It exhibits antiangiogenic and antiproliferative activity [40].

3.2. Panitumumab and cetuximab

The epidermal growth factor receptor (EGFR) is a target for the therapeutic monoclonal antibodies panitumumab and cetuximab the treatment of metastatic colorectal cancer. Panitumumab is a fully human Ig G2 mAb that binds the EGFR extracellular domain with high affinity and inhibits ligand-induced EGFR tyrosine phosphorylation, tumor cell activation, and tumor cell proliferation (**Figure 2**). Cetuximab is a chimeric human-mouse IgG1 mAb [41]. Cetuximab and panitumumab are both Food and Drug Administration (FDA) approved for advanced colorectal cancer therapy, and both have clear benefits for colon cancer treatment of most patients. The exception is those patients that carry *KRAS* mutations at codons 12 and 13 [42]. *KRAS* mutations occur in approximately 35–40% of colorectal tumors, and *KRAS* is a member of the rat sarcoma virus (Ras) gene family of oncogenes and is involved in integrating the signaling cascades controlling gene transcription, including many EGFR-mediated pathways [41]. The ligands of the EGFR transmembrane tyrosine kinase receptor include EGF, TGFα, epiregulin, amphiregulin, β-cellulin, and heparin. EGFR activates downstream signaling pathways such as the Ras/Raf/mitogen-activated protein kinase (MAPK) pathway, the phosphatidylinositol 3-kinase (PI3K)/AKT pathway, and the signal transducer and activator of transcription (STAT) pathway. These downstream pathways activate cellular survival, proliferation, invasion, metastasis, and angiogenesis. Abnormal activation of the EGFR signaling network due to excessive overexpression is common in colon cancer (**Figure 2**). EGFR is composed of an extracellular ligand-binding domain, a hydrophobic transmembrane region, and an intracellular domain with tyrosine kinase activity [41, 43].

Cetuximab competes with EGFR ligands, such as EGF or TGFα, with a high affinity ($K_d = 1 \times 10^{-10}$ M). This results in the inhibition of cell cycle progression and arrest of cell cycle in G1 phase, inhibition of angiogenesis, inhibition of metastasis by reduction of production of matrix metalloproteinase, inhibition of apoptosis, and potentiation of antitumor activities of chemotherapy and radiotherapy [43]. Panitumumab treatment results in improved clinical outcomes in patients with chemotherapy-refractory colon cancer [41]. Panitumumab also has a high affinity for EGFR ($K_d = 5 \times 10^{-11}$ M) and acts to arrest cell cycle progression and block cancer growth; however, it is an IgG2 and does not act through antibody-dependent cell cytotoxicity [43].

Using a single type of mAb to block a single transduction pathway may only have a limited effect, as tumors can shift to other alternate pathways. One solution is to combine monoclonal antibodies to block two signaling transduction pathways [44]. Use of multiple monoclonal antibodies has other advantages including limited overlapping toxicity and few to no pharmacokinetic interactions between antibodies. However, some studies indicate that certain combinations such as bevacizumab with cetuximab or panitumumab lead to shorter survival and increased toxicity in advanced colorectal cancer compared to therapy with a single antibody [44]. The addition of panitumumab to chemotherapy improves clinical outcomes among patients with wild-type *KRAS* [41]. Other biomarkers that affect the efficacy of panitumumab include mutations in the *BRAF* and *PIK3CA* genes [41]. An important side effect of panitumumab treatment is the occurrence of skin toxicity; however, occurrences of skin toxicity correlate with favorable outcomes for patients [41, 43].

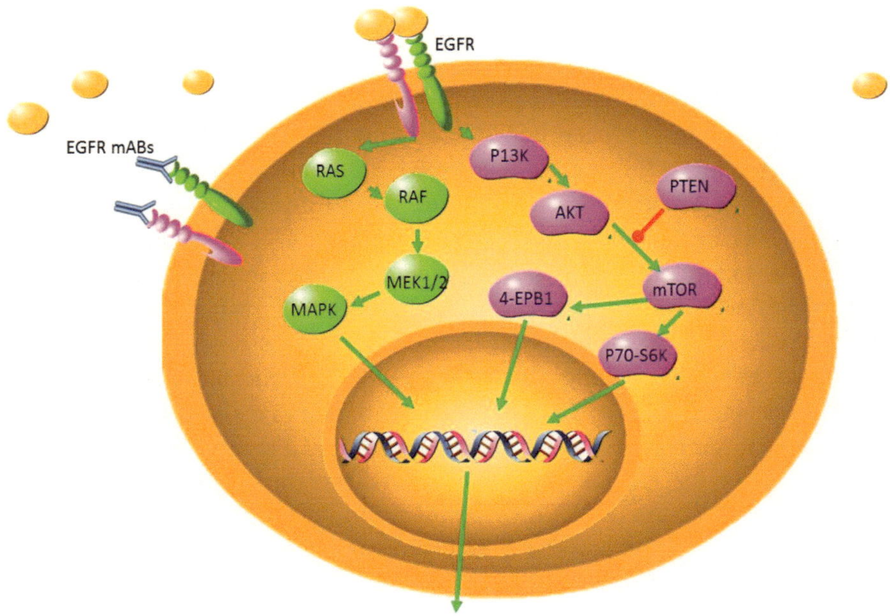

Figure 2. Mechanism of action of anti-EGFR mAbs. The binding of these mAbs on EGFR prevents the dimerization and the activation of EGFR.

4. Immune checkpoint inhibitors

During the progression of tumor development, the cancer cells undergo changes to escape immune surveillance. In order to accomplish this, a large enough number of the tumor cells must escape in order for there to be an equilibrium between tumor growth and tumor killing [1]. Normally, tumor-infiltrating lymphocytes (TIL) would control the progression of cancers; however, cancer cells can evade this response using a process known as T-cell exhaustion. This occurs due to the expression of inhibitory receptors. Blocking these receptors through the use of inhibitory molecules or monoclonal antibodies is known as immune checkpoint inhibition [45]. The immune system depends on multiple checkpoints to avoid overactivation in healthy cells. These inhibitory molecules expressed by the cancer cells take advantage of these checkpoints to escape detection by the immune system. They will often express molecules that serve as "immune checkpoints," by so doing; a message is sent to the immune system that an immune response is not necessary. Drugs are being developed to block immune checkpoint molecules from binding to their molecular partners, thus allowing the body to elicit an immune response and therefore attack cancer cells. An analysis of the expression patterns in colon cancers revealed a large overexpression of immune checkpoint-related proteins [46].

The programmed death-1 (PD-1) checkpoint is blocked in most cancers and blocking the pathway with antibodies to reactivate this checkpoint is a viable cancer therapy [47]. Recent insights indicate that blockade of the PD-1 checkpoint exists in many cancer patients and a repertoire of tumor-specific or tumor-selective T cells can be reactivated to achieve tumor therapy [48, 49]. Blocking the PD-1 pathway with antibodies results in durable tumor regression. Programmed death-ligand 1 (PD-L1) is a transmembrane receptor that plays a role in suppressing the immune system by suppressing the proliferation of CD8+ T cells and to lower the level of antigen particles by regulating apoptosis. PD-1, expressed on T cells, B cells, and other immune effector cells, interacts with this receptor, resulting in a negative signal to the T cell. Expression of PD-L1 in tumor biopsies shows that this pathway acts to block antitumor immune responses [46]. PD-1 has two ligands, PD-L1 and PD-L2. Tumor cells expressing PD-L1 are associated with poor outcomes for patients. Targeting these ligands prevent T-cell exhaustion and promotes T-cell recognition of tumors [45]. PD-L1 also binds to the co-stimulatory molecule CD80, implying that CD80 has the potential to facilitate antitumor immunity by inhibiting the PD-1 suppressive pathway [47].

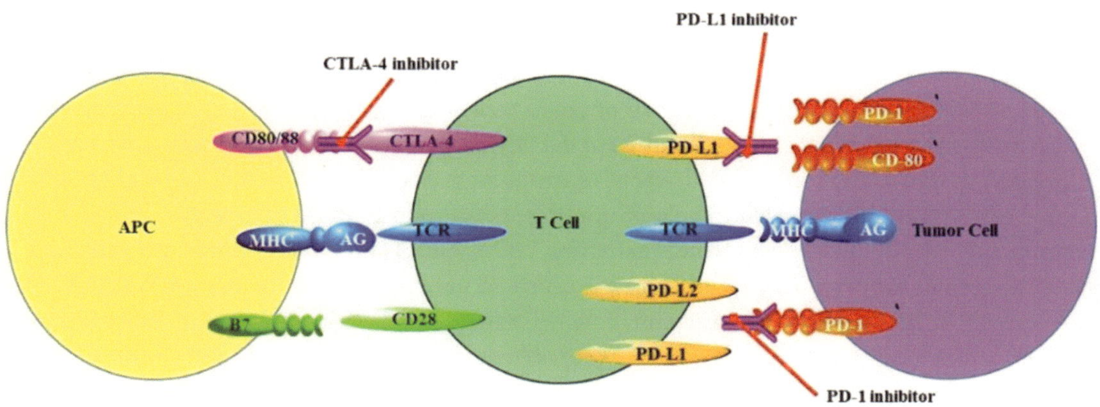

Figure 3. Immune checkpoint interactions and antibody-based inhibition on T cells. CTLA-4 inhibition can be performed by inhibiting CD28 co-stimulation (through binding with its ligands CD80 or CD86) that is required to complete T-cell activation. The PD-1/PD-L1 pathway can be inhibited by targeting its inhibitory role. Here it interacts with PD-L1 on the tumor cell. Inhibiting this interaction results in a more robust targeted antitumor immune response.

Ipilimumab is a mAb that targets CTLA-4 (cytotoxic T-lymphocyte-associated protein 4), which normally negatively regulates the activity of T cells. This antibody was the first checkpoint-blocking antibody to be approved by the US FDA for cancer treatment; CTLA-4 is a member of the Ig superfamily of receptors, which also includes PD-1, TIM-3 (T-cell Ig and mucin domain-containing protein 3), BTLA (B and T-lymphocyte attenuator), and VISTA (V domain Ig suppressor of T-cell activation). Use of this drug enhances the antitumor activity of

CD8 T cells and inhibits the suppressive function of Tregs [45]. This was followed by a second antibody, pembrolizumab, which targets the programmed death 1 (PD-1; CD279) molecule [50] (**Figure 3**). Trials of these antibody therapies have only shown modest clinical benefits, and this may indicate that tumors use multiple and nonoverlapping immunosuppressive mechanisms to evade the immune response [45]. Multiple studies indicate that effective therapy involves the targeting of multiple immunosuppressive pathways [51].

Tumor cells can also evade the immune system through the production of extracellular adenosine by CD73 which is expressed on lymphocytes and endothelial and epithelial cells. CD73 performs an endothelial cell barrier function, protecting cells from ischemia and regulating immune responses. This receptor is overexpressed in many types of cancer, with high CD73 expression being associated with poor outcomes for patients due to increases in tumor immune escape and metastasis [45]. Blocking CD73 can induce potent antitumor immune responses. Additionally the inhibition of molecular pathway components upstream of CD73 such as CD39 also has similar therapeutic effects. This treatment can also be used to supplement immune checkpoint therapies that make use of anti-CTLA-4 and anti-PD-1 mAbs, to increase the effectiveness of such therapies [45].

Another strategy to target immune checkpoints is the use of small molecule drugs that target critical survival pathways. These include Gleevec and ibrutinib, both of which are tyrosine kinase inhibitors. Ibrutinib is a covalent inhibitor of BTK (Bruton's tyrosine kinase), a key enzyme in B-cell receptor signaling [49].

Controlling the immune response to cancer cells through the use of anti-inflammatory drugs to control the inflammatory components reduces the risk of developing certain types of cancer. Aspirin is able to reduce the incidence of colon cancer and slow down tumor progression. Cyclooxygenase (Cox) enzymes 1 and 2 are the targets of aspirin. These enzymes are overexpressed in tumor cells. Immunosuppressive drugs such as cyclosporine A (CsA) and tacrolimus (FK506) inhibit the calcium/calmodulin-dependent phosphatase calcineurin, which acts upon members of the nuclear factor of activated T cells (NFAT) [52]. These transcription factors are important for cytokine production by T cells and are required for the normal function of B cells, DCs, and mast cells. Expression of NFAT family members leads to tumor suppression [53]. Treatment of tumor cells with CsA is capable of inducing necroptosis and a mild G0/G1 cell cycle arrest [52].

5. Cytokines

Cytokines are signaling proteins produced by white blood cells that help control the growth and activity of immune system cells. The two types of cytokines that are used in the treatment of cancer are IFNs and ILs. Cytokines stimulate a broad-based immune response as opposed to generating a targeted response to a specific antigen [54]. Tumors secrete factors to recruit inflammatory cells and/or activate stromal cells. Inflammation plays a major role in tumor promotion and progression. The soluble factors that drive inflammation are cytokines and chemokines produced by tumor cells themselves and by the cells recruited to the tumor microenvironment [55].

Several cytokines are capable of activating and recruiting specific immune cells that can enhance antitumor immunity; these include IL-2, IL-12, IL-15, TNFα, and GM-CSF. These cytokines can be used as single-agent therapies or in combination with other immunotherapeutic strategies. GM-CSF immunization leads to APC recruitment. Tumors activate Stat3 and Braf, which leads to the release of IL-10, inhibiting the tumoricidal activity of NK cells. Stat3 activation in DCs leads to these cells becoming tolerogenic DC [11].

Additionally, TNFα, hepatocyte growth factor, PDGF, and FGF19 activate Wnt/β-catenin signaling in tumor cells. This is the oncogenic pathway activated in the majority of colon cancers. This pathway results in β-catenin accumulation in the cytoplasm, which activates cell growth and differentiation pathways. IL-1β is a potent activator of Wnt signaling in colon cancer cells leading to increased survival of colon cancer cells [55].

Oncogenic signaling through the Wnt and NF-kB pathways is activated through TNFα. Pharmacological inhibition of TNFα by neutralizing TNFα antibodies has been used to treat both irritable bowel disorders and colon cancer. Results from trials using enbrel or remicade suggest that these neutralizing antibodies have activity against colon cancer cells. TNFα signaling initiates NF-kB signaling. NF-kB is continuously expressed in certain tumors, leading to enhanced survival by protecting the tumor cells from apoptosis. Treatment with the TNFα antagonist, etanercept led to inhibition of Wnt/β-catenin6 signaling as seen by the , reduced expression of active β-catenin [55].

5.1. Interleukins 1β, IL-6, and IL-1

The proinflammatory cytokine IL-1β is produced by activated macrophages. In turn, IL-1β induces the expression of TNFα, IL-6, IL-8, IL-17, Cox-2, and PGE2, promoters of tumor cell growth. Inducing the expression of IL-1β leads to increased incidence of cancer in wild-type mice. The IL-1β signaling pathway functions through the receptors IL-1RI and IL-1RII to induce NF-kB activity. The pathway involves the two adaptor proteins, MyD88 and IRAK. Macrophages are stimulated to release IL-1β and activate NF-kB and Wnt pathways, but IL-1β signaling requires STAT1. The silencing of STAT1 expression leads to decreased IL-1β release and prevented cancer cell growth [55].

IL-6 is secreted by stimulated monocytes, fibroblasts, and endothelial cells, macrophages, T cells, and B lymphocytes. Macrophages are stimulated by colon cancer cells to produce IL-6 and activate STAT3 in tumor cells. Inhibition of IL-6 signaling interferes with the growth of tumor cells and protects them from apoptosis. Research indicates that decreasing the expression or inhibiting the activity of STAT3 may have adverse effects on tumor promotion. Targeting STAT3 will affect the expression of β-catenin and the co-expression of STAT3 and β-catenin is associated with poor survival of colon cancer patients [55].

A subset of T-helper cells produces the cytokines IL-17, IL-22, and TNFα (Th17 cells). Paneth cells also produce IL-17. Th17 cells require IL-6, TGFβ, IL-1β, and IL-23, while IFN-γ and IL-4 negatively regulate differentiation of Th17 cells. IL-17 induces IL-6 and STAT3, promoting the survival of cancer cells. This cytokine may also have an anticancer function by enhancing antitumor immunity [55].

5.2. Tumor necrosis factor-related apoptosis-inducing ligand (TRAIL)

TRAIL (also known as Apo2L) activates the apoptotic cascade. Tumor cells can evade this apoptosis signal through the action of β-catenin. TRAIL's role in tumor surveillance has been confirmed in knockdown experiments and is a promising candidate to be used in cancer therapy, because it selectively kills cancer cells while leaving normal cells unharmed [55].

Sorafenib a Raf kinase inhibitor sensitized A TRAIL –resistant colon cancer line to TRAIL-induced apoptosis by preventing NF-kB-dependent expression of the antiapoptotic genes, IAP2 and MCl-1.

6. Oncolytic virus (OV) therapy

Over a century ago, researchers observed that viral infection both in human and animal models results in the expression of targets that can be recognized by T cells and/or antibodies. Subsequently, vaccination has been used to treat an array of diseases such as hepatitis B virus and human papillomavirus 15 which can cause liver and cervical cancer respectively. Vaccination against infections is used to induce neutralizing antibodies that act prophylactically. However, with regard to cancer vaccination, cancer vaccine candidates should induce and expand immune responses that can cause disruption of biological pathways that support cancer growth.

The concept of cancer immunotherapy is based on the ability of the immune system to recognize cancer cells and affect their growth and replication. Researchers have observed that cancer regression would occur spontaneously in patients after viral infection [56, 57]. For example, studies conducted by Lindeman and Klein 1967 showed that oncolysis of tumor cells by influenza virus increased immunogenicity of tumor cell antigens. The recent advances in successful sequencing of the cancer genome together with insights into how tumors evade the immune system have led cancer research to evolve from searching for a gene that causes individual cancer to one that blocks or disrupts biological pathways that support cancer growth [58, 59]. As a result, cancer vaccines are now being designed with the aim to boost the immune system to protect itself from carcinogenesis and progression of cancer. In 2010, the FDA approved Provenge which is a therapeutic vaccine for cancer [60]. It is designed to treat advances in prostate cancer and has shown to increase the survival rate. The success of Provenge resulted in stimulating the interest in the development of other therapeutic cancer vaccines.

In recent years, OV has been shown to be effective in treating cancer in both preclinical models and clinical trials. Toda and coworkers showed that genetically modified oncolytic HSV G207 is a potential cancer vaccine for induction of specific antitumor immunity in CT26 colon cancer cells [64, 61, 62]. This type of immunotherapy is largely dependent on the network of the host immune system to fight cancer by (i) boosting the patient's immune system, (ii) decreasing cancer-induced immunosuppression, and (iii) increasing the immunogenicity of the tumor itself [63, 64]; OVs can be RNA- or DNA-based virus derived from human or animals.

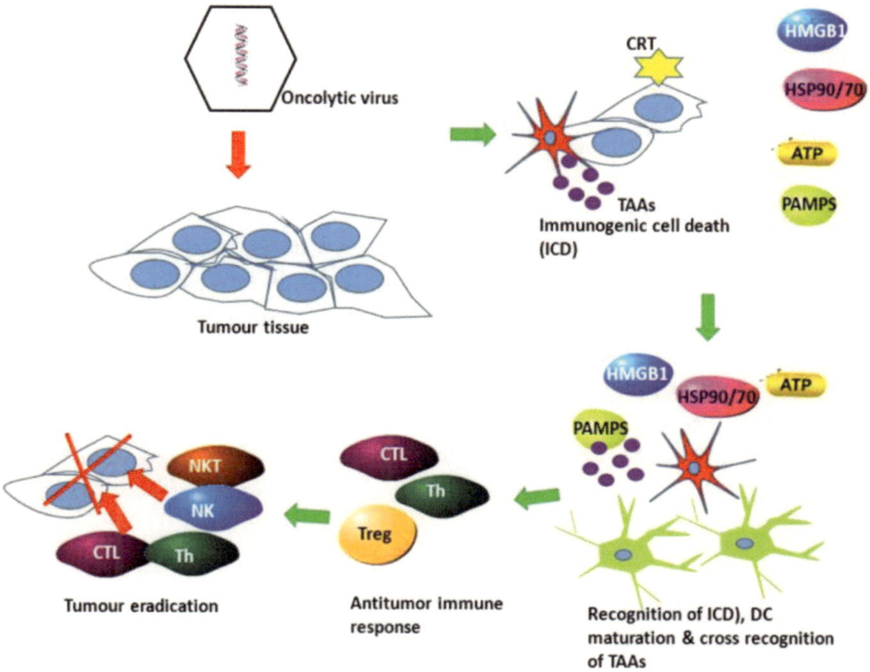

Figure 4. Immunogenic cell death of cancer cells induced by oncolytic viruses. An oncolytic virus selectively replicates in tumor cells, leading to induction of the death of these cells, presenting destruction signals on the cell surface and consequent release of danger signals from necrotic cells. Apoptotic bodies are engulfed by APC, and TAAs are processed and presented along with MHC complex and co-stimulatory molecules. The released DAMPs (and PAMPs) activate and mature DCs, and TAAs are cross-presented to naive T cells. This process can be further enhanced at different steps by other immunomodulatory agents (in a combination strategy). The resulting cytotoxic immune response against tumor and associated stromal cells, involving CD4+ and CD8+ T cells, may help in complete eradication of tumor mass. Additional immunotherapies targeting DCs, T cells, and the immunosuppressive TME can further enhance this antitumor immune response.

OV selectively infects and replicates in cancer and associated endothelial cells and subsequently kills these abnormal cells without harming the normal cells. The selectivity of OV can be an inherited feature of the virus or due to genetic engineering [56, 65]. OV therapy has multiple antitumoral activities including direct effect by cytotoxic cytokines released upon infection by tumor residents or infiltrating immune cells [66, 67]. The lysis-dependent cytoreductive activity activates innate immune receptors when immunogenic cell debris is taken up and cross presented by APCs (**Figure 4**).

OVs also directly affect various signaling pathways which are implicated in cancer such as Ras, Wnt, anti-apoptosis, and EGFR [66, 68, 69]. The altered signaling pathway creates a favorable environment for OV replication resulting in Cells infected with these viruses showing sustained proliferation, resisting cell death, evading growth suppressors and escaping immune surveillance. Cancer cells also show increased genomic instability and DNA damage stress, which is favorable to OV replication [70–72]. Genetic manipulation of OV enables these viruses to be (i) safe for use as a vaccine, (ii) highly selective for specific cancer type, and (iii) altering virus tropism. In comparison with current regimes for cancer treatment, OVs are advantageous because (i) they have a low chance for generation of resistance because they use multiple ways to exert cytotoxicity and (ii) virus dose in a tumor increases with time due to in situ virus replication whereas in the classical drug Pharmacokinetics, dose decreases with time [71, 73].

The major drawbacks in the use of OV include nonimmune human serum, development of anti-OV antibodies resulting from the use of human virus, and appropriate delivery into the tumor. Various delivery mechanisms have been explored to enable delivery of OV to tumor cells. For an example, cell carriers such as neural stem cells and myeloid-derived suppressor cells have been used to deliver OV to specific tumor cells. The cells protect the virus from anti-OV antibody neutralization, thereby facilitating virus deliver [71, 73]. In using OV to treat colon cancer, ONYX-015 has advanced to phase II clinical trials and is used in combination with chemotherapy [74, 75]. Recently, adenovirus 5 (PSE-EA1 and E deleted) has been approved to treat prostate cancer in China giving hope to development of OV as an alternative cancer treatment.

7. Bispecific antibody

Antibody-based therapy has been explored in treating a range of diseases and is promising to be a success with the FDA having approved more than 13 monoclonal antibodies for treatment of cancer (see Section 2). Furthermore, over 100 antibodies are at different stages of clinical trials. Medical researchers have explored the properties of antibodies which are (i) highly specific in binding their targets and (ii) are nontoxic for medical application using technologies such as hybridoma and phage display for antigen targeting [76–79]. Also, new technologies have been employed to manipulate antibodies for wide application. For example, the conventional antibody which is made up of two identical pairs of heavy and light chain linked together by disulfide bonds is monospecific and bivalent. Using a hybridoma technology, a fusion can be created between two hybridoma resulting in quadromas with two different heavy and light chains as a result of random pairing, thus forming molecules that do not occur in nature (**Figure 5A**). Antibodies produced by these methods have an ability to bind different species but could also be nonfunctional [77, 79, 80].

Conventional antibodies posed various challenges to therapeutic application due to inadequate exposure to the tumor as a result of their size (150 kDa) and impaired interactions with the immune system. Using enzyme-based antibody digestion, full antibodies may be truncated into Fc and Fab regions (**Figure 5A**). The Fab region which has the antigen-binding domain of the antibody is then used for therapeutic application. The drawback in using the Fab region of the antibody is its reduced half-life due to renal clearance [81, 82]. In addressing these

http://dx.doi.org/10.5772/63212

challenges, bispecific antibodies (BsAb) were developed in 1961 [83]. Just as their name implies, this class of antibodies binds two different antigens or two different epitopes on the same region.

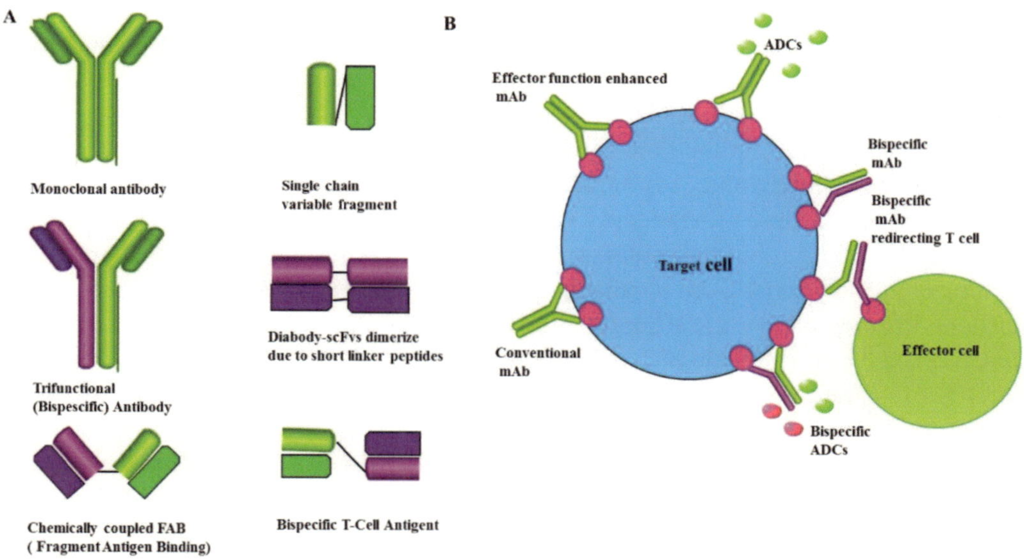

Figure 5. (A) Different forms of bispecific antibody. Trifunctional antibodies consist of two heavy and two light chains from two different antibodies. This results in an antibody with binding sites for two different antigens as well as an Fc region made up of two heavy chains forming a third binding site. A diabody consists of scFvs with very short linker peptides that force the closely positioned variable regions to fold together, forcing the scFvs to dimerize. Chemically coupled Fabs consist of the antigen-binding regions of two different monoclonal antibodies linked by a chemical means. Bispecific T-cell antigens are fusion proteins of two scFvs from four separate genes. (B) Development of bispecific compounds. Bispecific compounds enable simultaneous inhibition of two cell surface receptors, simultaneous blocking of two ligands, cross-linking of two receptors, and/or the recruitment of T cells to the proximity of tumor cells (redirected immune cell killing).

BsAb represent a class of antibodies that are yet to be fully explored in the treatment of cancer and other diseases. BsAb have a greater potential therapeutic efficiency than mono-targeted therapy, since they allow simultaneous engagements of two targets and limit potential escape pathways [84–86]. Numerous studies have shown that there is evidence of cross talk between receptor tyrosine kinases such as MET, VEGFR, and IGFR-IR which are known to promote cancer progression and drug resistance. And patients with colon cancer are known not to respond to anti-EGFR drugs with resistance emerging after initial usage [87, 88]. Engelman et al. showed that MET amplification leads to gefitinib resistance by activating the ERBB3 pathway, showing the complexity of tumor signaling pathways and a need to treat patients with drugs that target multiple targets [89].

In the use of BsAb, T cells are targeted because of their high cytotoxic retention, abundance in bloodstream, surveillance function, and proven ability to control malignant diseases [90, 91]. During cancer progression, cancer cells escape immune recognition by interfering with antigen presentation or T-cell activation or differentiation. In using the bispecific antibody, most targeted antigens for tumor therapy are differentiation antigens such as CD19, CD33, CEA, EpCAM Epithelial cell adhesion molecule, PMSA Prostate-specific membrane antigen , and EGF receptors. In most cases these antigens are overexpressed in cancer cells compared to the normal cells.

Blinatumomab is an example of a bispecific antibody that has shown great promise clinically in cancer patients. Blinatumomab is a 55 kDa-fusion protein comprised of two single-chain antibodies to CD19 and CD3, recombinantly joined by a flexible, non-glycosylated five-amino acid non-immunogenic linker that affords a very short distance between arms [92, 93]. Blinatumomab has high affinity for CD19 which is important in sustaining the malignant B-cell phenotype via mechanisms of proliferation, cell survival, and self-renewal [94, 95]. It draws malignant B cells in close proximity to CD3-positive T cells without regard to TCR specificity or reliance on MHC class I molecules on the surface of APCs for activation. The nonspecific binding of the polyclonal T-cell population prevents resistances to T-cell-based therapies as a result of downregulation of MHC molecules. CD19 and CD3 binding results in T-cell activation, marked by upregulation of T-cell activation markers CD25, CD69, CD2, IFN-γ, TNFα, and IL-2, IL-6, and IL-10 [96]. Cell lysis is mediated by secretion of perforin and various granzymes stored in the secretory vesicles of cytotoxic T cells [97]. In vitro data suggest that efficacy of blinatumomab is not compromised or dependent upon T cells, which may be limited in number in heavily pretreated patients [98]. Also blinatumomab-activated T cells appear to effectively induce serial target cell killing [92, 93].

8. Adoptive immunotherapy

In the wake of cancer treatment challenges or therapies, adoptive immunotherapy is one of the novel strategies being researched for cancer treatment. This concept was presented five decades ago [99–101] and is based on the transfer of ex vivo expanded antitumor CD8 T cells into affected patients (**Figure 6**). Delorme and Alexander [101] showed that the transfer of immune lymphocytes could inhibit the growth rate of carcinogen-induced sarcoma.

The immune system is responsible for the prevention of tumors or elimination of pathogens that can cause inflammation or an inflammatory environment for tumorigenesis or destroy tumor cells expressing TSAs or molecules induced by stress [102, 103]. Therefore, tumor development and progression are largely dependent on the patient's immune system to effectively inhibit cancer growth using its network of immune cell types. Each and every cell type has a specific function in inhibiting tumor growth (**Figure 7**). Consequently, the success of adoptive immunotherapy depends on approaches which will target different immune subsets.

Adoptive immunotherapies have explored the use of infiltrating T cells (CD8+ effector T cells and CD8+ effector memory cells), NK cells, and IL-2 for cancer-targeted therapies. The T cells are able to destroy tumor cells using cytotoxic granules containing perforin and granzymes and by using cell surface receptor such as TNF-related apoptosis-inducing ligand [104, 105]. Studies using mice have shown that adoptive transfer of T cells successfully induces antitumor

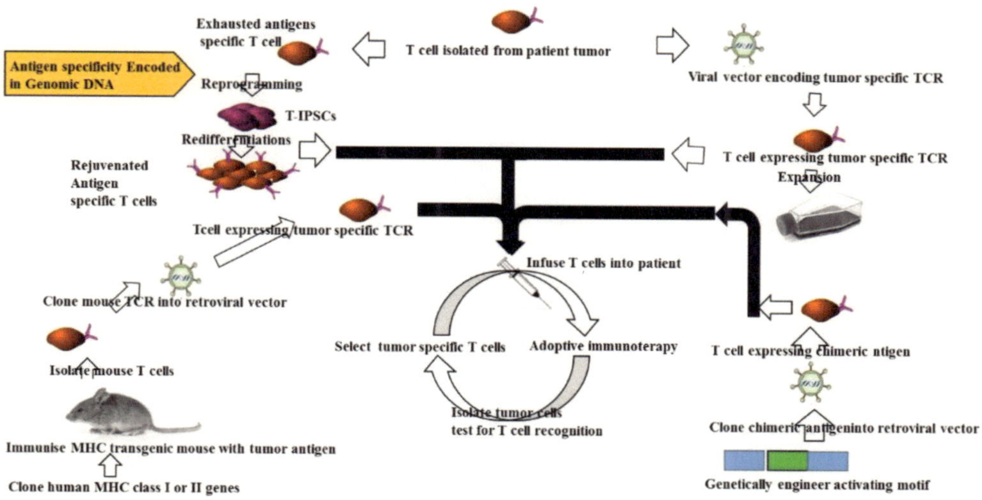

Figure 6. Different techniques used in adoptive immunotherapy. Adoptive immunotherapy with functional T cells can be performed in numerous ways. Exhaustion of antigen-specific T cells which can be a major problem in the practical application of this therapy can be solved through reprogramming clonally expanded antigen-specific $CD8^+$ T cells and then redirecting their redifferentiation into $CD8^+$ T cells possessing antigen-specific killing activity. T cells can be isolated from the patient. Isolated peptide antigens could be used to stimulate T cells that are already present in the patient's tumor or be used to prime tumor-specific T cells. If the T-cell populations generated are specific for the patient's tumor, they could be expanded and adoptively transferred if they are of human origin. T cells can be genetically engineered to recognize TAAs. TCRs from T cells that show a good antitumor response can be cloned and inserted into retroviruses, which are used to infect autologous T cells from the patient. Chimeric antigen receptors (CARs) can be generated through genetic engineering and then cloned into a retroviral vector and used to infect T cells from the patient. TCRs can also be isolated from humanized mice that express human MHC molecules and can be immunized with the tumor antigen of interest. Mouse T cells can then be isolated, and their TCR genes are cloned into recombinant vectors that can be used to genetically engineer autologous T cells from the patient.

response. Also, only a small number is required to mediate effective regression of tumor and survival [106–108]. Genetic modification of T cells has been successfully used to broaden their effective application by pairing with antigen receptors that recognize a range of different TAAs. Genetic engineering has also been employed to alter T cells so that they are able to avoid or be resistant to immune invasion strategies used by tumors such as the production of cytokines. Another modification of T cells involves attaching stimulatory signals for their activation [109, 110].

NK cells target and kill diseased cells using various mechanisms such as perforins and granzyme. The use of NK cells was first explored by Rosenberg et al. [111]. Lymphokine-activated killer cells were co-administered with IL-2 and resulted in a positive response in people with metastatic cancer [111]. Another combination of chemotherapy with transfer of allogeneic NK cells resulted in disease remission [112]. It is anticipated that a hybrid of T and NK cell will have great potential in the treatment of cancer using adoptive immunotherapy. However we are still a long way from the development of such a model treatment that can be developed for clinical trials and introduced into clinical practice.

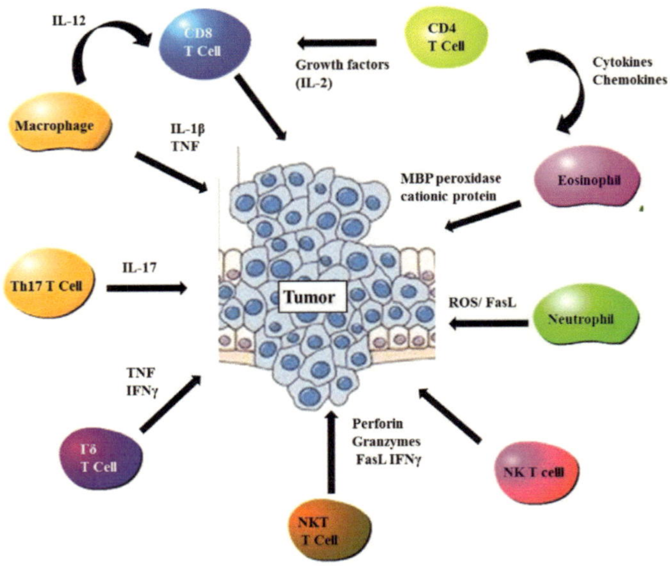

Figure 7. White blood cell types and mechanisms of response against tumors. The diagram illustrates all of the different immune-related cell types including T cells, NK, macrophages, eosinophils, and neutrophils that are able to respond against cancer cells. The method of response against the tumor cells is also indicated. In some cases these cell types can cooperate to produce additional responses.

9. Conclusion

The final goal of immunotherapeutic strategies to treat colon cancer would be the development of tumor-specific therapies that can be used in conjunction with standard chemotherapies with little side effects. The use of various combinations of different antibodies and OVs with synergistic antitumor activity and reduced toxicity will aim to achieve durable tumor eradication. One of the main obstacles is the identification of tumor-specific and essential tumor antigens. These antigens may differ with different tumors. In terms of checkpoint inhibition, it is important to establish the correct level of inhibition each patient requires to minimize toxicity. Another important goal is the identification and development of biomarkers to serve as prognostic markers for the monitoring of the individual patients response to immunotherapy, allowing for the identification of those patients who are most likely to benefit from these treatments. These goals require extensive further studies to refine immunotherapeutic strategies and combinatorial approaches.

Author details

Zodwa Dlamini*, Thandeka Khoza, Rodney Hull, Mpho Choene and Zilungile Mkhize-Kwitshana

*Address all correspondence to: dlaminiz@mut.ac.za

Research, Innovation & Engagements Portfolio, Mangosuthu University of Technology,
Durban, South Africa

References

[1] Cornelissen R, Heuvers ME, Maat AP, Hendriks RW, Hoogsteden HC, Aerts JG, Hegmans JP: New roads open up for implementing immunotherapy in mesothelioma. *Clinical and Developmental Immunology* 2012, 2012:927240.

[2] Evans C, Dalgleish AG, Kumar D: Review article: immune suppression and colorectal cancer. *Alimentary Pharmacology & Therapeutics* 2006, 24(8):1163–1177.

[3] Aptsiauri N, Cabrera T, Mendez R, Garcia-Lora A, Ruiz-Cabello F, Garrido F: Role of altered expression of HLA class I molecules in cancer progression. *Advances in Experimental Medicine and Biology* 2007, 601:123–131.

[4] Ma Y, Shurin GV, Peiyuan Z, Shurin MR: Dendritic cells in the cancer microenvironment. *Journal of Cancer* 2013, 4(1):36–44.

[5] Ma YJ, He M, Han JA, Yang L, Ji XY: A clinical study of HBsAg-activated dendritic cells and cytokine-induced killer cells during the treatment for chronic hepatitis B. *Scandinavian Journal of Immunology* 2013, 78(4):387–393.

[6] Roy S, Majumdar APN: Signaling in colon cancer stem cells. *Journal of Molecular Signaling* 2012, 7:11.

[7] Maccalli C, Pisarra P, Vegetti C, Sensi M, Parmiani G, Anichini A: Differential loss of T cell signaling molecules in metastatic melanoma patients' T lymphocyte subsets expressing distinct TCR variable regions. *Journal of Immunology* 1999, 163(12):6912–6923.

[8] Calon A, Espinet E, Palomo-Ponce S, Tauriello Daniele VF, Iglesias M, Céspedes María V, Sevillano M, Nadal C, Jung P, Zhang Xiang HF *et al*: Dependency of colorectal cancer on a TGF-β-driven program in stromal cells for metastasis initiation. *Cancer Cell* 2012, 22(5):571–584.

[9] Erdman SE, Poutahidis T: Cancer inflammation and regulatory T cells. *International Journal of Cancer* 2010, 127(4):768–779.

[10] Merika E, Saif MW, Katz A, Syrigos K, Morse M: Review. Colon cancer vaccines: an update. *In Vivo* 2010, 24(5):607–628.

[11] Bartnik A, Nirmal AJ, Yang S-Y: Peptide vaccine therapy in colorectal cancer. *Vaccines* 2013, 1(1):1.

[12] Beverley PCL: Immunology of vaccination. *British Medical Bulletin* 2002, 62(1):15–28.

[13] Heriot AG, Marriott JB, Cookson S, Kumar D, Dalgleish AG: Reduction in cytokine production in colorectal cancer patients: association with stage and reversal by resection. *British Journal of Cancer* 2000, 82(5):1009–1012.

[14] Galizia G, Lieto E, De Vita F, Romano C, Orditura M, Castellano P, Imperatore V, Infusino S, Catalano G, Pignatelli C: Circulating levels of interleukin-10 and interleukin-6 in gastric and colon cancer patients before and after surgery: relationship with radicality and outcome. *Journal of Interferon & Cytokine Research* 2002, 22(4):473–482.

[15] Yamaguchi S, Tatsumi T, Takehara T, Sasakawa A, Yamamoto M, Kohga K, Miyagi T, Kanto T, Hiramastu N, Akagi T *et al*: EphA2-derived peptide vaccine with amphiphilic poly(γ-glutamic acid) nanoparticles elicits an anti-tumor effect against mouse liver tumor. *Cancer Immunology, Immunotherapy* 2009, 59(5):759–767.

[16] Hazama S, Nakamura Y, Takenouchi H, Suzuki N, Tsunedomi R, Inoue Y, Tokuhisa Y, 7 Iizuka N, Yoshino S, Takeda K et al: A phase I study of combination vaccine treatment8 of five therapeutic epitope-peptides for metastatic colorectal cancer; safety, immuno–9 logical response, and clinical outcome. Journal of Translational Medicine 2014, 12:63.

[17] Begley J, Vo DD, Morris LF, Bruhn KW, Prins RM, Mok S, Koya RC, Garban HJ, Comin-Anduix B, Craft N *et al*: Immunosensitization with a Bcl-2 small molecule inhibitor. *Cancer Immunology, Immunotherapy* 2009, 58(5):699–708.

[18] Kaumaya PTP, Foy KC, Garrett J, Rawale SV, Vicari D, Thurmond JM, Lamb T, Mani A, Kane Y, Balint CR *et al*: Phase I active immunotherapy with combination of two chimeric, human epidermal growth factor receptor 2, B-cell epitopes fused to a promiscuous T-cell epitope in patients with metastatic and/or recurrent solid tumors. *Journal of Clinical Oncology* 2009, 27(31):5270–5277.

[19] Tan G-H, Li Y-N, Huang F-Y, Wang H, Bai R-Z, Jang J: Combination of recombinant xenogeneic endoglin DNA and protein vaccination enhances anti-tumor effects. *Immunological Investigations* 2007, 36(4):423–440.

[20] Saha A, Chatterjee SK, Foon KA, Celis E, Bhattacharya-Chatterjee M: Therapy of established tumors in a novel murine model transgenic for human carcinoembryonic antigen and HLA-A2 with a combination of anti-idiotype vaccine and CTL peptides of carcinoembryonic antigen. *Cancer Research* 2007, 67(6):2881–2892.

[21] Ali SA, Ahmad M, Lynam J, McLean CS, Entwisle C, Loudon P, Choolun E, McArdle SEB, Li G, Mian S *et al*: Anti-tumour therapeutic efficacy of OX40L in murine tumour model. *Vaccine* 2004, 22(27–28):3585–3594.

[22] Mukherjee P, Pathangey LB, Bradley JB, Tinder TL, Basu GD, Akporiaye ET, Gendler SJ: MUC1-specific immune therapy generates a strong anti-tumor response in a MUC1-tolerant colon cancer model. *Vaccine* 2007, 25(9):1607–1618.

[23] Miyagi Y, Imai N, Sasatomi T, Yamada A, Mine T, Katagiri K, Nakagawa M, Muto A, Okouchi S, Isomoto H *et al*: Induction of cellular immune responses to tumor cells and

peptides in colorectal cancer patients by vaccination with SART3 peptides. *Clinical Cancer Research* 2001, 7(12):3950–3962.

[24] Imai N, Harashima N, Ito M, Miyagi Y, Harada M, Yamada A, Itoh K: Identification of Lck-derived peptides capable of inducing HLA-A2-restricted and tumor-specific CTLs in cancer patients with distant metastases. *International Journal of Cancer* 2001, 94(2):237–242.

[25] Umansky V, Malyguine A, Shurin M: New perspectives in cancer immunotherapy and immunomonitoring. *Future Oncology* 2009, 5(7):941–944.

[26] Moulton HM, Yoshihara PH, Mason DH, Iversen PL, Triozzi PL: Active specific immunotherapy with a β-human chorionic gonadotropin peptide vaccine in patients with metastatic colorectal cancer: antibody response is associated with improved survival. *Clinical Cancer Research* 2002, 8(7):2044–2051.

[27] Morse MA, Bradley DA, Keler T, Laliberte RJ, Green JA, Davis TA, Inman BA: CDX-1307: a novel vaccine under study as treatment for muscle-invasive bladder cancer. *Expert Review of Vaccines* 2011, 10(6):733–742.

[28] Lynch TJ, Bell DW, Sordella R, Gurubhagavatula S, Okimoto RA, Brannigan BW, Harris PL, Haserlat SM, Supko JG, Haluska FG *et al*: Activating mutations in the epidermal growth factor receptor underlying responsiveness of non-small-cell lung cancer to gefitinib. *New England Journal of Medicine* 2004, 350(21):2129–2139.

[29] Watson SA, Gilliam AD: G17DT – a new weapon in the therapeutic armoury for gastrointestinal malignancy. *Expert Opinion on Biological Therapy* 2001, 1(2):309–317.

[30] Comeau JM, Labruzzo Mohundro B: From bench to bedside: promising colon cancer clinical trials. *American Journal of Managed Care* 2013, 19(1 Spec No):SP32–SP37.

[31] Rowe J, Cen P: TroVax in colorectal cancer. *Human Vaccines and Immunotherapeutics* 2014, 10(11):3196–3200.

[32] Wang X, Wang Q, Lin H, Li S, Sun L, Yang Y: HSP72 and gp96 in gastroenterological cancers. *Clinica Chimica Acta* 2013, 417:73–79.

[33] Walker KB, Keeble J, Colaco C: Mycobacterial heat shock proteins as vaccines – a model of facilitated antigen presentation. *Current Molecular Medicine* 2007, 7(4):339–350.

[34] Binder RJ, Han DK, Srivastava PK: CD91: a receptor for heat shock protein gp96. *Nature Immunology* 2000, 1(2):151–155.

[35] Liu B, Ye D, Song X, Zhao X, Yi L, Song J, Zhang Z, Zhao Q: A novel therapeutic fusion protein vaccine by two different families of heat shock proteins linked with HPV16 E7 generates potent antitumor immunity and antiangiogenesis. *Vaccine* 2008, 26(10):1387–1396.

[36] Huang C, Zhao J, Li Z, Li D, Xia D, Wang Q, Jin H: Multi-chaperone-peptide-rich mixture from colo-carcinoma cells elicits potent anticancer immunity. *Cancer Epidemiology* 2010, 34(4):494–500.

[37] Tol J, Punt CJ: Monoclonal antibodies in the treatment of metastatic colorectal cancer: a review. *Clinical Therapeutics* 2010, 32(3):437–453.

[38] Martins SF, Reis RM, Rodrigues AM, Baltazar F, Filho AL: Role of endoglin and VEGF family expression in colorectal cancer prognosis and anti-angiogenic therapies. *World Journal of Clinical Oncology* 2011, 2(6):272–280.

[39] Clarke JM, Hurwitz HI: Targeted inhibition of VEGF receptor 2: an update on ramucirumab. *Expert Opinion on Biological Therapy* 2013, 13(8):1187–1196.

[40] Saif MW: Anti-VEGF agents in metastatic colorectal cancer (mCRC): are they all alike? *Cancer Management and Research* 2013, 5:103–115.

[41] Peeters M, Cohn A, Köhne C-H, Douillard J-Y: Panitumumab in combination with cytotoxic chemotherapy for the treatment of metastatic colorectal carcinoma. *Clinical Colorectal Cancer* 2012, 11(1):14–23.

[42] Vale CL, Tierney JF, Fisher D, Adams RA, Kaplan R, Maughan TS, Parmar MKB, Meade AM: Does anti-EGFR therapy improve outcome in advanced colorectal cancer? A systematic review and meta-analysis. *Cancer Treatment Reviews* 2012, 38(6):618–625.

[43] You B, Chen EX: Anti-EGFR monoclonal antibodies for treatment of colorectal cancers: development of cetuximab and panitumumab. *Journal of Clinical Pharmacology* 2012, 52(2):128–155.

[44] Henricks LM, Schellens JHM, Huitema ADR, Beijnen JH: The use of combinations of monoclonal antibodies in clinical oncology. *Cancer Treatment Reviews* 2015, 41(10):859–867.

[45] Allard B, Pommey S, Smyth MJ, Stagg J: Targeting CD73 enhances the antitumor activity of anti-PD-1 and anti-CTLA-4 mAbs. *Clinical Cancer Research* 2013, 19(20):5626–5635.

[46] Llosa NJ, Cruise M, Tam A, Wicks EC, Hechenbleikner EM, Taube JM, Blosser RL, Fan H, Wang H, Luber BS *et al*: The vigorous immune microenvironment of microsatellite instable colon cancer is balanced by multiple counter-inhibitory checkpoints. *Cancer Discovery* 2015, 5(1):43–51.

[47] Ostrand-Rosenberg S, Horn LA, Alvarez JA: Novel strategies for inhibiting PD-1 pathway-mediated immune suppression while simultaneously delivering activating signals to tumor-reactive T cells. *Cancer Immunology, Immunotherapy* 2015, 64(10):1287–1293.

[48] Brahmer JR, Tykodi SS, Chow LQ, Hwu WJ, Topalian SL, Hwu P, Drake CG, Camacho LH, Kauh J, Odunsi K *et al*: Safety and activity of anti-PD-L1 antibody in patients with advanced cancer. *New England Journal of Medicine* 2012, 366(26):2455–2465.

[49] Brahmer JR, Pardoll DM: Immune checkpoint inhibitors: making immunotherapy a reality for the treatment of lung cancer. *Cancer Immunology Research* 2013, 1(2):85–91.

[50] Sagiv-Barfi I, Kohrt HEK, Czerwinski DK, Ng PP, Chang BY, Levy R: Therapeutic antitumor immunity by checkpoint blockade is enhanced by ibrutinib, an inhibitor of both BTK and ITK. *Proceedings of the National Academy of Sciences of the United States of America* 2015, 112(9):E966–E972.

[51] Curran MA, Montalvo W, Yagita H, Allison JP: PD-1 and CTLA-4 combination blockade expands infiltrating T cells and reduces regulatory T and myeloid cells within B16 melanoma tumors. *Proceedings of the National Academy of Sciences of the United States of America* 2010, 107(9):4275–4280.

[52] Werneck MB, Hottz E, Bozza PT, Viola JP: Cyclosporin A inhibits colon cancer cell growth independently of the calcineurin pathway. *Cell Cycle* 2012, 11(21):3997–4008.

[53] Mancini M, Toker A: NFAT proteins: emerging roles in cancer progression. *Nature Reviews Cancer* 2009, 9(11):810–820.

[54] Koido S, Ohkusa T, Homma S, Namiki Y, Takakura K, Saito K, Ito Z, Kobayashi H, Kajihara M, Uchiyama K *et al*: Immunotherapy for colorectal cancer. *World Journal of Gastroenterology : WJG* 2013, 19(46):8531–8542.

[55] Klampfer L: Cytokines, inflammation and colon cancer. *Current Cancer Drug Targets* 2011, 11(4):451–464.

[56] Kelly E, Russell SJ: History of oncolytic viruses: genesis to genetic engineering. *Molecular Therapy* 2007, 15(4):651–659.

[57] Lindenmann J, Klein PA: Viral oncolysis: increased immunogenicity of host cell antigen associated with influenza virus. *Journal of Experimental Medicine* 1967, 126(1):93–108.

[58] Bell J, McFadden G: Viruses for tumor therapy. *Cell Host & Microbe* 2014, 15(3):260–265.

[59] Hayden R, Pounds S, Knapp K, Petraitiene R, Schaufele RL, Sein T, Walsh TJ: Galactomannan antigenemia in pediatric oncology patients with invasive aspergillosis. *Pediatric Infectious Disease Journal* 2008, 27(9):815–819.

[60] Cheever MA, Higano CS: PROVENGE (Sipuleucel-T) in prostate cancer: the first FDA-approved therapeutic cancer vaccine. *Clinical Cancer Research* 2011, 17(11):3520–3526.

[61] Toda M, Martuza RL, Kojima H, Rabkin SD: In situ cancer vaccination: an IL-12 defective vector/replication-competent herpes simplex virus combination induces local and systemic antitumor activity. *Journal of Immunology* 1998, 160(9):4457–4464.

[62] Toda M, Rabkin SD, Kojima H, Martuza RL: Herpes simplex virus as an in situ cancer vaccine for the induction of specific anti-tumor immunity. *Human Gene Therapy* 1999, 10(3):385–393.

[63] Davis ID, Jefford M, Parente P, Cebon J: Rational approaches to human cancer immunotherapy. *Journal of Leukocyte Biology* 2003, 73(1):3–29.

[64] Bauzon M, Hermiston T: Armed therapeutic viruses – a disruptive therapy on the horizon of cancer immunotherapy. *Frontiers in Immunology* 2014, 5:74.

[65] Stanford MM, Barrett JW, Nazarian SH, Werden S, McFadden G: Oncolytic virotherapy synergism with signaling inhibitors: rapamycin increases myxoma virus tropism for human tumor cells. *Journal of Virology* 2007, 81(3):1251–1260.

[66] Prestwich RJ, Harrington KJ, Pandha HS, Vile RG, Melcher AA, Errington F: Oncolytic viruses: a novel form of immunotherapy. *Expert Review of Anticancer Therapy* 2008, 8(10): 1581–1588.

[67] Wongthida P, Diaz RM, Galivo F, Kottke T, Thompson J, Pulido J, Pavelko K, Pease L, Melcher A, Vile R: Type III IFN interleukin-28 mediates the antitumor efficacy of oncolytic virus VSV in immune-competent mouse models of cancer. *Cancer Research* 2010, 70(11):4539–4549.

[68] Guo ZS, Thorne SH, Bartlett DL: Oncolytic virotherapy: molecular targets in tumor-selective replication and carrier cell-mediated delivery of oncolytic viruses. *Biochimica et Biophysica Acta* 2008, 1785(2):217–231.

[69] Russell SJ, Peng K-W, Bell JC: Oncolytic virotherapy. *Nature Biotechnology* 2012, 30(7): 658–670.

[70] Cattaneo R, Miest T, Shashkova EV, Barry MA: Reprogrammed viruses as cancer therapeutics: targeted, armed and shielded. *Nature Reviews Microbiology* 2008, 6(7):529–540.

[71] Chiocca EA, Rabkin SD: Oncolytic viruses and their application to cancer immunotherapy. *Cancer Immunology Research* 2014, 2(4):295–300.

[72] Hanahan D, Weinberg Robert A: Hallmarks of cancer: the next generation. *Cell* 2011, 144(5):646–674.

[73] Casares N, Pequignot MO, Tesniere A, Ghiringhelli F, Roux S, Chaput N, Schmitt E, Hamai A, Hervas-Stubbs S, Obeid M *et al*: Caspase-dependent immunogenicity of doxorubicin-induced tumor cell death. *Journal of Experimental Medicine* 2005, 202(12): 1691–1701.

[74] Galanis E, Okuno SH, Nascimento AG, Lewis BD, Lee RA, Oliveira AM, Sloan JA, Atherton P, Edmonson JH, Erlichman C *et al*: Phase I–II trial of ONYX-015 in combination with MAP chemotherapy in patients with advanced sarcomas. *Gene Therapy* 2005, 12(5):437–445.

[75] Nemunaitis J, Khuri F, Ganly I, Arseneau J, Posner M, Vokes E, Kuhn J, McCarty T, Landers S, Blackburn A *et al*: Phase II trial of intratumoral administration of ONYX-015, a replication-selective adenovirus, in patients with refractory head and neck cancer. *Journal of Clinical Oncology* 2001, 19(2):289–298.

[76] Carter PJ: Potent antibody therapeutics by design. *Nature Reviews Immunology* 2006, 6(5):343–357.

[77] Hoogenboom HR: Selecting and screening recombinant antibody libraries. *Nature Biotechnology* 2005, 23(9):1105–1116.

[78] Kohler G, Milstein C: Continuous cultures of fused cells secreting antibody of predefined specificity. *Nature* 1975, 256(5517):495–497.

[79] Lonberg N: Human antibodies from transgenic animals. *Nature Biotechnology* 2005, 23(9):1117–1125.

[80] Staerz UD, Kanagawa O, Bevan MJ: Hybrid antibodies can target sites for attack by T cells. *Nature* 1985, 314(6012):628–631.

[81] Glennie MJ, McBride HM, Worth AT, Stevenson GT: Preparation and performance of bispecific F(ab' gamma)2 antibody containing thioether-linked Fab' gamma fragments. *Journal of Immunology* 1987, 139(7):2367–2375.

[82] Repp R, van Ojik HH, Valerius T, Groenewegen G, Wieland G, Oetzel C, Stockmeyer B, Becker W, Eisenhut M, Steininger H *et al*: Phase I clinical trial of the bispecific antibody MDX-H210 (anti-FcgammaRI × anti-HER-2/neu) in combination with Filgrastim (G-CSF) for treatment of advanced breast cancer. *British Journal of Cancer* 2003, 89(12):2234–2243.

[83] Nisonoff A, Rivers MM: Recombination of a mixture of univalent antibody fragments of different specificity. *Archives of Biochemistry and Biophysics* 1961, 93:460–462.

[84] Chan AC, Carter PJ: Therapeutic antibodies for autoimmunity and inflammation. *Nature Reviews Immunology* 2010, 10(5):301–316.

[85] Kontermann RE: Alternative antibody formats. *Current Opinion in Molecular Therapeutics* 2010, 12(2):176–183.

[86] Kontermann RE: Dual targeting strategies with bispecific antibodies. *MAbs* 2012, 4(2): 182–197.

[87] Dienstmann R, De Dosso S, Felip E, Tabernero J: Drug development to overcome resistance to EGFR inhibitors in lung and colorectal cancer. *Molecular Oncology* 2012, 6(1):15–26.

[88] Nahta R, Esteva FJ: HER2 therapy: molecular mechanisms of trastuzumab resistance. *Breast Cancer Research* 2006, 8(6):215.

[89] Engelman JA, Zejnullahu K, Mitsudomi T, Song Y, Hyland C, Park JO, Lindeman N, Gale CM, Zhao X, Christensen J *et al*: MET amplification leads to gefitinib resistance in lung cancer by activating ERBB3 signaling. *Science* 2007, 316(5827):1039–1043.

[90] Galon J, Costes A, Sanchez-Cabo F, Kirilovsky A, Mlecnik B, Lagorce-Pages C, Tosolini M, Camus M, Berger A, Wind P *et al*: Type, density, and location of immune cells within human colorectal tumors predict clinical outcome. *Science* 2006, 313(5795):1960–1964.

[91] Wahlin BE, Sander B, Christensson B, Kimby E: CD8+ T-cell content in diagnostic lymph nodes measured by flow cytometry is a predictor of survival in follicular lymphoma. *Clinical Cancer Research* 2007, 13(2 Pt 1):388–397.

[92] Hoffman L, Gore L: Blinatumomab, a bispecific anti-CD19/CD3 BiTE® antibody for the treatment of acute lymphoblastic leukemia: perspectives and current pediatric applications. *Frontiers in Oncology* 2014, 4.

[93] Hoffmann P, Hofmeister R, Brischwein K, Brandl C, Crommer S, Bargou R, Itin C, Prang N, Baeuerle PA: Serial killing of tumor cells by cytotoxic T cells redirected with a CD19-/CD3-bispecific single-chain antibody construct. *International Journal of Cancer* 2005, 115(1):98–104.

[94] Fujimoto M, Poe JC, Inaoki M, Tedder TF: CD19 regulates B lymphocyte responses to transmembrane signals. *Seminars in Immunology* 1998, 10(4):267–277.

[95] Rickert RC, Rajewsky K, Roes J: Impairment of T-cell-dependent B-cell responses and B-l cell development in CD19-deficient mice. *Nature* 1995, 376(6538):352–355.

[96] Brandl C, Haas C, d'Argouges S, Fisch T, Kufer P, Brischwein K, Prang N, Bargou R, Suzich J, Baeuerle PA *et al*: The effect of dexamethasone on polyclonal T cell activation and redirected target cell lysis as induced by a CD19/CD3-bispecific single-chain antibody construct. *Cancer Immunology, Immunotherapy* 2007, 56(10):1551–1563.

[97] Haas C, Krinner E, Brischwein K, Hoffmann P, Lutterbüse R, Schlereth B, Kufer P, Baeuerle PA: Mode of cytotoxic action of T cell-engaging BiTE antibody MT110. *Immunobiology* 2009, 214(6):441–453.

[98] Loffler A, Gruen M, Wuchter C, Schriever F, Kufer P, Dreier T, Hanakam F, Baeuerle PA, Bommert K, Karawajew L *et al*: Efficient elimination of chronic lymphocytic leukaemia B cells by autologous T cells with a bispecific anti-CD19//anti-CD3 single-chain antibody construct. *Leukemia* 2003, 17(5):900–909.

[99] Choi D, Kim T-G, Sung YC: The past, present, and future of adoptive T cell therapy. *Immune Network* 2012, 12(4):139–147.

[100] Rosenberg SA, Restifo NP, Yang JC, Morgan RA, Dudley ME: Adoptive cell transfer: a clinical path to effective cancer immunotherapy. *Nature Reviews Cancer* 2008, 8(4):299–308.

[101] Delorme EJ, Alexander P: Treatment of primary fibrosarcoma in the rat with immune lymphocytes. *Lancet* 1964, 2(7351):117–120.

[102] Dunn GP, Bruce AT, Ikeda H, Old LJ, Schreiber RD: Cancer immunoediting: from immunosurveillance to tumor escape. *Nature Immunology* 2002, 3(11):991–998.

[103] Swann JB, Smyth MJ: Immune surveillance of tumors. *Journal of Clinical Investigation* 2007, 117(5):1137–1146.

[104] Sallusto F, Lenig D, Forster R, Lipp M, Lanzavecchia A: Two subsets of memory T lymphocytes with distinct homing potentials and effector functions. *Nature* 1999, 401(6754):708–712.

[105] Darcy PK, Neeson P, Yong CSM, Kershaw MH: Manipulating immune cells for adoptive immunotherapy of cancer. *Current Opinion in Immunology* 2014, 27:46–52.

[106] Gattinoni L, Zhong XS, Palmer DC, Ji Y, Hinrichs CS, Yu Z, Wrzesinski C, Boni A, Cassard L, Garvin LM *et al*: Wnt signaling arrests effector T cell differentiation and generates CD8+ memory stem cells. *Nature Medicine* 2009, 15(7):808–813.

[107] Hacein-Bey-Abina S, Garrigue A, Wang GP, Soulier J, Lim A, Morillon E, Clappier E, Caccavelli L, Delabesse E, Beldjord K *et al*: Insertional oncogenesis in 4 patients after retrovirus-mediated gene therapy of SCID-X1. *Journal of Clinical Investigation* 2008, 118(9):3132–3142.

[108] Klebanoff CA, Gattinoni L, Torabi-Parizi P, Kerstann K, Cardones AR, Finkelstein SE, Palmer DC, Antony PA, Hwang ST, Rosenberg SA *et al*: Central memory self/tumor-reactive CD8+ T cells confer superior antitumor immunity compared with effector memory T cells. *Proceedings of the National Academy of Sciences of the United States of America* 2005, 102(27):9571–9576.

[109] Pule MA, Savoldo B, Myers GD, Rossig C, Russell HV, Dotti G, Huls MH, Liu E, Gee AP, Mei Z *et al*: Virus-specific T cells engineered to coexpress tumor-specific receptors: persistence and antitumor activity in individuals with neuroblastoma. *Nature Medicine* 2008, 14(11):1264–1270.

[110] Shook DR, Campana D: Natural killer cell engineering for cellular therapy of cancer. *Tissue Antigens* 2011, 78(6):409–415.

[111] Rosenberg SA, Lotze MT, Muul LM, Leitman S, Chang AE, Ettinghausen SE, Matory YL, Skibber JM, Shiloni E, Vetto JT *et al*: Observations on the systemic administration of autologous lymphokine-activated killer cells and recombinant interleukin-2 to patients with metastatic cancer. *New England Journal of Medicine* 1985, 313(23):1485–1492.

[112] Miller JS, Soignier Y, Panoskaltsis-Mortari A, McNearney SA, Yun GH, Fautsch SK, McKenna D, Le C, Defor TE, Burns LJ *et al*: Successful adoptive transfer and in vivo expansion of human haploidentical NK cells in patients with cancer. *Blood* 2005, 105(8): 3051–3057.

Chapter 11

The Management of the Primary Tumor in Patients with Metastatic Colorectal Cancer

Shahid Ahmed, Selliah Kanthan, Nayyer Iqbal,
Adnan Zaidi, Duc Le, Tahir Abbas and Kamal Haider

Additional information is available at the end of the chapter

http://dx.doi.org/10.5772/62867

Abstract

Over the past decade, the role of surgery in stage IV colorectal cancer (CRC) has evolved, yet the optimal surgical management of the primary tumor in patients with metastatic CRC that is not amenable to curative resection is unknown. A high rate of surgical resection of the primary tumor has been reported in patients with unresectable metastatic disease. Resection of the primary tumor in patients with metastatic CRC is often performed to deal with presenting primary tumor symptoms and or to prevent future primary tumor complications. Nevertheless, with access to novel agents and their efficacy in the primary tumor as well as lack of major complications related to an intact primary tumor, surgery is less commonly performed today. Although the data regarding survival advantages of resection of the primary tumor are inconsistent, overall the evidence suggests potential survival benefit of removal of the primary tumor in patients with both symptomatic and asymptomatic primary tumors even with access to more effective combination chemotherapy. However, the published literature favoring surgery mostly comprises retrospective observational studies. Consequently, the survival benefit related to surgery has been attributed to selection bias, and in the absence of randomized controlled trial no definite conclusion can be drawn. Currently, two randomized controlled trials are enrolling patients to answer this important question in the management of metastatic CRC.

Keywords: Primary tumor resection, stage IV colorectal cancer, palliative surgery, survival, metastatic colorectal cancer, primary tumor, colon cancer, rectal cancer, symptomatic tumor, chemotherapy

1. Introduction

The role of surgery in stage IV colorectal cancer (CRC) has evolved over the past two decades. Surgery has become an important treatment component in the management of patients with metastatic CRC [1–3]. Between 30 and 38% of patients diagnosed with stage IV CRC will undergo one or more major surgical procedures [4]. The known 5-year survival rate after liver and lung metastasectomy has been reported to be 25 to 51% and 30 to 73%, respectively [5]. Although administration of systemic therapy in patients with stage IV CRC may convert unresectable into resectable disease, in a majority of patients, the metastatic disease is not resectable. For most patients with advanced CRC, systemic chemotherapy is the primary treatment and the focus of management is on how best to palliate the symptoms and to prolong survival (**Figure 1**) [1]. With the availability of several novel agents and increasing use of liver-directed therapies, the median overall survival of patients with metastatic CRC has improved from 6 months with best supportive care alone to 30 months with the use of combination therapy [6].

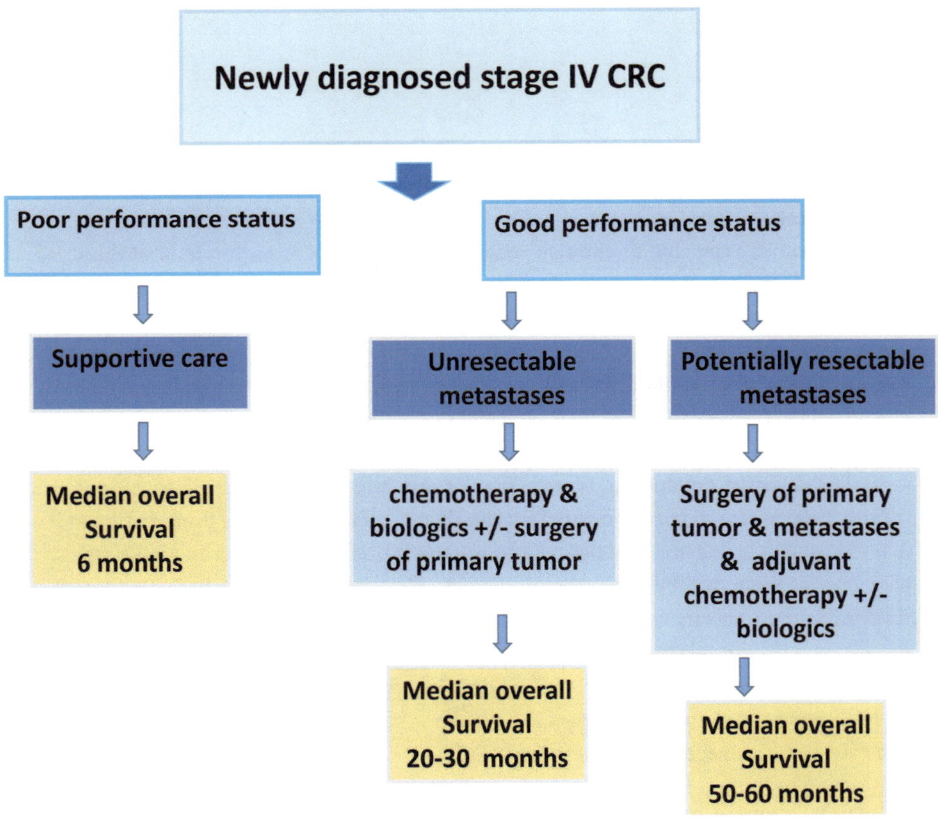

Figure 1. Framework of management of patients with stage IV CRC. Most patients are primarily treated with chemotherapy, nevertheless, a selected group of patients can be cured with primary tumor resection and metastasectomy. Currently, the role of resection of primary tumor in patients with unresectable metastatic disease is not well defined (Adapted with permission from Ahmed et al. [1]).

Even though enormous progress has been made in the treatment of patients with CRC within the past three decades, the optimal management of patients with metastatic disease not amenable to curative therapy who present without severe primary tumor-related symptoms has remained controversial. Resection of the primary tumor in patients with metastatic CRC is often performed to deal with presenting primary tumor symptoms and/or to prevent future primary tumor complications. Potential advantages of resection of the primary tumor in stage IV CRC are prevention of obstruction and major bleeding, better pain control, and potential reduction in serious adverse effects related to novel targeted therapy such as bleeding and perforation. Conversely, the newer generation chemotherapy in combination with targeted therapy has been associated with response rate of 40–60% [7]. Complications following resection of the primary tumor in patients with advanced CRC can delay or prevent initiation of systemic therapy and thereby precludes benefit associated with it. There is no evidence that response rates of the primary tumor are inferior to that of the metastases.

Recent data suggest that resection of the primary tumor in patients with stage IV CRC has been associated with a lower mortality risk [8]. Nevertheless, most studies failed to adjust for important prognostic variables such as performance status. In this chapter we will review the evidence regarding the benefit of resection of the primary tumor, limitations of the current evidence and future directions.

2. Argument for surgery

Resection of the primary tumor by lowering the tumor burden may maximize the benefit of chemotherapy and increase the potential for surgery with a curative intent. Evidence from other solid tumors such as renal cell cancer supports resection of the primary tumor in patients with metastatic disease. Two well-designed randomized trials demonstrated significant survival benefit for patients with metastatic renal cancer undergoing nephrectomy prior to systemic therapy. For example, Flanigan et al. reported median overall survival times of 11.1 compared with 8.1 months and Mickisch et al. of 17 versus 7 months in favor of nephrectomy [9, 10]. Surgical resection of the primary tumor in metastatic CRC may prevent complications caused by the primary tumor that may subsequently require emergency interventions which are associated with increased peri-operative mortality and unfavorable long-term outcome. Stillwell and others have shown that patients who were initially treated with chemotherapy were 7.3 times more likely to have a complication from the primary tumor and, when operated for such complications, were more likely to have a poor postoperative outcome [11–13].

3. Argument against surgery

Over the past decade, several highly active systemic agents, both cytotoxic and biologic, have become available for the treatment of patients with metastatic CRC. As a result, the median survival of patients with stage IV CRC has increased from 9 to 12 months with fluorouracil alone to up to 24 to 30 months with sequential modern cytotoxic and biologic treatments [1].

There remains concern of primary tumor–related complications during systemic therapy particularly with a risk of perforation when combining anti-VEGF (vascular endothelial growth factor) therapy to cytotoxic agents [14]. Recent studies, however, have demonstrated that combination chemotherapy and biological agents can be safely administered in patients with metastatic CRC with an in situ primary tumor [12, 15, 16]. A recent phase II trial utilizing bevacizumab containing regimen reported 14% primary tumor complications rate [17]. The author concluded that the survival is not compromised by leaving the primary colon tumor intact.

4. Evidence from the literature

The evidence regarding benefit of primary tumor resection, in patients with stage IV CRC and unresectable metastatic lesions is not conclusive. The published literature about survival advantages of removal of primary tumor is inconsistent; while some suggest benefit of surgery [8], others have failed to demonstrate survival benefit of non-curative resection of the primary tumor [18, 19].

Cirrochi and others performed a systematic review of seven non-randomized eligible studies involving 1086 patients. Of 1086 patients, 722 (66.4%) underwent primary tumor resection, and 364 (33.6%) were managed with chemotherapy alone [18]. The author concluded that resection of the primary tumor in asymptomatic patients with metastatic CRC was not associated with a consistent improvement in overall survival. Furthermore, primary tumor resection did not significantly reduce the risk of complications from the primary tumor. Another review by Scheer and others that specifically focused on complication rates of the primary tumor did not support surgery. Based upon the data on 850 patients from 7 papers published from 1999 to 2006 when first-line chemotherapy was administered in patients with unresectable stage IV CRC, obstruction and intestinal hemorrhage were observed in 13.9% and 3% of the patients, respectively. On the other hand, when upfront surgery of the primary tumor was performed, complications rates were 18.8–47%. Of note, two of 7 studies in this review did not have a surgical intervention group [19].

Our research group conducted a systematic review and meta-analysis of the current literature [8]. Of total of 3379 reports, 15 retrospective observational studies were selected with patients population of 12456 (**Table 1**) [12, 13, 20–31]. Six studies were exclusively done in minimally symptomatic patients and 10 studies met the criteria of using new generation anti-cancer therapy. All included studies were retrospective observational studies. No study met the criteria for good quality study using 'validity scoring for observational study' for any outcome of interest. Overall, 26% patients had rectal tumor, 21.9% in the resection group compared with 31% in the control. For the primary outcome "overall survival" 9 of 15 studies were of low quality and remaining 6 were fair quality. Among 12,456 patients, 8620 (69%) underwent surgery with a median overall survival of the 15.2 months (range: 10–30.7) compared with 11.4 months (range: 3–22) of the non-resection group. Quantitative meta-analysis utilizing the data of all 15 studies revealed that the primary tumor resection was associated with a significant improvement in survival compared with no surgery with a hazard ratio (HR) of 0.69 (95%

confidence interval [CI]: 0.61–0.79). Nine studies reported surgical mortality rate. Mean 30 days post-operative mortality rate in the intervention group was 4.9% (95% CI: 0–9.7%). Only seven studies reported non-fatal surgical complications including anastomic leak, surgical wound infection and other complications. The mean surgical morbidity rate was 25.9% (95% CI: 20.1–31.6). Mean primary tumor complications rate & non-surgical procedures rate in the control group were 29.7% (95% CI: 18.5–41.0) and 27.6% (95 CI: 15.4–39.9), respectively. No study provided quality of life data. In a sub-group analysis involving studies during the period of modern chemotherapy, the median overall survival of group with surgery was 18.7 months (range: 11–30.7) compared with 12.85 months (range: 5.8–22) in the control group. The HR for survival of the subgroup treated with irinotecan and or oxaliplatin based chemotherapy was in 0.68 (95% CI: 0.56-0.83) favoring the surgical intervention compared with HR of 0.73 (95% CI: 0.59–0.90) of the group treated with older regimen. Likewise, in a separate sub-group analysis of studies restricted to minimally symptomatic tumor from the primary tumor, the median overall survival of group with surgery was 18.5 months (range: 14.5–23) versus 13.15 months (range: 5.8–22) in the control group. The HR for survival of minimal symptomatic patients was 0.67 (95% CI: 0.48–0.94) favoring the intervention group compared with HR of 0.75 (95% CI: 0.67–0.84) of symptomatic patients. A substantial low quality studies, publications bias and selected reporting were the major limitations of the review. Consequently, the survival benefit related to surgery has been attributed to selection bias and selection of younger and healthier patients with good performance status.

To address some of the limitations reported in the literature our research group conducted a cohort study to evaluate survival benefit of surgery (**Table 2**) [32]. The study population was comprised of adult patients with histologically documented adenocarcinoma of colon and rectum, intact primary tumor and evidence of metastases, diagnosed between the period of 1992 and 2005, in the Canadian province of Saskatchewan. In this large population based cohort study individual medical records were reviewed to retrieve information about important prognostic variables including performance status. A total 1378 eligible patients with median age of 70 years were identified. Five hundred and forty four (39.5%) patients were symptomatic. Nine hundred and forty four (68.5%) patients underwent resection of the primary tumor. Of 1378 patients, 29.5% had rectal or recto-sigmoid tumor (rectal, 20.1%, recto-sigmoid, 9.4%). Among 1378 patients, 42.3% received chemotherapy and 45.1% received 2nd generation (irinotecan and/or oxaliplatin based) therapy. Patients who underwent primary tumor resection and received chemotherapy had median overall survival of 18.3 months (95%CI: 16.6–20) compared with 8.4 months (95% CI: 7.1–9.7) if they were treated with chemotherapy alone ($p<0.0001$). In a subgroup of patients who were treated with second generation chemotherapy, median survival of patients who underwent surgical resection of primary tumor was 24.6 months (95% CI: 20.2–29.0) versus 11.0 months (95% CI: 7.8–14.3) if they did not have surgery. Due to imbalance between the two groups with respect to important prognostic variables such as chemotherapy, metastasectomy, and performance status a Cox proportional multivariate analysis was performed. The analysis revealed that resection of the primary tumor was independently correlated with better survival after adjustment for important clinical and pathological variables. For example, use of chemotherapy (HR 0.47, 95% CI: 0.41–0.54), primary tumor resection (HR 0.49, 95% CI: 0.41–0.58), second line chemotherapy (0.47, 95% CI:

0.45-0.64), and metastasectomy (HR 0.54, 95% CI: 0.45-0.64) were correlated with superior survival whereas older age, poor performance status, low albumin, elevated bilirubin, elevated alkaline phosphatase, anemia, leukocytosis, colonic primary, and grade 3 tumor were correlated with inferior survival. The tests for interactions between the surgical resection of primary tumor and second line therapy or more than 2 metastatic sites, were significant suggesting greater benefit of surgery in patients who received further line of therapies or who had limited metastases. Since patients who undergo metastasectomy have potential to achieve long term survival, a secondary analysis, after excluding patients who underwent metastasectomy was performed. In the secondary analysis, surgical resection of primary tumor significantly correlated with better survival (adjusted HR of 0.43; 95% CI: 0.41–0.52).

Study and year of publication	Study design	Study duration	N	Patients	Co-interventions	Outcomes
Aslam et al. 2010 [26]	Retrospective multi-centers observational study	1998–2007	T: 647 I: 366 C: 281	Minimally symptomatic	Chemotherapy I: 63%, C: 36%	Median OS 14.5 (I) vs. 5.8 (C) months (p<0.05); post-operative mortality (I) 7%
Benoist et al. 2005 [12]	Retrospective single institutional case–control study	1997–2002	T: 59 I: 32 C: 27	Asymptomatic or minimally symptomatic	Chemotherapy I: 94%, C: 100%; metastasectomy I: 16%, C: 22%	Median OS 22 (I) vs. 23 (C) months (p=NS); post-operative mortality (I) 0%
Chan et al. 2010 [27]	Retrospective population based study	2000–2002	T: 411 I: 286 C: 125	Symptomatic & asymptomatic	Chemotherapy I: 61%, C: 58%; metastesectomy I: 10%, C: 0%	Median OS 14 (1) vs. 6 (C) months (p=<0.05)
Evans et al. 2009 [28]	Retrospective single institutional observational study	1999–2006	T: 97 I: 45 C: 52	Symptomatic & asymptomatic	Chemotherapy I: NP, C: 42%	Median OS 11 (I) vs. 7 (C) months (p=NS), post-operative mortality (I) 16%
Galizia G et al. 2008 [24]	Retrospective single institutional observational study	1995–2005	T: 65 I: 42 C: 23	Asymptomatic or minimally symptomatic	Chemotherapy I: 100%, C: 100%; metastasectomy I: 12%, C: 4%	Median OS 15.2 (I) vs. 12.3 (C) months (p=0.003); post-operative mortality (I) 0%
Karoui M et al. 2011 [21]	Retrospective multi-centers observational study	1998–2007	T: 208 I: 123 C: 85	Symptomatic & asymptomatic	Chemotherapy I: 100%, C: 99%; metastasectomy I: 23%, C: 29%	Median OS 30.7 (I) vs. 21.9 (C) months (p=0.004)
Konyalian et al. 2007 [29]	Retrospective single institutional cohort study	1991–2002	T: 109 I: 62 C: 47	Symptomatic & asymptomatic	Chemotherapy I: 71%,C: 60%;	Median OS 12.5 (I) vs. 4.6 (C) months (p<0.05); post-operative mortality (I) 5%
Michel et al. 2004 [30]	Retrospective single institutional observational study	1996–1999	T: 54 I: 31 C: 23	Asymptomatic or minimally symptomatic	Chemotherapy I: 97%,C: 100%; metastesectomy I: NP, C: 9%	Median OS 21 (I) vs. 14 (C) months (p=NS); post-operative mortality (I) 0%
Ruo et al. 2003 [13]	Single institutional retrospective observational study	1996–1999	T: 230 I: 127 C: 130	Asymptomatic or minimally symptomatic	Chemotherapy I: NP, C: 83%	Median OS 16 (I) vs. 9 (C) months (p=<0.05); post-operative mortality (I) 2%
Scoggins et al.1999 [22]	Single institutional retrospective observational study	1985–1997	T:89 I:66 C:23	Symptomatic & asymptomatic	NP	Median OS 14.5 (I) vs. 16.6 (C) months (p=NS)
Seo et al. 2010 [31]	Single institutional retrospective observational study	2001–2008	T:277 I:144 C:83	Asymptomatic or minimally symptomatic	Chemotherapy I: 100%, C: 100%;	Median OS 22 (I) vs. 14 (C) months (p=NS); post-operative mortality (I) 0%
Tebutt et al. 2003 [23]	Single institutional retrospective observational study	1990–2000	T:362 I:208 C:82	Symptomatic & asymptomatic	Chemotherapy I: 100%, C: 100%; metastasectomy I: 2%, C: 1%	Median OS 14 (I) vs. 8.2 (C) months (p=NS)
Temple et al. 2004 [25]	Population based study using SEERS & Medicare data	1991–1999	T:9011 I:6464 C: 2542	65 years or older symptomatic & asymptomatic	Chemotherapy I: 47%, C: 31%; metastasectomy I: 5.2%, C: 1.3%	Median OS 10 (I) vs. 3 (C) months (p<0.05); post-operative mortality (I) 9%
Venderbosch et al. 2011 (CAIRO) [20]	Retrospective multi-centers cohort of a RCT	2003–2004 (recruited period)	T:399 I:258 C: 141	Symptomatic & asymptomatic	100% chemotherapy in both groups	Median OS 16.7 (I) vs. 11.4 (C) months
Venderbosch et al. 2011 (CAIRO 2) [20]	Retrospective multi-centers cohort of a RCT	2005–2006 (recruited period)	T:488 I:289 C: 159	Symptomatic & asymptomatic	100% chemotherapy in both groups	Median OS 20.7 (I) vs. 13.4 (C) months

C=control group; I=intervention group; N=number; NP=not provided; NS=not significant; OS=overall survival; RCT=randomized controlled trial; T=total.

Table 1. Summary of studies that evaluated benefit of resection of primary tumor and were included in a systematic review and meta-analysis.

Study & year of publication	Study design	Study duration	N	Patients	Co-interventions	Outcomes*
Ahmed et al. 2013 [32]	Retrospective Population based cohort study	1992–2005	T: 1378 I: 944 C: 434	Symptomatic & asymptomatic	Chemotherapy I: 50%, C: 20% metastasectomy I: 19.4%, C: 3.5%	Median OS 18.3 (I) vs. 8.4 (C) months (p<0.001); post-operative mortality (I) 6.6%
Ahmed et al. 2015 [33]	Retrospective Population based cohort study	1992–2005	T: 834 I: 521 C: 313	Asymptomatic or minimally symptomatic	Chemotherapy I: 53%, C: 28%; metastasectomy I: 20.5%, C: 2.9%	Median OS 19.7 (I) vs. 8.4 (C) months (p<0.001); post-operative mortality (I) 4.8%
Ahmed et al. 2015–2016 [34]	Retrospective Population based cohort study	2006–2010	T:569 I:313 C:256	Symptomatic & asymptomatic	Chemotherapy I: 64%, C: 50%; metastasectomy I: 26%, C: 3%	Median OS 27 (I) vs. 14 (C) months(p<0.001); post-operative mortality (I) 5%

C=control group; I=intervention group; N=number; OS= overall survival; T=total.

Table 2. Summary of three population based cohort studies that used individual patients' data and evaluated survival benefit of surgery of primary tumor by controlling the important prognostic variables in stage IV CRC

Our study suggests that resection of the primary tumor in patients with stage IV CRC improves survival, independent of age, performance status, co-morbid illness and chemotherapy. Nevertheless, the study was inclusive of symptomatic patients who tend to get benefit from palliative resection of the primary tumor, we therefore conducted a sub-group analysis involving a cohort of patients with asymptomatic or minimally symptomatic primary tumor to confirm survival benefit of surgery (**Table 2**) [33]. A total of 834 patients with median age of 70 years were identified. Among them, 521 (63%) patients underwent surgery and 43.3% received chemotherapy. Patients who underwent surgery had median overall survival of 19.7 months (95% CI: 16.9–22.6) compared with 8.4 months (95% CI: 6.9–10.0) if they did not have surgery (p<0.0001). The study once more confirmed the survival benefit of surgery after adjustment of other important prognostic variables in a multivariate analysis. Among various prognostic variables, 5FU-based chemotherapy (HR 0.43; 95% CI: 0.36–0.53), surgery of primary tumor (HR 0.47; 0.39–0.57), metastasectomy (HR 0.48; 0.38–0.62), and 2nd line chemotherapy (HR 0.72; 0.58–0.92) were correlated with superior survival. Test for interaction between ≥1 metastatic sites and surgery was significant suggesting a larger benefit of surgery in patients with stage IVA disease.

4.1. Benefit of surgery in patients treated with combination chemotherapy and biologics

Our data revealed the potential benefit of resection of the primary tumor regardless of underlying symptoms and that patients with asymptomatic or minimally symptomatic primary tumor who underwent surgery had similar survival benefit with overall 53% reduction in mortality after adjustment for older age, comorbid illness, poor performance status, disease burden, chemotherapy, and metastasectomy. Of note, a larger benefit of surgery was noted in patients with stage IVA disease. However, only about 43% of patients were treated with systemic therapy. Among the treated patients about 45% received irinotecan- or oxaliplatin-based (FOLFIRI or FOLFOX) chemotherapy. Moreover, less than 5% received a biological agent. It is not known if similar benefit can be achieved with the use of more effective systemic therapy. Our research group undertook a study to validate our findings in a cohort of patients with stage IV CRC who were diagnosed during the period of modern systemic therapy. A cohort of 569 patients with stage 4 CRC diagnosed during 2006–2010 in the province of Saskatchewan was evaluated (**Table 2**) [34]. Their median age was 69 years (59–95), 57.3%

Variables	HR (95% confidence interval)
Use of any chemotherapy	
Yes	0.33 (0.26–0.43)
No	1
Metastasectomy	
Yes	0.43 (0.31–0.58)
No	1
Surgical resection of primary tumor	
Yes	0.44 (0.35–0.56)
No	1
Second-line treatment	
Yes	0.50 (0.35–0.70)
No	1
Third-line treatment	
Yes	0.58 (0.41–0.83)
No	1
Serum alkaline phosphatase >120 U/l	
Yes	1.50 (1.20–1.78)
No	1
Grade III tumors	
Yes	1.33 (1.10–1.62)
No	1
Leukocytosis	
Yes	1.32 (1.05–1.66)
No	1
Stage IVb CRC	
Yes	1.31 (1.10–1.56)
No	
ECOG performance status >1	
Yes	1.30 (1.04–1.57)
No	1

HR=hazard ratio; ECOG=Eastern Cooperative Oncology Group.

Table 3. Prognostic variables that correlate with survival in stage IV CRC in a multivariate analysis [34])

received chemotherapy, 91.4% received FOLFIRI or FOLFOX and 67% received a biologic agent. Median overall survival (OS) of patients who underwent surgical resection of primary tumor and received chemotherapy was 27 months compared with 14 months of the non-resection group (p<0.0001). Median OS of patients who received all active agents and had surgery was 39 months (95% CI: 25.1–52.9). Patients with asymptomatic primary tumor who underwent surgery and received systemic therapy had a median OS of 34 months (95% CI: 26.6–43.4) compared with median OS of 14 months (95% CI: 11.1–17.0) if they did not have surgery (p<0.001). Median duration of hospital stay of was 9 days (interquartile range: 7–13). Overall, 30 days mortality rate of the group who underwent surgery was 5.4%. Fifteen of 171 (8.8%) patients with symptomatic disease compared with 2 (1.4%) of 142 patients with asymptomatic or minimally symptomatic disease died within 30 days of surgery (p=0.003). Post-operative complications rates were not mutually exclusive and were as followed: post-operative wound infection, 7.3%, non-wound infection, 4.8%, anastomotic leak, 2.2%, wound dehiscence, 1.9%, bleeding, 1.6%, and pulmonary embolism, 1.8%.

On multivariate analysis, surgery of primary tumor, HR: 0.44 (95% CI: 0.35–0.56), use of chemotherapy, HR: 0.33 (95% CI: 0.26–0.43), metastasectomy, HR: 0.43 (95% CI: 0.31–0.58), second line therapy, HR: 0.50 (95% CI: 0.35–0.70), and third line therapy, HR: 0.58 (95% CI: 0.41–0.83) were correlated with superior survival (**Table 3**). After adjustment for other prognostic variables, only the interaction between surgical resection of primary tumor and subsequent line of therapy was significant suggesting a differential benefit of removal of primary tumor in patients who received other lines of therapies. In a subgroup of 345 patients with asymptomatic or relatively asymptomatic primary tumors, surgery was significantly correlated with better survival with HR 0.32 (95% CI: 0.22–0.45).

Other studies also supports potential advantage of resection of primary tumor in patients who are treated with modern chemotherapy regimens. A retrospective analysis of CAIRO study that compared combination versus sequential chemotherapy demonstrated a significantly better median OS of 16.7 months in patients who underwent resection of primary tumor compared with 11.4 months with no surgery (HR 0.61, 95% CI:49–0.76) [20]. Likewise, a pool analysis of four French phase 3 trials involving 850 patients indicated survival benefit of surgery [35]. More than two third of patients were treated with FOLFIRI or FOLFOX and about 12% received bevacizumab.

Since the publication of our meta-analysis, the resection of the primary tumor has become one of the key issues in the management of stage 4 CRC. Several recent studies have addressed this question in patients with symptomatic or minimally symptomatic tumors [36–39]. Ishihara and others retrospectively evaluated 1982 patients with stage 4 CRC from 1997 to 2007 [36]. Among the whole patient population, primary tumor resection significantly improved survival (HR: 0.46, 95% CI 0.32–0.66). However, primary tumor resection did not significantly improve survival in patients treated in the first 5 years of the study, patients aged >65 years, female patients, patients with right-sided colon cancer, and patients without nodal involvement. Gresham et al. [37] evaluated 517 patients with stage 4 CRC. Among them, 378 (73%) patients underwent palliative resection of their primary tumor. Palliative resection was associated with a longer median OS (17.9 vs. 7.9 months) and more favorable adjusted HR for death (0.56, 95 % CI: 0.40–0.78). In a propensity score-matched analysis, prognosis was also more favorable in the resected group (p = 0.0017). Tarantino and others used the Surveillance, Epidemiology, and End Results (SEER) database from 1998 to 2009 and identified 37,793 patients with stage IV CRC. Of those, 23,004 (60.9%) underwent palliative primary tumor resection. The primary cancer resection was associated with a significantly improved OS (HR: 0.40, 95% CI: 0.39–0.42) and cancer-specific survival (HR: 0.39, 95% CI: 0.38–0.40) [38]. Yun and others assessed 416 patients with asymptomatic unresectable stage IV CRC from year 2000 to 2008 [39]. Among 416 patients, 218 (52.4%) underwent palliative resection of the primary tumor. Their data revealed that palliative resection was not associated with a significant increase in survival compared with non-resection. Clancy and others performed an updated meta-analysis of 21 eligible studies involving a total of 44,226 patients [40]. Resection of the primary tumor in patients with unresectable metastases compared with chemotherapy alone was associated with a lower mortality risk (odd ratio [OR] 0.28; 95% CI: 0.165–0.474; P<0.001), translating into a difference in mean survival of 6.4 months in favor of resection (95% CI: 5.025–7.858). Patients who underwent resection of the primary tumor were more likely to have liver metastasis only (OR 1.551; 95% CI: 1.247–1.929), were less likely to have ≥2 metastasis (OR 0.653; 95% CI: 0.508–0.839), and were less likely to have rectal cancer (OR 0.495; 95% CI: 0.390–0.629).

5. Time trend in surgery of the primary tumor

In spite of uncertain survival benefit, a high rate of surgical resection has been reported in patients with unresectable metastatic disease. Nevertheless, with access to novel agents and their efficacy in the primary tumor as well as lack of major complications related to an intact primary tumor, surgery is less commonly performed [16, 17, 41]. Hu and others performed a retrospective cohort study using data from the National Cancer Institute's Surveillance, Epidemiology, and End Results CRC registry involving 64,157 patients diagnosed with stage IV colon or rectal cancer from January, 1988, through December, 2010. Of the 64,157 patients, 43,273 (67.4%) had undergone primary tumor resection [42]. The annual rate of primary tumor resection significantly decreased from 74.5% in 1988 to 57.4% in 2010, and a significant annual percentage change occurred between 1998–2001 and 2001–2010 (−0.41% vs −2.39%). Among various prognostic variables age younger than 50 years, female sex, being married, higher tumor grade, and presence of colon tumors were correlated with primary tumor resection.

6. Mechanisms of potential survival advantages of surgery

The underlying mechanism of potential survival benefit related to the removal of primary tumor is mostly hypothetical. It is well recognized that surgical resection of primary tumor with or without debulking of metastatic lesions, in some malignant diseases such as ovarian and renal cell cancer, has been associated with better survival [43, 10]. Non-curative resection of the primary tumor in patients with advanced cancer may prevent local tumor complications and improve disease control by simply reducing the tumor bulk. The host-tumor interaction plays an important role in cancer progression [44]. It is plausible that the primary tumor may secrete cytokines that promote tumor growth and reduce response to cytotoxic agents [46]. Turner and others examined the effect of primary tumor resection on systemic inflammation and survival in patients with stage IV CRC using the neutrophil-lymphocyte ratio (NLR) as a biomarker of systemic inflammation [46]. The reversal of an elevated NLR following the primary tumor resection was associated with significantly improved OS (hazard ratio, 0.53).

Hence, resection of the primary tumor by affecting the tumor-host relationship may slow the cancer progression. Furthermore, removal of primary tumor may restore the host immune system and may improve response to systemic therapy [47].

7. Limitations of the published literature

Most studies obtained data retrospectively. Many studies failed to provide baseline prognostic information of resection and non-resection groups while others showed significant imbalance in baseline characteristics of the two groups and did not make adjustment for that. Only few studies provided detail information about the use and type of chemotherapy in each group. In addition, to our knowledge no study have adjusted for BRAF mutation which has been reported in about 5-11% stage IV CRC and is an important prognostic marker [48]. Although our cohort studies were good quality studies, imbalance of several known and unknown prognostic variables between the two groups suggests bias [32–34]

8. Future directions

At least two randomized clinical trials are currently evaluating the survival benefit of removal of primary tumor in patients with metastatic CRC [49, 50]. The SYNCHRNOUS trial is a multicenter German study comparing resection of the primary tumor and systemic therapy to systemic therapy alone in patients with metastatic colon cancer which is not amenable to curative therapy [49]. The investigators estimated that resection of the primary tumor will prolong survival from 20 to 26 months. In addition to survival, the study is evaluating short- and long-term safety of both treatment strategies, subsequent curative procedures, and patients' quality of life. In this trial, 694 patients (347 per group) will be enrolled to test the hypothesis that removal of the primary tumor has been associated with superior survival.

The CAIRO trial is a multicenter Dutch trial which is evaluating benefit of resection of the primary tumor in patients with synchronous unresectable metastatic CRC [50]. Patients with synchronous metastatic colon cancer with asymptomatic or minimally symptomatic primary tumor will be randomized to systemic treatment or resection of the primary tumor followed by systemic treatment. Unlike SYNCHRONOUS, trial patients with colon or rectal cancer are included in this study. A total of 360 patients will be enrolled to detect a difference in median overall survival of 13 compared with 19 months.

9. Conclusions

Although evidence suggests possible survival benefits with surgery despite the availability of effective chemotherapeutic agents, due to a lack of prospective clinical trials, no firm conclusions can be drawn with respect to whether surgical resection of the primary tumor should be routinely offered to all patients with newly diagnosed metastatic CRC. Currently, two randomized controlled trials are evaluating this important question in the management of metastatic CRC. If the magnitude of survival benefits is confirmed in future randomized clinical trials, surgical resection of the primary tumor could potentially be a more cost effective intervention compared with novel systemic therapy in the management of stage IV CRC.

Author details

Shahid Ahmed[1,2,3*], Selliah Kanthan[4], Nayyer Iqbal[1,2], Adnan Zaidi[1,2], Duc Le[1,2], Tahir Abbas[1,2] and Kamal Haider[1,2]

*Address all correspondence to: shahid.ahmed@saskcancer.ca

1 Saskatchewan Cancer Agency, University of Saskatchewan, Saskatoon, Canada

2 Department of Oncology, University of Saskatchewan, Saskatoon, Canada

3 Department of Community Health and Epidemiology, University of Saskatchewan, Saskatoon, Canada

4 Department of Surgery, University of Saskatchewan, Saskatoon, Canada

References

[1] Ahmed S, Johnson K, Ahmed O, et al. Advances in the management of colorectal cancer: from biology to treatment. Int J Colorectal Dis. 2014; 29: 1031–1042.

[2] Rees M, Tekkis PP, Welsh FK, et al. Evaluation of long-term survival after hepatic resection for metastatic colorectal cancer: a multifactorial model of 929 patients. Ann Surg. 2008; 247: 125–135.

[3] Tomlinson JS, Jarnagin WR, DeMatteo RP, et al. Actual 10-year survival after resection of colorectal liver metastases defines cure. J Clin Oncol. 2007; 25: 4575–4580.

[4] Zhao Z, Pelletier E, Barber B, et al. Major surgery in patients with metastatic colorectal cancer in Western Europe. J Gastrointest Canc. 2012; 43: 456–461.

[5] Shah S, Haddad R, Al-Sukhni W, et al. Surgical resection of hepatic and pulmonary metastases from colorectal carcinoma. J Am Coll Surg. 2006; 202: 468–475.

[6] Kanthan R, Senger JL, Ahmed S, et al. Recent Advances in the Management of Stage IV Colon Cancer. J Cancer Ther. 2012; 3: 1104–1118.

[7] Loupakis F, Cremolini C, Masi G, et al. Initial therapy with FOLFOXIRI and bevacizumab for metastatic colorectal cancer. N Engl J Med. 2014; 371: 1609–1618.

[8] Ahmed S, Shahid RK, Leis A, et al. Should non-curative resection of primary tumor be performed in patients with stage IV colorectal cancer? A systematic review and meta-analysis. Curr Oncol. 2013; 20: e420–e441.

[9] Flanigan RC, Salmon SE, Blumenstein BA, et al. Nephrectomy followed by interferon alfa-2b compared with interferon alfa-2b alone for metastatic renal-cell cancer. N Engl J Med. 2001; 345: 1655–1659.

[10] Mickisch GH, Garin A, van PH, de PL, et al. Radical nephrectomy plus interferon-alfa-based immunotherapy compared with interferon alfa alone in metastatic renal-cell carcinoma: a randomised trial. Lancet. 2001; 358: 966–970.

[11] Stillwell AP, Buettner PG, Ho YH. Meta-analysis of survival of patients with stage IV colorectal cancer managed with surgical resection versus chemotherapy alone. World J Surg. 2010; 34: 797–807.

[12] Benoist S, Pautrat K, Mitry E, et al. Treatment strategy for patients with colorectal cancer and synchronous irresectable liver metastases. Br J Surg. 2005; 92: 1155–1160.

[13] Ruo L, Gougoutas C, Paty PB, et al. Elective bowel resection for incurable stage IV colorectal cancer: prognostic variables for asymptomatic patients. J Am Coll Surg. 2003; 196: 722–72.

[14] Saif MW, Elfiky A, Salem RR. Gastrointestinal perforation due to bevacizumab in colorectal cancer. Ann Surg Oncol. 2007; 14: 1860–1869.

[15] Damjanov N, Weiss J, Haller DG. Resection of the primary colorectal cancer is not necessary in non-obstructed patients with metastatic disease. Oncologist. 2009; 14: 963–969.

[16] Poultsides GA, Servais EL, Saltz LB, et al. Outcome of primary tumor in patients with synchronous stage IV colorectal cancer receiving combination chemotherapy without surgery as initial treatment. J Clin Oncol. 2009; 27: 3379–3384.

[17] McCahill LE, Yothers G, Sharif S, et al. Primary mFOLFOX6 plus bevacizumab without resection of the primary tumor for patients presenting with surgically unresectable metastatic colon cancer and an intact asymptomatic colon cancer: definitive analysis of NSABP trial C-10. J Clin Oncol. 2012 10; 30: 3223–3228.

[18] Cirocchi R, Trastulli S, Abraha I, et al. Non-resection versus resection for an asymptomatic primary tumour in patients with unresectable stage IV colorectal cancer. Cochrane Database Syst Rev. 2012; 15:8:CD008997.

[19] Scheer MG, Sloots CE, van der Wilt GJ, et al. Management of patients with asymptomatic colorectal cancer and synchronous irresectable metastases. Ann Oncol. 2008; 19: 1829–1835.

[20] Venderbosch S, Wilt JH, Teerenstra S, et al. Prognostic value of resection of primary tumor in patients with stage IV colorectal cancer: Retrospective analysis of two randomized studies and a review of the literature. Ann Surg Oncol. 2011; 18: 3252–3260.

[21] Karoui M, Roudot-Thoraval F, Mesli F, et al. Cancer and Unresectable Distant Metastases Improves Overall Survival: Results of a Multicentric Study. Dis Colon Rectum. 2011; 54: 930–938.

[22] Scoggins CR, Meszoely IM, Blanke CD et al. Nonoperative management of primary colorectal cancer in patients with stage IV disease. Ann Surg Oncol 1999; 6: 651–657.

[23] Tebbutt NC, Norman AR, Cunningham D, et al. Intestinal complications after chemotherapy for patients with unresected primary colorectal cancer and synchronous metastases. Gut. 2003; 52: 568–573.

[24] Galizia G, Lieto E, Orditura M et al. First-line chemotherapy vs bowel tumor resection plus chemotherapy for patients with unresectable synchronous colorectal hepatic metastases. Arch Surg. 2008; 143: 352–358.

[25] Temple LK, Hsieh L, Wong WD, et al. Use of surgery among elderly patients with stage IV colorectal cancer. J Clin Oncol. 2004; 22: 3475–3484.

[26] Aslam MA, Kelkar A, Sharpe D. Ten years experience of managing the primary tumours in patients with stageIV CRC. Int J Surg. 2010; 8: 305–313.

[27] Chan TW, Brown C, Ho CC, et al. Primary tumor resection in patients presenting with metastatic colorectal cancer. Am J Clin Oncol. 2010; 33: 52–55.

[28] Evans MD, Escofet X, Karandikar SS, et al. Outcomes of resection and non-resection strategies in management of patients with advanced colorectal cancer. World J Surg Oncol. 2009; 7: 28.

[29] Konyalian VR, Rosing DK, Haukoos JS, et al. The role of primary tumour resection in patients with stage IV colorectal cancer. Colorectal Dis. 2007; 9: 430–437.

[30] Michel P, Roque I, Di Fiore F, et al. Colorectal cancer with non-resectable synchronous metastases: should the primary tumor be resected? Gastroenterol Clin Biol. 2004; 28: 434–437.

[31] Seo GJ, Park JW, Yoo SB, et al. Intestinal complications after palliative treatment for asymptomatic patients with unresectable stage IV colorectal cancer. J Surg Oncol. 2010; 102: 94–99.

[32] Ahmed S, Leis A, Fields A, et al. Survival impact of surgical resection of primary tumor in patients with stage IV colorectal cancer: Results from a large population-based cohort study. Cancer. 2014; 120: 683–691.

[33] Ahmed S, Fields A, Pahwa P, et al. Surgical resection of primary tumor in asymptomatic or minimally symptomatic patients with stage IV colorectal cancer: A Canadian Province Experience. Clin Colorectal Cancer. 2015; 14: e41–e47.

[34] Ahmed S, Pahwa P, Kanthan S, et al. Surgical management of the primary tumor in stage IV colorectal cancer: A validation study. J Clin Oncol. 2015; 33 (suppl 3; abstr 675).

[35] Faron M, Bourredjem A, Pignon J, et al. Impact on survival of primary tumor resection in patients with colorectal cancer and unresectable metastasis: Pooled analysis of individual patients' data from four randomized trials. J Clin Oncol 30, 2012 (suppl; abstr 3507)

[36] Ishihara S, Nishikawa T, Tanaka T, et al. Benefit of primary tumor resection in stage IV colorectal cancer with unresectable metastasis: a multicenter retrospective study using a propensity score analysis. Int J Colorectal Dis. 2015; 30: 807–812.

[37] Gresham G, Renouf DJ, Chan M, et al. Association between palliative resection of the primary tumor and overall survival in a population-based cohort of metastatic colorectal cancer patients. Ann Surg Oncol. 2014; 21(12): 3917–3923.

[38] Tarantino I, Warschkow R, Worni M, et al. Prognostic relevance of palliative primary tumor removal in 37,793 metastatic colorectal cancer patients: A population-based, propensity score-adjusted trend analysis. Ann Surg 2015; 262: 112–120.

[39] Yun JA, Huh JW, Park YA, et al. The role of palliative resection for asymptomatic primary tumor in patients with unresectable stage IV colorectal cancer. Dis Colon Rectum. 2014; 57: 1049–1058.

[40] Clancy C, Burke JP, Barry M, et al. A meta-analysis to determine the effect of primary tumor resection for stage IV colorectal cancer with unresectable metastases on patient survival. Ann Surg Oncol. 2014; 21: 3900–3908.

[41] Cercek A, Weiser MR, Goodman KA, et al. Complete pathologic response in the primary of rectal or colon cancer treated with FOLFOX without radiation. J Clin Oncol. 2010; 28 (suppl 15; abstr 3649).

[42] Hu C, Bailey C, You Y, et al. Time trend analysis of primary tumor resection for stage IV colorectal cancer: less surgery, improved survival. JAMA Surg. 2015; 150: 245–51.

[43] Vergote I, van Gorp T, Amant F, et al. Timing of debulking surgery in advanced ovarian cancer. Int J Gynecol Cancer. 2008; 18: 11–19.

[44] McAllister SS, Weinberg RA. Tumor-Host Interactions: A Far-Reaching Relationship. JCO 2010; 28: 4022–4028.

[45] Merogi AJ, Ramesh R, Robinson WR, et al. Tumor-host interaction: analysis of cytokines, growth factors, and tumor –infiltrating lymphocytes in ovarian carcinomas. Hum Pathol. 1997; 28: 321–331.

[46] Turner N, Tran B, Tran PV, et al. Primary tumor resection in patients with metastatic colorectal cancer is associated with reversal of systemic inflammation and improved survival. Clin Colorectal Cancer. 2015; 14: 185–191.

[47] Danna EA, Sinha P, Gilbert M, et al. Surgical removal of primary tumor reverses tumor-induced immunosuppression despite the presence of metastatic disease. Cancer Res 2004; 64: 2205–2211.

[48] Yokota T, Ura T, Shibata N, et al. BRAF mutation is a powerful prognostic factor in advanced and recurrent colorectal cancer. Br J Cancer. 2011; 104: 856–886.

[49] Rahbari NN, Lordick, F, Fink C, et al. Resection of the primary tumour versus no resection prior to systemic therapy in patients with colon cancer and synchronous unresectable metastases (UICC stage IV): SYNCHRONOUS - a randomised controlled multicentre trial (ISRCTN30964555). BMC Cancer 2012; 12: 142.

[50] Dutch Colorectal Cancer Group. CAIRO 4. http://www.dccg.nl/dccg-trials/cairo-4/ (Accessed on December 14, 2015).

Chapter 12

Simultaneous Surgery for Synchronous Colorectal Liver Metastases

Nikola Kolev, Valentin Ignatov, Anton Tonev,
Aleksandar Zlatarov, Boryana Naydenova,
Georgi Ivanov, Dilyan Petrov and Krasimir Ivanov

Additional information is available at the end of the chapter

http://dx.doi.org/10.5772/64317

Abstract

Colon cancer is one of the leading malignant diseases in the Western world, leading to significant morbidity and has significant predilection for liver metastases. Synchronous metastases account for approximately 15–25% of the newly discovered liver lesions. The only curative treatment for colon cancer liver metastases (CLM) remains surgery. Several strategies have been developed for the treatment of synchronous CLM, including simultaneous resection, two-stage liver surgery, and liver-first approach. The timing of surgery is not universally determined. Even more reports support the simultaneous resection strategy with results showing similar morbidity, length of hospital stay, and perioperative mortality comparable to staged resection. In conclusion, SCLM patients can successfully be treated with simultaneous approach or stages, both having similar perioperative and long-term outcomes. With the advance of liver surgery techniques, minor and major liver surgeries can be performed safely with low morbidity and mortality as part of either a simultaneous or a staged operative strategy.

Keywords: colon cancer, simultaneous resection, hepatectomy, liver metastases, adjuvant therapy

1. Introduction

Colon cancer remains one of the leading causes of cancer-related death in the Western world. The most common site for metastases from colon cancer is the liver [1]. According to studies, liver metastases develop in almost half of the colon cancer patients. Approximately 15–25% of them are synchronous metastases. Surgical therapy for liver metastases remains the only potentially curative therapy for patients with colon liver metastases (CLMs) [1, 2]. The resection of synchronous CLMs, also known as SCLMs, appears to have survival rates similar to those of metachronous metastases [3]. The most appropriate moment for surgery in SCLM and primary tumor is not completely determined. The most common approach is resection of the primary tumor and consequent liver resection after 2–4 months later [4–7]. The advocates of this approach consider the probability of increased morbidity associated with the simultaneous procedure. This issue has been addressed in many studies comparing the simultaneous and staged approach. The results show similar morbidity, length of hospital stay, and perioperative mortality between the two [8–11]. Moreover, since a second laparotomy can be avoided by the simultaneous removal of the primary tumor and liver metastasis of colon may be preferred, it allows sooner completion of surgery, thereby permitting faster initiation of adjuvant therapy. However, there is no consensus on when to perform surgical resection of liver metastases and primary colon for patients with SCLM.

This chapter is aimed to present the efficacy and safety of simultaneous resections for synchronous colon cancer liver metastases.

2. Definition of resectability

As we know, the criteria defining when to perform the resection have significantly changed in recent years. Older criteria include patients with less than four unilobular metastases, resection margins over 1 cm and lack of extrahepatic disease. The main consideration for resectability is the ability to complete curative (*R*0) resection with adequate liver remnant. Modern definitions of resectability of liver metastatic disease criteria were presented by the Consensus Conference on the Multidisciplinary Treatment of Liver Metastases of colorectal cancer in 2012 [12].

The preoperative staging is aimed at the determination of surgical resectability. With the improved accuracy of combined computed tomography, positron emission tomography, liver contrast-enhanced magnetic resonance imaging and high-resolution CT, the ability to detect small-volume disease has been significantly enhanced [13]. Patients with positive celiac and/or paraaortic lymph nodes may not benefit from liver resection [14]. Although positive retropancreatic lymph nodes are suggestive of poor prognosis, the survival is proven to be better in patients with positive celiac lymph nodes and therefore these patients may benefit from liver surgery especially when they are subjected to perioperative chemotherapy [15]. Considering the individual characteristics of each case, all patients must be referred to specialized centers with multidisciplinary team to determine the proper timing of resection for primary tumor and SCLM [1].

3. Perioperative results

The specialization of general surgeons in hepatobiliary surgery training, development of hepatobiliary techniques, and up-to-date anesthetic and intensive care management has made hepatic resection safer [16]. Nowadays, the major liver resections are showing minimal morbidity and mortality [11, 17]. According to a meta-analysis, patients undergoing staged resection had more postoperative complications, which are attributed to the need of two or more laparotomies. More incisions result in a greater risk of wound complications [2]. Staged resections are preferred to synchronous colonic resection and hepatic resections in some centers. A perceived increase in perioperative risk with simultaneous resection has traditionally provided the rationale for performing the resection in stages. On theory, the staged resection must have the advantage of better perioperative outcomes. The supporting evidence states that staged resection has significantly lower morbidity and mortality, and thus leads to better long-term results [5, 18–20]. On the other hand, more and more reports emerge in support of simultaneous resection without significant change of mortality and morbidity rates [21, 22]. Chua et al. [11] analyzed retrospectively 96 patients with synchronous colorectal cancer and liver metastases. These patients have been subjected to synchronous or staged resection. The analysis of postoperative results demonstrates that the two groups did not differ significantly in terms of postoperative complications and both lacked operative mortality.

Simultaneous and staged resections for SCLM have comparable morbidity and mortality and close long-term oncologic outcomes. In a study on this topic, the overall morbidity and mortality were 19.6 and 3.0%, respectively. Perioperative outcomes show no difference in patients treated with a staged or simultaneous approach.

Morbidity and mortality rate is similar between patients with major or minor liver resection and does not depend on the operative strategy. In a study by Martin et al. on patients with SCRLM, the reported morbidity and mortality were similar in the groups of staged and simultaneous approach [23]. Another study by Brouqet et al. had similar findings but it should be noted that the results were not stratified for major or minor liver resection [46]. According to the study by Reddy et al. [25], the major liver resection is associated with an increase of morbidity and mortality, although minor liver resection has similar perioperative results with the staged approach.

In conclusion, the safety of staged and simultaneous approach for minor and major hepatectomy is equal. The two strategies have similar operative time and no difference in blood loss. Analysis shows that patients with the staged resection have longer recovery period in the hospital and these with simultaneous resection have lower morbidity rate. A meta-analysis by Chen et al. on 14 studies compares concomitant resection to staged resection in patients with resectable synchronous hepatic metastases. The study includes 2204 patients who were divided into two groups—with simultaneous resection and with staged resection. In analysis, attention to quality of life (QoL) was turned. There are indicators for QoL such as operative time, intraoperative blood loss, and hospital stay. Postoperative morbidity rate is lower in groups of patients with simultaneous resection of the primary tumor and the synchronous liver metastases. And with other study on this topic is improved that simultaneous resection can play a role in better outcome [27]. After searching and analyzing the literature, there is review that deserved attention. It shows that results for patients with simultaneous and delayed resections are similar, and this meta-analysis is in agreement with studies [28]. Fukami et al. reported a series of 158 patients, 63 patients with synchronous colorectal liver metastases.

Of those with synchronous colorectal liver metastases, 41 patients (65%) underwent synchronous resection, and 22 (35%) underwent delayed resection. They noticed shorter total postoperative hospital stay in the synchronous resection group [29].

Synchronous		**Staged**	
Benefit	Risk	Benefit	Risk
Reduced complications due to single operation	Increased infectious liver complications due to bacterial contamination from intestinal resection		Increased morbidity associated with multiple procedures
Reduced length of hospital stay	Risk of complications from unresected primary	Reduced complications from unresected primary	Risk of hepatotoxicity from chemotherapy given between colorectal and hepatic resections
	Increased anastomotic complications due to impaired liver function		
	Extent of hepatic resection limited due to concomitant intestinal resection	Larger hepatic resections may be performed without increased morbidity	
No delay in initiating systemic treatment	Chemotherapy-associated hepatotoxicity may limit extent of liver resection		Risk of complications following colorectal resection may delay chemotherapy prior to liver resection
Opportunity to observe tumor response to neoadjuvant chemotherapy	No opportunity to assess tumor response if resection precedes systemic therapy		

Table 1. Potential risks and benefits of synchronous versus staged resection [34].

A new challenge for the surgeon is the laparoscopic simultaneous resection of synchronous colorectal metastases and the primary tumor. The studies have discussed the technical feasibility and short-come outcomes of the procedure. Tranchart et al. reported a preliminary series questioning the feasibility of combined laparoscopic resection of colorectal cancer (CRC) and synchronous colorectal liver metastases (SCRLM). The aim of this study was to compare the short- and long-term outcomes for matched patients undergoing combined resections. A total number of 89 patients were matched in the analysis. There was no difference in global operative time, blood loss, and transfusion rates between the two groups. A conversion was required in 7% of the laparoscopic procedures. Morbidity rates were similar in the two groups ($p = 1.0$). Their conclusion is that in patients without severe comorbidities presenting with one, small (≤3 cm), CRLM resectable by a wedge resection or a left lateral sectionectomy, combined laparoscopic resection of CRC and SCRLM allows similar short- and long-term outcomes compared with the open approach [30]. Another international large study was published by Feretti et al., comparing the duration of the intervention, blood loss, transfusion rate, conversion rate, resection margin, specific and overall morbidity, perioperative mortality, length of hospital stay, and survival. Univariate and multivariate analyses were performed examining postoperative morbidity in all cohorts of patients. The combined data show that in experienced centers, simultaneous laparoscopic approach is technically feasible, safe, and associated with good oncological outcomes [31]. Miyamoto et al. reported earlier 13 patients who underwent simultaneous laparoscopic colectomy and hepatic resection. The primary sites were right colon in four, left colon in six, and rectum in three. The liver procedures included 14 partial resections or three left lateral hepatectomies. The results of the study conclude that the combined approach is feasible and safe in selected patients with primary CRC and synchronous liver metastases [32]. Other authors such as Muangkaew et al., Miyamoto et al., and Inoue et al. confirm that the feasibility of simultaneous laparoscopic colectomy and hepatectomy for primary colorectal cancer with synchronous liver metastases appears feasible with low morbidity and favorable outcomes [27, 33, 51] (**Table 1**).

4. Long-term oncological results

One of the studies is aimed at the long-term oncologic outcomes in patients with sCLM submitted to resection of both the primary CRC and CRLM. Results show that 57% of patients experienced a recurrence. Other conclusion is that operative strategy for sCLM had no connection with long-term outcomes. In a much smaller, single institution cohort, Brouqet et al. had similarly reported comparable overall survival among patients treated with the classic, simultaneous, or liver-first approach [46]. Rather than operative strategy, tumor-specific factors were associated with long-term oncologic success. These data serve to underline the importance of biology and not technique in the prognosis of patients with SCLM [23].

While the presence of synchronous metastases has been demonstrated to be a negative prognostic factor, it is not a contraindication to hepatectomy if a hepatic resection with curative intent can be achieved. The reported 5-year survival rates after liver resection for patients with SCLM range from 20 to 40%. Although some authors reported poorer prognosis for simultaneous resections compared with staged resections [5, 18], more recent studies demonstrated that the strategy to simultaneously resect the primary tumor and the synchronous metastases yielded no difference in survival compared to staged liver resection [8–10, 21, 35, 36]. Nonetheless, some authors argued that a waiting period of 2–6 months is necessary between the resection of primary tumor and liver resection, to make for subclinical metastases to become evident, in order to enable a better clearance of the tumor [19]. According to the "cascade" theory, in which cancer cells must first form metastases in the liver and then cells from these metastases migrate to the lungs, subsequently disseminated in an arterial pattern, dissemination of cancer cells toward the lungs may occur during the period between the resection of the primary tumor and the resection of the synchronous liver metastases [37].

At Zhongshan Hospital, Shanghai performed an analysis in 154 patients with consecutive synchronous colorectal liver metastasis who underwent simultaneous resection. The study for 10 years shows that this approach to simultaneous resection is safe and has significantly better outcomes in short and long term [38].

Tranchart et al. presented a propensity score-matching analysis of 142 patients who underwent combined laparoscopic resection of CRC and SCRLM, which were compared to a database of 241 patients treated by open during the same period. The 3-year-old overall survival in the laparoscopy and open groups was similar [30]. Another study by Ferreti et al. reported large international multicenter series of laparoscopic simultaneous resection of CRC and SCRLM. The results showed that overall 1-, 3-, and 5-year survival were 98.8, 82.1, and 71.9%, respectively [28]. Fukami et al. [29] compared two groups of simultaneous resection and delayed resection of SCRLM and found similar survival rate between the two groups (p = 0.054). Another study published by Wang et al. reports that there are no significant differences in postoperative complication rate and long-term survival between curative simultaneous and staged resection [39].

There is effective adjuvant therapies for colorectal cancer and simultaneous resection provides sooner completion of surgical therapy and earlier initiation of adjuvant therapy in patients with high risk of additional microscopic disease, which is of advantage to the patients [1].

5. Strategies in the treatment of synchronous colon cancer liver metastases

The most discussed topic for surgeons is the management of sCLM and how to balance between operative timing and strategy. The situation is complicated because of efficacious systemic chemotherapy regimens, targeted biological agents, and adjunctive strategies (e.g., ablative therapies) [1]. Regardless of the information, surgeons need to answer three important questions, summed up by Castellanos et al. in their review [2]:

1. Should the primary and metastatic lesions be resected at the same time?
2. If surgical resection is staged, should the primary or metastatic lesion be resected first?
3. What is the role of perioperative chemotherapy with surgical resection?

Simultaneous resections for primary tumor and liver metastases have technical and oncological specifics. According to standard guidelines, treatment plan is decided by regular tumor board plus hepatobiliary surgeon. Simultaneous resection is the choice for right colon primary cancers and smaller and fewer metastases. In patients with synchronous metastases, operation is done only when safe and good resection margins can be achieved. Simultaneous resection could be done independently of location of the primary cancer and the extent of liver metastasis without fatal postoperation complications [1]. Four prognostic factors were identified in a study by Capussoti et al., which have no effect on survival in the staged resections: more than three liver metastases, T4-primary colorectal tumor, liver metastases infiltrating surrounding structures, and male sex. The optimal timing of surgery should be based on patient's characteristics such as the extent of disease, comorbidities, body habitus, and surgical experience [40]. Simultaneous resections for patients with peritoneal carcinomatosis are not advised [41].

While there is an abundance of evidence demonstrating the benefit of hepatectomy for CLM, there is only limited evidence available to empirically guide the timing of resection for sCLMs. The conventional paradigm has been to first resect the primary tumor, and then perform a hepatectomy. This approach is suggested to avoid complications associated with a major combined surgery. Another argument in favor of this approach is related to the tumor biology —the time windows between surgeries allow the aggressive disease to manifest and thus spare the patient the risk of major liver surgery. This has been supported by observations that staged resection does not result in increased risk of unresectability due to growth of CLM, but rather to appearance of new liver and/or extrahepatic disease. The time window between the staged resections provides the option for systemic treatment, which may decrease the risk of new metastatic lesions and thus improve overall survival. On the other hand, staged resection for SCRLM may result in increased hospitalization, additional cost, as well as increased pain, stress for patients subjected to staged approach instead of one single procedure [1, 2]. Considering the increasing number of studies showing decreased morbidity associated with simultaneous approach for SCRLM, it could be used in selected patients. The evidence for similar short-term and long-term outcomes after simultaneous or delayed resection is growing, even for major liver resection [1]. On the other hand, other groups of authors suggest that perioperative mortality is significantly higher for simultaneous resection, especially after major liver resections [1]. A multicenter retrospective analysis of 1004 patients with SCRLM treated between 1982 and 2011 demonstrates no difference in postoperative complications or a 90-day postoperative mortality between staged and simultaneous approaches for SCRLM [1]. The authors defined the major liver resection as resection of more than three segments. This procedure was more frequently performed in a staged strategy (39%) versus simultaneous approach. A meta-analysis by Slesser et al. compares the outcomes of simultaneous and staged resections for SCRLM of 3159 patients from studies from 1991 to 2010. They found no significant difference in operative blood loss, duration of operation, postoperative complications, overall survival, and disease-free survival. The total number of 1778 (56.3%) patients underwent delayed resection and had significantly larger liver metastases with increased bilobar distribution, and most of those patients underwent major liver resection [42]. Yin et al. presented a meta-analysis of studies including 2880 patients. The findings were similar although significantly lower incidence of postoperative complications was noted in the simultaneous resection group. This meta-analysis recommended the following criteria for the selection of patients for simultaneous approach: metastases in less than four liver segments, age <70 years, and exclusion of severe comorbidities [34].

This analysis confirmed that treatment strategy can change because of the clinical condition of the patient, surgeon, or on the recommendation of a multidisciplinary committee [2].

New retrospective analysis about mortality and morbidity after hepatectomy, colorectal resection, and synchronous resection for colorectal cancer in 43,408 patients shows reliable results that morbidity after synchronous hepatic and colorectal resections is variable and risk is similar. Comparison of outcomes leads to conclusion that there is potential benefit for synchronous resections with minor hepatectomy [44].

The timing of the procedure has also been questioned by Feng et al. in a meta-analysis. Their conclusion is balanced and gives no clear advantage to the simultaneous approach in comparison to the delayed approach. According to the authors, the number of liver metastases was the major confounding factor for postoperative morbidity, especially in staged resections. Without baseline imbalances, simultaneous resection took no statistical significant advantage in safety and efficacy [43].

Over the past years with establishing of laparoscopic technology, there are studies about laparoscopic approach in the simultaneous resection of colorectal primary tumor and liver metastases. Results of studies show that there are 142 patients with laparoscopic liver resection for synchronous colorectal liver metastases. In conclusion, from these data, this approach is safe and offers good outcomes from an oncological view of point [44].

6. The role of perioperative chemotherapy

Despite the improvements in surgical approaches of liver resection, recurrence of disease has been reported in up to two-thirds of patients, with half of these occurring in the remnant liver. In patients with SCRLM who appear resectable on diagnosis, the National Comprehensive Cancer Network guidelines recommend simultaneous resection followed by adjuvant therapy (FOLFOX or CapeOx (capecitabine, oxaliplatin)) or neoadjuvant therapy for 2–3 months before surgery. The recommendations for neoadjuvant chemotherapy are toward FOLFIRI, FOLFOX, or CapeOx with or without bevacizumab. The KRAS status of the tumor defines whether panitumumab or cetuximab will be combined with FOLFOX or FOLFIRI [1, 2].

7. Conclusion

The role of surgery for synchronous colorectal liver metastases is well established. The remaining issue addresses the timing of the procedure. The choice between staged or simultaneous resection of SCRLM is a matter of careful selection of patients, based on tumor characteristics—extent of disease, degree of liver involvement, and patient's factors—performance status, age, and comorbidities. The sequence of actions considering systemic therapy and surgery is also open to discussion. Some authors reported poorer short-term results for synchronous resections compared with staged resections [5]. Conversely, more recent studies have shown that simultaneous colorectal and liver surgery are feasible and safe [8, 9]. Resection of synchronous colorectal cancer liver metastases is a safe and effective procedure compared to minor hepatic resection alone.

In conclusion, SCRLM patients may benefit from both approaches, which are supported by the short-term and long-term outcomes reported in various studies. Both minor and major liver surgeries are feasible with comparable morbidity and mortality for staged and simulta-

http://dx.doi.org/10.5772/64317

neous surgery. Despite the promising results, major liver surgery should be approached with caution as a simultaneous procedure with primary tumor resection. Laparoscopic simultaneous resections also present a feasible option with similar short-term and long-term outcomes. The key to the selection of strategy might be found in the tumor biology because survival in patients with SCRLM is more or less independent of the surgical strategy.

Author details

Nikola Kolev[1], Valentin Ignatov[1], Anton Tonev[1*], Aleksandar Zlatarov[1], Boryana Naydenova[2*], Georgi Ivanov[1], Dilyan Petrov[1] and Krasimir Ivanov[1]

*Address all correspondence to: teraton@abv.bg and dr_b_naydenova@yahoo.com

1 Department of General and Operative Surgery, Medical University Varna, Varna, Bulgaria

2 Department of Anesthesiology, Emergency, Intensive and Maritime Medicine, Medical University Varna, Bulgaria

References

[1] Jinggui Chen QL. Simultaneous vs. staged resection for synchronous colorectal liver metastases: a metaanalysis. Int J Colorectal Dis. Int J Colorectal Dis. 2011;26(2):191–9.

[2] Castellanos JA, Merchant NB. Strategies for management of synchronous colorectal metastases. Curr Surg Rep. 2014;2(8):62.

[3] Bockhorn M, Frilling A, Frühauf NR, Neuhaus J, Molmenti E, Trarbach T, et al. Survival of patients with synchronous and metachronous colorectal liver metastases--is there a difference? J Gastrointest Surg Off J Soc Surg Aliment Tract. 2008 Aug;12(8):1399–405.

[4] Schlag P, Hohenberger P, Herfarth C. Resection of liver metastases in colorectal cancer – competitive analysis of treatment results in synchronous versus metachronous metastases. Eur J Surg Oncol. 1990 Aug;16(4):360–5.

[5] Nordlinger B, Guiguet M, Vaillant JC, Balladur P, Boudjema K, Bachellier P, et al. Surgical resection of colorectal carcinoma metastases to the liver. A prognostic scoring system to improve case selection, based on 1568 patients. Association Française de Chirurgie. Cancer. 1996 Apr 1;77(7):1254–62.

[6] Vogt P, Raab R, Ringe B, Pichlmayr R. Resection of synchronous liver metastases from colorectal cancer. World J Surg. 1991 Jan;15(1):62–7.

[7] Jaeck D, Bachellier P, Weber JC, Mourad M, Walf P, Boudjema K, Surgical treatment of synchronous hepatic metastases of colorectal cancers. Simultaneous or delayed resection? Ann Chir. 1995 Dec;50(7):507–12; discussion 13–6.

[8] Fujita S, Akasu T, Moriya Y. Resection of synchronous liver metastases from colorectal cancer. Jpn J Clin Oncol. 2000 Jan 1;30(1):7–11.

[9] Elias D, Detroz B, Lasser P, Plaud B, Jerbi G. Is simultaneous hepatectomy and intestinal anastomosis safe? Am J Surg. 1995 Feb;169(2):254–60.

[10] Lyass S, Zamir G, Matot I, Goitein D, Eid A, Jurim O. Combined colon and hepatic resection for synchronous colorectal liver metastases. J Surg Oncol. 2001 Sep;78(1):17–21.

[11] Chua HK, Sondenaa K, Tsiotos GG, Larson DR, Wolff BG, Nagorney DM. Concurrent vs. staged colectomy and hepatectomy for primary colorectal cancer with synchronous hepatic metastases. Dis Colon Rectum. 2004 Aug;47(8):1310–6.

[12] Weber DM. Laparoscopic surgery: an excellent approach in elderly patients. Arch Surg Chic Ill 1960. 2003 Oct;138(10):1083–8.

[13] Adams RB, Aloia TA, Loyer E, Pawlik TM, Taouli B, Vauthey J-N. Selection for hepatic resection of colorectal liver metastases: expert consensus statement. HPB. 2013;15(2): 91–103.

[14] Alberts SR, Poston GJ. Treatment advances in liver-limited metastatic colorectal cancer. Clin Colorectal Cancer. 2011;10(4):258–65.

[15] Adam R, de Haas RJ, Wicherts DA, Aloia TA, Delvart V, Azoulay D, et al. Is hepatic resection justified after chemotherapy in patients with colorectal liver metastases and lymph node involvement? J Clin Oncol. 2008 Aug 1;26(22):3672–80.

[16] Jaeck D, Nakano H, Bachellier P, Inoue K, Weber J-C, Oussoultzoglou E, et al. Significance of hepatic pedicle lymph node involvement in patients with colorectal liver metastases: a prospective study. Ann Surg Oncol. 9(5):430–8.

[17] Martin RCG, Augenstein V, Reuter NP, Scoggins CR, McMasters KM. Simultaneous versus staged resection for synchronous colorectal cancer liver metastases. J Am Coll Surg. 2009 May;208(5):842–50; discussion 850–2.

[18] Reddy SK, Pawlik TM, Zorzi D, Gleisner AL, Ribero D, Assumpcao L, et al. Simultaneous resections of colorectal cancer and synchronous liver metastases: a multi-institutional analysis. Ann Surg Oncol. 2007 Dec;14(12):3481–91.

[19] Bolton JS, Fuhrman GM. Survival after resection of multiple bilobar hepatic metastases from colorectal carcinoma. Ann Surg. 2000 May;231(5):743–51.

[20] Jenkins LT, Millikan KW, Bines SD, Staren ED, Doolas A. Hepatic resection for metastatic colorectal cancer. Am Surg. 1997 Jul;63(7):605–10.

[21] Scheele J. Hepatectomy for liver metastases. Br J Surg. 1993;80(3):274–6.

[22] Weber JC, Bachellier P, Oussoultzoglou E, Jaeck D. Simultaneous resection of colorectal primary tumour and synchronous liver metastases. Br J Surg. 2003 Aug;90(8):956–62.

[23] Siegel R, Naishadham D, Jemal A. Cancer statistics, 2012. CA Cancer J Clin. 2012 Feb; 62(1):10–29.

[24] Capussoti L, Ferrero A, Vigano L, Ribero D, Lo Tesoriere R, Polastri R. Neoadjuvant therapy of colorectal liver metastases: lessons learned from clinical trials, major liver resections synchronous with colorectal surgery. Ann Surg Oncol. 2007;14:195–201.

[25] Martin RCG, Scoggins CR, McMasters KM. Safety and efficacy of microwave ablation of hepatic tumors: a prospective review of a 5-year experience. Ann Surg Oncol. 2010 Jan;17(1):171–8.

[26] C. Land, Alex C. Michalos, Joseph Sirgy. Handbook of Social Indicators and Quality of Life Research edited by Kenneth.

[27] Miyamoto Y, Beppu T, Sakamoto Y, Imai K, Hayashi H, Nitta H, Ishiko T, Watanabe M, Baba H. Simultaneous laparoscopic resection of primary tumor and liver metastases for colorectal cancer: surgical technique and short-term outcome. Hepatogastroenterology. 2015 Jun;62(140):846–52.

[28] Yin Z, Liu C, Chen Y, Wang J. Timing of hepatectomy in resectable synchronous colorectal liver metastases (SCRLM): Simultaneous or delayed? Article in Hepatol. 57(6) June 2013 with 6 Reads; Impact Factor: 11.06. DOI: 10.1002/hep.26283. Source: PubMed

[29] Fukami Y, Kaneoka Y, Maeda A, Takayama Y, Onoe S, Isogai M. Simultaneous resection for colorectal cancer and synchronous liver metastases. Surg Today. 2016 Feb;46(2):176–82. DOI: 10.1007/s00595-015-1188-1. Epub 2015 May 26

[30] Tranchart H, Fuks D, Vigano L, Ferretti S, Paye F, Wakabayashi G, et al. Laparoscopic simultaneous resection of colorectal primary tumor and liver metastases: a propensity score matching analysis. Surg Endosc. 2016 May;30(5):1853–62.

[31] Ferretti S, Tranchart H, Buell JF, Eretta C, Patriti A, Spampinato MG, Huh JW, Vigano L, Han HS, Ettorre GM, Jovine E, Gamblin TC, Belli G, Wakabayashi G, Gayet B, Dagher I. Laparoscopic simultaneous resection of colorectal primary tumor and liver metastases: results of a multicenter international study. World J Surg. 2015 Aug;39(8):2052–60. DOI: 10.1007/s00268-015-3034-4.

[32] Tranchart H, Fuks D, Vigano L, Ferretti S, Paye F, Wakabayashi G, Ferrero A, Gayet B, Dagher I. Laparoscopic simultaneous resection of colorectal primary tumor and liver metastases: a propensity score matching analysis. Surg Endosc. 2015 Aug 15. [Epub ahead of print]

[33] Muangkaew P, Cho JY, Han HS, Yoon YS, Choi Y, Jang JY, Choi H, Jang JS, Kwon SU. Outcomes of simultaneous major liver resection and colorectal surgery for colorectal

liver metastases. J Gastrointest Surg. 2016 Mar;20(3):554–63. DOI: 10.1007/s11605-015-2979-9. Epub 2015 Oct 15.

[34] Fahy B, Fischer C. Synchronous resection of colorectal primary and hepatic metastasis. J Gastrointest Oncol. 2012;3:48–58. DOI: 10.3978/j.issn.2078-6891.2012.004

[35] Dimick JB, Wainess RM, Cowan JA, Upchurch GR, Knol JA, Colletti LM. National trends in the use and outcomes of hepatic resection. J Am Coll Surg. 2004 Jul;199(1):31–8.

[36] Scheele J, Stangl R, Altendorf-Hofmann A, Gall FP. Indicators of prognosis after hepatic resection for colorectal secondaries. Surgery. 1991 Jul;110(1):13–29.

[37] Tanaka K, Shimada H, Matsuo K, Nagano Y, Endo I, Sekido H, et al. Outcome after simultaneous colorectal and hepatic resection for colorectal cancer with synchronous metastases. Surgery. 2004 Sep;136(3):650–9.

[38] Wei Y, Lin Q, Tang W, Xu P, Xu J. Analysis of long-term outcomes and risk factors in patients undergoing simultaneous resection of synchronous colorectal liver metastasis (Article), – Department of General Surgery, Zhongshan Hospital, Fudan University, Shanghai, China.

[39] Wang L, Yan X, Wang K, Bao Q, Sun Y, Wang H, Jin K, Xing B, Wakabayashi G, Ferrero A, Gayet B, Dagher I. Simultaneous versus staged liver resection of synchronous liver metastasis from colorectal cancer. Surg Endosc. 2015 Aug 15. [Epub ahead of print], Zhonghua Wei Chang Wai Ke Za Zhi. 2014 Oct;17(10):1009–13.

[40] Adam R, de Haas RJ, Wicherts DA, Vibert E, Salloum C, Azoulay D, et al. Concomitant extrahepatic disease in patients with colorectal liver metastases: when is there a place for surgery? Ann Surg. 2011 Feb;253(2):349–59.

[41] Slesser AAP, Simillis C, Goldin R, Brown G, Mudan S, Tekkis PP. A meta-analysis comparing simultaneous versus delayed resections in patients with synchronous colorectal liver metastases. Surg Oncol. 2013 Mar;22(1):36–47.

[42] Yin Z, Liu C, Chen Y, et al. Timing of hepatectomy in resectable synchronous colorectal liver metastases (SCRLM): simultaneous or delayed? Hepatology. 2013;57:2346–57.

[43] Feng Q, Wei Y, Zhu D, Ye L, Lin Q, Li W, Qin X, Lyu M, Xu J. Timing of hepatectomy for resectable synchronous colorectal liver metastases: for whom simultaneous resection is more suitable – a meta-analysis. PLoS One. 2014 Aug 5;9(8):e104348. DOI: 10.1371/journal.pone.0104348. eCollection 2014.

[44] Shubert CR, Habermann EB, Bergquist JR, Thiels CA, Thomsen KM, Kremers WK, Kendrick ML, Cima RR, Nagorney DM, Brouquet A, Nordlinger B. A NSQIP review of major morbidity and mortality of synchronous liver resection for colorectal metastasis stratified by extent of liver resection and type of colorectal resection. J Surg Oncol. 102:932–36. DOI: 10.1002/jso.21657.

[45] Martin R, Paty P, Fong Y, Grace A, Cohen A, DeMatteo R, et al. Simultaneous liver and colorectal resections are safe for synchronous colorectal liver metastasis. J Am Coll Surg. 2003 Aug;197(2):233–41; discussion 241–2.

[46] Brouquet A, Mortenson MM, Vauthey J-N, Rodriguez-Bigas MA, Overman MJ, Chang GJ, et al. Surgical strategies for synchronous colorectal liver metastases in 156 consecutive patients: classic, combined or reverse strategy? J Am Coll Surg. 2010 Jun;210(6): 934–41.

[47] Jarnagin WR, Gonen M, Fong Y, DeMatteo RP, Ben-Porat L, Little S, et al. Improvement in perioperative outcome after hepatic resection: analysis of 1,803 consecutive cases over the past decade. Ann Surg. 2002 Oct;236(4):397–406; discussion 406–7.

[48] Inoue A, Uemura M, Yamamoto H, Hiraki M, Naito A, Ogino T, Nonaka R, Nishimura J, Wada H, Hata T, Takemasa I, Eguchi H, Mizushima T, Nagano H, Doki Y, Mori M. Short-term outcomes of simultaneous laparoscopic colectomy and hepatectomy for primary colorectal cancer with synchronous liver metastases. Int Surg. 2014 Jul–Aug; 99(4):338–43. DOI: 10.9738/INTSURG-D-14-00019.1.

Chapter 13

Adjuvant Treatment in Colon Cancer

Ivan Shterev Donev, Nikola Kolev, Valentin Ignatov,
Anton Tonev, Aleksandar Zlatarov,
Assia Konsoulova, Elitza Entcheva,
Plamena Drenakova and Krasimir Ivanov

Additional information is available at the end of the chapter

http://dx.doi.org/10.5772/64101

Abstract

Worldwide, more than 1 million people develop colorectal cancer (CRC) annually. CRC is a major health problem in the Western world and the second most common cause of cancer mortality. To improve performance, the role of chemotherapy for CRC has increased dramatically over the last decade. The vast majority of CRC patients now receive chemotherapy with multiple agents that are currently approved for the treatment in the appropriate setting [1]. However, it is a complex process to select the optimal chemotherapy for each patient and practice evidence gap is still a problem. Some guidelines for the treatment of CRC have been developed to promote the standardization of CRC treatment. Postoperative, or "adjuvant," systemic therapy has become standard for stage III colon cancer. Adjuvant therapy should also be strongly considered in stage II patients. It is generally recommended for any medically fit patient with stage II cancer with unfavorable factors. The hypothesis that the antitumor activity of the combination agent, including oxaliplatin, irinotecan, bevacizumab, cetuximab in metastatic cure rates, would result in increased adjuvant proved to be often wrong. Although new drug development takes years, targeted drug use can occur more quickly with advanced tests and will be a focus of future work. In addition, efforts will focus on identifying biomarkers that predict response to systemic therapy so that tailored therapy can be initiated. The future of oncology will come with the better understanding of the biology and genetics of the tumor and its host. This will help to develop tailored approach to the patients, including more specific systemic therapy, aimed at molecular targets of the malignant tumor, thus reducing the negative effects. At that time, the treatment of oncological diseases will experience a new era, comparable to the introduction of antibiotics.

Keywords: Chemotherapy, Adjuvant treatment, Colon cancer

1. Introduction

Colorectal cancer develops in more than 1 million people every year. This is a major health problem and a second of frequency cause of mortality by cancer. The mortality from CRC has decreased by almost 35% for 17 years and the reasons are early diagnosis, new screening programs and treatment principles. Surgery is the basic of the initial treatment, but the next step on treatment in most of patients with CRC is adjuvant chemotherapy. Adjuvant chemotherapy decreases the risk of following metastatic dissemination. This systemic treatment aims eradication of disseminated microscopic tumor cells, control of development of the primary tumor and the tumor extension. The histologic stage of the tumor at the time of resection determined the 5-year survival rate of CRC patients. The most important factor for survival in patients with CRC and without metastatic disease is the stage of the tumor. The stage of the tumor responds to depth of the tumor penetration through the intestinal wall (*T*) and the number of lymph nodes with invasion (*N*). 14% decrease of overall survival is because of systemic treatment. Because of this it is considered to start adjuvant chemotherapy as soon as possible.

Oral fluoropyrimidines, oxaliplatin, and irinotecan added to 5-FU chemotherapy (CT) led to good results about progression-free survival (PFS), response rate, and overall survival (OS) in patients with metastatic colorectal cancer. This statement is subject to the clinical trial about the adjuvant setting of non-metastatic disease in patients with stage III tumors. The adjuvant CT regimens used often in oncology are shown in **Table 1**.

Name	Protocol
5FU/LV (bolus)	Mayo clinic regimen
LV5FU2	LV 200 mg/m^2, 5FU 400 mg/m^2 bolus followed by 5FU 600 mg/m^2 22-h infusion, given every 14 days for 12 cycles
Capacetabine	Capacetabine 1250 mg/m^2 twice daily for 14 days every 3 weeks
FLOX	5FU 500 mg/m^2 bolus every week for 6 weeks, LV 500 mg/m^2 every week for 6 weeks of 8 week cycle, for 3 cycles + oxaliplatin 85 mg/m^2 on week 1, 3, 5 of each cycle
mFOLFOX6	LV 400 mg/m^2 IV on day 1, 5 FU 400 mg/m^2 IV bolus on day 1 followed by 2400 mg/m^2 by continuous infusion over 46 h (day 1 and 2); oxaliplatin 85 mg/m^2 IV day 1;every 14 days for 12 cycles
FOLFOX4	LV5FU2 + oxaliplatin 85 mg/m^2 on day 1 (with LV)

Abbreviations: 5FU = 5 fluorouracil; IV = intravenous; LV = leucovorin

Table 1. Different regimens used for adjuvant chemotherapy in colorectal cancer.

In patients with stage II colon cancer surgery alone is usually curative but in 20–30% of them there is tumor recurrence and metastatic disease. The chemotherapy has side effects in patients and some of them change survival rate. The studies found markers for prediction of return the disease. This marker is useful in stage II colorectal cancer. The studies about adjuvant therapy and stage of the tumor show that cytotoxic therapy has more in stage II of CRC. In the future, should be handled with the direction to find more specific markers for precise selection [1].

Data for colon cancer genesis and metastasis in lymph node show that CXC chemokine receptor type 7 (CXCR7) had role in these processes. The study about this in group of 34 patients at age between 34 and 79 years with malignant colon pathology and second group of 18 patients with normal colon tissue. CXCR7 levels were higher in group with colon tumors, 20 cause of this group was presented with lymph node metastases. There are an evidence for involvement of the upregulated CXCR7 expression in colon cancer and lymph node metastasis [10].

MSI is a change in the length of DNA microsatellites caused by insertion or deletion of repeated units (1–5 nucleotides), due to defects in mismatch repair genes or methylation of their promoters. Tumors with MSI are proximal, poorly differentiated, and mucinous. This tumors show marked lymphocyte infiltration. Colon cancers with high-frequency of MSI have clinical and pathological differences from microsatellite-stable tumors; thus colon cancer patients stage II or III with microsatellite-stable tumors or tumors exhibiting high-frequency microsatellite instability have favorable outcome. Therefore MSI is a predictor for decreased benefit of Fluorouracil-based adjuvant chemotherapy. MMR protein deficiency and MSI can cause by silencing or mutation of mismatch repair (MMR) genes [2]. This condition occurs in patients with Lynch syndrome and is a rare cause for hereditary colon cancer: 2–4% of all cases. Somatic mutation can found in 19% of CRC and 52% of sporadic colon cancer has silencing of MMR genes. There are three groups in sporadic CRC—microsatellite stable (MSS), low-frequency MSI (MSI-L), and high-frequency MSI (MSI-H). MSI-H is frequently found in stage II disease. This confirms a data about the decreased use from 5FU adjuvant chemotherapy in patients with colon cancer stage II disease.

In contrast to this, it was shown in recent studies of more than 2000 patients. This study proved that MSI-H status was prognostic but not predictive of benefit or detrimental impact of adjuvant chemotherapy [3]. Tests for discovery MSI in colorectal cancer for ≤70 years:

1. immunohistochemical tests for MMR protein producing;
2. for changes in the length of repetitive DNA elements in tumor tissue due to insertion or deletion [4, 5].

Starting a development of several multigenes such as Oncotype DX with purpose to identify which patient would have a great help from adjuvant CT. In this trial patient's chance of recurrence was classified in three groups—low, intermediate and high. Recurrence score was calculated by the evaluation of a panel of 12 genes—7 recurrences cancer-related and 5 reference genes [1, 8]. The statistical analysis clarifies that recurrence DFS and OS score of recurrence of disease correlated with disease relapse. Relapse of disease depends of TNM staging, MSI, number of histologically examined lymph nodes and tumor grade.

That result of multigene analysis could not predict a help for patient of adjuvant CT.

2. Treatment guidelines for adjuvant chemotherapy

2.1. 5 FU

The value of adjuvant CT in patients with stage III colon cancer is first reported in 1990 by Moertel and colleagues (Dukes C, TxN+M0). Comparing between adjuvant 5-FU/levamisole chemotherapy for 1 year, levamisole alone and without chemotherapy showed an increase in OS and PFS in patients receiving first model of chemotherapy. 5FU is a pyrimidine analog, inhibitor of enzyme thymidylate synthase (TS) (involved in de novo synthesis of thymidine) and is involved in the process of incorporation of nucleotides into RNA and DNA, leading to inhibition of DNA synthesis and function. Continuous infusion of 5FU is 100–1000 times lower than the concentrations if injected i.v. bolus. In second way 5FU reaches a maximum plasma and bone marrow concentration [7, 9].

There is information that the expression of E2F1, which control the transcription of genes encoding proteins engaged in DNA synthesis including TS. A study examined the relationship between E2F1 and TS expression in patients with colon cancer and the effect of 5 FU. It showed that the combined E2F1/TS immunophenotype could be a potential indicator for sensitivity of patients on adjuvant chemotherapy with 5FU [11].

Over 85% of the drug is inactivated in metabolic processes by the enzyme dihydropyrimidine dehydrogenase (DPD). DPD synthesize by the liver. Some mutations in DPD can found in approximately 2% of the general population. This can cause serious life-threatening toxicity in patients. Leucovorin (LV, folic acid) intensifies the antitumor activity of 5FU. Treatment without LV is still a reasonable option.

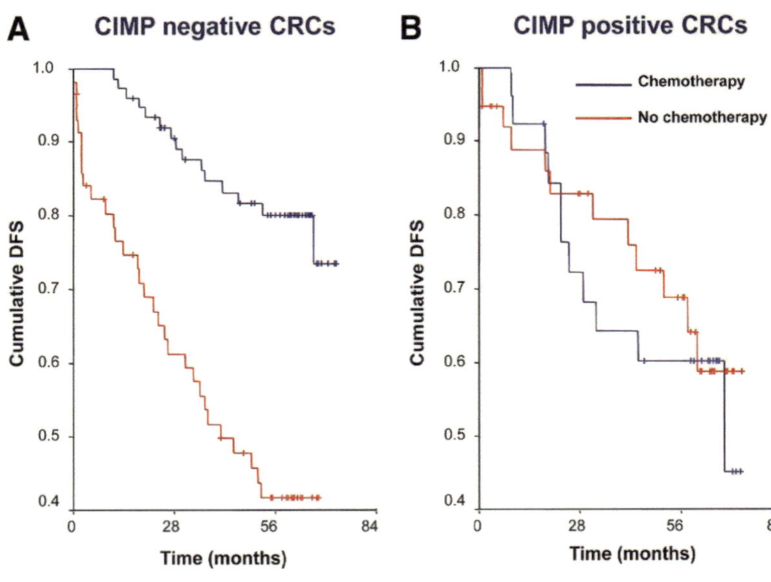

Figure 1. Comparison between CIMP negative and CIMP positive in relation to the effects of chemotherapy [12].

Rodrigo Jover and all explored effect of 5FU chemotherapy in patients with CRC. Their study included group of patients with CpG island methylator phenotype (CIMP) colorectal cancer and analyze a response of patients with this mutation. CIMP status was determined by analysis of the CACNAG1, SOCS1, RUNX3, NEUROG1, and MLH1 promoters. Tumors were CIMP positive when they had 3 promoters methylated. Result of study shows that patients with CIMP positive colorectal cancer do not have a benefit from adjuvant chemotherapy with 5-fluorouracil regarding to survival time [12] **Figure 1**.

Analysis of the data from several trials in which patients randomly received only tumor resection or tumor resection and adjuvant 5FU/LV, showed that benefit of adjuvant CT was observed in stage III patients [1]. These patients have higher risk because of the metastatic regional node.

In patients with stage T3 or T4 resectable rectal cancer treatment is with preoperative radiotherapy with or without simultaneous chemotherapy. In randomized study in patients with rectal cancer after surgery they start adjuvant chemotherapy or are on dispensary and monitored. Radiotherapy including 45 Gy to the posterior pelvis in 25 fractions of 18 Gy over 5 weeks and the courses of chemotherapy had fluorouracil and folinic acid. For preoperative chemotherapy, two courses were given (during weeks 1 and 5 of radiotherapy). Adjuvant chemotherapy was given in four cycles, every 3 weeks. Conclusion of this study can show that adjuvant fluorouracil-based chemotherapy after preoperative radiotherapy (with or without chemotherapy) does not affect disease-free survival or overall survival [13].

5FU/LV plus oxaliplatin as adjuvant treatment is used in stage II colorectal cancer. The study on group of elderly patients show no importance DPS or OS benefit even in this causes with high risk characteristics—T4 tumors, bowel obstruction, venous invasion etc. 5FU/LV stay the preferred adjuvant chemotherapy regimen.

5-Fluorouracil (5FU)-based chemotherapy (CT) remains the mainstay treatment of CRC and activates executioner caspases in target cells. Executioner caspases are key proteins involved in cell disassembly during apoptosis. Their activation also has a role in tissue regeneration and repopulation by stimulating signal transduction and cell proliferation. A study about this proteins and 5FU-based chemotherapy shows that patients with low levels of active caspase-3 had an increased disease-free survival time. Lower serum levels of active caspase-3 were found in patients with metastasized CRC. This indicates that low levels of active caspase-3 may be a new predictor of CT responsiveness. Inhibition of caspase-3 may be a marker for improve patient outcomes following CT in advanced CRC [14].

2.2. Oral fluoropyrimidines

Two oral prodrugs of 5FU—capecitabine and Uracil/tegafur (UFT) showed efficacy in the metastatic setting, as compared to 5FU/LV bolus regimens. Capecitabine is oral administration, rapidly absorbed with peak blood levels after 1.5 h [1]. Capecitabine is contraindicated in patients with severe renal impairment (creatinine clearance below 30 mL/min).

Adjuvant therapy for patients with resected stage III colon cancer includes i.v. bolus regimen of 5FU/LV, and oral capecitabine is unsuitable. Taking a capecitabine has rarely occurring symptoms of diarrhea, stomatitis, nausea, alopecia, neutropenia, and febrile neutropenia [6].

3. Combination adjuvant therapies

The benefits of adjuvant chemotherapy by combinations with drugs—oxaliplatin, irinotecan, bevacizumab, or cetuximab in the metastatic disease—were not confirmed. Oxaliplatin is a third-generation platinum compound and reported that its safety administration with evidence for clinical activity, because ability to develop a covalent adducts with cellular DNA. Study for oxaliplatin examined platinum in the body for 8–75 months after treatment with cisplatin and oxaliplatin, because of time to excretion. Therapeutic index of oxaliplatin is limited. Adverse reactions from this treatment are symptoms in the peripheral nerves, the hematopoietic and the gastrointestinal system.

In the adjuvant chemotherapy the addition of oxaliplatin can improve patient outcomes. The MOSAIC trial explores 2246 patients with stage II or III CRC. They take LV/5FU2 or FOLFOX-4 (LV/5FU2 + oxaliplatin).

The results are summarized in **Table 2**.

	FOLFOX (%)	5FULV2 (%)	P value
5-year DPS (sage II + III)	73.3	67.4	0.003
6-year OS (stage II + III)	78.5	76.0	0.046
6-years OS (stage III only)	72.9	68.7	0.023
6-years OS (stage II only)	85	83.3	0.65
Grade 3-4 neutropenia	41	5	
Grade 3-4 diarrhea	11	7	
Grade 3 neuropathy	12	0	

Unfortunately the side effects are more frequent.

Table 2. The FOLFOX regimen has significantly better oncological results compared to 5FULV2.

In conclusion, FOLFOX-4 is more toxic than separately LV/5FU2. The mortality in the first 60 days has close rate [2].

Multicenter AGEO Study assessed the efficacy of adjuvant chemotherapy with fluoropyrimidine with and without oxaliplatin. And results support other conclusion that there is a benefit from the combined application of fluoropyrimidine and oxaliplatin in patients with colon cancer stage III with deficient mismatch repair (dMMR).

The NSABP C-07 and the MOSAIC trials had a similar purpose, but used different plans to treatment. In one of trials used FLOX regimen—oxaliplatin was given on weeks 1, 3, and 5

http://dx.doi.org/10.5772/64101

plus weekly and bolus 5FU/LV on weeks 1 through 6. This is 8 weeks cycle. The results compared with standard use of 5FU/LV. More than 2000 patients received FLOX or 5FU/LV treatment. All of patients were classified into two groups—stage II patients (29%) and stage III patients (71%). The research is for 34 months. Results of this study showed benefit in the short 7-year term, but then in long term, there was no difference in the results between the two groups.

The MOSAIC and NSABP C-07 trials make research for oxaliplatin but with different doses. Their small positive results improved a benefit of oxaliplatin to chemotherapy in patients with stage II disease. But this is not enough to justify given outcomes and the risk of neurotoxicity.

Phase III of trial, which aim was to comparing capecitabine plus oxaliplatin (XELOX) with bolus 5FU/LV as adjuvant therapy for stage III colon cancer proved that XELOX had an improved 3-year DFS rate compared with 5FU/LV. Patients with XELOX had less frequently diarrhea or alopecia but occurred more vomiting, neurosensory toxicity, and hand–foot syndrome. All trials showed that FOLFOX, FLOX and XELOX could all be with equal value when they used in the adjuvant setting [3].

Irinotecan is a semisynthetic analog of camptothecin, first isolated from the Chinese/Tibetan ornamental tree Camptotheca acuminata. It is a chemotherapy agent that causes S-phase-specific cell killing by poisoning the enzyme topoisomerase I in the cell [4].

PETACC-3 investigators also investigate how add of irinotecan to adjuvant LV/5FU2 would improve status of patients with colon cancer. They observed that patients with irinotecan to LV/5FU2 had an increased frequency of adverse reaction and neutropenia. In conclusion of this trial, irinotecan in combination with LV/5FU2 as adjuvant therapy did not show benefits in patients with stage III colon cancer [5]. Using irinotecan in the adjuvant setting in stage II and III patients did not support with data. Analysis of PETACC-3 trial could not justify the expected benefit from administration of irinotecan to LV/5FU2. Bevacizumab is a recombinant, humanized monoclonal antibody against the vascular endothelial growth factor (VEGF), inhibitor of VEGF function in vascular endothelial cells and thereby inhibits the tumor neoangiogenesis, upon which solid tumors depend on growth and metastasis [3, 6]. Bevacizumab demonstrated positive impact added to standard CT in the metastatic disease.

Cetuximab is a monoclonal antibody which upon binding to the transmembrane epidermal growth factor receptor (EGFR). EGFR controls many important tumor cell functions including tumor growth, neoangiogenesis, inhibition of the apoptotic response to chemotherapy, and radiotherapy. Cetuximab realize inhibition and degradation [3].

There are reports from last years about drug screening system, which is based on nanoimprinting 3-dimensional (3D) culture. It is use to predict effectiveness of new chemotherapeutic drugs. Also with this system can find the most effective agent for colon cancer. A research in this area examines the benefit from treatment with regorafenib on a mouse model in vivo. Result from this study was based on new nanoimprinting 3D culture and it shows that regorafenib is on track to be the most effective drug. In study were compared this agent and 5 FU and in conclusion regorafenib may be the most effective adjuvant therapy for colon cancer in the future [15].

4. Adjuvant therapy for resectable metastatic disease

Patients with metastatic disease who are subjected to liver or lung resection is first submitted to active systemic chemotherapy. The therapy should not be more than 6 months.

Regimens recommended that resectable metastatic disease and non-metastatic disease had a similar adjuvant setting.

5. Adjuvant CT for elderly patients

Colon cancer in most of the cases is diagnosed in patients >70 years in USA. The purpose and aim of oncology is to give patients aged >75 years longer life than they expected. Adjuvant therapy gave a survival advantage in younger and older patients. There is a discussion about safety and efficacy of the treatment in elderly and younger patients, but analysis showed that there are certain toxicity rates and similar advantage for survival. The most of data about adjuvant therapy is from trial on elderly patients and without new therapeutic agents such as oxaliplatin [3].

The study which purpose is to show benefits from adjuvant chemotherapy for patients ≥75 years of age with resected stage III colon cancer (CC) presented that adjuvant chemotherapy does not show the expected result. Oxaliplatin offers small incremental. The use of adjuvant chemotherapy after the age of 75 years should be assessed individually [16].

The results of a study indicate that patients aged >75 years represent nearly 20% of all cases with lymph node-positive colon cancer although the majority of recommendations limit colorectal cancer screening to individuals aged u years. Older age was associated with much lower rates of adjuvant chemotherapy administration, whereas the survival benefits of such treatment remain comparable to those of younger patients with stage III colon cancer. This statement is established on large population-based study. There are a lot of trials and data for adjuvant chemotherapy, but optimal and efficient strategy is not established. More research needed to understand which benefit is bigger from administration of adjuvant treatment after surgical resection.

6. Recommendation in summary

1. Application of target treatment (bevacizumab, cetuximab or panitumumab) to standard CT is not confirmed in the adjuvant setting.

2. Patients with stage I disease require observation without any adjuvant treatment.

3. Patients with low-risk stage II disease have some treatment options: capecitabine or 5-FU/leucovorin regimen, observation without adjuvant treatment or enrollment in a clinical trial.

4. Patients with high-risk stage II disease and poor prognostic features (T4 tumors, lymphovascular invasion, Nx lymph node status, poor differentiation bowel obstruction, positive resection margins) are considered for more aggressive adjuvant approach like 5-FU/leucovorin, capecitabine, FOLFOX, capecitabine/oxaliplatin, FLOX. This group of patients needs an observation like alternative, but there is a certain risk of disease relapse. This risk is higher without adjuvant treatment. Patients with stage III disease can receive surgical treatment followed by 6 months of adjuvant treatment with FOLFOX, capecitabine/oxaliplatin, FLOX, 5-FU/leucovorine or capecitabine only (in patients contraindicated for oxaliplatin-based chemotherapy) [6].

Author details

Ivan Shterev Donev[1], Nikola Kolev[2], Valentin Ignatov[2], Anton Tonev[2*], Aleksandar Zlatarov[2], Assia Konsoulova[4], Elitza Entcheva[3], Plamena Drenakova[2] and Krasimir Ivanov[2]

*Address all correspondence to: teraton@abv.bg

1 Department of Medical Oncology, Medical University Varna, Varna, Bulgaria

2 Department of General and Operative Surgery, Medical University Varna, Varna ,Bulgaria

3 Department of Radiotherapy, Medical University Varna, Varna, Bulgaria

4 Department of Medical Oncology, Medical University, Varna, Bulgaria

References

[1] Ivanov K, Kolev N, Shterev I, Tonev A, Ignatov V, Bojkov V, et al. Adjuvant treatment in colorectal cancer. In: Khan J, editor. Colorectal cancer—surgery, diagnostics and treatment [Internet]. InTech; 2014 [cited 2016 Mar 1]. http://www.intechopen.com/books/colorectal-cancer-surgery-diagnostics-and-treatment/adjuvant-treatment-in-colorectal-cancer

[2] Haller DG, Tabernero J, Maroun J, Braud F de, Price T, Cutsem EV, et al. Capecitabine plus oxaliplatin compared with fluorouracil and folinic acid as adjuvant therapy for stage III colon cancer. J Clin Oncol. 2011;29(11):1465–71.

[3] Twelves C, Wong A, Nowacki MP, Abt M, Burris H, Carrato A, et al. Capecitabine as adjuvant treatment for stage III colon cancer. N Engl J Med. 2005;352(26):2696–704.

[4] Xu Y, Villalona-Calero MA. Irinotecan: mechanisms of tumor resistance and novel strategies for modulating its activity. Ann Oncol. 2002;13(12):1841–51.

[5] Sulzyc-Bielicka V, Domagala P, Bielicki D, Safranow K, Rogowski W, Domagala W. E2F1/TS immunophenotype and survival of patients with colorectal cancer treated with 5FU-based adjuvant therapy. Pathol Oncol Res. 2016;1–8.

[6] The NCCN Guidelines. Clinical Practice Guidelines in Oncology (NCCN Guidelines) Colon Cancer. 2015. http://wenku.baidu.com/view/c4a06f301711cc7931b716fa.html

[7] Clinical Practice Guidelines in Oncology (NCCN Guidelines) Colon Cancer Version 2.2015, 10/03/14 National Comprehensive Cancer Network, Inc. 2014 The NCCN Guidelines NCCN Guidelines for Patients available at www.nccn.org; NCCN Guidelines Version 2.2015 Panel MembersColon Cancer. http://wenku.baidu.com/view/c4a06f301711cc7931b716fa.html

[8] Oncotype DX®. Colon cancer assay improves recurrence risk stratification in stage II colon cancer patients. http://obroncology.com/obrgreen/print/Oncotype-DX-Colon-Cancer-Assay-Improves-Recurrence-Risk-Stratification-in-Stage-II-Colon-Cancer-Patients

[9] Moertel CG, Fleming TR, Macdonald JS, Haller DG, Laurie JA, Goodman PJ, et al. Levamisole and fluorouracil for adjuvant therapy of resected colon carcinoma. N Engl J Med 1990;322(6):352–8.

[10] Chris Twelves, Alfred Wong, Marek P. Nowacki, Markus Abt, Howard Burris, III, Alfredo Carrato, Jim Cassidy, Andrés Cervantes, Jan Fagerberg, Vassilis Georgoulias, Fares Husseini, Duncan Jodrell, Piotr Koralewski, Hendrik Kröning, Jean Maroun, Norbert Marschner, Joseph McKendrick, Marek Pawlicki, Riccardo Rosso, Johannes Schüller, Jean-François Seitz, Borut Stabuc, Jerzy Tujakowski, Guy Van Hazel, Jerzy Zaluski, Werner Scheithauer. Capecitabine as adjuvant treatment for stage III colon cancer. N Engl J Med 2005;352:2696–2704. doi:10.1056/NEJMoa043116. http://www.nejm.org/doi/full/10.1056/NEJMoa043116

[11] Marshall JL, Haller DG, de Gramont A, Hochster HS, Lenz HJ, Ajani JA, Goldberg RM. Adjuvant therapy for stage II and III colon cancer: consensus report of the International Society of Gastrointestinal Oncology. http://www.ncbi.nlm.nih.gov/pmc/articles/PMC2632523/

[12] International Multicentre Pooled Analysis of B2 Colon Cancer Trials (IMPACT B2) Investigators. Efficacy of adjuvant fluorouracil and folinic acid in B2 colon cancer. J Clin Onc 1999;17(5):1356–63.

[13] Daniel G. Haller, Josep Tabernero, Jean Maroun, Filippo de Braud, Timothy Price, Eric Van Cutsem, Mark Hill, Frank Gilberg, Karen Rittweger and Hans-Joachim Schmoll. Capecitabine plus oxaliplatin compared with fluorouracil and folinic acid as adjuvant therapy for stage III colon cancer. http://jco.ascopubs.org/content/29/11/1465.long

[14] Chris Twelves, Alfred Wong, Marek P. Nowacki, Markus Abt, Howard Burris III, Alfredo Carrato, Jim Cassidy, Andrés Cervantes, Jan Fagerberg, Vassilis Georgoulias, Fares Husseini, Duncan Jodrell, Piotr Koralewski, Hendrik Kröningk, Jean Maroun, Norbert Marschner, Joseph McKendrick, Marek Pawlicki, Riccardo Rosso, Johannes Schüller, Jean-François Seitz, Borut Stabuc, Jerzy Tujakowski, Guy Van Hazel, Jerzy Zaluski, Werner Scheithauer. Capecitabine as adjuvant treatment for stage III colon cancer. N Engl J Med 2005; 352:2696–2704. doi:10.1056/NEJMoa043116. http://www.nejm.org/doi/full/10.1056/NEJMoa043116

[15] Xu Y, Villalona-Calero MA. Irinotecan: mechanisms of tumor resistance and novel strategies for modulating its activity. Ann Oncol 2002;13(12):1841

Section 4

New Therapies

Chapter 14

Robot-Assisted Colonic Resections for Cancer

Monica Ortenzi, Giovanni Lezoche,
Roberto Ghiselli and Mario Guerrieri

Additional information is available at the end of the chapter

http://dx.doi.org/10.5772/62416

Abstract

Minimally invasive surgery for colon cancer, if compared with open surgery, has shown similar oncologic outcomes, and it has become the standard management for malignant colonic disease. Its benefits appear yet in early post-operative period such as less postoperative pain, earlier recovery of gastrointestinal functions and shorter hospital stay. Robotic surgery was born in the attempt to overcome the intrinsic limitations of laparoscopic technique. It offers the possibility to have a tridimensional magnified view of surgical field and to use wristed instrument to perform an accurate dissection and lymphadenectomy. It provides the possibility to rotate at 360 degrees the instruments, facilitating considerably the performance of intracorporeal ileo-colic anastomosis in right colectomy. We want to illustrate the feasibility and technique to carry out right and left colectomy in a robotic-assisted way and its advantages with respect to laparoscopic surgery.

Keywords: robot-assisted, surgery, laparoscopy, colon, cancer

1. Introduction

Colon cancer has always been a hot topic, and a revolution has come about in its surgical management in the past 20 years with the introduction of laparoscopic surgery. This progress has culminated with the advent of robotic surgery.

Robotic surgery came about in an attempt to overcome the limitations of laparoscopy mainly because of long rigid instruments, poor ergonomics, and two-dimensional visualization [1–3].

Robotic system was introduced in the surgical field more than 25 years ago [4].

Laparoscopic and robotic surgeries have walked along a parallel path. When Semm reported the first laparoscopic appendectomy in 1983, the "Arthrobot" was first applied in orthopedic operations, which marked the beginning of robotic surgery [5].

Robotic technology applied to surgical procedures has had a rapid growth since then. PUMA (Programmable Universal Machine for Assembly), SARP (Surgeon-Assistant Robot for Prostatectomy) systems, PROBOT (Prostate robot), VRobot (Urology robot), and SPUD (Surgeon Programmable Urological Device) have been introduced and applied in urologic surgery [6–9].

The first robotic device approved by the US Food and Drug Administration (FDA) in 1994 was the AESOP (Automated Endoscopic System for Optimal Positioning) system followed by the ZEUS system (Computer Motion Inc.) in 1998 [10].

The ZEUS robotic system consisted of two separate components: a surgeon control center and three robotic arms attached to the operating table that provided four degrees of freedom and were able to hold various instruments, telemanipulated with joysticks at distance from the surgical console [11].

In 1998, this system was the one used for the first abdominal robotic procedure for fallopian tube anastomosis at Cleveland Clinic [12].

In 2001, Jacques Marescaux used the ZEUS system to perform the transatlantic robot-assisted cholecystectomy known as "Operation Lindbergh", between New York and Strasburg giving a great demonstration of telepresence surgery [13].

In 2001, 10 years after the first laparoscopic colectomy, Weber described the first robot-assisted colectomy [14].

The first fully robotic system that was approved by FDA in 2000 for its application in laparoscopic surgery was the da Vinci™ Surgical System.

It derives its name from military medical research and was initially developed in a project funded by the Pentagon's Defense Advanced Research Projects Agency with the aim of allowing remote operations on wounded soldiers [15].

This system was developed by Intuitive Surgical (Mountain View, CA). Later, Intuitive Surgical introduced the da Vinci S system, the da Vinci Si system, and the da Vinci Xi system in 2006, 2009, and 2014, respectively [16].

The da Vinci Si system consists of a remote surgeon's console, a patient cart, and a vision cart.

The console is composed of a stereo viewer, which provides a three-dimensional visualization of the operative field with 10× magnification, a touchpad, which allows for arms and control selection, and joysticks to control the instrument arms remotely. The footswitch panel is located at the base of the console and is composed of two groups of footswitches. The three switches on the left control the functions of the system such as camera control, master clutch, and arm swap. The four pedals on the right side of the footswitch panel are used for power supply.

The four arms of the column hold the robotic instruments.

They are wrapped in sterile drapes for operations and have clutch buttons used to vary arm joint angulation to adjust the instrument arms even during the procedure.

EndoWrist instruments are installed onto the instrument arms after the system is docked to ports that are inserted into the patient's abdominal wall. Most instruments offer seven degrees of freedom and 90° of articulation in the wrist.

The system provides for tremor filtration and scaled motion, translating larger movements of the surgeon's hands into finer motions of the instruments.

The vision cart includes a 24-inch touch screen monitor and provides shelves for optional surgical equipment such as insufflators and electrosurgical generators [16–18].

2. Right colectomy

This procedure is carried out in a three-arm technique.

The patient is placed in the supine position under general anesthesia with the arms alongside the body and in a mild reverse Trendelenburg position with a left tilt. This position allows the surgeon to expose the patient's right and transverse colon by moving the small bowel aside under gravity. Final positioning is adjusted according to the operative field exposure before robot docking.

Pneumoperitoneum is induced with a supraumbilical incision and the pressure is maintained between 12 and 15 mmHg.

A 12-mm port for the air sealer is positioned on the left midclavicular line, on transverse umbilical line. A 30° laparoscope is used in this procedure.

Once the 12-mm port for the laparoscope and the camera is inserted in the supraumbilical incision, the other port is placed under vision.

A total of four ports (three robotic ports and one assistant port) are set.

We usually place an 8-mm port for instrument arm 1 on the axillary line, 2 cm below the left costal margin, and another suprapubic 8 mm port for instrument arm 2. An assistant 10–12 mm port is placed on the left of the camera port.

The surgical cart is positioned cranial to the patient's head.

The bipolar vessel sealer, used to coagulate and dissect tissues, and the fenestrated grasper are mounted on arms 1 and 2.

The bed-assistant surgeon introduces a laparoscopic grasper used to give tension and facilitate the dissection.

The ileocolic vessels are identified, and the peritoneum is opened just below their prominence. Ileocolic vessels are divided, and the dissection is continued in an avascular plane under the right colon flexure to expose the duodenum between Gerota's fascia posteriorly and Toldt's fascia anteriorly.

Right colic vessels (if present), right colic veins, and the right branch of the middle colic artery are dissected with a bipolar vessel sealer. Parietal peritoneum is incised, and the dissection is carried out in a craniocaudal way till the cecum is reached. Once the specimen is totally mobilized, the transverse colon is resected with a mechanical stapler. In the case of intracorporeal anastomosis, the ileum is approximated to the transverse colon, and one sero-serosal stitch of suspension is positioned between the ileal loop and the transverse colon where the isoperistaltic side-to-side anastomosis is confectioned (**Figure 1**).

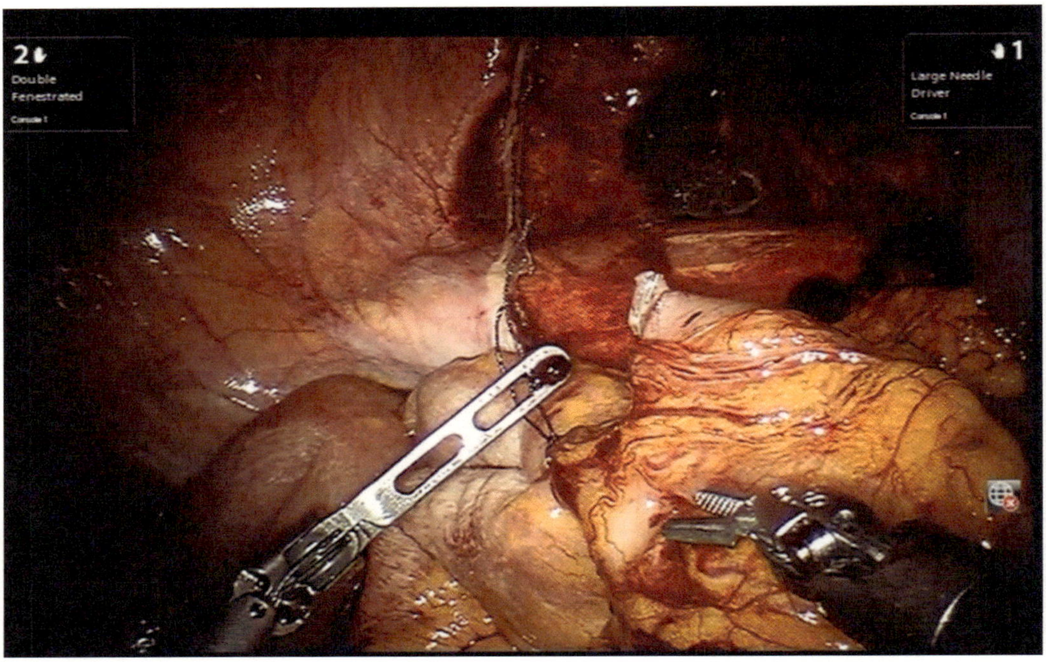

Figure 1. Suspension stitch between the ileal loop and the transverse colon.

Monopolar scissors are mounted on arm 1 and used to create enterotomies.

The surgeon-assistant introduces the larger part of the cartridge inside the colostomy and then the smaller part into the ileum (**Figure 2**). Intracorporeal latero-lateral isoperistaltic anastomosis is done. The enterotomies are then closed with a two-layer suture: the first layer of continuous suture and a second layer of interrupted sero-serosal suture with Vicryl 3/0 (**Figure 3**). A surgical specimen is extracted through the McBurney incision in the right iliac fossa.

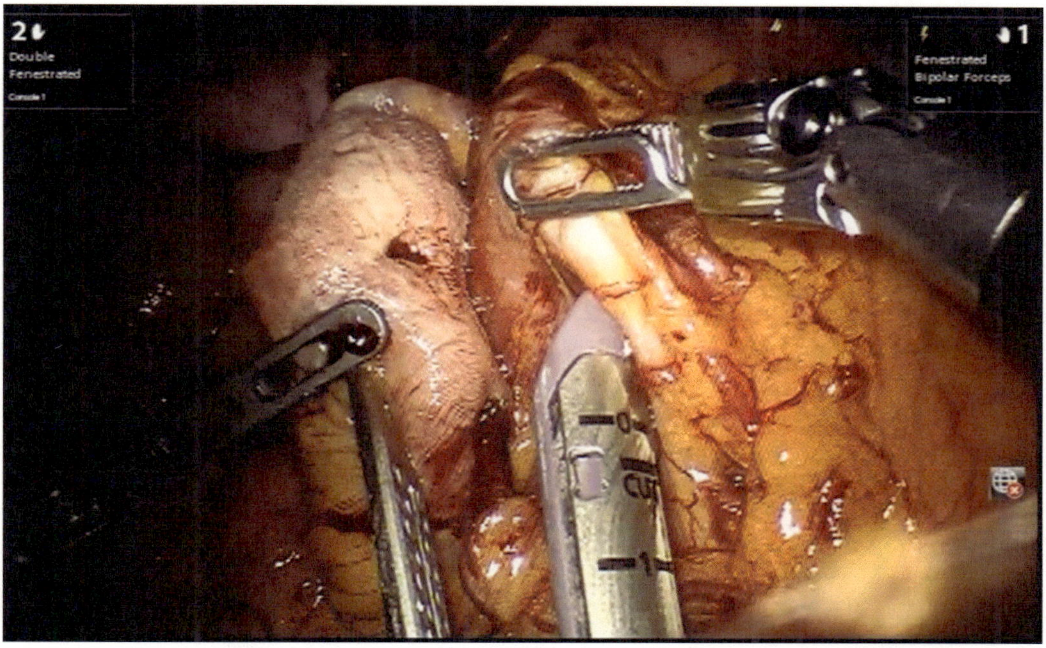

Figure 2. Insertion of the mechanical cartridge into the enterotomies.

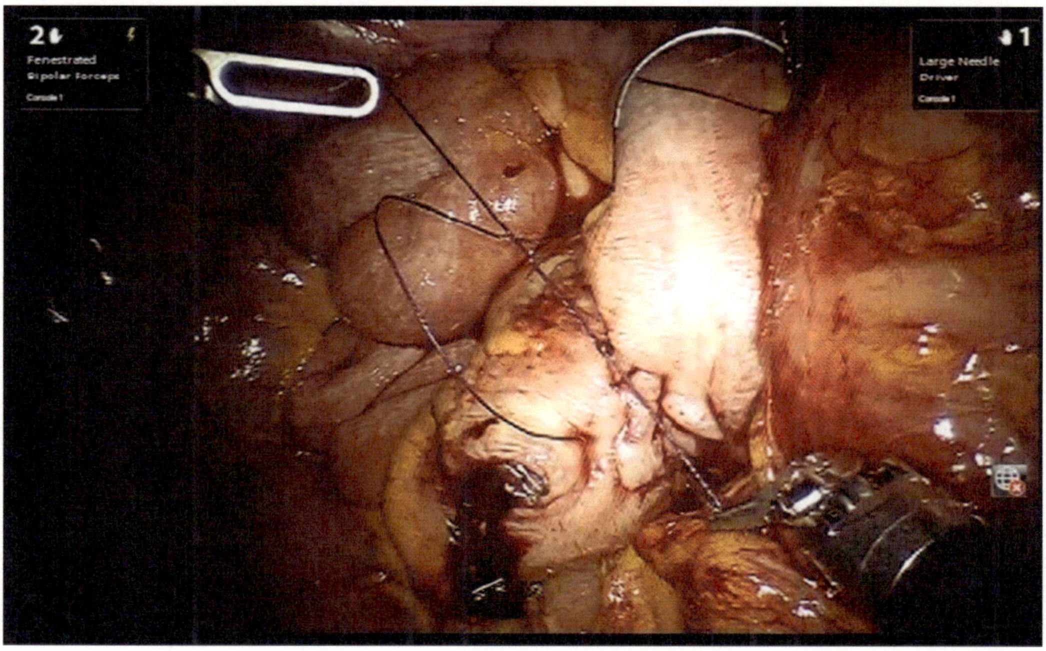

Figure 3. Closure of the enterotomies with a double layer manual suture with Vicryl 3/0.

3. Left colectomy

The patient is placed in a lithomy position with the left arm adducted.

A mild Trendelenburg position and a right tilt are set to expose the operative field. A 12-mmHg pneumoperitoneum is induced through a supraumbilical incision, and the 12-mm port for the camera is placed.

The other three 8-mm robotic ports are positioned under the vision, one on the right midclavicular line 2 cm below the right costal margin and the other in the midline under the xiphoid process. Two 10 mm trocars for the bed-assistant surgeon are added. A total of five ports are positioned. The robotic cart is on the patient's left side. The bipolar vessel sealer is mounted on arm 1. Arm 2 hosts the double fenestrated forceps. The dissection begins from the inferior mesenteric vein that is dissected by a bipolar vessel sealer once it is identified at the level of the inferior border of the pancreas.

The gastrocolic, splenocolic, and coloepiploic ligaments are dissected (**Figure 4**).

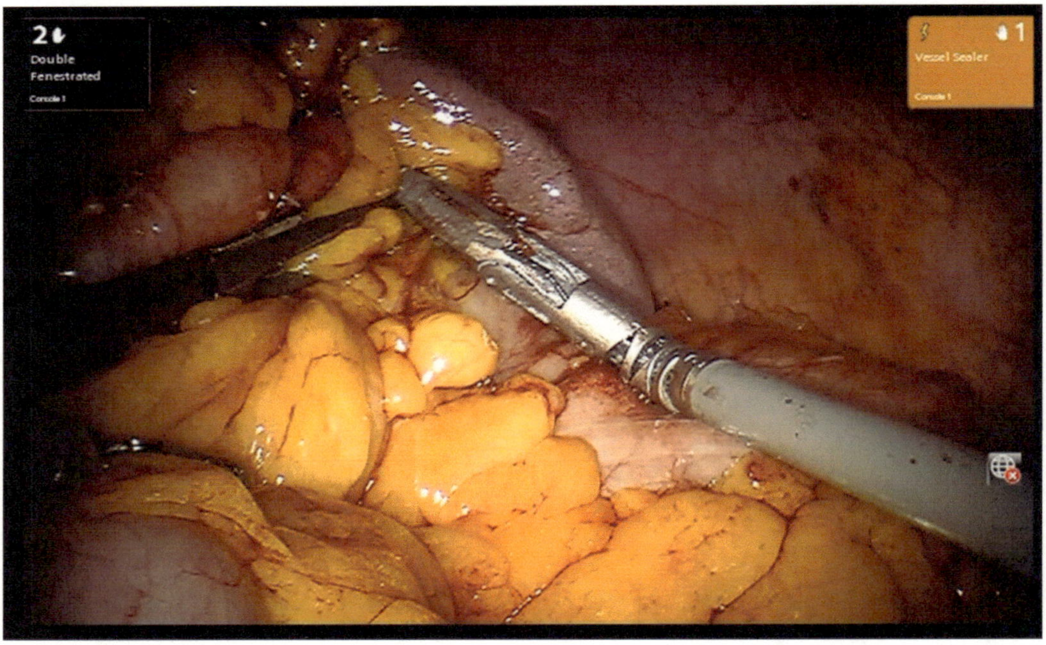

Figure 4. Division of the splenocolic ligament with electothermal bipolar vessel sealer.

The root of the transverse mesocolon is exposed by the assistant and dissected by bipolar electrocautery to expose the pancreas and allow for a full mobilization of the splenic flexure.

Then, the parietal peritoneum is incised, and the dissection is made on the avascular plane between the two folds of Toldt's fascia.

http://dx.doi.org/10.5772/62416

The assistant pulls up the dissected inferior mesenteric vein with a grasper, and the arch of the inferior mesenteric artery is lifted up.

Once the artery is identified, it is divided between the clips placed by the assistant.

A careful locoregional lymphadenectomy is carried out by preserving the paraaortic nerves and the superior hypogastric plexus.

The colon is resected at the level of the promontory with a mechanical stapler (**Figure 5**).

The anastomosis is fashioned according to the Knight & Griffen technique.

During this step, the robot is usually undocked.

The surgical specimen is extracted through a minilaparotomy in the left iliac fossa. The descending colon is extracted through the protected incision and transected proximally. The anvil of a circular stapler is inserted into the colon stump and fixed by a manual purse-string suture. The colon is then reintroduced into the abdomen and the minilaparotomy is closed. A laparoscopy is carried out to perform the transanal end-to-end mechanical colorectal anastomosis.

Sometimes, we did not undock the robot, and once the colon is reintroduced into the abdomen, robotic instruments are used to perform the end-to-end anastomosis (**Figure 6**).

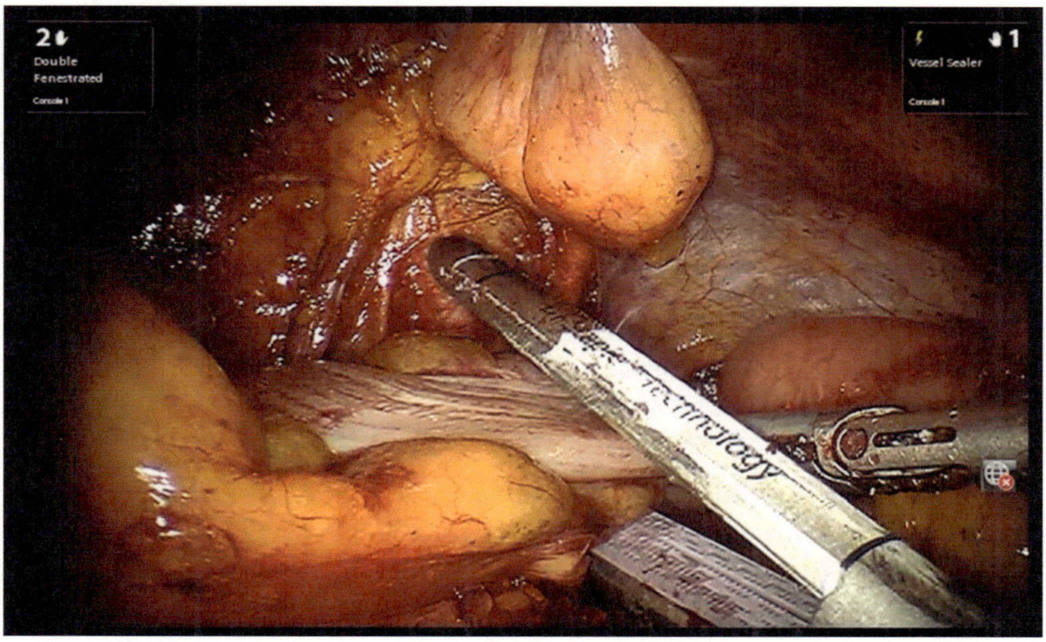

Figure 5. Section of the sigmoid colon at the level of the promontory with the mechanical cartridge.

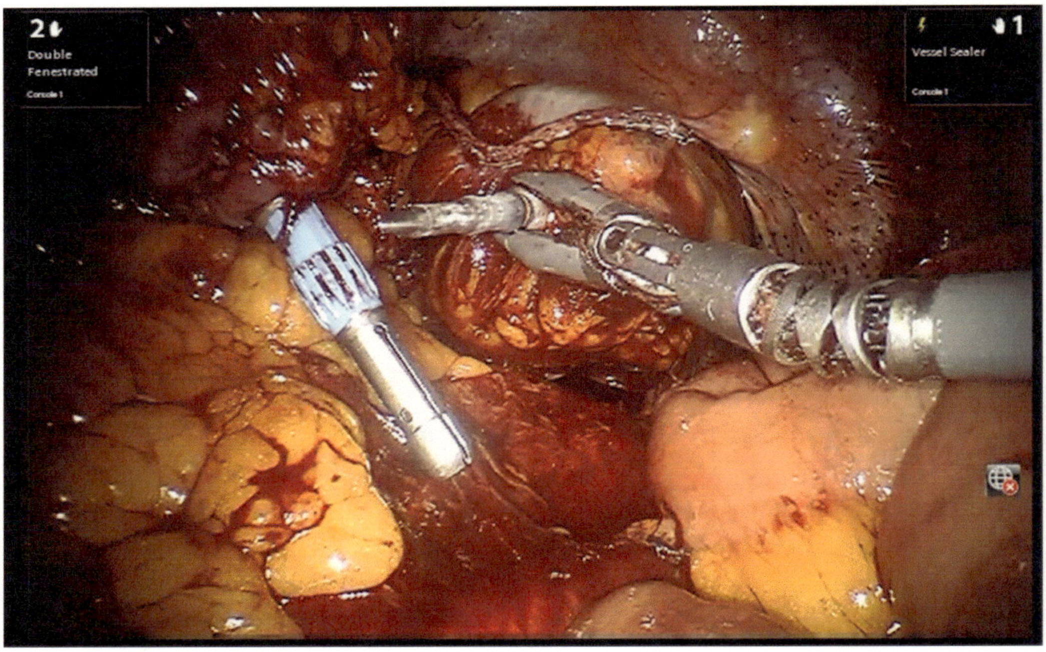

Figure 6. Confection of the end-to-end anastomosis without undocking the robotic system.

4. Advantages

Findings from the literature show how robot-assisted right and left hemicolectomies are comparable to conventional laparoscopic procedures in terms of short-term post-operative outcomes [18].

Patients undergoing robotic procedures typically return to normal activity faster and experience very low mortality and morbidity events [19–25].

The indications for robotic colectomy are well described and include benign conditions, such as inflammatory bowel disease, volvulus, diverticular disease, arteriovenous malformations, ischemic colitis, and polyps not amenable to endoscopic removal [26]. There are also emergent indications such as nearly obstructing lesions, ischemic colitis, and hemorrhage [27, 28].

Patients with contraindications for pneumoperitoneum, with an advanced disease invading adjacent organ and tumor greater than 8 cm in diameter, are contraindicated for robotic colectomy [26].

Colorectal robotic surgery also seems to be feasible for malignant disease comparable results in terms of oncologic radicality and surgical accuracy and in terms of short-term outcomes with respect to standard laparoscopy [18].

http://dx.doi.org/10.5772/62416

In a study of 50 consecutive right colectomies for cancer, D'Annibale et al. did not notice any statistically significant difference between laparoscopic and robotic groups in pathologic parameters and lymph node harvest. They concluded that robotic right colectomy was safe and provided adequate oncologic resection with acceptable short-term results [29].

However, if laparoscopic and robotic colectomies could be compared in terms of post-operative course and oncological outcomes, the robotic system offers several undoubtable technical advantages in performing colon surgery.

Robotic surgery allows an enhanced stabilized three-dimensional stereoscopic vision of the operative field and depth perception beyond the standard two-dimensional laparoscopic monitor [29, 30].

The da Vinci Si system provides hand stabilization, eliminating surgeon tremor and allowing for the refinement of scaled movements [29, 30]. This gives the surgeon the possibility to obtain greater precision in the surgical field.

In addition, the surgeon can work in a more ergonomic position compared with laparoscopic procedures that sometimes require maintaining a difficult posture even in long-lasting procedures [3, 20].

This improved surgical dexterity makes the switch to an intracorporeal anastomosis easier, which may lead to a higher adoption rate for intracorporeal anastomosis for right colectomies.

The potential benefits of intracorporeal anastomosis have been described in several studies and were known from laparoscopy.

Hanna et al. [31] recently concluded that intracorporeal anastomosis in laparoscopic right hemicolectomy is associated with similar post-operative and non-inferior oncologic outcomes compared with extracorporeal anastomosis, but it offers several advantages including freedom of specimen extraction sites, smaller incisions, and a lower risk of conversion to open resection especially in morbidly obese patients.

Hellan et al. [32] have found similar outcomes with intracorporeal and extracorporeal anastomosis but shorter incisions with intracorporeal anastomosis. Grams et al. [33] have reported an earlier return of bowel function, shorter length of hospital stay, and fewer complications.

Better outcomes are achieved when an intracorporeal anastomosis is performed. This is probably because of less traction and tension applied to the colon and the mesentery during an intracorporeal anastomosis as well as because of less trauma to the incision, which may result in less post-operative ileus and fewer complications [31, 34].

Another advantage in performing an intracorporeal anastomosis is the possibility to choose where to make the incision for extraction. In fact, keeping the extraction site far from the midline results in decreased risk of incisional hernia [35, 36].

The three-dimensional vision also provides advantages in mobilizing the left colic flexure with an accurate identification of the flexure borders and its relation to the spleen, while a gentle traction on the spleen is granted by the robotic arm, avoiding the risk of splenic rupture or laceration [14, 27, 36–38, 42].

Authors (years)	Patients (n)	OT (min)	HLN (n)	IC (%)	CR (%)	HS (days)	PC (%)	MR (%)
Rawling et al. [23]	LRC: 15	169.2			13.3	5.5	13.3	
	RRC: 17	189.9			0	5.2	11.7	
Park et al. [19]	LRC: 35	130	30.8	0	0	8.3	17.1	0
	RRC: 35	195	29.9	0	0	7.9	20	0
Deutsch et al. [20]	LRC: 47	214.4	18.7		0	6.3	42.55	2.12
	RRC: 18	219.2	21.1		11.1	4.3	33.33	0
Halabi et al. [21]	LRC: 53413					6	0.04	0.51
	RRC: 670					6	0	0
Casillas et al. [22]	LRC: 110	79	24	0	9.90	29	35	1
	RRC: 52	143	28	0	4.17	19	17	0

LRC, laparoscopic right colectomy; RRC, robotic right colectomy; OT, operative time; IC, intraoperative complications; HLN, harvested lymph node; CR, conversion rate; HS, hospital stay; PC, post-operative complications; MR, mortality rate.

Table 1. Robotic right colectomy data review.

Authors (years)	Patients (n)	OT (min)	HLN(n)	IC (%)	CR (%)	HS (days)	PC (%)	MR (%)
Rawling et al. [23]	LLC: 27	199.4		0	0	6.6	15.38	
	RLC: 30	225.2		7.7	15.38	6	23.07	
Deutsch et al. [20]	LLC: 45	254.7	30		0	4.2	17.7	0
	RLC: 61	289.7	10		3.33	4.1	18.03	0
Casillas et al. [22]	LLC: 68	188	14	0	5.88	32	12	0
	RLC: 82		14	0	5.88	32	12	0
Halabi et al. [21]	LLC: 62235					6	0.04	0.51
	RLC: 1473					6	0	0
Lim et al. [24]	LLC: 34	217.6	16.5			6.2	10.3	0
	RLC: 146	252.5	12			5.5	5.9	0

LLC, laparoscopic left colectomy; RLC, robotic left colectomy; OT, operative time; IC, intraoperative complications; HLN, harvested lymph node; CR, conversion rate; HS, hospital stay; PC, post-operative complications; MR, mortality rate.

Table 2. Robotic left colectomy review data.

The improved dexterity of the instruments favors precise tissue dissection and facilitates lymph node dissection.

Some authors have also reported lower conversion rates for laparoscopic colonic resections [16, 35, 36, 43], ranging from 0 to 4%, compared with 16.7–25%.

In our experience of 42 robotic colectomies, conversion was needed in three patients (7.1%). Two patients, who underwent right colectomy, required conversion to open surgery, one for excessive visceral obesity and the other for adhesions because of previous abdominal surgery. The mean number of lymph nodes in right colectomies (34 cases) and left colectomies (8 cases) was 17.7 and 13.9, respectively. Leak rate and 30-day mortality were 0%.

We recently conducted a retrospective analysis to compare operative measures and post-operative outcomes between laparoscopic 3D and robotic colectomy for cancer.

There were no differences between robotic colonic resections and 3D laparoscopic ones in terms of the number of lymph nodes removed and post-operative outcomes, but we found intracorporeal anastomosis easier to perform in robotic right colectomies than in the laparoscopic ones. In left colectomies, we observed that the robotic technique provided better outcomes, with earlier solid food intake registered in patients [39] (**Tables 1** and **2**).

5. Limitations

The high cost of robotic surgery because of the purchase and maintenance of the equipment is the main limitation to the widespread diffusion of this technology [39]. We estimated a cost of €4,950 for robotic procedures versus €1,950 needed for laparoscopic ones [36]. The cost factor can be prohibitive to the availability of robotic technology restricting it only to bigger centers.

Moreover, a higher number of complications have been observed in the low volume centers when compared with medium- and high-volume centers and surgeons [40].

Furthermore, robotic procedures are associated with a significantly longer operating time. Most of the authors have reported that the docking time was the main cause of longer operating time [3, 18, 41, 44].

There are also some practical and technical disadvantages. The major technical drawback of robotic surgery is the lower tensile feedback. The surgeon must rely on visual clues through the monitor to guide the instrumentation and ensure that appropriate and safe manipulation is preserved by trying to estimate the tension placed on tissues by da Vinci's powerful robotic arms [3, 38]. Performing robotic surgery requires two equally experienced surgeons, one working from the console and the other one staying at the operating table. The risk of system malfunction, inability to reposition the patient once the robot is docked, external and internal collision of the bulky robotic arms, and limited access to the patient by the anesthesia team when the tower is placed have also been observed [3, 20].

6. Conclusions

As was the case with laparoscopy, robotic technology will certainly undergo substantial development in the near future. It has proven to be safe and feasible also in the case of cancer and comparable to laparoscopy, but it still presents some drawbacks.

However, the real benefit to the patient must be carefully proven before this technology can become widely accepted in clinical practice.

Author details

Monica Ortenzi*, Giovanni Lezoche, Roberto Ghiselli and Mario Guerrieri

*Address all correspondence to: monica.ortenzi@gmail.com

Polytechnic University of Marche, Surgical Clinic, United Hospitals, Ancona, Italy

References

[1] Ballantyne GH. (2002). Robotic surgery, telerobotic surgery, telepresence, and telementoring: review of early clinical results. Surg Endosc. 10: 1389–1402.

[2] Yohannes P, Rotariu P, Pinto P, Smith AD, Lee BR. (2002). Comparison of robotic versus laparoscopic skills: is there a difference in the learning curve? Urology. 1: 39–45.

[3] Corcione F, Esposito C, Cuccurullo D, Settembre A, Miranda N, Amato F, Pirozzi F, Caiazzo P. (2005). Advantages and limits of robot-assisted laparoscopic surgery: preliminary experience. Surg Endosc. 19(1): 117–119.

[4] Kwoh YS, Hou J, Jonckheere EA, Hayati S. (1988). A robot with improved absolute positioning accuracy for CT guided stereotactic brain surgery. IEEE Trans Biomed Eng. 35(2): 153–160.

[5] Semm K. (1983). Endoscopic appendectomy. Endoscopy. 15: 59–64.

[6] Davies BL, Hibberd RD, Coptcoat MJ, Wickham JE. (1989). A surgeon robot prostatectomy–a laboratory evaluation. I Med Eng Tech. 13: 273–277.

[7] Harris SJ, Arambula-Cosio F, Mei Q, Hibberd RD, Davies BL, Wickham JEA, Nathan MS, Kundu B. (1997). The Probot—an active robot for procedures. Proc Inst Mech Eng H. 211: 317–325.

[8] Ho G, Ng WS, Teo MY. (2001). Experimental study of transurethral robotic laser resection of the prostate using the laser Trode lightguide. J Biomed Opt. 6: 244–251.

[9] Ho G, Ng WS, Teo MY, Cheng WS. (2001). Computer-assisted transurethral laser resection of the prostate (CALRP): theoretical and experimental motion plan. IEEE Trans Biomed Eng. 48: 1125–1133.

[10] Unger SW, Unger HM, Bass RT. (1994). AESOP robotic arm. Surg Endosc. 8: 1131.

[11] Kalan S, Chauhan S, Coelho RF, et al. (2010). History of robotic surgery. JRS. 4(3): 141–147.

[12] Falcone T, Goldberg J, Garcia-Ruiz A, Margossian H, Stevens L. (1999). Full robotic for laparoscopic tubal anastomosis: a case report. J Laparoendosc Adv Surg Tech A. 9: 107–113.

[13] Marescaux J, Leroy J, Rubino F, et al. (2002). Transcontinental robot-assisted remote telesurgery: feasibility and potential applications. Ann Surg. 235(4): 487–492.

[14] Weber P, Merola S, Wasielewski A, Ballantyne GH. (2002). Telerobotic-assisted laparoscopic right and sigmoid colectomies for benign disease. Dis Colon Rectum. 45(12): 1689–1696.

[15] Ballantyne GH, Moll F. (2003). The da Vinci telerobotic surgical system: the virtual operative field and telepresence surgery. Surg Clin North Am. 6: 1293–1304.

[16] Spinoglio G, Marano A, Priora F, Melandro F, Formisano G. (2015). History of robotic surgery. In: Spinoglio G. Editor. Robotic Surgery: Current Applications and New Trends. Springer-Verlag Italia, 2–12.

[17] Hagen ME, Curet MJ. (2014). The da Vinci Surgical® Systems. In: Watanabe G. Robotic Surgery. Springer Edition, 9–19.

[18] Spinoglio G, Summa M, Priora F, Quarati R, Testa S. (2008). Robotic colorectal surgery: first 50 cases experience. Dis Colon Rectum. 51(11): 1627–1632.

[19] Park JS, Choi GS, Park SY, Kim HJ, Ryuk JP. (2012). Randomized clinical trial of robot assisted *versus* standard laparoscopic right colectomy. Br J Surg. 99: 1219–1226.

[20] Deutsch GB, Sathyanarayana SA, Gunabushanam V, Mishra N, Rubach E, Zemon H, Klein JD, Denoto G, 3rd. (2012). Robotic vs. laparoscopic colorectal surgery: an institutional experience. Surg Endosc. 26(4): 956–963.

[21] Halabi WJ, Kang CY, Jafari MD, Nguyen VQ, Carmichael JC, Mills S, Stamos MJ, Pigazzi A. (2013). Robotic-assisted colorectal surgery in the United States: a nationwide analysis of trends and outcomes. World J Surg. 37(12): 2782–2790.

[22] Casillas MA, Jr., Leichtle SW, Wahl WL, Lampman RM, Welch KB, Wellock T, Madden EB, Cleary RK. (2014). Improved perioperative outcomes of robotic versus conventional laparoscopic colorectal operations. Am J Surg. 208(1): 33–40.

[23] Rawlings AL, Woodland JH, Vegunta RK, Crawford DL. (2007). Robotic versus laparoscopic colectomy. Surg Endosc. 21(10): 1701–1708.

[24] Lim DR, Min BS, Kim MS, Alasari S, Kim G, Hur H, Baik SH, Lee KJ, Kim NK. (2013). Robotic versus laparoscopic anterior resection of sigmoid colon cancer: comparative study of long-term oncologic outcomes. Surg Endosc. 27(4): 1379–1385.

[25] Delaney CP, et al. (2003). Comparison of robotically performed and traditional laparoscopic colorectal surgery. Dis Colon Rectum. 46:1633–1639.

[26] NCCN Clinical Practice Guidelines in Oncology: Colon Cancer. (2013). The National Comprehensive Cancer Network. http://www.nccn.org. Accessed 10 December 2012.

[27] Mutch M, Cellini C. (2011). Surgical management of colon cancer. In: Beck DE, Roberts PL, Saclarides TJ, Senagore AJ, Stamos MJ, Wexner SD. Editors. The ASCRS Textbook of Colon and Rectal Surgery. Second Edition, New York, NY: Springer Science + Business Media, LLC. 711–720.

[28] Lujan HJ, Plasencia G. (2014). Robotic right colectomy: three-arm technique. In: Kim KC. Editor, Springer Edition.

[29] D'Annibale A, Pernazza G, Morpurgo E, Monsellato I, Pende V, Lucandri G, Termini B, Orsini C, Sovernigo G. (2010). Robotic right colon resection: evaluation of first 50 consecutive cases for malignant disease. Ann Surg Oncol. 17: 2856–2862.

[30] D'Annibale A, A, Morpurgo E, Fiscon V, Trevisan P, Sovernigo G, Orsini C, Guidolin D. (2004). Robotic and laparoscopic surgery for treatment of colorectal diseases. Dis Colon Rectum. 47(12): 2162–8.

[31] Hanna MH, Hwang GS, Phelan MJ, Bui TL, Carmichael JC, Mills SD, Stamos MJ, Pigazzi A. (2015). Laparoscopic right hemicolectomy: short- and log-term outcomes of intracorporeal versus extracorporeal anastomosis. Surg Endosc. Dec 29

[32] Hellan M, Stein H, Pigazzi A. (2009). Totally robotic low anterior resection with total mesorectal excision and splenic flexure mobilization. Surg Endosc. 23: 447–451.

[33] Grams J, Tong W, Greenstein AJ, Salky B. (2010) Comparison of intracorporeal versus extracorporeal anastomosis in laparoscopic-assisted hemicolectomy. Surg Endosc. 24(8): 1886–1891.

[34] Scatizzi M, Kroning KC, Borrelli A, Andan G, Lenzi E, Feroci F. (2010). Extracorporeal versus intracorporeal anastomosis after laparoscopic right colectomy for cancer: a case controlled study. World J Surg. 34: 2902–2908.

[35] Samia H, Lawrence J, Nobel T, Stein S, Champagne BJ, Delaney CP. (2013). Extraction site location and incisional hernias after laparoscopic colorectal surgery: should we be avoiding the midline? Am J Surg. 205: 264–226.

[36] Campagnacci R, Baldoni A, Ghiselli R, Cappelletti-Trombettoni MM, Guerrieri M. (2015). Prevention of hernia incision in laparoscopic left colon resection. Minerva Chir. 70(3): 155–160.

[37] Anvari M, Birch DW, Bamehriz F, Gryfe R, Chapman T. (2004). Robotic-assisted laparoscopic colorectal surgery. Surg Laparosc Endosc Percutan Tech. 14: 311–315.

[38] Rawlings AL, Woodland JH, Crawford DL. (2006). Telerobotic surgery for right and sigmoid colectomies: 30 consecutive cases. Surg Endosc. 20: 1713–1718.

[39] Guerrieri M, Campagnacci R, Sperti P, Belfiori G, Gesuita R, Ghiselli R. (2015). Totally robotic vs 3D laparoscopic colectomy: a single centers preliminary experience. World J Gastroenterol. 21(46): 13152–13159.

[40] Keller DS, Hashemi L, Lu M, Delaney CP. (2013). Short-term outcomes for robotic colorectal surgery by provider volume. J Am Coll Surg. 217: 1063–1069.

[41] Cirocchi R, Cochetti G, Randolph J et al. (2014). Laparoscopic treatment of colovesical fistulas due to complicated colonic diverticular disease: a systematic review. Tech Coloproctol. doi:10.1007/s10151-014-1157-5

[42] DeSouza AL, Prasad LM, Park JJ, Marecik SJ, Blumetti J, Abcarian H. (2010). Robotic assistance in right hemicolectomy: is there a role? Dis Colon Rectum. 53: 1000–1006.

[43] Jayne DG, Thorpe HC, Copeland J, Quirke P, Brown JM, Guillou PJ. (2010). Five-year follow-up of the Medical Research Council CLASICC trial of laparoscopically assisted versus open surgery for colorectal cancer. Br J Surg. 97: 1638–1645.

[44] Zimmern A, Prasad L, Desouza A. (2010). Robotic colon and rectal surgery: a series of 131 cases. World J Surg. 34: 1954–1958.

Chapter 15

Immunotherapy in Colorectal Cancer

Gabriel Mak, Michele Moschetta and
Hendrik-Tobias Arkenau

Additional information is available at the end of the chapter

http://dx.doi.org/10.5772/63136

Abstract

Colorectal cancer (CRC) remains one of the most common malignancies and the second leading cause of cancer-related death worldwide; treatment algorithms include surgery, chemotherapy and targeted therapies. Immunotherapy has recently emerged as an effective treatment approach in several types of cancer, including non–small cell lung cancer, melanoma and kidney cancer. In CRC, novel immune-checkpoint inhibitors such as anti-CTLA4 and PD1/PDL1 monoclonal antibodies have shown limited efficacy, although ongoing trials in mismatch repair-deficient CRC have shown significant and promising results. Here, we review the role of immune-microenvironment in colorectal cancer and current clinical data about therapeutic activity of immunotherapy in the treatment of CRC.

Keywords: colorectal cancer, immunotherapy, drug development, checkpoint inhibition, mismatch repair

1. Introduction

Colorectal cancer (CRC) is the fourth most common cancer and the second leading cause of cancer-related death worldwide. Surgery, chemotherapy, radiation therapy and targeted agents including anti-angiogenic and anti-epidermal growth factor receptor (EGFR) therapies form the backbone of treatment for CRC in various stages. Unfortunately, when diagnosed at advanced stage, CRC is still inevitably fatal. More than 50% of patients diagnosed with CRC eventually develop metastases, and almost 90% of these patients have unresectable disease [1–3]. In some patients with metastatic disease, metastectomy is still possible and can result in a cure in appropriately selected patients [2, 3]. The almost totality of metastatic CRC patients eventually develops resistance to all available standard therapies leading to cancer progression and death [4].

As we will discuss here, immunotherapy and immunomodulatory drugs may represent future therapeutic options to be included in the therapeutic armamentarium in the treatment of CRC. The importance of inflammation in CRC is partially supported by the evidence that patients with inflammatory bowel diseases, i.e., patients with ulcerative colitis and Crohn's disease are at increased risk for developing CRC [5]. It is assumed that chronic inflammation is a significant contributor to cancer development. This is supported by the fact that colon cancer risk increases with longer duration of colitis, greater anatomic extent of colitis, the concomitant presence of other inflammatory manifestations like primary sclerosing cholangitis [6] and the fact that certain drugs used to treat inflammation, such as 5-aminosalicylates and steroids, may prevent the development of CRC in this clinical setting [7]. It may be thus possible that by shaping the immune composition of the CRC microenvironment through novel immunotherapies, this may ultimately lead to a therapeutic effect in CRC.

2. The immune-cell microenvironment in colorectal cancer

An important step in tumour progression is the evasion and suppression of the host immune system [8, 9], as shown in **Figure 1**. In the normal microenvironment, the effector cells, including the natural killer (NK) cells and cytotoxic T lymphocytes (CTLs), are capable of driving potent anti-tumour suppressive activities. Tumour cells are often able to induce an

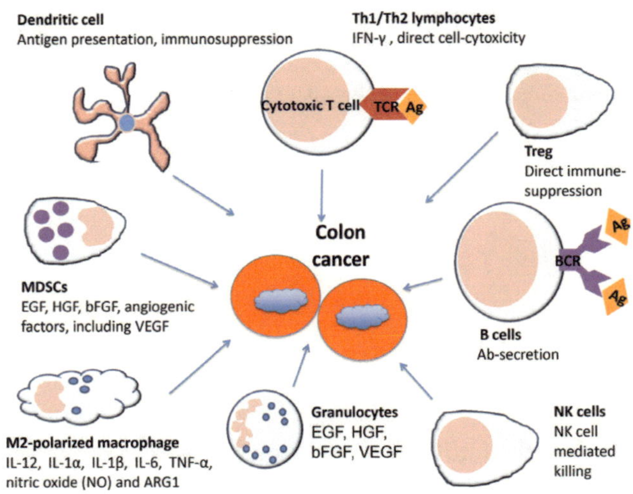

Figure 1. Immune-cell microenvironment in colorectal cancer. The evasion and suppression of the host immune system is an important step of colorectal cancer (CRC) progression. In physiologic conditions, effector cells, including the natural killer (NK) cells and cytotoxic T lymphocytes (CTLs), exert tumour surveillance and tumour suppressive activities. Tumour cells are able to induce an immunosuppressive microenvironment that protects them from the host immune system through the expansion of regulatory immune cells (i.e., myeloid-derived suppressor cells (MDSCs) and regulatory T cells (Tregs)) and alternative activation of other immune cells, including macrophages, granulocytes and dendritic cells.

immunosuppressive microenvironment that protects them from the host immune system. Overall, tumour cells are able to shape the host microenvironment, which is rich of immune cell populations, in a suitable way for them to survive to the host immune system recognition [10, 11]. The two major immunosuppressive mechanisms in cancer are (1) expansion of regulatory immune cells (i.e., myeloid-derived suppressor cells (MDSCs) and regulatory T cells (Tregs)) and (2) activation of the inhibitory T-cell pathways—programmed cell death-1/ programmed cell death-ligand 1 pathways (PD-1/PD-L1 pathways).

3. Myeloid-derived suppressor cells

Myeloid-derived suppressor cells are a heterogeneous and immature subset of circulating cells of myeloid derivation that can differentiate into, macrophages, granulocytes or dendritic cells (DCs) under physiologic conditions. However, under pathological conditions such as cancer or inflammation, the differentiation of these immature myeloid cells is inhibited resulting in accumulation of MDSCs in the tumour microenvironment or in the sites of inflammation [12]. For example, in cancer patients and tumour models, MDSCs accumulate in the tumour microenvironment because of the release of soluble factors by tumour cells or by other cells of the microenvironment, i.e., granulocyte macrophage colony stimulating factor (GM-CSF), interleukin-1 β and stromal-derived growth factor 1-α [13, 14]. MDSCs can then suppress T-cell proliferation through expression of several immune suppressive factors, including arginase, reactive oxygen species (ROS) and nitric oxide (NO). MDSCs can also promote the development of Treg cells *in vivo*, which are anergic and immune-suppressive [15]. Several studies have consistently shown that cancer patients with higher MDSC levels have shorter survival compared to patients with lower MDSC levels [16, 17]. Moreover, depletion of MDSCs in tumour-bearing mice using anti Gr-1 antibody [18, 19] or MDSC-targeting specific peptides have shown anti-tumour activities [20] suggesting that MDSCs can be a good target for future anti-tumour treatments. Two main subsets of MDSCs have been described, namely, granulocytic MDSC (G-MDSC) or polymorphonuclear (PMN)-MDSCs and monocytic MDSC (Mo-MDSC). G-MDSCs have granulocyte-like morphology characterised by increased levels of ROS and low levels of NO, whereas Mo-MDSCs have monocyte-like morphology with increased level of NO, but low levels of ROS. Human G-MDSCs and Mo-MDSCs are classically defined as $CD11b^{+}$ $CD33^{+}$ HLA-$DR^{-/low}CD14^{-}$ and $CD11b^{+}$ $CD33^{+}$ HLA-$DR^{-/low}$ $CD14^{+}$, respectively. In tumour-bearing mice, G-MDSCs are the major MDSC subset that expands in the peripheral lymphoid organs after tumour engraftment pointing to a different biology of these cells in human and mice [21].

MDSCs promote metastasis development and primary tumour growth both in CRC patients and CRC murine models [22]. Importantly, MDSCs have also been implicated in the resistance to anti-angiogenic therapies used for the treatment CRC [23] via their ability to stimulate the expression of genes, whose products promote leukocyte recruitment, alternative angiogenic mechanisms, tumour migration, wound healing and formation of premetastatic niches in distal metastatic organs [23].

4. Regulatory T cells (Tregs)

Treg cells are a subset of $CD4^+$ T lymphocytes characterised by the expression of Forkhead Box P3 (FOXP3) transcription factor [24]. Tregs are able to suppress the function of antigen presenting cells (APCs), i.e., dendritic cells, and effector T cells by direct contact or by release of anti-inflammatory cytokines (IL-10 and TGF- β). Tregs are major players in the development of tumour immunosuppressive microenvironment; these cells accumulate both in the tumour microenvironment and the peripheral blood of patients with cancer [25, 26]. The increased frequency of Tregs both in the peripheral blood and especially in the sites of tumour growth has generally been considered a marker of poor prognosis due to Treg-mediated suppression of anti-tumour immunity [27, 28]. In transgenic mouse models, it has been shown in mice that Treg depletion induces regression of solid tumours and lymphomas, following increased intratumoural accumulation of activated $CD8^+$ cytotoxic T cells [29–31]. These data indicate that targeting Tregs can represent a potential anti-tumour strategy; however, the development of autoimmune diseases following administration of Treg cells has been described in these preclinical studies and may represent a limitation in the pursue of novel anti-Treg treatments in patients. In CRC, several studies have shown that Treg density in tumour specimens represents an independent negative prognostic factor [32–34]. Low-dose cyclophosphamide has been shown to reduce the numbers and function of Tregs and to induce anti-tumour, immune-mediated effects [35, 36]; this has been shown to be true in preclinical models of CRC [37], but no studies have been carried out in CRC patients so far.

5. Dendritic cells

Dendritic cells are cells of bone marrow origin defined as professional antigen presenting cells, which have the ability to present self and non-self antigens to T cells, thus promoting immunity or immune-tolerance [38]. Antigen presentation by DCs is able to induce naive T cells differentiation into effector and memory T cells; however, it can also lead to different forms of T-cell tolerance, depending on the local microenvironment stimuli and the functional status of the DCs. Myeloid-DCs (mDCs) and plasmacytoid-DCs (pDCs) are two major DC subsets that have been identified based on their origin, immune-phenotype and functional status [39]. In human, mDCs are usually defined as $Lin^-HLADR^+CD11c^+CD123^{dim}$ cells, whereas pDCs are $Lin^-CD11c^-CD4^+CD45RA^+CD123^+ILT3^+$. Several studies have documented accumulation of DCs in tumour sites, which often correlated with poor prognosis [40–42]. The loss of tumour-derived antigen presentation ability by tumour-infiltrating DCs has been shown to be the consequence of the suppressive effects of the tumour microenvironment mediated by various cytokines [43]. For example, it has been demonstrated that tumour-infiltrating pDCs from solid tumours express high levels of inducible T-cell co-stimulator ligand (ICOS-L), which explains their ability to induce Tregs proliferation [44, 45], thus leading to local immunosuppression. Moreover, TGF- β secreted by DCs from breast cancer patients is able to induce Treg-cell proliferation and accumulation, thus leading to tumour growth [46]. The role of DCs in CRC has been controversial mostly due to the technical difficulties associated with their quantification and identification. For these reasons, it is difficult to draw a conclusion about the role of DCs and performance of DCs as a predictor of outcome for CRC [47, 48].

6. Natural killer cells

NK cells represent a heterogeneous lymphocyte population with direct-cytotoxic anti-tumour capacity and multiple immunoregulatory properties. Natural killer group 2D (NKG2D) is one of the NK cell activating receptors that recognises various proteins expressed on the surface of target cells in response to several forms of cellular stress. One of the ligand of NKG2D is the MHC class I polypeptide-related sequence A (MICA); target tumour cells that express MICA are efficiently killed via NKG2D despite the expression of MHC class I molecules, describing a pathway of anti-tumour activity mediated by NK cells [49]. Several preclinical studies have shown the susceptibility of CRC cells to the NK cell–mediated killing [50–52], which can be enhanced by the contemporary treatment with anti-CRC drugs like anti-EGFR inhibitors [53].

Interestingly Gharagozloo et al. [54] have recently shown that metastatic CRC patients present a significant reduction in the percentage of circulating NKG2D^{+}NK cells as well as NKG2D mRNA expression in peripheral blood as compared to healthy controls, suggesting a specific defect of NK cell–mediated natural immunity in CRC patients.

7. Macrophage in colorectal cancer

Cells of the monocyte–macrophage lineage are one of the major components of the leukocyte infiltration in tumours; there is strong evidence that these cells promote inflammatory circuits that ultimately lead to tumour progression, tumour cell invasion and metastasis [55].

Macrophages recruited to the tumour-associated microenvironment may exist both in a classically activated inflammatory phenotypes (M1) with anti-tumour capacity or an alternatively activated, immunosuppressive (M2) phenotype with tumour supporting ability [56]; M1-polarised macrophage secretes a large amount of IL-12, IL-1α, IL-1β, IL-6, TNF-α, nitric oxide (NO) and ARG1, and stimulate secretion of IFN-γ by Th1 lymphocytes, thus activating Th1 immune response which in turn stimulate the tumour specific-CTL cytotoxicity. However, during tumour progression, macrophages shift towards a M2-polarised phenotype induced by the exposure of these cells to IL-4, IL-13, M-CSF/CSF-1, IL-10 and TGF-β1, among other factors present in the tumour microenvironment. In this state, macrophages are defined as tumour-associated macrophages (TAMs) and are able to support tumour growth, survival and metastasis. TAMs mostly derived by circulating monocyte which are recruited to the tumour bed by the secretion from tumour cells and the other cells of the tumour microenvironment of inflammatory cytokines such as M-CSF/CSF-1, SDF-1/CCL12 and MCP-1/CCL2. M2 macrophages then are able to secrete large amount of growth factors, such as EGF, HGF, bFGF, inflammatory factors (such as COX2) and angiogenic factors, including VEGF and angiogenic chemokines, which in turn all together promote progression of tumours (reviewed in [55, 57]).

In general, higher densities of TAMs in tumours and overexpression of key stimulators of M2 differentiation are considered markers of poor prognosis in a number of cancers [55, 57]. TAMs are associated with tumour progression and poor survival in CRC patients [58, 59], in line with *in vitro* and *in vivo* studies showing that macrophages are able to promote survival and induce proliferation of CRC cells via activation of Wnt pathway in CRC cells [60–62]. However, some other studies have shown that macrophages actually exert a tumour-suppressive activity in CRC via direct inhibition of tumour cell proliferation and via production of chemokines that attract T cells, stimulate proliferation of allogeneic T cells and activate type-1 T cells associated with anti-tumour immune responses [63]. In CRC, the role of macrophages may be ultimately context and stage dependent with implications for the design of future therapies aiming to target these cells.

8. Immune therapy in CRC

Given the complexity of the immune microenviroment and immune-cell composition of CRC, targeting this type of cancer via novel immunotherapies has been proved challenging. However, as described in the following paragraphs, recent advanced in the immunotherapy drug-development together with a better understanding of the genetic basis of immune stimulation have finally lead to the proof of concept demonstration that immunotherapy may represent an important therapeutic tool in the treatment of CRC.

9. Immune-cytokine therapy in CRC

Non-specific immunotherapy utilising cytokines such as interferon (IFN), interleukins and granulocyte macrophage colony-stimulating factor (GM-CSF) have been studied because of the potential ability to modulate and promote host immunity against tumour antigens. A Phase II trial of 29 patients with metastatic CRC using gemcitabine, oxaliplatin and 5-fluorouracil (GOLF) in combination with IL-2 and GM-CSF immune adjuvant regimen (GOLFIG) yielded promising results, with an overall response rate of 56.5%, disease control rate of 96% and median time to progression of 12.5 months [64]. A Phase III study comparing the GOLFIG regimen against the control arm of FOLFOX-4 in first line treatment of metastatic CRC was terminated early due to poor recruitment into the control arm. However, the experimental arm did show superiority in Progression Free Survival and Overall Response Rate with a trend towards improvement of overall survival; this trial does provide proof-of-concept that GOLFIG chemoimmunotherapy may represent a novel reliable option for first-line treatment of metastatic CRC [65].

10. Vaccines as therapeutic tools in CRC

Vaccine-based therapy can be delivered as whole-tumour-cell vaccines, peptide vaccines, viral vector vaccines or dendritic call vaccines, each with its inherent advantages and disadvantages

http://dx.doi.org/10.5772/63136

(reviewed in [66, 67]). Overall in the treatment of CRC, there have been only small Phase I and Phase II studies with suggestions that vaccines may have a role in the adjuvant setting, and limited efficacy in metastatic disease. [68].

11. Rationale of checkpoint receptor pathway as a target in colorectal cancer

Immune checkpoints refer to a very complex and articulated series of inhibitory pathways that intricate into the immune system and that are crucial for regulating self-tolerance and modulating the duration and extent of physiological immune responses in peripheral tissues in order to avoid excessive immune-activation and subsequent collateral tissue damage (**Figure 2**) [69]. It is now well established that tumour cells can co-opt certain immune-checkpoint pathways; this represents a novel and important mechanism of immune resistance, particularly against T cells that are specific for tumour antigens. Consequently, the blockade of immune checkpoints is able to unleash T-cell–mediated anti-tumour immune response in a potent and sometime curative way [69].

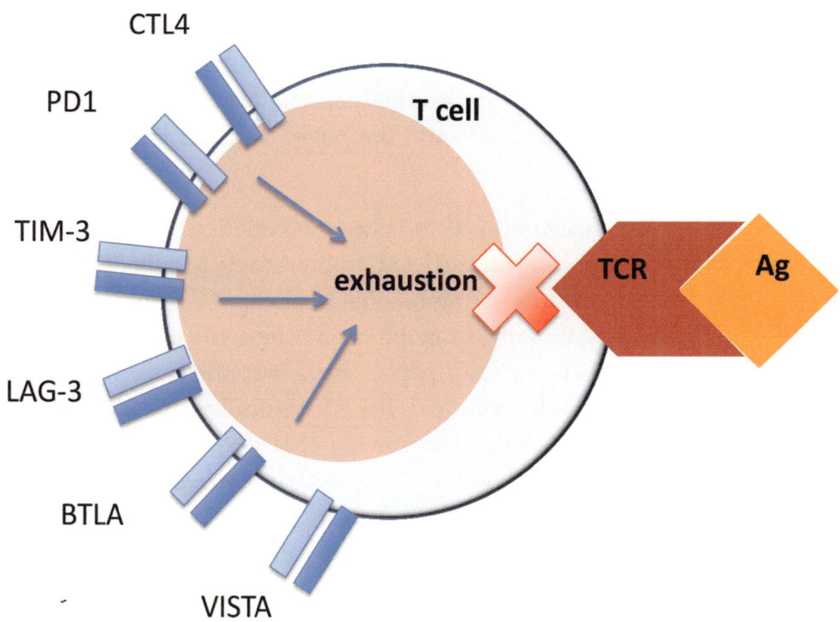

Figure 2. Immune checkpoint and immunosuppression in CRC. Immune checkpoints activate inhibitory pathways in T cell that ultimately lead to T-cell–mediated immunity suppression. Tumour cells can co-opt these immune-checkpoint pathways thus leading to T-cell exhaustion and tumour immunotolerance.CTLA4: cytotoxic T-lymphocyte-associated antigen 4; PD1: programmed cell death protein 1; TIM3: T-cell membrane protein 3; LAG3: lymphocyte activation gene 3; BTLA: B- and T-lymphocyte attenuator; VISTA: V-domain Ig suppressor of T-cell activation.

The two immune-checkpoint receptors that have been most studied in the context of clinical cancer immunotherapy, cytotoxic T-lymphocyte-associated antigen 4 (CTLA4; also known as CD152) and programmed cell death protein 1 (PD1; also known as CD279) are both inhibitory receptors and have both shown to be appropriate targets (**Figure 2**). Importantly, several other checkpoint immune pathways have recently emerged to be additional targets for the development of new immunotherapy drugs mostly in preclinical studies (**Figure 2**); these include lymphocyte activation gene 3 (LAG3; also known as CD223), 2B4 (also known as CD244), B- and T-lymphocyte attenuator (BTLA; also known as CD272), T-cell membrane protein 3 (TIM3; also known as HAVcr2), adenosine A2a receptor (A2aR) to name a few [70].

Programmed cell death 1 is a Type I transmembrane protein, which belongs to the CD28 family [71]. PD-1 is expressed on activated and exhausted T and B cells and has two ligands PD-L1 and PD-L2. Importantly, PD-L1 is not expressed on normal epithelial tissues, but can aberrantly be expressed on a variety of solid tumours [72]. On the other hand, PD-L2 is more broadly expressed on normal healthy tissues. Binding of PD-L1 to PD-1 reduces cytokine production and activation of the target T cells, leading to an immunosuppressive microenvironment.

Clinical trials targeting PD-1/PD-L1 pathway to overcome tumour-associated immune suppression have shown promising results for a variety of solid tumours. Checkpoint inhibitor immunotherapy is currently FDA-approved for the treatment of melanoma, kidney cancer and NSCLC. However, it has been shown active in many other types of solid, including gastric, ovarian cancer, and bladder cancer, and hematologic cancers, particularly Hodgkin lymphoma [73–76]. It is currently unclear what determines response to this type of treatment and this is an area of active research giving the costs and the potential toxicity associated with these treatments.

The accumulation of somatic mutations accompanies the initiation and progression of most cancers conferring to the tumour cells unrestricted proliferative capacity [77]. The analysis of cancer genomes has revealed that tumour mutational landscapes [78] are extremely variable among patients, among different tumours from the same patient and even among the different regions of a single tumour. Two separate papers have recently shown that response to checkpoint inhibitors, i.e., anti-CTL4 and anti-PDL1 Ab, critically depend on the mutational load of the specific tumours. The first study by Snyder et al. [79] found that mutational load associates with exceptional response to the anti-CTLA-4 Ab ipilimumab in melanoma patients. Using genome-wide somatic neoepitope analysis and patient-specific HLA-typing, they identified candidate tumour neoantigens for each patient predicted to be able to activate a T-cell response in anti-CTLA-4 treated patients.

Interestingly, the probability for a tumour to carry such neoantigens was dependent on the mutational load of the specific tumour, as it was the probability to respond to anti-CTLA-4 Ab. Similar results were obtained in NSCLC patients treated with pembrolizumab, an antibody-targeting PD-1 [80]. A higher non-synonymous mutation burden in tumours was associated with improved objective response, durable clinical benefit and progression-free survival. Therapeutic benefit in these patients correlated with the molecular smoking signature, higher neoantigen burden and DNA repair pathway mutations. All these factors were associated with increased mutation burden [80].

Both studies suggest for the first time a genomic-based mechanism to the response to novel immunotherapy drugs that can potentially help with designing rational combination treatments, i.e., DNA-damaging agents plus immune-checkpoint inhibitors.

12. PD1/PDL1—immune-checkpoint inhibitors

In unselected colon cancer, the response to immune-checkpoint inhibitors has shown limited efficacy [73]. In tumours that have shown response, predictive markers to checkpoint inhibition are being evaluated—with microsatellite insufficiency (MSI) or mismatch-repair (MMR) status being the most promising thus far [81].

Pembrolizumab (MK-3475)—a highly selective humanised IgG4 monoclonal antibody that blocks the interaction of PD-1 with its ligands PD-L1 and PD-L2—has undergone extensive testing in multiple tumour types. In the KEYNOTE-028 study—a multicohort, Phase Ib trial of pembrolizumab for programmed death-ligand 1 (PD-L1) positive advanced solid tumours; there were 156 screened patients with advanced colorectal cancer, with 33 (21%) of these being PD-L1 positive and 23 went on to receive treatment. Although the safety profile was acceptable with only one patient experiencing a grade ≥3 treatment-related adverse events with elevated bilirubin; it was felt there was overall minimal anti-tumour activity. One patient who had microsatellite instability high disease experienced a partial response, with four patients (17%) having the best response of stable disease, and progressive disease in 16 patients (70%) [82].

The initial Phase I study of anti-PD-1 antibody nivolumab included 17 colorectal patients, who were heavily pre-treated; the majority of these patients had PD-L1 negative tumours and thus overall, this study showed limited clinical efficacy [83]. However, one patient with colorectal cancer treated with five doses in this study experienced a complete response at 6 months, which was ongoing after 3 years; it was noted that the patient's tumour was MSI-high, and evidence of PD-L1 expression by infiltrating macrophages and lymphocytes [84].

Based on the previous reports associating mutational load to response to checkpoint inhibitors, Le et al. hypothesised that mismatch repair–deficient tumours and mismatch repair (MMR)–deficient tumours are more responsive to PD-1 blockade than are MMR-proficient tumours. A Phase II study of 41 patients evaluating the clinical activity of pembrolizumab in metastatic carcinoma with or without MMR-deficiency showed hazard ratios for disease progression or death (0.10; 95% CI, 0.03–0.37; $P < 0.001$) and for death (0.22; 95% CI, 0.05–1.00; $P = 0.05$) that favoured patients with mismatch repair-deficient colorectal cancer [85]. Thus, ongoing studies are exploring this particular subset.

The KEYNOTE-164 study (NCT02460198) is a Phase II study currently recruiting patients with previously treated locally advanced unresectable or metastatic mismatched repair-deficient or MSI-high colorectal carcinoma to assess efficacy of pembrolizumab monotherapy [85]. In the same patient population of MSI-high colorectal cancers, the Phase III KEYNOTE-177 (NCT02563002) study will compare pembrolizumab monotherapy against standard of care chemotherapy in first line treatment of advanced CRC [86].

Regarding anti-PD-L1 compounds, atezolizumab (MPDL3280A) has shown activity in Phase I studies—with one of four patients with colorectal cancer having a durable partial response [87]. In the Phase Ib study of atezolizumab in combination with bevacizumab in refractory metastatic CRC, and that of atezolizumab and bevacizumab with FOLFOX in the oxaliplatin naïve population, this confirmed acceptable safety and clinical activity—unconfirmed ORR 8% (1/13) and 44% (8/18) in the two arms respectively [88]. However, the Phase I study of BMS936559, which included 18 colorectal patients showed no response in this tumour type [89]. There are ongoing studies with other anti-PD-L1 compounds including durvalumab/ MEDI4736 (NCT01693562) and avelumab (NCT01772004).

13. Anti-CTLA4 Therapy

Tremilimumab, a fully human immunoglobulin (Ig) G2 monoclonal antibody that blocks inhibitory signalling from CTLA4 was studied as monotherapy treatment in a Phase II single arm study, of 47 patients with refractory metastatic CRC. Tremelimumab was intended to be administered every 90 days. Clinical activity was unable to be demonstrated, with 43 of 45 evaluable patients unable to receive a second dose—with a median duration on study of 2.3 months [90]. However, a Phase I combination study of tremelimumab with durvalumab (NCT01975831) is ongoing; and ipilimumab is also being studied in combination with nivolumab (NCT02060188).

14. Other immune-checkpoint inhibitors

In MSI-high colon cancers, it has been shown that up-regulation of PD-1, PD-L1, CTLA-4, LAG-3 and IDO immune checkpoints enables evasion from Th1 response [91]. As described, PD-L1, PD-1, CTLA-4 have been and are being investigated in the treatment of CRC. Anti-LAG-3 monoclonal antibodies (BMS-986016), alone and in combination with nivolumab are also being evaluated (NCT01968109).

15. Other combined immunotherapy strategies

As there has been limited efficacy from current immunotherapy strategies, it has been proposed that combination of immunotherapy with conventional chemotherapy, radiotherapy and targeted agents should be trialled [92]. The use of DNA damaging agents may increase the mutation burden, thus increase the efficacy of checkpoint inhibition.

16. Conclusion

Advanced CRC remains inevitably lethal despite optimal management, thus novel therapeutic approaches are urgently needed. Immunotherapy, particularly novel immune-checkpoint inhibitors, is transforming the therapeutic landscape of many types of cancer. Although in CRC the clinical data have been disappointing so far, this is probably due to the lack of knowledge of biomarkers/clinical features that can allow us the optimal selection of patients likely to respond to the specific immunotherapies. This has been proved by the identification of MMR status as a specific marker of response to anti-PD1/PDL1 treatment in CRC. In the future, a deeper understanding of immunobiology of CRC together with the development of novel immunotherapeutic agents will surely lead to new successful treatments for advanced CRC patients. This will be followed by further studies of combination of novel immunotherapies together with the present standard of care, i.e., surgery, chemotherapy and target therapies that will additionally improve the prognosis of advanced metastatic CRC.

Author details

Gabriel Mak[1], Michele Moschetta[1] and Hendrik-Tobias Arkenau[1,2*]

*Address all correspondence to: Tobias.Arkenau@hcahealthcare.co.uk

1 Sarah Cannon Research Institute, London, UK

2 University College London, London, UK

References

[1] Lee WS, Yun SH, Chun HK, Lee WY, Yun HR, Kim J, et al. Pulmonary resection for metastases from colorectal cancer: prognostic factors and survival. Int J Colorectal Dis. 2007;22(6):699–704.

[2] Choti MA, Sitzmann JV, Tiburi MF, Sumetchotimetha W, Rangsin R, Schulick RD, et al. Trends in long-term survival following liver resection for hepatic colorectal metastases. Ann Surg. 2002;235(6):759–766.

[3] Kanas GP, Taylor A, Primrose JN, Langeberg WJ, Kelsh MA, Mowat FS, et al. Survival after liver resection in metastatic colorectal cancer: review and meta-analysis of prognostic factors. Clin Epidemiol. 2012;4:283–301.

[4] Bergers G, Hanahan D. Modes of resistance to anti-angiogenic therapy. Nat Rev Cancer. 2008;8(8):592–603.

[5] Itzkowitz SH, Yio X. Inflammation and cancer IV. Colorectal cancer in inflammatory bowel disease: the role of inflammation. Am J Physiol Gastrointest Liver Physiol. 2004;287(1):G7–G17.

[6] Kim ER, Chang DK. Colorectal cancer in inflammatory bowel disease: the risk, pathogenesis, prevention and diagnosis. World J Gastroenterol. 2014;20(29):9872–9881.

[7] Stolfi C, De Simone V, Pallone F, Monteleone G. Mechanisms of action of non-steroidal anti-inflammatory drugs (NSAIDs) and mesalazine in the chemoprevention of colorectal cancer. Int J Mol Sci. 2013;14(9):17972–17985.

[8] Quail DF, Joyce JA. Microenvironmental regulation of tumor progression and metastasis. Nat Med. 2013;19(11):1423–1437.

[9] Swann JB, Smyth MJ. Immune surveillance of tumors. J Clin Invest. 2007;117(5):1137–1146.

[10] Smyth MJ, Ngiow SF, Ribas A, Teng MW. Combination cancer immunotherapies tailored to the tumour microenvironment. Nat Rev Clin Oncol. 2016 Mar;13(3):143–58. doi: 10.1038/nrclinonc.2015.209. Epub 2015 Nov 24.

[11] Kawano Y, Moschetta M, Manier S, Glavey S, Gorgun GT, Roccaro AM, et al. Targeting the bone marrow microenvironment in multiple myeloma. Immunol Rev. 2015;263(1): 160–172.

[12] Gabrilovich DI, Nagaraj S. Myeloid-derived suppressor cells as regulators of the immune system. Nat Rev Immunol. 2009;9(3):162–174.

[13] Almand B, Clark JI, Nikitina E, van Beynen J, English NR, Knight SC, et al. Increased production of immature myeloid cells in cancer patients: a mechanism of immunosuppression in cancer. J Immunol. 2001;166(1):678–689.

[14] Diaz-Montero CM, Salem ML, Nishimura MI, Garrett-Mayer E, Cole DJ, Montero AJ. Increased circulating myeloid-derived suppressor cells correlate with clinical cancer stage, metastatic tumor burden, and doxorubicin-cyclophosphamide chemotherapy. Cancer Immunol Immunother. 2009;58(1):49–59.

[15] Huang B, Pan PY, Li Q, Sato AI, Levy DE, Bromberg J, et al. Gr-1+CD115+ immature myeloid suppressor cells mediate the development of tumor-induced T regulatory cells and T-cell anergy in tumor-bearing host. Cancer Res. 2006;66(2):1123–1131.

[16] Walter S, Weinschenk T, Stenzl A, Zdrojowy R, Pluzanska A, Szczylik C, et al. Multipeptide immune response to cancer vaccine IMA901 after single-dose cyclophosphamide associates with longer patient survival. Nat Med. 2012;18(8):1254–1261.

[17] Solito S, Falisi E, Diaz-Montero CM, Doni A, Pinton L, Rosato A, et al. A human promyelocytic-like population is responsible for the immune suppression mediated by myeloid-derived suppressor cells. Blood. 2011;118(8):2254–2265.

[18] Serafini P, Meckel K, Kelso M, Noonan K, Califano J, Koch W, et al. Phosphodiesterase-5 inhibition augments endogenous antitumor immunity by reducing myeloid-derived suppressor cell function. J Exp Med. 2006;203(12):2691–2702.

[19] Li H, Han Y, Guo Q, Zhang M, Cao X. Cancer-expanded myeloid-derived suppressor cells induce anergy of NK cells through membrane-bound TGF-beta 1. J Immunol. 2009;182(1):240–249.

[20] Qin H, Lerman B, Sakamaki I, Wei G, Cha SC, Rao SS, et al. Generation of a new therapeutic peptide that depletes myeloid-derived suppressor cells in tumor-bearing mice. Nat Med. 2014;20(6):676–681.

[21] Youn JI, Nagaraj S, Collazo M, Gabrilovich DI. Subsets of myeloid-derived suppressor cells in tumor-bearing mice. J Immunol. 2008;181(8):5791–5802.

[22] Inamoto S, Itatani Y, Yamamoto T, Minamiguchi S, Hirai H, Iwamoto M, et al. Loss of SMAD4 promotes colorectal cancer progression by accumulation of myeloid-derived suppressor cells through the CCL15-CCR1 chemokine axis. Clin Cancer Res. 2016;22(2): 492–501.

[23] Ichikawa M, Williams R, Wang L, Vogl T, Srikrishna G. S100A8/A9 activate key genes and pathways in colon tumor progression. Mol Cancer Res. 2011;9(2):133–148.

[24] Fontenot JD, Gavin MA, Rudensky AY. Foxp3 programs the development and function of CD4+CD25+ regulatory T cells. Nat Immunol. 2003;4(4):330–336.

[25] Nishikawa H, Sakaguchi S. Regulatory T cells in tumor immunity. Int J Cancer. 2010;127(4):759–767.

[26] Mougiakakos D, Choudhury A, Lladser A, Kiessling R, Johansson CC. Regulatory T cells in cancer. Adv Cancer Res. 2010;107:57–117.

[27] Curiel TJ, Coukos G, Zou L, Alvarez X, Cheng P, Mottram P, et al. Specific recruitment of regulatory T cells in ovarian carcinoma fosters immune privilege and predicts reduced survival. Nat Med. 2004;10(9):942–949.

[28] Bates GJ, Fox SB, Han C, Leek RD, Garcia JF, Harris AL, et al. Quantification of regulatory T cells enables the identification of high-risk breast cancer patients and those at risk of late relapse. J Clin Oncol. 2006;24(34):5373–5880.

[29] Lahl K, Loddenkemper C, Drouin C, Freyer J, Arnason J, Eberl G, et al. Selective depletion of Foxp3+ regulatory T cells induces a scurfy-like disease. J Exp Med. 2007;204(1):57–63.

[30] Klages K, Mayer CT, Lahl K, Loddenkemper C, Teng MW, Ngiow SF, et al. Selective depletion of Foxp3+ regulatory T cells improves effective therapeutic vaccination against established melanoma. Cancer Res. 2010;70(20):7788–7799.

[31] Teng MW, Ngiow SF, von Scheidt B, McLaughlin N, Sparwasser T, Smyth MJ. Conditional regulatory T-cell depletion releases adaptive immunity preventing carcinogenesis and suppressing established tumor growth. Cancer Res. 2010;70(20):7800–7809.

[32] Vlad C, Kubelac P, Fetica B, Vlad D, Irimie A, Achimas-Cadariu P. The prognostic value of FOXP3+ T regulatory cells in colorectal cancer. J BUON. 2015;20(1):114–119.

[33] Wang Q, Feng M, Yu T, Liu X, Zhang P. Intratumoral regulatory T cells are associated with suppression of colorectal carcinoma metastasis after resection through overcoming IL-17 producing T cells. Cell Immunol. 2014;287(2):100–105.

[34] Lin YC, Mahalingam J, Chiang JM, Su PJ, Chu YY, Lai HY, et al. Activated but not resting regulatory T cells accumulated in tumor microenvironment and correlated with tumor progression in patients with colorectal cancer. Int J Cancer. 2013;132(6):1341–1350.

[35] Lutsiak ME, Semnani RT, De Pascalis R, Kashmiri SV, Schlom J, Sabzevari H. Inhibition of CD4(+)25+ T regulatory cell function implicated in enhanced immune response by low-dose cyclophosphamide. Blood. 2005;105(7):2862–2868.

[36] Ghiringhelli F, Larmonier N, Schmitt E, Parcellier A, Cathelin D, Garrido C, et al. CD4+CD25+ regulatory T cells suppress tumor immunity but are sensitive to cyclophosphamide which allows immunotherapy of established tumors to be curative. Eur J Immunol. 2004;34(2):336–344.

[37] Son CH, Bae JH, Shin DY, Lee HR, Jo WS, Yang K, et al. Combination effect of regulatory T-cell depletion and ionizing radiation in mouse models of lung and colon cancer. Int J Radiat Oncol Biol Phys. 2015;92(2):390–398.

[38] Banchereau J, Steinman RM. Dendritic cells and the control of immunity. Nature. 1998;392(6673):245–252.

[39] O'Doherty U, Peng M, Gezelter S, Swiggard WJ, Betjes M, Bhardwaj N, et al. Human blood contains two subsets of dendritic cells, one immunologically mature and the other immature. Immunology. 1994;82(3):487–493.

[40] Bell D, Chomarat P, Broyles D, Netto G, Harb GM, Lebecque S, et al. In breast carcinoma tissue, immature dendritic cells reside within the tumor, whereas mature dendritic cells are located in peritumoral areas. J Exp Med. 1999;190(10):1417–1426.

[41] Treilleux I, Blay JY, Bendriss-Vermare N, Ray-Coquard I, Bachelot T, Guastalla JP, et al. Dendritic cell infiltration and prognosis of early stage breast cancer. Clin Cancer Res. 2004;10(22):7466–7474.

[42] Sandel MH, Dadabayev AR, Menon AG, Morreau H, Melief CJ, Offringa R, et al. Prognostic value of tumor-infiltrating dendritic cells in colorectal cancer: role of maturation status and intratumoral localization. Clin Cancer Res. 2005;11(7):2576–2582.

[43] Zou W. Immunosuppressive networks in the tumour environment and their therapeutic relevance. Nat Rev Cancer. 2005;5(4):263–274.

[44] Conrad C, Gregorio J, Wang YH, Ito T, Meller S, Hanabuchi S, et al. Plasmacytoid dendritic cells promote immunosuppression in ovarian cancer via ICOS costimulation of Foxp3(+) T-regulatory cells. Cancer Res. 2012;72(20):5240–5249.

[45] Faget J, Bendriss-Vermare N, Gobert M, Durand I, Olive D, Biota C, et al. ICOS-ligand expression on plasmacytoid dendritic cells supports breast cancer progression by

promoting the accumulation of immunosuppressive CD4+ T cells. Cancer Res. 2012;72(23):6130–6141.

[46] Ramos RN, Chin LS, Dos Santos AP, Bergami-Santos PC, Laginha F, Barbuto JA. Monocyte-derived dendritic cells from breast cancer patients are biased to induce CD4+CD25+Foxp3+ regulatory T cells. J Leukoc Biol. 2012;92(3):673–682.

[47] Malietzis G, Lee GH, Jenkins JT, Bernardo D, Moorghen M, Knight SC, et al. Prognostic value of the tumour-infiltrating dendritic cells in colorectal cancer: a systematic review. Cell Commun Adhes. 2015;22(1):9–14.

[48] Legitimo A, Consolini R, Failli A, Orsini G, Spisni R. Dendritic cell defects in the colorectal cancer. Hum Vaccin Immunother. 2014;10(11):3224–3235.

[49] Groh V, Rhinehart R, Secrist H, Bauer S, Grabstein KH, Spies T. Broad tumor-associated expression and recognition by tumor-derived gamma delta T cells of MICA and MICB. Proc Natl Acad Sci USA. 1999;96(12):6879–6884.

[50] Kim GR, Ha GH, Bae JH, Oh SO, Kim SH, Kang CD. Metastatic colon cancer cell populations contain more cancer stem-like cells with a higher susceptibility to natural killer cell-mediated lysis compared with primary colon cancer cells. Oncol Lett. 2015;9(4):1641–1646.

[51] Taglia L, Matusiak D, Benya RV. GRP-induced up-regulation of Hsp72 promotes CD16+/94+ natural killer cell binding to colon cancer cells causing tumor cell cytolysis. Clin Exp Metastasis. 2008;25(4):451–463.

[52] Helms RA, Bull DM. Natural killer activity of human lymphocytes against colon cancer cells. Gastroenterology. 1980;78(4):738–744.

[53] Bae JH, Kim SJ, Kim MJ, Oh SO, Chung JS, Kim SH, et al. Susceptibility to natural killer cell-mediated lysis of colon cancer cells is enhanced by treatment with epidermal growth factor receptor inhibitors through UL16-binding protein-1 induction. Cancer Sci. 2012;103(1):7–16.

[54] Gharagozloo M, Kalantari H, Rezaei A, Maracy MR, Salehi M, Bahador A, et al. The decrease in NKG2D+ natural killer cells in peripheral blood of patients with metastatic colorectal cancer. Bratisl Lek Listy. 2015;116(5):296–301.

[55] Cook J, Hagemann T. Tumour-associated macrophages and cancer. Curr Opin Pharmacol. 2013;13(4):595–601.

[56] Sica A, Schioppa T, Mantovani A, Allavena P. Tumour-associated macrophages are a distinct M2 polarised population promoting tumour progression: potential targets of anti-cancer therapy. Eur J Cancer. 2006;42(6):717–727.

[57] Pollard JW. Tumour-educated macrophages promote tumour progression and metastasis. Nat Rev Cancer. 2004;4(1):71–78.

[58] Nagorsen D, Voigt S, Berg E, Stein H, Thiel E, Loddenkemper C. Tumor-infiltrating macrophages and dendritic cells in human colorectal cancer: relation to local regulatory

T cells, systemic T-cell response against tumor-associated antigens and survival. J Transl Med. 2007;5:62.

[59] Ohnishi K, Komohara Y, Saito Y, Miyamoto Y, Watanabe M, Baba H, et al. CD169-positive macrophages in regional lymph nodes are associated with a favorable prognosis in patients with colorectal carcinoma. Cancer Sci. 2013;104(9):1237–1244.

[60] Kaler P, Galea V, Augenlicht L, Klampfer L. Tumor associated macrophages protect colon cancer cells from TRAIL-induced apoptosis through IL-1beta-dependent stabilization of Snail in tumor cells. PLoS One. 2010;5(7):e11700.

[61] Kaler P, Augenlicht L, Klampfer L. Macrophage-derived IL-1beta stimulates Wnt signaling and growth of colon cancer cells: a crosstalk interrupted by vitamin D3. Oncogene. 2009;28(44):3892–902.

[62] Kaler P, Godasi BN, Augenlicht L, Klampfer L. The NF-kappaB/AKT-dependent induction of Wnt signaling in colon cancer cells by macrophages and IL-1beta. Cancer Microenviron. 2009;2(1):69–80.

[63] Ong SM, Tan YC, Beretta O, Jiang D, Yeap WH, Tai JJ, et al. Macrophages in human colorectal cancer are pro-inflammatory and prime T cells towards an anti-tumour type-1 inflammatory response. Eur J Immunol. 2012;42(1):89–100.

[64] Correale P, Cusi MG, Tsang KY, Del Vecchio MT, Marsili S, Placa ML, et al. Chemo-immunotherapy of metastatic colorectal carcinoma with gemcitabine plus FOLFOX 4 followed by subcutaneous granulocyte macrophage colony-stimulating factor and interleukin-2 induces strong immunologic and antitumor activity in metastatic colon cancer patients. J Clin Oncol. 2005;23(35):8950–8958.

[65] Correale P, Botta C, Rotundo MS, Guglielmo A, Conca R, Licchetta A, et al. Gemcitabine, oxaliplatin, levofolinate, 5-fluorouracil, granulocyte-macrophage colony-stimulating factor, and interleukin-2 (GOLFIG) versus FOLFOX chemotherapy in metastatic colorectal cancer patients: the GOLFIG-2 multicentric open-label randomized phase III trial. J Immunother. 2014;37(1):26–35.

[66] Halama N, Zoernig I, Jaeger D. Advanced malignant melanoma: immunologic and multimodal therapeutic strategies. J Oncol. 2010;2010:8.

[67] Singh PP, Sharma PK, Krishnan G, Lockhart AC. Immune checkpoints and immunotherapy for colorectal cancer. Gastroenterol Rep. 2015;3(4):289–297.

[68] Nagorsen D, Thiel E. Clinical and immunologic responses to active specific cancer vaccines in human colorectal cancer. Clin Cancer Res. 2006;12(10):3064–3069.

[69] Pardoll DM. The blockade of immune checkpoints in cancer immunotherapy. Nat Rev Cancer. 2012;12(4):252–264.

[70] Dong ZY, Wu SP, Liao RQ, Huang SM, Wu YL. Potential biomarker for checkpoint blockade immunotherapy and treatment strategy. Tumour Biol. 2016 Apr;37(4):4251–61. doi: 10.1007/s13277-016-4812-9. Epub 2016 Jan 16.

[71] Ishida Y, Agata Y, Shibahara K, Honjo T. Induced expression of PD-1, a novel member of the immunoglobulin gene superfamily, upon programmed cell death. EMBO J. 1992;11(11):3887–3895.

[72] Dong H, Strome SE, Salomao DR, Tamura H, Hirano F, Flies DB, et al. Tumor-associated B7-H1 promotes T-cell apoptosis: a potential mechanism of immune evasion. Nat Med. 2002;8(8):793–800.

[73] Topalian SL, Hodi FS, Brahmer JR, Gettinger SN, Smith DC, McDermott DF, et al. Safety, activity, and immune correlates of anti-PD-1 antibody in cancer. N Engl J Med. 2012;366(26):2443–2454.

[74] Brahmer JR, Tykodi SS, Chow LQ, Hwu WJ, Topalian SL, Hwu P, et al. Safety and activity of anti-PD-L1 antibody in patients with advanced cancer. N Engl J Med. 2012;366(26):2455–2465.

[75] Powles T, Eder JP, Fine GD, Braiteh FS, Loriot Y, Cruz C, et al. MPDL3280A (anti-PD-L1) treatment leads to clinical activity in metastatic bladder cancer. Nature. 2014;515(7528):558–562.

[76] Ansell SM, Lesokhin AM, Borrello I, Halwani A, Scott EC, Gutierrez M, et al. PD-1 blockade with nivolumab in relapsed or refractory Hodgkin's lymphoma. N Engl J Med. 2015;372(4):311–319.

[77] Hanahan D, Weinberg RA. Hallmarks of cancer: the next generation. Cell. 2011;144(5): 646–674.

[78] Kandoth C, McLellan MD, Vandin F, Ye K, Niu B, Lu C, et al. Mutational landscape and significance across 12 major cancer types. Nature. 2013;502(7471):333–339.

[79] Snyder A, Makarov V, Merghoub T, Yuan J, Zaretsky JM, Desrichard A, et al. Genetic basis for clinical response to CTLA-4 blockade in melanoma. N Engl J Med. 2014;371(23):2189–2199.

[80] Rizvi NA, Hellmann MD, Snyder A, Kvistborg P, Makarov V, Havel JJ, et al. Cancer immunology. Mutational landscape determines sensitivity to PD-1 blockade in non-small cell lung cancer. Science. 2015;348(6230):124–128.

[81] Ciombor KK, Wu C, Goldberg RM. Recent therapeutic advances in the treatment of colorectal cancer. Annu Rev Med. 2015;66:83–95.

[82] B.H. O'Neil JW, D. Lorente, E. Elez, J. Raimbourg, C. Gomez-Roca, S. Ejadi, S.A. Piha-Paul, R.A. Moss, L.L. Siu, K. Dotti, A. Santoro, M. Gould, S.S. Yuan, M. Koshiji, S.W. Han. Pembrolizumab (MK-3475) for patients (pts) with advanced colorectal carcinoma (CRC): preliminary results from KEYNOTE-028. Eur J Cancer. 2015;51:S3–S103.

[83] Brahmer JR, Drake CG, Wollner I, Powderly JD, Picus J, Sharfman WH, et al. Phase I study of single-agent anti–programmed death-1 (MDX-1106) in refractory solid tumors: safety, clinical activity, pharmacodynamics, and immunologic correlates. J Clin Oncol. 2010;28(19):3167–3175.

[84] Lipson EJ, Sharfman WH, Drake CG, Wollner I, Taube JM, Anders RA, et al. Durable cancer regression off-treatment and effective reinduction therapy with an anti-PD-1 antibody. Clin Cancer Res. 2013;19(2):462–468.

[85] Dung T, Le NSA, Laheru D, Browner IS, Wang H, Uram JN, Kemberling H, Zheng L, Iannone R, Friedman E, Meister A, Donehower RC, De Jesus-Acosta A, Diaz LA. Phase 2 study of programmed death-1 antibody (anti-PD-1, MK-3475) in patients with microsatellite unstable (MSI) tumors. J Clin Oncol 2014;32:5s:(suppl; abstr TPS3128).

[86] Luis A, Diaz DTL, Yoshino T, Andre T, Bendell JC, Zhang Y, Lam B, Koshiji M, Jäge D. KEYNOTE-177: first-line, open-label, randomized, phase III study of pembrolizumab (MK-3475) versus investigator-choice chemotherapy for mismatch repair deficient or microsatellite instability-high metastatic colorectal carcinoma. J Clin Oncol. 2016;34:(suppl 4S; abstr TPS789).

[87] Herbst R, Gordon MS, Fine G, Sosman J, Soria J, Hamid O, et al. A study of MPDL3280A, an engineered PD-L1 antibody in patients with locally advanced or metastatic tumors. J Clin Oncol (Meeting Abstracts) May 2013;31(15_suppl 3000).

[88] Bendell J, Powderly JD, Lieu C, Eckhardt SG, Hurwitz H, Hochster H, et al. Safety and efficacy of MPDL3280A (anti-PDL1) in combination with bevacizumab (bev) and/or FOLFOX in patients (pts) with metastatic colorectal cancer (mCRC). Journal of Clinical Oncology, 2015 Gastrointestinal Cancers Symposium (January 15-17, 2015);33(3_suppl) (January 20 Supplement), 2015: 704.

[89] Brahmer JR, Tykodi SS, Chow LQM, Hwu W-J, Topalian SL, Hwu P, et al. Safety and activity of anti–PD-L1 antibody in patients with advanced cancer. N Engl J Med. 2012;366(26):2455–2465.

[90] Chung KY, Gore I, Fong L, Venook A, Beck SB, Dorazio P, et al. Phase II study of the anti-cytotoxic T-lymphocyte-associated antigen 4 monoclonal antibody, tremelimumab, in patients with refractory metastatic colorectal cancer. J Clin Oncol. 2010;28(21): 3485.

[91] Llosa NJ, Cruise M, Tam A, Wicks EC, Hechenbleikner EM, Taube JM, et al. The vigorous immune microenvironment of microsatellite instable colon cancer is balanced by multiple counter-inhibitory checkpoints. Cancer Discov. 2015;5(1):43–51.

[92] Markman JL, Shiao SL. Impact of the immune system and immunotherapy in colorectal cancer. J Gastrointestinal Oncol. 2014;6(2):208–223.

Chapter 16

New Chemotherapeutic Agents: Monoterpenes and Fatty Acid Synthase Inhibitors

Soichiro Murata

Additional information is available at the end of the chapter

http://dx.doi.org/10.5772/62283

Abstract

Colorectal cancer (CRC) is one of the most common cancers in the world. Around 90% of CRC deaths are caused by metastasis, and systemic chemotherapy is the last hope for patients with unresectable metastases of CRC. Although recent systemic chemotherapy advances have prolonged survival in patients with unresectable CRC, the effectiveness, cost, and side effects of the chemotherapeutic agents still need to improve. The use of plant-, microbial-, or fungal-derived natural products for medical benefits is playing an important role globally, such as in anti-cancer drugs and antibiotics.

The cancer cells are different from normal cells in many points. In contrast to normal cells, most of the fatty acids in malignant cells are derived from *de novo* lipogenesis that emphasizes the importance of up-regulation of endogenous lipid biosynthesis in malignant transformation.

Several anti-cancer drugs available on the market today, such as Taxol, Oncovin, Navelbine, and Vumon, trace their origins to plants. Monoterpenes of several essential oils from plants possess medical benefits. Various monoterpenes such as d-limonene, geraniol, 1,8-cineole, and perillyl alcohol (POH) are effective for CRC in in vitro and animal experiments.

Fatty acid synthase (FASN), the key enzyme of *de novo* lipogenesis, is significantly up-regulated in many cancers including CRC. In normal adults, FASN is mainly expressed in cells with lipid metabolisms such as liver and adipose tissues. The expression of FASN has been found to be up-regulated in various human cancer cells including CRC. Lipogenesis by cancer cells provides proliferative and survival advantages and drug resistance against chemotherapeutic agents. Inhibition of lipogenesis targeting FASN induces apoptosis selectively in human cancer cells both in vitro and in vivo. The differential expression of FASN between cancer cells and normal cells makes FASN a suitable target for cancer treatment. The pharmacological FASN inhibitors are cerulenin, C75, C93, orlistat, luteolin, epigallocatechin-3-gallate (EGCG), triclosan, capsaicin, curcumin, and so on.

In this chapter, we discuss the usefulness of monoterpenes and FASN inhibitors against CRC for the novel chemotherapeutic agents.

Keywords: fatty acid synthase inhibitor, monoterpene, colorectal cancer, chemotherapy, cerulenin

1. Introduction

Colorectal cancer (CRC) is one of the most common cancers in the world, and about 90% of CRC deaths are caused by metastasis, not by primary solid tumors [1]. Despite recent advances, systemic chemotherapy for metastatic disease is considered palliative, and long-term survivors are rarely seen treated only by chemotherapy [2]. Natural products are the most successful strategy to discover new agents used in anti-cancer therapy and more than two-thirds of the drugs used in cancer treatment [3]. A large number of studies have focused on the efficacy of essential oils and their chemical constituents as bioactive new products [4], especially cancer treatment [5, 6]. The essential oils are a mixture of volatile lipophilic substances: monoterpenes, sesquiterpenes, and phenylpropanoids. These substances have many biological activities such as analgesic, anti-convulsant, anti-inflammatory [6, 7, 9], and anti-tumor activities [10–14]. Monoterpenes of several essential oils from plants possess medical benefits. The various monoterpenes, such as limonene, geraniol, 1,8-cineole, and perillyl alcohol (POH), are effective for CRC in in vitro and animal experiments [15].

2. Monoterpenes

Terpenes are the largest class of plant-derived secondary metabolites, and they are the main component of essential oils [16, 17]. Monoterpenes are the largest class of terpenes [18]. The therapeutic properties of monoterpenes are anti-allergic, anti-inflammatory, anti-cancer, and so on [19]. The basic structure of monoterpenes consists of two isoprene units $(C5H8)_2$. Monoterpenes exist in many forms in nature, such as hydrocarbons, alcohols and their glycosides, ethers, aldehydes, ketones, carboxylic acids, and esters [15]. Monoterpenes are classified as acyclic, monocyclic, and bicyclic according to the ring formation. The important acyclic monoterpenes, which have anti-tumor effects, are myrcene and geraniol [20]. The important monocyclic monoterpenes with anti-tumor effects are linalyl acetate, camphor, thymol, carvacrol, POH, d-limonene, and many others. POH and d-limonene are said to inhibit the development of several types of carcinomas as they were in Phase I and II clinical testing, respectively [21, 22]. The bicyclic monoterpenes that have anti-tumor effects are 1,8-cineole (eucalyptol), and α- and β-pinene [23, 24].

3. Monoterpene and colorectal cancer

In this chapter, we reviewed monoterpenes with anti-CRC activity. The monoterpenes presented in this chapter were selected with reference to effects shown in specific experimental models for evaluation of anti-tumor activity and/or by complementary studies aimed to elucidate mechanisms of action shown in **Table 1**.

Compound	**Mechanism**	**Animal/cell line tested**	**IC50, etc**	**Reference**
Acyclic				
Geraniol	Cell cycle arrest/5FU synergy	Caco-2	200 μM (Caco-2 IC30)	[26]
	Cell cycle arrest	Caco-2	400 μM(70% inhibition)	[27]
	ERK1/2 inactivation	Caco-2	400 μM(60% reduction of PKC activity)	[28]
	Synergistic with 5FU	TC-118/Swiss nu/nu mouse	5FU 20 mg/kg, geraniol 150 mg/kg	[29]
	Thymidylate synthase reduction		53% tumor reduction	
Monocyclic				
Alpha terpineol	Cell cycle arrest, apoptosis	HCT-116 (p53+/+, −/−)	1 mM	[30]
Linalyl acetate			Alpha terpineol + linalyl acetate + camphor	
Camphor				
Carvacrol	Anti-oxidant activity	Caco-2, K562, HepG2	150–200 μM (IC50 of K562)	[31, 32]
	Cytotoxic effect	Caco-2	600 μM (IC50)	[34]
	Anti-oxidant activity	DMH/DSS carcinogenesis rat	50 mg/kg	[35]
Thymol	Cytotoxic effect	Caco-2	700 μM (IC 50))	[34]
	Apoptosis	HL60	75 μM(12 h), 50 μM(24 h)	[36]
Thymoquinone (TQ)	Apoptosis, Wnt signal	Apc^{Min} rat	375 mg/kg BW 12 w (polyp decrease)	[38]
	Apoptosis	HCT-116 xenograft	5 mg/kg (3 times/week ip)	[39]
	ERK JNK, apoptosis by ROS	Caco-2	15.0 μM (IC50 24 h)	[40]
		HCT-116	30 μM (IC50 24 h)	
		LoVo	38 μM (IC50 24 h)	[40]
		DLD-1	42 μM (IC50 24 h)	

Compound	Mechanism	Animal/cell line tested	IC50, etc	Reference
		HT-29	110 μM (IC50 48 h)	
	Nanoparticle with poly(sodium *N*-undecylenyl-valinate)	MDA-MB-231	viability 16.0 ± 5.6%(96 h)	[41]
	Protection from Doxorubicin	Mouse with DOX(20 mg/kg)	TQ (8 mg/kg p.o.) protect cardiotoxicity	[42]
	Synergistic with Doxorubicin	HT-29	46.8 μM to 39.0 μM (with DOX)	[43]
D-limonene	Blood orange volatile	SW480, HT-29	100 ppm, 74.2% reduction of SW480	[44]
	Ornithine decarboxylase (ODC)	Azoxymethane, F344 rat	0.5% d-limonene decreases ACF formation	[45]
	Apoptosis by Akt inactivation	colon cancer (LS174T)	3.2 mM viability 30% decrease	[46]
	Clinical trial phase I and II	CRC patients	0.5 mg/m^2/day	[47, 48]
Perillyl alcohol	Protein isoprenylation	HT-29	50 μM (IC50)	[49]
	Apoptosis	Azoxymethane	2 g/kg decrease cancer incidence to 1/3	[50]
	G1 arrest	HCT-116	0.5 mM (IC50)	[51]
	Clinical trial	CRC patients	1200–1600 mg/m^2/day	[52–56]
Bicyclic				
1,8-cineole	Akt inactivation	RKO	50 mg/kg reduced tumor weight as 1/3	[24]

Table 1. Monoterpene and colorectal cancer.

3.1. Geraniol

Geraniol is an acyclic monoterpenes. Geraniol is one of the main components of geranium oil, and its content is about 20% [25]. Geraniol shows a cytotoxic effect in Caco-2 colon cancer cells [26–28]. Geraniol decreases the expression of p44/p42 ERK and has an anti-tumor effect in Caco-2 cells [28]. In addition, geraniol has a synergistic anti-tumor effect combined with 5-fluorouracil in TC-118 human colorectal tumors [29].

3.2. Alpha terpineol, linalyl acetate, and camphor

Alpha terpineol, linalyl acetate, and camphor are monocyclic monoterpenes, and they are the bioactive components of Lebanese sage (*Salvia libanotica*) essential oil [30]. Linalyl acetate is found in many flowers and spice plants. Camphor is found in the wood of the camphor laurel.

http://dx.doi.org/10.5772/62283

These three components cause inhibition of the growth of the human colon cancer cell lines (HCT-116 p53+/+ and p53−/−) and were inactive on FHs74 Int normal human intestinal cell lines [30]. It has been demonstrated that alpha terpineol, linalyl acetate, and camphor synergize to induce cell cycle arrest and apoptosis, mainly through mitochondrial damage (cytochrome c release), caspase activation, and PARP cleavage in human CRC cells [30].

3.3. Carvacrol

Carvacrol is a monocyclic monoterpene constituent of essential oils produced from the aromatic plant *Oreganum vulgarea* sp. Carvacrol has a cytotoxic effect in K562, HepG2, and Caco-2 cells [31, 32]. It inhibits the proliferation and migration of the two-colon cancer cell lines HCT-116 and LoVo. Cell invasion was suppressed after carvacrol treatment by decreasing the expression of matrix metalloprotease-2 (MMP-2) and MMP-9. Carvacrol treatment also caused cell cycle arrest in the G2/M phase and decreased cyclin B1 expression. Finally, carvacrol-induced cell apoptosis in a dose-dependent manner [33]. Carvacrol promotes the endogenous anti-oxidant system and suppresses inflammation in DMH/DSS-induced rats and reduces the tumor formation of colitis-associated CRC [34].

3.4. Thymol

Thymol is a monocyclic monoterpene and can be found in the oil of thyme. Thymol presents a cytotoxic effect in several cell lines, such as HepG2, V79, and Caco-2 human colon cancer cells [35]. The cytotoxic effect of thymol on human leukemia cell HL-60 appears to be associated with induction of cell cycle arrest at sub G0/G1 phase and apoptotic cell death. Thymol induced apoptosis in HL-60 cells involves both caspase-dependent and caspase-independent pathways [36].

3.5. Thymoquinone

Thymoquinone (2-methyl-5-isopropyl-1,4-benzoquinone) is a monocyclic monoterpene present in the seed oil of the plant *Nigella sativa* L. (Renunculaceae family), commonly known as black cumin or black seed that is widely consumed as a condiment in many societies [37]. Thymoquinone possesses anti-proliferative and pro-apoptotic activities in several cancer cell lines [37]. Thymoquinone decreased the number of large polyps in the intestine, activated GSK-3-β, increased membrane localization of β-catenin, and reduced nuclear expression of c-myc in in vivo experiments of Apc^{Min+} mice [38]. Thymoquinone reduced the size of xenograft tumors, induced apoptosis, and inhibited tumor cell proliferation in HCT-116 human colon cancer cell xenograft tumor growth in NMRI mice [39]. Reactive oxygen species and activation of ERK and JNK signaling were involved in thymoquinone-induced apoptosis in a panel of human colon cancer cells (Caco-2, HCT-116, LoVo, DLD-1, and HT-29) [40]. Encapsulation of thymoquinone into nanoparticles enhances the anti-proliferative effect in HT-29 cells [41]. Thymoquinone boosted the effect of doxorubicin by reducing its cardiotoxicity in several cancer cell lines including the CRC cell line HT29 [42, 43].

3.6. D-limonene

Limonene is a monocyclic monoterpene, and it is a major constituent of citrus oils. It has optical isomers, d-limonene and l-limonene, and d-limonene has a more lemon-like odor and therapeutic effects. D-limonene is contained in citrus volatile oil, and the citrus volatile oil induces apoptosis and has an anti-angiogenic effect against colon cancer SW480 and HT-29 [44]. D-limonene also inhibited the development of colonic aberrant crypt foci (ACF) induced by azoxymethane in F344 rats, which suggests that this monoterpenoid might be a chemopreventive agent for colonic carcinogenesis in rats [45]. D-limonene suppressed the viability of LS174T colon cancer cells in a dose-dependent manner and caused a dose-dependent apoptotic cell death. D-limonene decreased the levels of Akt pathway, activated caspase-3 and caspase-9 and PARP cleavage in a dose-dependent manner [46]. A group of 32 patients with solid tumors registered and completed Phase I study of administration of d-limonene orally. The maximum tolerated dose was 8 g/m^2 per day, and nausea, vomiting, and diarrhea were dose-limiting factors [47]. Three individuals with colorectal carcinoma with d-limonene suspended progression of the disease for over 6 months [47]. D-limonene at a dosage of 0.5 g/m^2/day was able to halt progression of cancer for 9 months in a patient diagnosed with locally advanced mucinous cystadenocarcinoma of the appendix. A patient with presacral recurrence of an adenocarcinoma in the sigmoid colon experienced a minor reduction (<50%) in tumor size at a dose of 0.5 g/m^2/day for 12 months. Another patient with local retrovesical recurrence of colorectal adenocarcinoma remained stabilized on 1 g/m^2/day (2 g/day) for 7.5 months [47, 48].

3.7. Perillyl alcohol (POH)

POH is a monocyclic monoterpene, and it is derived from limonene. POH is a naturally occurring dietary monoterpene isolated from the essential oils of lavender, peppermint, and other plants. It has an anti-tumor effect in several cancer cell lines including the HT-29 colon cancer cell line [49]. Dietary POH at 1 or 2 g/kg greatly reduced the incidence and the number of invasive adenocarcinomas of the colon of rats injected with azoxymethane [50]. To establish the molecular mechanisms of POH, cell cycle and cell cycle regulatory proteins were studied in HCT-116 human colon cancer cells. POH exerted a dose-dependent inhibitory effect on cell growth correlated with a G1 arrest [51]. Phase I and II clinical trials using POH were started [21, 22, 52–55]. In seven Phase I clinical trials, POH was administered orally to cancer patients with advanced malignancy. POH was given in divided doses ranging from 2,400 to 16,200 mg per day (equivalent to approximately 40–270 mg/kg). Treatment duration varied with each patient but was generally between 2 and 9 months. Nausea, vomiting, eructation, and satiety were dose-limiting factors in several of these trials [21]. Meadows et al. conducted Phase II study in patients with metastatic CRC [56]. The authors found that oral POH administration did not have clinical anti-tumor activity when used for patients with advanced colorectal carcinoma, despite preclinical evidence of anti-cancer activity. Instead of oral administration, POH was administered through nasal inhalation to recurrent glioma patients, and these studies not only demonstrated clinical activity of POH but also revealed that long-term intranasal inhalation of the compound was very well tolerated over several years of daily use [21, 57, 58].

http://dx.doi.org/10.5772/62283

3.8. 1,8-cineole (eucalyptol)

1,8-cineole (eucalyptol) is a bicyclic monoterpene, which comprises up to 90% of the essential oil of some species of the generic product Eucalyptus oil. 1,8-cineole has several effects such as anti-inflammatory, anti-oxidant, and anti-atherosclerotic activity in vitro and in vivo. 1,8-cineole has a cytotoxic effect in Hep G2, HeLa, MOLT-4, K-562, and CTVR-1 cell lines [59]. 1,8-cineole was reported to have moderate anti-oxidant and cytotoxic properties and pronounced analgesic and anti-tumor activity [60]. Murata et al. showed that the human CRC cell line RKO expressed phosphoserine 473-Akt constitutively and treatment with 1,8-cineole dephosphorylated Akt. 1,8-cineole treatment activated p38 and dephosphorylated Akt, which induced caspase-3 cleavage and resultant cleavage of PARP and finally caused apoptosis. In a xenograft mouse model, 1,8-cineole therapy showed tumor shrinkage [24].

3.9. α- and β-pinene

α- and β-pinene are bicyclic monoterpenes. They are natural compounds isolated from pine needle oil. Bhattacharjee and Chatterjee [61] promoted the identification of proapoptotic, anti-inflammatory, anti-proliferative, anti-invasive, and potential anti-angiogenic activities of α-pinene, β-pinene, d-limonene, and geraniol by employing a dual reverse virtual screening protocol. The anti-tumor activity of α-pinene on the BEL-7402 hepatoma cell line in vitro and in vivo and the mechanisms involved were investigated. The results showed that liver cancer cell growth was inhibited obviously in vitro and in vivo: Chk1 and Chk2 levels were up-regulated; and Cyclin B, CDC25, and CDK1 levels were down-regulated [62].

3.10. Conclusion of monoterpenes

Several studies have shown in vitro and in vivo anti-tumor activity of monoterpenes derived from many essential oils obtained from plants. This chapter shows that many monoterpenes are being examined for in vitro and in vivo anti-tumor activity of CRC. In addition, two of the monoterpenes, d-limonene and POH, were moved on to Phase I and II clinical trials, which indicates the safety of monoterpenes for clinical use. There are many monoterpenes that show anti-tumor effects in vitro and in vivo, and with additional research some monoterpenes act to inhibit the proliferation and to induce tumor cell death in clinical use.

4. Fatty acid synthase (FASN) inhibitors

Fatty acid synthase (FASN), the key enzyme of *de novo* lipogenesis, is significantly up-regulated in many cancers including CRC [63, 64]. In normal adults, FASN is mainly expressed in cells with lipid metabolisms, such as liver and adipose tissues [65]. Under a usual diet, the *de novo* fatty acid synthesis in normal cells is rarely needed and the FASN protein level is low [66]. FASN is a 270-kDa cytosolic enzyme containing seven catalytic domains [67]. FASN synthesizes palmitate from one acetyl-CoA, seven malonyl-CoAs, and seven NADPHs [65, 66]. The expression of FASN has been found to be up-regulated in various human cancer cells including

CRC [68–70]. FASN is elevated in ACF compared with normal colonic mucosa [71]. Lipogenesis by cancer cells gives proliferative and survival advantages and drug resistance against chemotherapeutic drugs [72]. An increased expression of lipogenic enzymes is associated with a more aggressive metastatic phenotype in CRC [73]. Inhibition of lipogenesis targeting FASN induces apoptosis selectively in human cancer cells both in vitro and in vivo [74–76]. The differential expression of FASN, together with the different responses to FASN inhibition between cancer cells and normal cells, makes FASN a suitable target for cancer treatment. The pharmacological FASN inhibitors are cerulenin, C75, C93, orlistat, luteolin, and epigallocatechin-3-gallate (EGCG). Triclosan [77], capsaicin [78], and curcumin [79] are reported to inhibit FASN and have anti-tumor effect. There are several newly developed agents, such as TVB-3567 [80], TVB-3166 [81], and GSK2194069 [82].

Compound	Mechanism	Animal/cell line tested	IC50, etc	Reference
Cerulenin	Akt inhibition	Colon 26 liver metastasis/Balb-c mouse	30 mg/kg reduces 50% of liver metastasis	[93]
	Akt inhibition, synergistic with oxaliplatin	RKO/xenograft in SCID mouse	Cerulenin 15 mg/kg, oxaliplatin 2.5 mg/kg	[94]
	Malonyl-co A independent apoptosis	RKO	10 μg/ml	[101]
C75	Malonyl-co A independent apoptosis	RKO	10 μg/ml	[101]
Orlistat	ER stress, synergistic with thapsigargin	HT-29	Orlistat 25 μM, thapsigargin 25 nM	[114]
Luteolin	Cell cycle arrest, apoptosis	HT-29	60 μM 83% decrease of survival at 72 h	[121]
	S1P, ceramide, Akt inhibition	Caco-2	100 μM more than 50% decrease at 48 h	[122]
	Synergic effect with aspirin	DMH rat carcinogenesis	0.2 mg/kg/weekly for 15 weeks	[123]
	iNOS, COX2 inhibition	Mouse, azoxymethane administration	1.2 mg/kg orally	[124]
	β-catenin, GSK-3-β, cyclin D1 inhibition	HCT-15	100 μM (IC50)	[125]
EGCG	Cell proliferation, apoptosis	HCT-116	100 μM 98.4% decrease of survival at 48 h	[131]
	VEGF/VEGFR axis	SW837 mouse xenograft	0.01% EGCG drinking	[133]
	HES1, Notch 2	HT-29 mouse xenograft	5 mg/kg intragastrically	[135]
	Clinical trials	Polyp relapse decreasing	1.5~2.5 g green tea extract/daily	[137]

Table 2. FASN inhibitors and colorectal cancer.

In this chapter, we reviewed FASN inhibitors with anti-CRC activity. The FASN inhibitors presented in this chapter were selected with reference to effects shown in specific experimental models for evaluation of anti-tumor activity and/or by complementary studies aimed to elucidate mechanisms of action shown in **Table 2**.

4.1. Cerulenin

Cerulenin is the first-known FASN inhibitor, which is isolated from the culture filtrate of the fungus *Cephalosporum caerulens* [83–86]. It was originally used as an anti-fungal antibiotic and is a potent non-competitive irreversible inhibitor of FASN by binding to the active site of the KS domain [87–89]. Cerulenin treatment significantly decreases fatty acid synthesis and induces selective cytotoxicity in various types of cancer cells [90–92]. Murata et al. [93] revealed the anti-tumor activities of cerulenin in murine colon cancer cell lines Colon 26 and CMT 93. Shiragami et al. [94] evaluated the anti-tumor effect of cerulenin in human CRC cell lines HCT-116 and RKO. The overexpression of FASN has been seen to cooperate with survival pathways, including the phosphatidylinositol-3-kinase (PI3K)/Akt pathway. CRC cell lines expressed FASN and phosphorylated Akt constitutively, and the treatment of CRC cells with cerulenin suppressed FASN expression, dephosphorylated constitutive activated Akt, and increased cleaved caspase-3 in murine CRC cell lines Colon 26 and CMT 93, and in human CRC cell line HCT-116 and RKO cells [93, 94]. FASN has a major role in the synthesis of phospholipids including phosphatidylinositol trisphosphate (PIP3) [95]. PIP3 binds to Akt and activates kinase phosphoinositide-dependent protein kinase-1 (PDK-1) with high affinity, and the phosphorylation of Akt is dependent on PIP3 [95]. In an in vivo experiment, Murata et al. [93] evaluated the potential effectiveness of cerulenin for metastatic liver tumors of the CRC cell line. Shiragami et al. [94] revealed the synergistic effect of cerulenin in combination with oxaliplatin, which means that reduction is possible when combined with cerulenin in the CRC treatment. Recently, Chang et al. revealed cerulenin down-regulated energy metabolism and PI3K/Akt/mTOR signaling pathway using human CRC cell lines HT-29 and LoVo [96]. Bauerschlag et al. [97] revealed that relative to normal fallopian tube tissue, ovarian cancer tissue had 1.8-fold FASN overexpression and cell lines had around 100-fold protein overexpression. In the ovarian cancer cell lines, cerulenin markedly decreased FASN expression and cell viability and induced apoptosis. Unlike concomitant administration, sequential cerulenin/cisplatin treatment reduced cisplatin's half-maximal inhibitory concentration up to 54% in a cisplatin-resistant cell line [97].

4.2. C75

C75 is a cerulenin-derived, semi-synthetic FASN inhibitor lacking cerulenin' s reactive epoxy group [98], and C75 is more chemically stable than cerulenin [98]. C75 has significant anti-tumor effects against many types of cancer cells, such as the human breast [98], prostate [91], and ovary [99] as well as renal carcinoma in xenograft animal models [100]. Li et al. reported that both C75 and cerulenin produce rapid, potent inhibition of DNA replication and S-phase progression in human cancer cells, as well as apoptotic death. They also revealed that these

FASN inhibitors reduce cyclin A-, B1-associated kinase activities, and p53, p21 accumulation which cause growth arrest at G1 and G2 [101]. Cerulenin and C75 were useful against p53 mutations [101]. They discussed that accumulation of malonyl-CoA was independent of apoptosis induction, and they estimated that the effect of these agents has resulted from product depletion [101].

4.3. C93

In addition to inhibiting FASN, C75 stimulates fatty acid oxidation by activating carnitine *O*-palmitoyltransferase-1 (CPT1) [102]. Activation of CPT1 contributes to the reduction of neuropeptide Y expression in the hypothalamus [102, 103]. The limiting toxicity of C75 is due to this stimulation of fatty acid oxidation rather than the inhibition of FASN. C93, which was designed to specifically inhibit FAS without affecting CPT1 activity [104]. Orita et al. revealed that C93 inhibited FASN of four human lung cancer cell lines: LX7, H1975, H460, and A549. Moreover, C93 inhibited subcutaneous and orthotopic H460 xenograft tumor without causing anorexia and weight loss in the treated animals [105]. They found that higher levels of FAS expression were observed in 77% of the squamous cancers, 96% of the adenocarcinomas, and 94% of Barrett's lesions with high-grade dysplasia, when compared with the levels in normal esophageal epithelium and non-dysplastic Barrett's mucosa. Mice with Colo680N esophageal squamous cell carcinoma cell xenograft were treated C93, which significantly inhibited the growth of orthotopic xenograft tumors without causing anorexia and weight loss in the treated animals [106].

4.4. Orlistat

Orlistat is an anti-obesity drug approved by the US Food and Drug Administration. Orlistat is also reported to inhibit FASN [107]. Orlistat is the only long-term option for obesity treatment in the United States, and it is the only approved weightloss drug in Europe [108]. Orlistat is a synthetic hydrogenated derivative of lipstatin, produced by the fungus *Streptomyces toxytricini* [109]. It partially inhibits gastric lipase, pancreatic lipase, and carboxyl ester lipase enzymes that work by hydrolyzing the dietary triglycerides into fatty acids and monoglycerides, which are absorbed by the mucosa of the gastrointestinal tract [110]. Orlistat reduces the absorption of ingested fat and increasing its excretion in the feces [111]. The main anti-obesity action of orlistat is in helping to reduce caloric intake in individuals [112]. Orlistat also helps individuals to reduce the fat content of their diet, as diets rich in fatty products will lead to more adverse effects, such as diarrhea and fecal incontinence [108, 112]. Several studies have shown that orlistat exhibits anti-tumor effects in many cancer cells including human CRC cell line HT-29 in vitro and in vivo by inhibiting FASN activity [107, 113–115]. Treatment of tumor cells with orlistat-induced ER stress, which is further confirmed by the increased expression of the ER stress–regulated genes CHOP, ATF4, and GRP78. FAS inhibitors cooperate with the ER stress inducer thapsigargin to enhance tumor cell killing. These results provide the first evidence that FASN inhibitors induce ER stress and establish an important mechanistic link between FASN activity and ER function [114]. Yang et al. revealed that orlistat induced an ATF4-

dependent transcriptional induction of REDD1 (also known as Rtp801 or DDIT4), a known mTOR inhibitor and works as a novel caspase-2 regulator in the ovarian cancer. REDD1 positively controls caspase-2-dependent cell death of ovarian cancer cells by inhibiting mTOR, and this is the main pathway of orlistat-induced cell death in ovarian cancer [116]. Agostini et al. revealed that orlistat inhibited the orthotopic tongue squamous cell carcinoma in the BALB/c nude mice. In in vivo experiment, the drug was able to decrease both the volume and proliferation indexes of the tongue orthotopic tumors and, importantly, reduced the number of metastatic cervical lymph nodes by 43% [117].

4.5. Luteolin

Luteolin, 3′,4′,5,7-tetrahydroxyflavone, is found in a variety of vegetables, fruits, and medicinal herbs. Luteolin has been shown to function as an anti-oxidant, anti-inflammatory, and anti-cancer agent [118]. Additionally, luteolin induces cell cycle arrest and apoptosis in the liver and lung cancer cell lines [119, 120]. Lim do et al. indicated that luteolin inhibited HT-29 cell proliferation by inducing cell cycle arrest and apoptosis [121]. Luteolin exerts toxic effects on colon cancer cells by inhibiting both S1P biosynthesis and ceramide traffic, inhibiting Akt activation [122]. The supplementations of luteolin in addition to aspirin in the treatment of DMH-induced carcinogenesis in rats reflect a better effect than the use of aspirin alone [123]. Luteolin suppresses both iNOS and COX-2 expressions and plays an anti-inflammatory role during the administration of azoxymethane in mice [124]. Luteolin decreased the expressions of β-catenin, phospho GSK-3-β, and cyclin D in HCT-15 cells. Luteolin also promoted cell cycle arrest at the G2/M phase and induced apoptosis in HCT-15 cells. Furthermore, Western blot analysis showed that luteolin treatment enhanced the expression of Bax and caspase-3, whereas the expression of Bcl-2 was suppressed [125].

4.6. Epigallocatechin gallate (EGCG)

EGCG, which is green tea polyphenol, inhibits the activity of FASN [126, 127]. EGCG induces apoptosis in human breast and prostate cancer cells [128–130]. It is also the major biologically active component that inhibits cell proliferation and induces apoptosis in HCT-116 and SW-480 human CRC cells [131]. EGCG suppresses FASN expression and downstream PI3K/Akt pathway [132]. EGCG activates stress signals, such as c-Jun N-terminal kinase (JNK) and p38 mitogen-activated protein kinase (MAPK), and induces apoptosis in CRC cell lines [131]. EGCG has also been reported to inhibit the growth of human CRC cells in subcutaneous xenograft models [133–135]. Maruyama et al. revealed that EGCG strongly reduces liver metastasis of human CRC in SCID mice [136].

Epidemiologically, green tea consumption of >10 cups daily reduced CRC risk in Japanese [137]. A double-blind, placebo-controlled study with green tea in Italian patients showed a successful prevention of prostate cancer. The progression of prostate cancer in men with high-grade prostate intraepithelial neoplasia, the main premalignant lesion of prostate cancer, was significantly prevented by oral administration of green tea catechins, 600 mg/d for 1 year [138]. Shimizu et al. conducted a randomized trial to determine the preventive effect of green tea extract (GTE) supplements on metachronous colorectal adenomas by raising green tea consumption in the target population from an average of 6 cups (1.5 g GTE) daily to 10 cups equivalent (2.5 g GTE) by supplemental GTE tablets. To 136 patients with colorectal polyp resection, they performed colonoscopy to confirm no polyps in the colorectum 1 year later. Then they randomized into two groups, i.e., GTE group and control group. The incidence of metachronous adenomas at the endpoint colonoscopy was 31% (20 of 65) in the control group and 15% (9 of 60) in the GTE group (relative risk, 0.49; 95% confidence interval, 0.24–0.99; $P < 0.05$). The size of relapsed adenomas was also smaller in the GTE group than in the control group ($P < 0.001$). No serious adverse events occurred in the GTE group. They concluded that GTE is an effective supplement for the chemoprevention of metachronous colorectal adenomas [137]. The multicenter RCT trial to investigate EGCG for reducing colon polyp recurrence in elderly people was performed, which was called minimizing the risk of metachronous adenomas of the colorectum with GTE (MIRACLE). The clinical trial was a randomized, placebo-controlled, multicenter trial to investigate the effect of diet supplementation with GTE containing 300 mg of EGCG on the recurrence of colon adenomas. Patients who had undergone polypectomy for colonic polyps were randomized to receive either GTE containing 150 mg of EGCG two times daily or a placebo over the course of 3 years. Incidence, number, and histology of adenoma at endpoint colonoscopy at 3 years will be compared in both groups [139].

4.7. Triclosan

Triclosan has the U.S. Food and Drug Administration approval as a bactericide in personal hygiene products (toothpaste, mouth rinse, hand wash, soaps, and deodorant) and has been used since 1968 [77]. Triclosan has an established safety profile with minimal toxicity in rats, dogs, baboons, and humans; no significant weight loss is associated with triclosan treatment; and triclosan is not a genotoxic or mutagenic compound [77]. Triclosan has excellent oral bioavailability and stability in plasma [140]. Triclosan also acts as a FASN inhibitor to inhibit enoyl reductase of FASN [141], and it showed chemo-preventative activity in a rat mammary carcinogenesis model [142]. Similarly, treatment of male rats with triclosan did not induce significant changes in body weight at any of the test doses [143]. Recently, Sadowski et al. evaluated triclosan as a repurposed drug against prostate cancer cells and compared its activity to C75 and orlistat, two well-known FASN inhibitors [77, 144]. In this comparative study, Sadowski et al. discovered that triclosan is a superior alternative to C75 and orlistat in inducing cell death of prostate cancer cells through inhibition of FASN [77].

4.8. Capsaicin

Capsaicin (trans-8-methyl-*N*-vanillyl-6-non-enamide) is the major component in hot chili peppers and several types of red peppers of the genus *Capsicum*. It constitutes approximately 40–60% of the six natural capsaiciniod contents of this herb [145, 146]. It is commonly and frequently consumed worldwide as a spice, food additive, and as a drug for traditional medications. Capsaicin is a specific and potent anti-carcinogenic agent through the apoptosis pathway in both in vitro and in vivo cancer models, whereas it does not induce cytotoxicity in normal cells [147–151]. Impheng et al. revealed that capsaicin also acts as FASN inhibitor [78]. Capsaicin decreased FASN expression and inducing apoptosis in HepG2 cells. The lipogenic enzyme FASN, not ACC and ACLY, is proposed to be the particular target of capsaicin to induce apoptosis in HepG2 cells. This study also suggests that an accumulation of malonyl-CoA, as a result of a reduction of fatty acid synthesis, is a critical proapoptotic factor that inhibits CPT-1 activity, leading to accumulation of ceramide which in turn induces apoptosis [78].

4.9. Curcumin

Curcumin is a hydrophobic polyphenol derived from the rhizome of *Curcuma longa*. It possesses various pharmacological activities, such as respiratory conditions, inflammation, liver disorders, diabetic wounds, and certain tumors [152]. Curcumin has chemopreventive and therapeutic properties against many tumors in both in vitro and in vivo models [153–158]. Curcumin suppresses cell proliferation and inflammation, induces apoptosis, and sensitizes tumor cells to cancer therapies, and it also suppresses invasion, angiogenesis, and metastasis of cancer cells [159]. It was found that curcumin showed both fast-binding and slow-binding inhibitions to FASN in vitro. Curcumin inhibited FASN with an IC50 value of 10.5 μg/ml non-competitively with respect to NADPH and partially competitively against both substrates Ac-CoA and Mal-CoA [160]. Compared with the known FASN inhibitors14, C75 and EGCG, curcumin was generally more potent [126]. Curcumin-induced HepG2 cell apoptosis by inhibiting intracellular FASN activity and down-regulating FASN expression and mRNA level. Sodium palmitate-rescued, curcumin-induced apoptosis in HepG2 cells confirmed that apoptosis related to inhibition of FASN [79].

4.10. Newly developed agents

TVB-3567 [80] and TVB-3166 [81] are newly developed FASN inhibitors provided from 3-V Biosciences, which inhibit many kinds of cancer cell lines, such as CRC cell lines, COLO-205, and HT-29 [81]. GSK2194069 was identified from a high-throughput screen of the GSK compound collection, and this agent inhibits cell growth of A549 cells [82].

4.11. Conclusion of FASN inhibitors

Several studies have shown in vitro and in vivo anti-tumor activity of FASN inhibitors. This chapter shows that many FASN inhibitors are being examined for in vitro and in vivo anti-tumor activity of CRC. In addition, one of the FASN inhibitors, EGCG, has moved on to clinical trials aimed at preventing Colon polyp recurrence, which indicates the safety of monoterpenes for clinical use. Other FASN inhibitors are effective in in vitro/in vivo researches, and the clinical trials of using these reagents are expected, but still need more research. Newly developed agents, such as TVB-3166, TVB-3567, and GSK2194069, are expected to become new candidates for chemotherapeutic agents against unresectable cancers.

Author details

Soichiro Murata

Address all correspondence to: soichiro@yokohama-cu.ac.jp

Department of Regenerative Medicine, Yokohama City University, Yokohama, Japan

References

[1] Gupta GP and Massague J. Cancer metastasis: building a framework. Cell 127: 679–695, 2006.

[2] Tachimori A, Yamada N, Amano R, et al. Combination therapy of S-1 with selective cyclooxygenase-2 inhibitor for liver metastasis of colorectal carcinoma. Anticancer Res 28: 629–638, 2008.

[3] Efferth T. Cancer therapy with natural products and medicinal plants. Planta Medica 76: 1035–1036, 2010.

[4] De Sousa DP. Medicinal Essential Oils: Chemical, Pharmacological and Therapeutic Aspects. 1st edition. New York, NY: Nova Science Publishers, 2012.

[5] Rasoanaivo P, Randriana RF, Maggi F, et al. Chemical composition and biological activities of the essential oil of *Athanasia brownie* Hochr. (Asteraceae) endemic to Madagascar. Chem Biodivers 10: 1876–1886, 2013.

[6] Zapata B, Betancur LG, Duran C, and Stashenko E. Cytotoxic activity of Asteraceae and Verbenaceae family essential oils. J Essential Oil Res 6: 50–57, 2014.

[7] de Sousa DP. Analgesic-like activity of essential oils constituents. Molecules 16: 2233–2252, 2011.

[8] de Almeida RN, de Fátima Agra M, Maior FNS, and de Sousa DP. Essential oils and their constituents: anticonvulsant activity. Molecules 16: 2726–2742, 2011.

[9] da Silveira e SáRita de Cássia, Nalone AndradeLuciana, de OliveiraRafael dos Reis Barreto, and de SousaDamião Pergentino. A review on anti-inflammatory activity of phenylpropanoids found in essential oils. Molecules 19: 1459–1480, 2014.

[10] Su YC, and Ho CL. Composition, in-vitro anticancer, and antimicrobial activities of the leaf essential oil of Machilus mushaensis from Taiwan. Nat Prod Commun 8: 273–275, 2013.

[11] Manjamalai A, and Grace VMB. The chemotherapeutic effect of essential oil of *Plectranthus amboinicus* (Lour) on lung metastasis developed by B16F-10 cell line in C57BL/6 mice. Cancer Invest 31: 74–82, 2013.

[12] Ashour HM. Antibacterial, antifungal, and anticancer activities of volatile oils and extracts from stems, leaves, and flowers of *Eucalyptus sideroxylon* and *Eucalyptus torquata*. Cancer Biol Therap 7: 399–403, 2008.

[13] Medina-Holguín AL, Holguín FO, Micheletto S, Goehle S, Simon JA, and O'Connell MA. Chemotypic variation of essential oils in the medicinal plant, *Anemopsis californica*. Phytochemistry 69: 919–927, 2008.

[14] Kathirvel P, and Ravi S. Chemical composition of the essential oil from basil (*Ocimum basilicum* Linn.) and its in vitro cytotoxicity against HeLa and HEp-2 human cancer cell lines and NIH 3T3 mouse embryonic fibroblasts. Nat Prod Res 26: 1112–1118, 2012.

[15] Sobral MV, Xavier AL, Lima TC, and de Sousa DP. Antitumor activity of monoterpenes found in essential oils. Sci World J 953451, 2014.

[16] Balcerzak L, Lipok J, Strub D, and Lochyński S. Biotransformations of monoterpenes by photoautotrophic micro-organisms. J Appl Microbiol 117: 1523–1536, 2014.

[17] Velankar HR, and Heble MR. Biotransformation of (L)-citronellal to (L)-citronellol by free and immobilized *Rhodotorula minuta*. Electron J Biotechnol 6: 90–130, 2003.

[18] Gounaris Y. Biotechnology for the production of essential oils, flavours and volatile isolates. A review. Flavour Fragr J. 25: 367–386, 2010.

[19] Schewe H, Mirata MA, Holtmann D, and Schrader J. Biooxidation of monoterpenes with bacterial monooxygenases. Process Biochem 46: 1885–1899, 2011.

[20] Mitić-CulafićD, Zegura B, NikolićB, Vuković-GacićB, Knezević-VukcevićJ, and Filipic M. Protective effect of linalool, myrcene and eucalyptol against t-butyl hydroperoxide induced genotoxicity in bacteria and cultured human cells. Food Chem Toxicol 47: 260–266, 2009.

[21] Chen TC, Da Fonseca CO, and Schönthal AH. Preclinical development and clinical use of perillyl alcohol for chemoprevention and cancer therapy. Am J Cancer Res 5: 1580–1593, 2015.

[22] Wang G, Tang W, and Bidigare RR. Terpenoids as therapeutic drugs and pharmaceutical agents. In: ZhangL, DemainAL (Eds.), Natural Products: Drug Discovery and Therapeutic Medicine. Totowa: Humana Press, pp. 197–227, 2005.

[23] Girola N, Figueiredo CR, Farias CF, Azevedo RA, Ferreira AK, Teixeira SF, Capello TM, Martins EG, Matsuo AL, Travassos LR, and Lago JH. Camphene isolated from essential oil of *Piper cernuum* (Piperaceae) induces intrinsic apoptosis in melanoma cells and displays antitumor activity in vivo. Biochem Biophys Res Commun 467: 928–934, 2015.

[24] Murata S, Shiragami R, Kosugi C, Tezuka T, Yamazaki M, Hirano A, Yoshimura Y, Suzuki M, Shuto K, Ohkohchi N, and Koda K. Antitumor effect of 1, 8-cineole against colon cancer. Oncol Rep 30: 2647–2652, 2013.

[25] Maruyama N, Takizawa T, Ishibashi H, Hisajima T, Inouye S, Yamaguchi H, and Abe S. Protective activity of geranium oil and its component, geraniol, in combination with

vaginal washing against vaginal candidiasis in mice. Biol Pharm Bull 31: 1501–1506, 2008.

[26] Carnesecchi S, Langley K, Exinger F, Gosse F, and Raul F. Geraniol, a component of plant essential oils, sensitizes human colonic cancer cells to 5-Fluorouracil treatment. J Pharmacol Exp Therap 301: 625–630, 2002.

[27] Carnesecchi S, Schneider Y, Ceraline J, et al. Geraniol, a component of plant essential oils, inhibits growth and polyamine biosynthesis in human colon cancer cells. J Pharmacol Exp Therap 298: 197–200, 2001.

[28] Carnesecchi S, Bradaia A, Fischer B, et al. Perturbation by geraniol of cell membrane permeability and signal transduction pathways in human colon cancer cells. J Pharmacol Exp Therap 303: 711–715, 2002.

[29] Carnesecchi S, Bras-Gonçalves R, Bradaia A, Zeisel M, Gossé F, Poupon MF, and Raul F. Geraniol, a component of plant essential oils, modulates DNA synthesis and potentiates 5-fluorouracil efficacy on human colon tumor xenografts. Cancer Lett. 215: 53–59, 2004.

[30] Itani WS, El-Banna SH, Hassan SB, et al. Anti-colon cancer components from Lebanese sage (*Salvia libanotica*) essential oil: mechanistic basis. Cancer Biol Therap 7: 1765–1773, 2008.

[31] Horváthová E, Sramková M, Lábaj J, and Slamenová D. Study of cytotoxic, genotoxic and DNA-protective effects of selected plant essential oils on human cells cultured in vitro. Neuro Endocrinol Lett 27: 44–47, 2006.

[32] Horvathova E, Turcaniova V, and Slamenova D. Comparative study of DNA-damaging and DNA-protective effects of selected components of essential plant oils in human leukemic cells K562. Neoplasma 54: 478–483, 2007.

[33] Fan K, Li X, Cao Y, Qi H, Li L, Zhang Q, and Sun HD. Carvacrol inhibits proliferation and induces apoptosis in human colon cancer cells. Anticancer Drugs 26: 813–823, 2015.

[34] Arigesavan K, and Sudhandiran G. Carvacrol exhibits anti-oxidant and anti-inflammatory effects against 1, 2-dimethyl hydrazine plus dextran sodium sulfate induced inflammation associated carcinogenicity in the colon of Fischer 344 rats. Biochem Biophys Res Commun 461: 314–320, 2015.

[35] Slamenová D, Horváthová E, Sramková M, and Marsálková L. DNA-protective effects of two components of essential plant oils carvacrol and thymol on mammalian cells cultured in vitro. Neoplasma 54: 108–112, 2007.

[36] Deb DD, Parimala G, Saravana Devi S, and Chakraborty T. Effect of thymol on peripheral blood mononuclear cell PBMC and acute promyelotic cancer cell line HL-60. Chem Biol Interact 193: 97–106, 2011.

[37] Kundu J, Chun KS, Aruoma OI, and Kundu JK. Mechanistic perspectives on cancer chemoprevention/chemotherapeutic effects of thymoquinone. Mutat Res 768: 22–34, 2014.

[38] Lang M, Borgmann M, Oberhuber G, Evstatiev R, Jimenez K, Dammann KW, Jambrich M, Khare V, Campregher C, Ristl R, and Gasche C. Thymoquinone attenuates tumor growth in ApcMin mice by interference with Wnt-signaling. Mol Cancer 12: 41, 2013.

[39] Gali-Muhtasib H, Ocker M, Kuester D, Krueger S, El-Hajj Z, Diestel A, Evert M, El-Najjar N, Peters B, Jurjus A, Roessner A, and Schneider-Stock R. Thymoquinone reduces mouse colon tumor cell invasion and inhibits tumor growth in murine colon cancer models. J Cell Mol Med 12: 330–342, 2008.

[40] El-Najjar N, Chatila M, Moukadem H, et al. Reactive oxygen species mediate thymoquinone-induced apoptosis and activate ERK and JNK signaling. Apoptosis 15: 183–195, 2010.

[41] Ganea GM, Fakayode SO, Losso JN, Van Nostrum CF, Sabliov CM, and Warner IM. Delivery of phytochemical thymoquinone using molecular micelle modified poly(D, L lactide-co-glycolide) (PLGA) nanoparticles. Nanotechnology 21: 285104, 2010.

[42] Al-Shabanah OA, Badary OA, Nagi MN, Al-Gharably NM, Al-Rikabi AC, and Al-Bekairi AM. Thymoquinone protects against doxorubicin-induced cardiotoxicity without compromising its antitumor activity. J Exp Clin Cancer Res 17: 193–198, 1998.

[43] Effenberger-Neidnicht K, and Schobert R. Combinatorial effects of thymoquinone on the anti-cancer activity of doxorubicin. Cancer Chemotherap Pharmacol 67: 867–874, 2011.

[44] Chidambara Murthy KN, Jayaprakasha GK, and Patil BS. D-limonene rich volatile oil from blood oranges inhibits angiogenesis, metastasis and cell death in human colon cancer cells. Life Sci 91: 429–439, 2012.

[45] Kawamori T, Tanaka T, Hirose Y, Ohnishi M, and Mori H. Inhibitory effects of d-limonene on the development of colonic aberrant crypt foci induced by azoxymethane in F344 rats. Carcinogenesis 17: 369–372, 1996.

[46] Jia SS, Xi GP, Zhang M, Chen YB, Lei B, Dong XS, and Yang YM. Induction of apoptosis by D-limonene is mediated by inactivation of Akt in LS174T human colon cancer cells. Oncol Rep 29: 349–354, 2013.

[47] Vigushin DM, Poon GK, Boddy A, et al. Phase I and pharmacokinetic study of d-limonene in patients with advanced cancer. Cancer Research Campaign Phase I/II Clinical Trials Committee. Cancer Chemother Pharmacol 42: 111–117, 1998.

[48] Sun J. D-Limonene: safety and clinical applications. Altern Med Rev 12: 259–264, 2007.

[49] Crowell PL, Ren Z, Lin S, Vedejs E, and Gould MN. Structure-activity relationships among monoterpene inhibitors of protein isoprenylation and cell proliferation. Biochem Pharmacol 47: 1405–1415, 1994.

[50] Reddy BS, Wang CX, Samaha H, Lubet R, Steele VE, Kelloff GJ, and Rao CV. Chemoprevention of colon carcinogenesis by dietary perillyl alcohol. Cancer Res 57: 420–425, 1997.

[51] Bardon S, Foussard V, Fournel S, and Loubat A. Monoterpenes inhibit proliferation of human colon cancer cells by modulating cell cycle-related protein expression. Cancer Lett 181: 187–194, 2002.

[52] Ripple GH, Gould MN, Stewart JA, et al. Phase I clinical trial of perillyl alcohol administered daily. Clin Cancer Res 4: 1159–1164, 1998.

[53] Ripple GH, Gould MN, Arzoomanian RZ, et al. Phase I clinical and pharmacokinetic study of perillyl alcohol administered four times a day. Clin Cancer Res 6: 390–396, 2000.

[54] Azzoli CG, Miller VA, Kenneth KNG, et al. A phase I trial of perillyl alcohol in patients with advanced solid tumors. Cancer Chemotherap Pharmacol 51: 493–498, 2003.

[55] Hudes GR, Szarka CE, Adams A, et al. Phase I pharmacokinetic trial of perillyl alcohol (NSC 641066) in patients with refractory solid malignancies. Clin Cancer Res 6: 3071–3080, 2000.

[56] Meadows SM, Mulkerin D, Berlin J, et al. Phase II trial of perillyl alcohol in patients with metastatic colorectal cancer. Int J Gastrointest Cancer 32: 125–128, 2002.

[57] da Fonseca CO, Simao M, Lins IR, Caetano RO, Futuro D, and Quirico-Santos T. Efficacy of monoterpene perillyl alcohol upon survival rate of patients with recurrent glioblastoma. J Cancer Res Clin Oncol 137: 287–293, 2011.

[58] Da Fonseca CO, Teixeira RM, Silva JC, De Saldanha DA, Gama Fischer J, Meirelles OC, Landeiro JA, and Quirico-Santos T. Long-term outcome in patients with recurrent malignant glioma treated with perillyl alcohol inhalation. Anticancer Res 33: 5625–5631, 2013.

[59] Hayes AJ, Leach DN, Markham JL, and Markovic B. In vitro cytotoxicity of Australian tea tree oil using human cell lines. J Essential Oil Res 9: 575–582, 1997.

[60] Asanova ZK, Suleimenov EM, Atazhanova GA, et al. Biological activity of 1,8-cineole from levant wormwood. Pharma Chem J 37: 28–30, 2003.

[61] Bhattacharjee B, and Chatterjee J. Identification of proapoptopic, anti-inflammatory, anti-proliferative, anti-invasive and anti-angiogenic targets of essential oils in cardamom by dual reverse virtual screening and binding pose analysis. Asian Pacific J Cancer Prev 14: 3735–3742, 2013.

[62] Chen W, Liu Y, Li M, Mao J, Zhang L, Huang R, Jin X, and Ye L. Anti-tumor effect of α-pinene on human hepatoma cell lines through inducing G2/M cell cycle arrest. J Pharmacol Sci 127: 332–338, 2015.

[63] Wu X, Qin L, Fako V, and Zhang JT. Molecular mechanisms of fatty acid synthase (FASN)-mediated resistance to anti-cancer treatments. Adv Biol Regul 54: 214–221, 2014.

[64] Furuta E, Okuda H, Kobayashi A, and Watabe K. Metabolic genes in cancer: their roles in tumor progression and clinical implications. Biochim Biophys Acta 1805: 141–152, 2010.

[65] Kusakabe T, Maeda M, Hoshi N, et al. Fatty acid synthase is expressed mainly in adult hormone-sensitive cells or cells with high lipid metabolism and in proliferating fetal cells. J Histochem Cytochem 48: 613–622, 2000.

[66] Weiss L, Hoffmann GE, Schreiber R, et al. Fatty-acid biosynthesis in man, a pathway of minor importance. Purification, optimal assay conditions, and organ distribution of fatty-acid synthase. Biol Chem Hoppe-Seyler 367: 905–912, 1986.

[67] Smith S, Witkowski A, and Joshi AK. Structural and functional organization of the animal fatty acid synthase. Prog Lipid Res 42: 289–317, 2003.

[68] Nguyen PL, Ma J, Chavarro JE, et al. Fatty acid synthase polymorphisms, tumor expression, body mass index, prostate cancer risk, and survival. J Clin Oncol 28: 3958–3964, 2010.

[69] Zhou Y, Niu C, Li Y, et al. Fatty acid synthase expression and esophageal cancer. Mol Biol Rep 39: 9733–9739, 2012.

[70] Long QQ, Yi YX, Qiu J, Xu CJ, and Huang PL. Fatty acid synthase (FASN) levels in serum of colorectal cancer patients: correlation with clinical outcomes. Tumour Biol 35: 3855–3859, 2014.

[71] Kearney KE, Pretlow TG, and Pretlow TP. Increased expression of fatty acid synthase in human aberrant crypt foci: possible target for colorectal cancer prevention. Int J Cancer 125: 249–252, 2009.

[72] Ong ES, Zou L, Li S, Cheah PY, Eu KW, and Ong CN. Metabolic profiling in colorectal cancer reveals signature metabolic shifts during tumorigenesis. Mol Cell Proteomics 2010 Feb 10 Epub.

[73] Luque-García JL, Martínez-Torrecuadrada JL, Epifano C, Cañamero M, Babel I, and Casal JI. Differential protein expression on the cell surface of colorectal cancer cells associated to tumor metastasis. Proteomics 10: 940–952, 2010.

[74] Kuhajda FP. Fatty-acid synthase and human cancer: new perspectives on its role in tumor biology. Nutrition 16: 202–208, 2000.

[75] Kuhajda FP. Fatty acid synthase and cancer: new application of an old pathway. Cancer Res 66: 5977–5980, 2006.

[76] Yoshii Y, Furukawa T, Oyama N, et al. Fatty acid synthase is a key target in multiple essential tumor functions of prostate cancer: uptake of radiolabeled acetate as a predictor of the targeted therapy outcome. PLoS One 8: e64570, 2013.

[77] Sadowski MC, Pouwer RH, Gunter JH, Lubik AA, Quinn RJ, and Nelson CC. The fatty acid synthase inhibitor triclosan: repurposing an anti-microbial agent for targeting prostate cancer. Oncotarget 5: 9362–9381, 2014.

[78] Impheng H, Pongcharoen S, Richert L, Pekthong D, and Srisawang P. The selective target of capsaicin on FASN expression and de novo fatty acid synthesis mediated through ROS generation triggers apoptosis in HepG2 cells. PLoS One 9: e107842, 2014.

[79] Fan H, Tian W, and Ma X. Curcumin induces apoptosis of HepG2 cells via inhibiting fatty acid synthase. Target Oncol 9: 279–286, 2014.

[80] Benjamin DI, Li DS, Lowe W, Heuer T, Kemble G, and Nomura DK. Diacylglycerol metabolism and signaling is a driving force underlying FASN inhibitor sensitivity in cancer cells. ACS Chem Biol 10: 1616–1623, 2015.

[81] Ventura R, Mordec K, Waszczuk J, Wang Z, Lai J, Fridlib M, Buckley D, Kemble G, and Heuer TS. Inhibition of de novo palmitate synthesis by fatty acid synthase induces apoptosis in tumor cells by remodeling cell membranes, inhibiting signaling pathways, and reprogramming gene expression. EBio Med 2: 806–822, 2015.

[82] Hardwicke MA, Rendina AR, Williams SP, Moore ML, Wang L, Krueger JA, Plant RN, Totoritis RD, Zhang G, Briand J, Burkhart WA, Brown KK, and Parrish CA. A human fatty acid synthase inhibitor binds β-ketoacyl reductase in the keto-substrate site. Nat Chem Biol 10: 774–779, 2014.

[83] Nomura S, Horiuchi T, Hata T, and Omura S. Inhibition of sterol and fatty acid biosyntheses by cerulenin in cell-free systems of yeast. J Antibiot (Tokyo) 25: 365–368, 1972.

[84] Nomura S, Horiuchi T, Omura S, and Hata T. The action mechanism of cerulenin. I. Effect of cerulenin on sterol and fatty acid biosynthesis in yeast. J Biochem 71: 783–796, 1972.

[85] Vance D, Goldberg I, Mitsuhashi O, and Bloch K. Inhibition of fatty acid synthetases by the antibiotic cerulenin. Biochem Biophys Res Commun 48: 649–656, 1972.

[86] D'Agnolo G, Rosenfeld IS, Awaya J, Omura S, and Vagelos PR. Inhibition of fatty acid synthesis by the antibiotic cerulenin. Specific inactivation of beta-ketoacyl-acyl carrier protein synthetase. Biochim Biophys Acta 326: 155–156, 1973.

[87] Goldberg I, Walker JR, and Bloch K. Inhibition of lipid synthesis in *Escherichia coli* cells by the antibiotic cerulenin. Antimicrob Agents Chemother 3: 549–554, 1973.

[88] Omura S. The antibiotic cerulenin, a novel tool for biochemistry as an inhibitor of fatty acid synthesis. Bacteriol Rev 40: 681–697, 1976.

[89] Omura S. Cerulenin. Methods Enzymol 72: 520–532, 1981.

[90] Jeong NY, Lee JS, Yoo KS, et al. Fatty acid synthase inhibitor cerulenin inhibits topoisomerase I catalytic activity and augments SN-38-induced apoptosis. Apoptosis 18: 226–237, 2013.

[91] Chen HW, Chang YF, Chuang HY, Tai WT, and Hwang JJ. Targeted therapy with fatty acid synthase inhibitors in a human prostate carcinoma LNCaP/tk-luc-bearing animal model. Prostate Cancer Prostatic Dis 15: 260–264, 2012.

[92] Zhao W, Kridel S, Thorburn A, et al. Fatty acid synthase: a novel target for antiglioma therapy. Br J Cancer 95: 869–878, 2006.

[93] Murata S, Yanagisawa K, Fukunaga K, et al. Fatty acid synthase inhibitor cerulenin suppresses liver metastasis of colon cancer in mice. Cancer Sci 101: 1861–1865, 2010.

[94] Shiragami R, Murata S, Kosugi C, et al. Enhanced antitumor activity of cerulenin combined with oxaliplatin in human colon cancer cells. Int J Oncol 43: 431–438, 2013.

[95] Denley A, Gymnopoulos M, Kang S, Mitchell C, and Vogt PK. Requirement of phosphatidylinositol(3,4,5) trisphosphate in phosphatidylinositol 3-kinase-induced oncogenic transformation. Mol Cancer Res 7: 1132–1138, 2009.

[96] Chang L, Wu P, Senthilkumar R, Tian X, Liu H, Shen X, Tao Z, and Huang P. Loss of fatty acid synthase suppresses the malignant phenotype of colorectal cancer cells by down-regulating energy metabolism and mTOR signaling pathway. J Cancer Res Clin Oncol 142: 59–72, 2016.

[97] Bauerschlag DO, Maass N, Leonhardt P, Verburg FA, Pecks U, Zeppernick F, Morgenroth A, Mottaghy FM, Tolba R, Meinhold-Heerlein I, and Bräutigam K. Fatty acid synthase overexpression: target for therapy and reversal of chemoresistance in ovarian cancer. J Transl Med 13: 146, 2015.

[98] Kuhajda FP, Pizer ES, Li JN, Mani NS, Frehywot GL, and Townsend CA. Synthesis and antitumor activity of an inhibitor of fatty acid synthase. Proc Natl Acad Sci U S A 97: 3450–3454, 2000.

[99] Rahman MT, Nakayama K, Rahman M, et al. Fatty acid synthase expression associated with NAC1 is a potential therapeutic target in ovarian clear cell carcinomas. Br J Cancer 107: 300–307, 2012.

[100] Horiguchi A, Asano T, Asano T, Ito K, Sumitomo M, and Hayakawa M. Pharmacological inhibitor of fatty acid synthase suppresses growth and invasiveness of renal cancer cells. J Urol 180: 729–736, 2008.

[101] Li JN, Gorospe M, Chrest FJ, Kumaravel TS, Evans MK, Han WF, and Pizer ES. Pharmacological inhibition of fatty acid synthase activity produces both cytostatic and cytotoxic effects modulated by p53. Cancer Res 61:1493–1499, 2001.

[102] Thupari JN, Landree LE, Ronnett GV, and Kuhajda FP. C75 increases peripheral energy utilization and fatty acid oxidation in diet-induced obesity. Proc Natl Acad Sci U S A 99: 9498–9502, 2002.

[103] Loftus TM, Jaworsky DE, Frehywot GL, et al. Reduced food intake and body weight in mice treated with fatty acid synthase inhibitors. Science 288: 2379–2381, 2000.

[104] McFadden JM, Medghalchi SM, Thupari JN, et al. Application of a flexible synthesis of (5R)-thiolactomycin to develop new inhibitors of type I fatty acid synthase. J Med Chem 48: 946–961, 2005.

[105] Orita H, Coulter J, Lemmon C, Tully E, Vadlamudi A, Medghalchi SM, Kuhajda FP, and Gabrielson E. Selective inhibition of fatty acid synthase for lung cancer treatment. Clin Cancer Res 13: 7139–7145, 2007.

[106] Orita H, Coulter J, Tully E, Abe M, Montgomery E, Alvarez H, Sato K, Hino O, Kajiyama Y, Tsurumaru M, and Gabrielson E. High levels of fatty acid synthase expression in esophageal cancers represent a potential target for therapy. Cancer Biol Ther 10: 549–554, 2010.

[107] Kridel SJ, Axelrod F, Rozenkrantz N, and Smith JW. Orlistat is a novel inhibitor of fatty acid synthase with antitumor activity. Cancer Res 64: 2070–2075, 2004.

[108] Halpern B, and Halpern A. Safety assessment of FDA-approved (orlistat and lorcaserin) anti-obesity medications. Expert Opin Drug Saf 14: 305–315, 2015.

[109] Borgström B. Mode of action of tetrahydrolipstatin: a derivative of the naturally occurring lipase inhibitor lipstatin. Bioch Biophys Acta 962: 308–316, 1988.

[110] Zhi J, Melia AT, Eggers H, et al. Review of limited systemic absorption of orlistat, a lipase inhibitor, in healthy human volunteers. J Clin Pharmacol 35: 1103–1108, 1995.

[111] Ballinger A, and Peikin SR. Orlistat: its current status as an anti-obesity drug. Eur J Pharmacol 440: 109–117, 2002.

[112] Mancini MC, and Halpern A. Orlistat in the prevention of diabetes in the obese patient. Vasc Health Risk Manag 4: 325–336, 2008.

[113] Menendez JA, Vellon L, and Lupu R. Anti-tumoral actions of the anti-obesity drug orlistat (Xenical TM) in breast cancer cells: blockade of cell cycle progression, promotion of apoptotic cell death and PEA3-mediated transcriptional repression of Her2/neu (erbB-2) oncogene. Ann Oncol 16: 1253–1267, 2005.

[114] Little JL, Wheeler FB, Fels DR, Koumenis C, and Kridel SJ. Inhibition of fatty acid synthase induces endoplasmic reticulum stress in tumor cells. Cancer Res 2007; 67: 1262–1269.

http://dx.doi.org/10.5772/62283

[115] Carvalho MA, Zecchin KG, Seguin F, et al. Fatty acid synthase inhibition with Orlistat promotes apoptosis and reduces cell growth and lymph node metastasis in a mouse melanoma model. Int J Cancer 123: 2557–2565, 2008.

[116] Yang CS, Matsuura K, Huang NJ, Robeson AC, Huang B, Zhang L, and Kornbluth S. Fatty acid synthase inhibition engages a novel caspase-2 regulatory mechanism to induce ovarian cancer cell death. Oncogene 34: 3264–3272, 2015.

[117] Agostini M, Almeida LY, Bastos DC, Ortega RM, Moreira FS, Seguin F, Zecchin KG, Raposo HF, Oliveira HC, Amoêdo ND, Salo T, Coletta RD, and Graner E. The fatty acid synthase inhibitor orlistat reduces the growth and metastasis of orthotopic tongue oral squamous cell carcinomas. Mol Cancer Ther 13: 585–595, 2014.

[118] Lin Y, Shi R, Wang X, and Shen HM. Luteolin, a flavanoid with potential for cancer prevention and therapy. Curr Cancer Drug Target 8: 634–646, 2008.

[119] Chang J, Hsu Y, Kuo P, Kuo Y, Chiang L, and Lin C. Increase of Bax/Bcl-XL ratio and arrest of cell cycle by luteolin in immortalized human hepatoma cell line. Life Sci 76: 1883–1893, 2005.

[120] Leung HW, Wu CH, Lin CH, and Lee HZ. Luteolin induced DNA damage leading to human lung squamous carcinoma CH27 cell apoptosis. Eur J Pharmacol 508: 77–83, 2005.

[121] Lim do Y, Jeong Y, Tyner AL, and Park JH. Induction of cell cycle arrest and apoptosis in HT-29 human colon cancer cells by the dietary compound luteolin. Am J Physiol Gastrointest Liver Physiol 292: G66–G75, 2007.

[122] Abdel Hadi L, Di Vito C, Marfia G, Ferraretto A, Tringali C, Viani P, and Riboni L. Sphingosine kinase 2 and ceramide transport as key targets of the natural flavonoid luteolin to induce apoptosis in colon cancer cells. PLoS One 10: e0143384, 2015.

[123] Osman NH, Said UZ, El-Waseef AM, and Ahmed ES. Luteolin supplementation adjacent to aspirin treatment reduced dimethylhydrazine-induced experimental colon carcinogenesis in rats. Tumour Biol 36: 1179–1190, 2015.

[124] Pandurangan AK, Kumar SA, Dharmalingam P, and Ganapasam S. Luteolin, a bioflavonoid inhibits azoxymethane-induced colon carcinogenesis: Involvement of iNOS and COX-2. Pharmacogn Mag 10(Suppl. 2): S306–S310, 2014.

[125] Pandurangan AK, Dharmalingam P, Sadagopan SK, Ramar M, Munusamy A, and Ganapasam S. Luteolin induces growth arrest in colon cancer cells through involvement of Wnt/β-catenin/GSK-3β signaling. J Environ Pathol Toxicol Oncol 32: 131–139, 2013.

[126] Wang X, and Tian W. Green tea epigallocatechin gallate: a natural inhibitor of fatty-acid synthase. Biochem Biophys Res Commun 288: 1200–1206, 2001.

[127] Wang X, Song KS, Guo QX, and Tian WX. The galloyl moiety of green tea catechins is the critical structural feature to inhibit fatty-acid synthase. Biochem Pharmacol 66: 2039–2047, 2003.

[128] Vergote D, Cren-Olivé C, Chopin V, et al. (−)-Epigallocatechin (EGC) of green tea induces apoptosis of human breast cancer cells but not of their normal counterparts. Breast Cancer Res Treat 76: 195–201, 2002.

[129] Khan N, Bharali DJ, Adhami VM, et al. Oral administration of naturally occurring chitosan-based nanoformulated green tea polyphenol EGCG effectively inhibits prostate cancer cell growth in a xenograft model. Carcinogenesis 35: 415–423, 2014.

[130] Yeh CW, Chen WJ, Chiang CT, Lin-Shiau SY, and Lin JK. Suppression of fatty acid synthase in MCF-7 breast cancer cells by tea and tea polyphenols: a possible mechanism for their hypolipidemic effects. Pharmacogenom J 3: 267–276, 2003.

[131] Du GJ, Zhang Z, Wen XD, Yu C, Calway T, Yuan CS, and Wang CZ. Epigallocatechin gallate (EGCG) is the most effective cancer chemopreventive polyphenol in green tea. Nutrients 4: 1679–1691, 2012.

[132] Pan MH, Lin CC, Lin JK, and Chen WJ. Tea polyphenol (−)-epigallocatechin 3-gallate suppresses heregulin-beta1-induced fatty acid synthase expression in human breast cancer cells by inhibiting phosphatidylinositol 3-kinase/Akt and mitogen-activated protein kinase cascade signaling. J Agricult Food Chem 55: 5030–5037, 2007.

[133] Shimizu M, Shirakami Y, Sakai H, et al. (−)-Epigallocatechin gallate inhibits growth and activation of the VEGF/VEGFR axis in human colorectal cancer cells. Chem Biol Interact 185: 247–252, 2010.

[134] Tran PL, Kim SA, Choi HS, Yoon JH, and Ahn SG. Epigallocatechin-3-gallate suppresses the expression of HSP70 and HSP90 and exhibits anti-tumor activity in vitro and in vivo. BMC Cancer 10: 276, 2010.

[135] Jin H, Gong W, Zhang C, and Wang S. Epigallocatechin gallate inhibits the proliferation of colorectal cancer cells by regulating Notch signaling. Onco Targets Ther 6: 145–153, 2013.

[136] Maruyama T, Murata S, Nakayama K, et al. (−)-Epigallocatechin-3-gallate suppresses liver metastasis of human colorectal cancer. Oncol Rep 31: 625–633, 2014.

[137] Shimizu M, Fukutomi Y, Ninomiya M, Nagura K, Kato T, Araki H, Suganuma M, Fujiki H, and Moriwaki H. Green tea extracts for the prevention of metachronous colorectal adenomas: a pilot study. Cancer Epidemiol Biomark Prev 17: 3020–3025, 2008.

[138] Bettuzzi S, Brausi M, Rizzi F, Castagnetti G, Peracchia G, and Corti A. Chemoprevention of human prostate cancer by oral administration of green tea catechins in volunteers with high-grade prostate intraepithelial neoplasia: a preliminary report from a one-year proof-of-principle study. Cancer Res 66: 1234–1240, 2006.

[139] Stingl JC, Ettrich T, Muche R, Wiedom M, Brockmöller J, Seeringer A, and Seufferlein T. Protocol for minimizing the risk of metachronous adenomas of the colorectum with green tea extract (MIRACLE): a randomised controlled trial of green tea extract versus placebo for nutriprevention of metachronous colon adenomas in the elderly population. BMC Cancer 11: 360, 2011.

[140] Rodricks JV, Swenberg JA, Borzelleca JF, Maronpot RR, and Shipp AM. Triclosan: a critical review of the experimental data and development of margins of safety for consumer products. Crit Rev Toxicol 40: 422–484, 2010.

[141] Liu B, Wang Y, Fillgrove KL, and Anderson VE. Triclosan inhibits enoyl-reductase of type I fatty acid synthase in vitro and is cytotoxic to MCF-7 and SKBr-3 breast cancer cells. Cancer Chemother Pharmacol 49: 187–193, 2002.

[142] Lu S, and Archer MC. Fatty acid synthase is a potential molecular target for the chemoprevention of breast cancer. Carcinogenesis 26: 153–157, 2005.

[143] Kumar V, Chakraborty A, Kural MR, and Roy P. Alteration of testicular steroidogenesis and histopathology of reproductive system in male rats treated with triclosan. Reprod Toxicol 27: 177–185, 2009.

[144] Pandey PR, Liu W, Xing F, Fukuda K, and Watabe K. Anti-cancer drugs targeting fatty acid synthase (FAS). Recent Pat Anticancer Drug Discov 7: 185–197, 2012.

[145] Aza-Gonzalez C, Nunez-Palenius HG, and Ochoa-Alejo N. Molecular biology of capsaicinoid biosynthesis in chili pepper (*Capsicum* spp.). Plant Cell Rep 30: 695–706, 2011.

[146] Reilly CA, Ehlhardt WJ, Jackson DA, et al. Metabolism of capsaicin by cytochrome P450 produces novel dehydrogenated metabolites and decreases cytotoxicity to lung and liver cells. Chem Res Toxicol 16: 336–349, 2003.

[147] Huang SP, Chen JC, Wu CC, et al. Capsaicin induced apoptosis in human hepatoma HepG2 cells. Anticancer Res 29: 165–174, 2009.

[148] Skrzypski M, Sassek M, Abdelmessih S, et al. Capsaicin induces cytotoxicity in pancreatic neuroendocrine tumor cells via mitochondrial action. Cell Signal 26: 41–48, 2014.

[149] Lau JK, Brown KC, Dom AM, et al. Capsaicin induces apoptosis in human small cell lung cancer via the TRPV6 receptor and the calpain pathway. Apoptosis 19: 1190–1201, 2014.

[150] Pramanik KC, Boreddy SR, and Srivastava SK. Role of mitochondrial electron transport chain complexes in capsaicin mediated oxidative stress leading to apoptosis in pancreatic cancer cells. PLoS One 6: e20151, 2011.

[151] Zhang JH, Lai FJ, Chen H, et al. Involvement of the phosphoinositide 3-kinase/Akt pathway in apoptosis induced by capsaicin in the human pancreatic cancer cell line PANC-1. Oncol Lett 5: 43–48, 2013.

[152] Braga ME, Leal PF, Carvalho JE, et al. Comparison of yield, composition, and antioxidant activity of turmeric (*Curcuma longa* L.) extracts obtained using various techniques. J Agric Food Chem 51: 6604–6611, 2002.

[153] Khor TO, Keum YS, Lin W, et al. Combined inhibitory effects of curcumin and phenethyl isothiocyanate on the growth of human PC-3 prostate xenografts in immune deficient mice. Cancer Res 66: 613–621, 2006.

[154] Kunnumakkara AB, Anand P, and Aggarwal BB. Curcumin inhibits proliferation, invasion, angiogenesis and metastasis of different cancers through interaction with multiple cell signaling proteins. Cancer Lett 269: 199–225, 2008.

[155] Kunnumakkara AB, Guha S, Krishnan S, et al. Curcumin potentiates antitumor activity of gemcitabine in an orthotopic model of pancreatic cancer through suppression of proliferation, angiogenesis, and inhibition of nuclear factor-kappaB regulated gene products. Cancer Res 67: 3853–3861, 2007.

[156] Ravindran J, Prasad S, and Aggarwal BB. Curcumin and cancer cells: how many ways can curry kill tumor cells selectively? AAPS J 11: 495–510, 2009.

[157] Wu SH, Hang LW, Yang JS, et al. Curcumin induces apoptosis in human non-small cell lung cancer NCI-H460 cells through ER stress and caspase cascade and mitochondria-dependent pathways. Anticancer Res 30: 2125–233, 2010.

[158] Xu Y, Zhang J, Han J, et al. Curcumin inhibits tumor proliferation induced by neutrophil elastase through the upregulation of α1-antitrypsin in lung cancer. Mol Oncol 6: 405–417, 2012.

[159] Ruby AJ, Kuttan G, Babu KD, et al. Anti-tumour and antioxidant activity of natural curcuminoids. Cancer Lett 94: 79–83, 1995.

[160] Zhao J, Sun X, Ye F, et al. Suppression of fatty acid synthase, differentiation and lipid accumulation in adipocytes by curcumin. Mol Cell Biochem 351: 19–28, 2011.

Chapter 17

Anti-Epidermal Growth Factor Receptor (EGFR) Treatment in Patients with Metastatic Colorectal Cancer

Rumeysa Ciftci and Deniz Tural

Additional information is available at the end of the chapter

http://dx.doi.org/10.5772/62304

Abstract

Colorectal cancer is one of the most common cancer types and still a major public health problem. Approximately a half of the patients develop metastasis during the course of disease. Prognosis of metastatic colorectal cancer (mCRC) is poor with best supportive care alone (median survival: 6 months). Fortunately, combination chemotherapy has significantly improved survival up to 17–22 months. Cetuximab and panitumumab, the two monoclonal antibodies (mAbs) against epidermal growth factor receptor (EGFR), provide significant clinical benefit in only RAS wild (WT) mCRC. Major side effects are skin toxicity, infusion reactions, fatigue, and electrolyte imbalances. When these mAbs are combined with chemotherapy, overall survival could be as long as 24 months. However, RAS WT status does not ensure response to anti-EGFR mAbs. In addition, RAS WT patients consequently develop resistance to these agents after an initial responsive period. Therefore, understanding the primary and secondary resistance mechanisms apart from RAS status is very important to improve outcomes of mCRC patients. Oncogenic activation of EGFR downstream signaling effectors (KRAS, BRAF, PTEN, and PIK3CA) appears to be the main components of resistance. In future, a comprehensive biomarker analysis will probably help to identify the mCRC patients who will truly benefit from anti-EGFR mAbs.

Keywords: cetuximab, metastatic colorectal cancer, panitumumab, RAS, survival

1. Introduction

Colorectal cancer (CRC) is one of the most commonly diagnosed cancers in both genders (second in females and third in males) [1]; and it is also the third common cause of cancer-related death in both genders [2, 3]. Although the mortality rate of CRC has been decreasing in Western countries, its incidence has been increasing worldwide [1].

CRC can spread by lymphatic, hematogenous and transperitoneal dissemination. The most common metastatic sites are the regional lymph nodes, liver, lungs, and peritoneum. Approximately 50–60% of patients with CRC develop metastasis, and local recurrence is included in 15% of the patients who have first relapse [4].

Survival of metastatic colorectal cancer (mCRC) is approximately 5–6 months with best supportive care (BSC) alone, and chemotherapeutic agents have been shown to provide significant survival benefit. Fluoropyrimidines have been the mainstay of the systemic treatment of mCRC for several years. Median survival of patients with mCRC increased up to 12–14 months and 17–22 months with fluoropyrimidines alone and its combinations with irinotecan and/or oxaliplatin, respectively [5–7]. Also, addition of target-directed cancer drugs, such as monoclonal antibodies (mAbs) against VEGF (e.g., bevacizumab, aflibercept) and EGFR (e.g., cetuximab and panitumumab), have remarkably improved the outcomes of mCRC [8–13]. Unfortunately, targeted therapies, including anti-EGFR drugs, are active only in a fraction of patients and most of them subsequently become resistant to the treatment. Therefore, identification of the genetic alterations associated with the clinical response and resistance to anti-EGFR mAbs is important to improve outcomes of patients with mCRC.

2. Epidermal growth factor receptor and KRAS mutation

Epidermal growth factor receptor (EGFR) is a transmembrane tyrosine kinase receptor that presents on the surface of normal epithelium. It is over-expressed in up to 80% of colorectal tumors [14, 15] and mediates cell differentiation, proliferation, migration, angiogenesis and apoptosis [16].

The EGFR signaling acts through at least two parallel intracellular pathways: mitogen-activated protein kinases (MAPK) and phosphor-inositol kinases (PI3K). MAPK form the major cell proliferation signaling pathways from the cell surface to the nucleus through a series of genes, including RAS, RAF, and MEK. Various signals, such as EGF, amphiregulin, amphiregulin, and heparin-binding EGF, could stimulate EGFR. After dimerization and phosphorylation of the stimulated EGFR, RAS is activated [17]. RAS activation, which starts the PI3K and RAF cascades, is the central distributor of the signal. Activation of PI3K/AKT pathway inhibits apoptosis, whereas RAF activation stimulates cellular proliferation. Hence, mutations in the KRAS gene may result in an independent activation of the downstream signaling of tumor growth [17]. Prospective randomized trials elucidated that presence of mutation in KRAS gene leads to non-response to anti-EGFR–based treatment in mCRC [8–12, 18–20].

Incidence of KRAS mutations is approximately 28.7% in all human cancers, thus it is considered one of the causal cancer genes [17]. RAS mutations occur in the early phases of cancer development and are preserved during tumor progression. KRAS mutation rate in CRC is 36%

and most common point mutations are located in codons 12 (80%) and 13 (15%) of exon 2, while codon 61, 117, and 146 mutations are less common [17, 21]. Unusual KRAS mutations affecting more than one codon and insertions are rare. The discordance of KRAS status between primary tumor and synchronous metastasis in the same patient tends to be low (ranging from 0 to 31%) [22]. In addition, KRAS status is not different between CRC biopsies before and after neoadjuvant therapy [23], or the biopsy and resection specimens of CRC [21, 24]. Because the data are limited, routine rebiopsy of metastases for RAS mutation analysis in recurrent disease is not recommended currently. In contrast, RAS mutations vary significantly between synchronous primary CRC lesions, therefore the mutation status of the metastasis is unpredictable [21].

3. Anti-EGFR mAbs in mCRC

Cetuximab (Erbitux) and panitumumab (Vectibix) are the two anti-EGFR mAbs active for the treatment of mCRC. Both are effective only in the wild type (WT) RAS (NRAS and KRAS) tumors (approximately 40% of all mCRCs) [8–12, 18–20]. Therefore, it is well established that KRAS and NRAS mutation status (exons 2, 3, and 4) should be known before initiating anti-EGFR based treatment for mCRC [25].

3.1. Mechanism of action

Cetuximab and panitumumab keep EGFR in an inactive state by binding to the extracellular ligand-binding site of EGFR when the ligand is unbound (acting as competitive antagonists). Consequently, intracellular signaling pathways of EGFR (RAS/RAF/MAPK and PI3K/PTEN/AKT) related to cell proliferation, invasion, and survival are inhibited [26][**Figure 1**]. Both cetuximab, an IgG1 type chimeric monoclonal antibody, and panitumumab, an IgG2 type fully human monoclonal antibody, induce apoptosis by inhibiting EGFR. Also, these molecules, especially cetuximab, activate antibody-dependent cellular cytotoxicity, inhibit metastasis and angiogenesis by blocking ligand-induced phosphorylation of EGFR on endothelial cells [16, 27, 28].

3.2. Predictive markers for response

The identification of patients with mCRC who are most likely to respond to the anti-EGFR mAbs is an important clinical question. Although there are no accepted predictive markers of response to bevacizumab or to chemotherapeutics, there are some analyses to select individuals who might benefit from anti-EGFR mAbs.

3.3. RAS mutations

Activating KRAS mutations cause constitutive activation of the RAS-RAF-ERK pathway, even in the absence of EGFR ligands. Consequently, tumor becomes resistant to anti-EGFR therapy [16, 17, 21, 29]. Prospective randomized studies showed that KRAS mutations are negative predictors of the response to anti-EGFR–based treatment [8–12, 18–20]. Thus, panitumumab and cetuximab are approved only for patients with WT KRAS tumors.

All KRAS mutations may not be similar for prediction of anti-EGFR therapy [30–33]. Although some retrospective studies suggest that patients with KRAS p.G13D mutation benefit more from cetuximab than those with KRAS codon 12 mutations [32], this benefit could not be confirmed in a prospective trial [33]. Therefore, data are not enough to change the clinical practice or to draw any firm conclusions about the effectiveness of anti-EGFR mAbs in mCRC with KRAS p.G13D mutation.

Almost 60% of CRC patients with WT KRAS mutation also have poor response to anti-EGFR–based treatment [34], suggesting the possibility of other molecular determinants of response. Heterogeneity of neoplastic cells that harbor specific RAS mutations within a single tumor may also influence response to EGFR-targeted agents [35]. Lower frequency mutations in KRAS apart from exon 2 or in NRAS may also cause resistance to anti-EGFR therapies [18, 36–41]. NRAS mutations in mCRC are less common than KRAS mutations (approximately 5%) and develop most often in codons 61, 12, and 13 [21]. The PRIME trial, in which patients with mCRC were randomly assigned to first-line FOLFOX with or without panitumumab, revealed that 17% of the patients with KRAS exon 2 WT tumors had other mutations in KRAS exons 3 and 4 and in NRAS exons 2, 3, and 4 [38]. These additional mutations were also associated

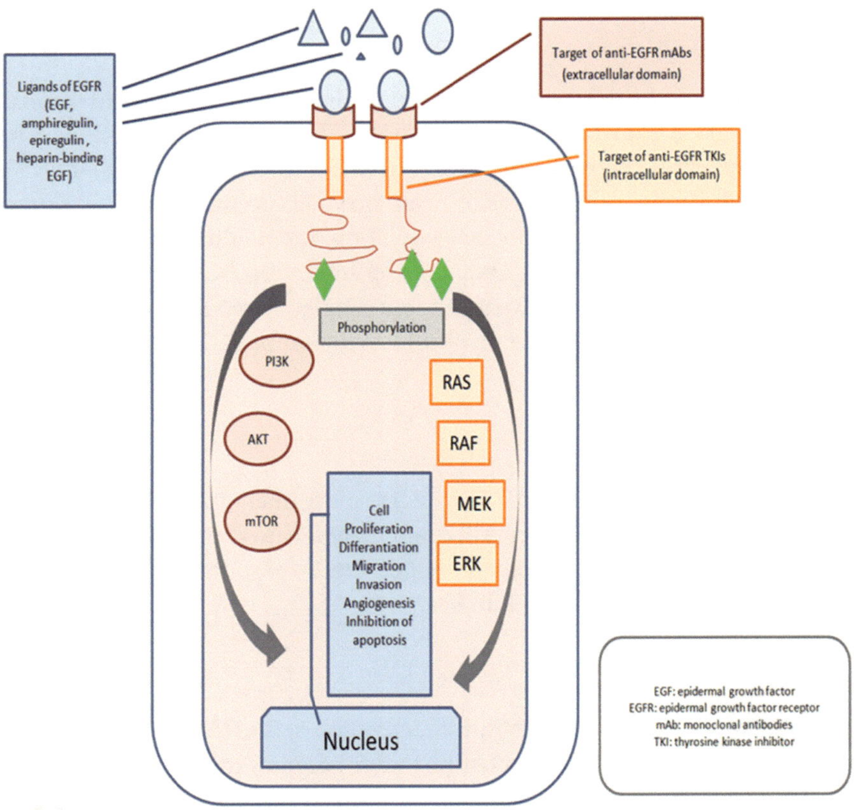

Figure 1. Epidermal growth factor receptor pathway as a therapeutic target for metastatic colorectal cancer.

http://dx.doi.org/10.5772/62304

with unresponsiveness to panitumumab, and poorer progression-free and overall survival in the panitumumab arm. Currently, testing for all RAS mutations (KRAS and NRAS exons 2, 3, and 4) rather than just those in KRAS exon 2 is the preferred approach to select appropriate patients with mCRC for anti-EGFR mAbs, since anti-EGFR mAbs are neither beneficial nor recommended for mCRC with any KRAS or NRAS mutations [42].

3.4. Other biomarkers

As mentioned before, WT RAS status does not ensure a response to EGFR-targeted therapies. Interestingly, the expression of the EGFR protein has not been strongly associated with clinical response to cetuximab in mCRC [43]. Majority of patients with EGFR-positive mCRC do not respond to anti-EGFR therapies [44, 45], while objective response is possible with EGFR-negative tumors [46–48]. Therefore, selection of patients for anti-EGFR mAbs based upon EGFR expression is not recommended. Likewise, EGFR mutations are rare in mCRC, and somatic mutations in the EGFR tyrosine kinase domain are not associated with cetuximab sensitivity [49]. However, it has been reported that over-expression of genes encoding amphiregulin and epiregulin, the two EGFR ligands, is strongly associated with better response to cetuximab in patients with mCRC [43].

Results of studies about association between EGFR copy number and response to anti-EGFR therapy are conflicting [44, 50–53]. Thus, EGFR amplification test to select patients for therapy is not standard in clinical practice.

BRAF mutations, which are mutually exclusive with KRAS mutations, are found in about 5 to 10% of mCRCs. BRAF mutations are associated with poor prognosis [54] and resistance to anti-EGFR agents in the second-line setting and beyond [50, 55]. Although randomized trials confirm the prognostic value of BRAF mutations, it does not have predictive role for anti-EGFR agents in first-line setting [56, 57]. Currently, BRAF mutation analysis should not be used for the selection of patients with WT RAS mCRC for anti-EGFR therapy.

Mutations of other genes, including phosphatidylinositol-4,5-bisphosphate 3-kinase, catalytic subunit alpha (PIK3CA) [58], p53 [59], PTEN [50] and genes involved in the insulin-like growth factor 1 (IGF1) signaling pathway [60, 61], or polymorphisms in EGF [62] may also have an impact on response to anti-EGFR mAbs. However, these biomarkers are not mature enough to be incorporated into clinical practice.

4. Clinical efficacy of anti-EGFR mAbs in mCRC

4.1. Cetuximab

4.1.1. Cetuximab monotherapy

In a randomized phase III trial, cetuximab monotherapy and BSC were compared in patients with mCRC who had failed or were intolerant of all standard therapies (n = 572) [63]. Partial response rate was 8% with cetuximab and overall survival (OS) was significantly improved with cetuximab (6.1 vs. 4.6 months). Subgroup analysis revealed that only patients with KRAS WT tumor provided survival benefit from cetuximab [19, 64]. Among patients with mutated KRAS, survival was similar in cetuximab and BSC arms.

4.1.2. Cetuximab combinations

4.1.2.1. Combination with irinotecan

A phase II study compared efficacy of cetuximab plus irinotecan and single agent irinotecan in 138 patients with irinotecan-refractory mCRC [65]. Partial response rate and time to tumor progression (TTP) were 15% and 6.5 months, respectively.

The BOND trial, a larger randomized phase II trial, compared irinotecan plus cetuximab versus cetuximab alone in 329 patients with irinotecan-refractory mCRC [9]. Combination therapy was significantly better than single agent cetuximab in terms of response rate (22.9% vs. 10.8%) and TTP (4.1 vs. 1.5 months); however, median survival was similar (8.6 vs. 6.9 months). In addition, benefit of adding cetuximab to irinotecan in patients with oxaliplatin-refractory mCRC has been reported in the EPIC trial [66]. Both objective response rates (16 vs. 4%) and PFS (4 vs. 2.6 months) were significantly higher with irinotecan plus cetuximab compared with single agent irinotecan. However, OS was similar (10.7 vs. 10 months), probably because of cross-over.

Study	**Year**	**Population**	**Patient number**	**Regimen**	**Median PFS (month)**	***p****	**Median OS (month)**	***p****	**Response rate (%)**	***p****
CRYSTAL[57]	2009	All	599	FOLFIRI	8	**0.048**	18.6	0.31	38.7	**0.0038**
			599	FOLFIRI + Cetuximab	8.9		19.9		46.9	
		KRAS WT subgroup	350	FOLFIRI	8.4	**0.0012**	20	**0.0093**	39.7	**<0.001**
			316	FOLFIRI + Cetuximab	9.9		23.5		57.3	
		KRAS MT subgroup	183	FOLFIRI	7.7	0.26	16.7	0.75	36.1	0.35
			214	FOLFIRI + Cetuximab	7.4		16.2		31.3	
OPUS[18]	2009	All	168	FOLFOX4	7.2	0.62	18	0.91	36	0.064
			169	FOLFOX4 + Cetuximab	7.2		18.3		46	
		KRAS WT subgroup	97	FOLFOX4	7.2	**0.0064**	18.5	0.39	34	**0.0027**
			82	FOLFOX4 + Cetuximab	8.3		22.8		57	
		KRAS	59	FOLFOX4	8.6	0.0153	17.5	0.2	53	0.029

Study	Year	Population	Patient number	Regimen	Median PFS (month)	*p**	Median OS (month)	*p**	Response rate (%)	*p**
		MT subgroup	77	FOLFOX4 + Cetuximab	5.5		13.4		34	
COIN[67]	2011	KRAS WT group	367	FOLFOX/ XELOX	8.6	0.60	17.9	0.68	57	0.049
			362	FOLFOX/ XELOX + Cetuximab	8.6		17		64	
		KRAS WT group	127	FOLFOX	9.2	0.056	–	–	–	–
			117	FOLFOX + Cetuximab	9.0		–		–	
		KRAS WT group	240	XELOX	8.0	0.56	–	–	–	–
			245	XELOX + Cetuximab	8.4		–		–	
		KRAS MT group	268	FOLFOX/ XELOX	-	-	14.8	0.80	-	-
			297	FOLFOX/ XELOX + Cetuximab	–		13.6		–	
NORDIC-VII[68]	2012	All	185	Nordic FLOX (control group)	7.9	–	20.4	–	41	–
			194	FLOX + Cetuximab	8.3	0.31	19.7	0.67	49	0.15
			187	intermittent FLOX + Cetuximab	7.3	N/A	20.3	0.79	47	N/A
		KRAS WT subgroup	97	Nordic FLOX (control group)	8.7	–	22	–	47	–
			97	FLOX + Cetuximab	7.9	0.66	20.1	0.48	46	0.89
			109	intermittent FLOX + Cetuximab	7.5	N/A	21.4	0.66	51	N/A
		KRAS MT	58	Nordic FLOX (control	7.8	–	20.4	–	40	–

Study	Year	Population	Patient number	Regimen	Median PFS (month)	p*	Median OS (month)	p*	Response rate (%)	p*
		subgroup		group)						
			72	FLOX + Cetuximab	9.2	**0.07**	21.1	0.89	49	0.31
			65	intermittent FLOX + Cetuximab	7.2	N/A	20.5	0.84	42	N/A
CALGB /SWOG[69] 80405 (study is ongoing)	2014	KRAS WT group	578	FOLFIRI or mFOLFOX6 + Cetuximab	10.45	N/A	29.93	0.34	–	–
			559	FOLFIRI or mFOLFOX6 + Bevacizumab	10.84		29.04		–	

*95% confidence interval.
PFS, progression-free survival; OS, overall survival; All, all patients group; WT, wild type; MT, mutant type; N/A, not available; KRAS, KRAS exon 2, codons 12 and 13; FOLFIRI, irinotecan, fluorouracil, and leucovorin; FOLFOX, fluorouracil, leucovorin, and oxaliplatin; XELOX, capecitabine and oxaliplatin; FLOX, fluorouracil, leucovorin, and oxaliplatin.

Table 1. Clinical trials of cetuximab plus chemotherapy as first-line treatment for metastatic colorectal cancer.

The CRYSTAL trial enrolled 1200 patients with mCRC and investigated the role of adding cetuximab to FOLFIRI as first-line therapy [8]. Response rate (47 vs. 39%) and median PFS (8.9 vs. 8 months), the primary end point of the study, were significantly better with FOLFIRI plus cetuximab compared with FOLFIRI alone, while OS was not significantly different between groups. An updated analysis of the CRYSTAL trial also demonstrated that adding cetuximab to FOLFIRI significantly improves OS (23.5 vs. 20 months), PFS (9.9 vs. 8.4 months), and response rate (57.3% vs. 39.7%) in patients with WT KRAS tumor. Perhaps more importantly, the rate of surgery for metastasis (7.9 vs. 4.6%, $p = 0.06$) and the rate of R0 resection (5.1 vs. 2%, $p = 0.02$) were both higher in patients with KRAS WT tumors who received cetuximab plus FOLFIRI compared with FOLFIRI alone [57]. Adverse effects that were more frequent with cetuximab were grade 3 or 4 diarrhea, skin toxicity, and infusion reactions. Based in large part on these data, cetuximab was approved for use in combination with FOLFIRI for first-line treatment of patients with KRAS WT mCRC [**Table 1**].

4.1.2.2. Combination with oxaliplatin

Randomized trials revealed conflicting results about benefits of adding cetuximab to oxaliplatin-based regimens. Three trials have evaluated the addition of cetuximab to oxaliplatin-based chemotherapy (FOLFOX/CAPOX) in first-line treatment of KRAS WT mCRC [18, 67, 68]. In randomized multicenter phase II OPUS study, FOLFOX4 plus cetuximab was compared with FOLFOX4 alone. Cetuximab provided significantly better response rate (61 vs. 37 %) and PFS (7.7 vs. 7.2 months) among patients with KRAS exon 2 WT tumors. However, median OS did not improve with addition of cetuximab (22.8 vs. 18.5) [18].

In randomized phase III MRC COIN study, adding cetuximab to oxaliplatin-based chemotherapy in patients with KRAS exon 2 WT mCRC increased response rate (64 vs. 57%) with no benefit in PFS (8.6 months in both groups) or OS (17.9 vs. 17) [67]. Likewise, another phase III study (NORDIC-VII) showed no survival benefit with the addition of cetuximab to FLOX regimen even in the KRAS WT group [68].

On the other hand, recently published randomized phase III CALGB/SWOG 80405 trial, in which 73% of the enrolled patients received FOLFOX as chemotherapy backbone, demonstrated that FOLFOX plus cetuximab can be effective as first-line treatment of patients with KRAS WT mCRC [69].

Converting initially unresectable isolated liver metastases to resectable status is another important issue for patients with mCRC, as R0 resection of isolated metastasis provide significant survival benefit. In the OPUS trial, addition of cetuximab to FOLFOX4 significantly increased ability for R0 resection of isolated liver metastasis [18]. In addition, the randomized phase II CELIM trial demonstrated that adding cetuximab to either irinotecan or oxaliplatin-based chemotherapy has similar efficacy in patients with initially unresectable liver metastases [70]. However, the efficacy of cetuximab-oxaliplatin combination for downstaging patients with isolated CRC liver metastases is unsettled. Recently, the randomized EPOC trial demonstrated that adding cetuximab to FOLFOX in patients with KRAS WT and potentially resectable isolated liver metastases was associated with worse PFS (14.8 vs. 24.2 months) [71]. Therefore, FOLFOX plus cetuximab should be used with caution in perioperative metastatic setting.

4.2. Panitumumab

4.2.1. Panitumumab monotherapy

In a multicenter trial ($n = 463$) adding panitumumab to BSC provided a 10% objective response rate in patients with mCRC refractory to standard treatment options [12, 72]. However, there was no significant PFS benefit, probably because of cross-over. Re-analysis according to KRAS status demonstrated that benefit of panitumumab monotherapy was restricted to KRAS WT tumors. Partial response rates in patients with KRAS WT and mutant tumors were 17% and 0%, respectively [73]. Although efficacy of panitumumab is similar to cetuximab monotherapy [63, 74], there is no data supporting to switch the anti-EGFR mAbs cetuximab and panitumumab after one of them fails.

4.2.2. Panitumumab combinations

There are increasing data supporting the efficacy of panitumumab in combination with oxaliplatin- or irinotecan-based regimens in patients with WT RAS tumors [10, 75–80].

4.2.2.1. Combination with irinotecan

The efficacy of first-line FOLFIRI-panitumumab combination in mCRC was evaluated in a single-arm phase II study. This regimen was well tolerated and response rates were 48% and 29% in the KRAS WT and mutant subsets, respectively [81]. Except this study, data regarding to FOLFIRI-panitumumab combination at first-line setting is mainly based on extrapolation from data in the second-line treatment. As an example, in a randomized phase III study (Study 181) the combination of panitumumab and FOLFIRI provide significant PFS benefit (5.9 vs. 3.9 months), but there was no difference in OS in patients with WT KRAS mCRC [11].

4.2.2.2. Combination with oxaliplatin

The phase III PRIME study compared panitumumab plus FOLFOX and FOLFOX alone as first-line treatment of patients with pan-RAS WT mCRC. Addition of panitumumab to FOLFOX significantly improved both PFS (10.1 vs. 9.2 months) and OS (23.8 vs. 19.4 months) [38]. Importantly, addition of panitumumab deteriorated PFS (7.3 vs. 8.9 months) in patients with KRAS mutation, consistent with other trials testing the addition of panitumumab or cetuximab to oxaliplatin-based chemotherapy [**Table 2**]. In addition, 17% of those with non-mutated KRAS exon 2 had other RAS mutations. These mutations were associated with worse PFS and OS with adding panitumumab to FOLFOX, similar to KRAS exon 2 mutations [38].

Study	Year	Population	Patient number	Regimen	Median PFS (month)	p^*	Median OS (month)	p^*	Response rate (%)	p^*
PRIME[10]	2010	KRAS WT group	331	FOLFOX4	8.0	**0.02**	19.7	0.072	48	0.068
			325	FOLFOX4 + Panitumumab	9.6		23.9		55	
		KRAS MT group	219	FOLFOX4	8.8	**0.02**	19.3	0.068	40	–
			221	FOLFOX4 + Panitumumab	7.3		15.5		40	

*95% Confidence interval.

PFS, progression-free survival; OS, overall survival; All, all patients group; WT, wild type; MT, mutant type; N/A, not available; KRAS, KRAS exon 2, codons 12 and 13; FOLFOX, fluorouracil, leucovorin, and oxaliplatin.

Table 2. Selected phase III trial of panitumumab plus chemotherapy as first-line treatment for metastatic colorectal cancer.

4.2.3. Cetuximab versus panitumumab

Data are limited about head-to-head comparison of panitumumab and cetuximab in mCRC. The ASPECCT trial, a randomized non-inferiority phase III study, showed that median OS was similar in patients with chemorefractory KRAS exon 2 WT mCRC who were treated with panitumumab (6 mg/kg once every 2 weeks) alone and with cetuximab (initial dose 400 mg/m^2, 250 mg/m^2 once a week thereafter) alone [82]. In addition, the incidence of any grade and grade 3–4 adverse events was similar in both treatment groups. However, the incidence of grade 3–4 infusion reactions was lower and grade 3–4 hypomagnesemia is higher with panitumumab compared with cetuximab [83]. Currently, there are no data supporting to use panitumumab or cetuximab beyond progression under an anti-EGFR mAb or to switch to cetuximab or panitumumab after one of them fails.

4.2.4. Bevacizumab versus cetuximab or panitumumab in combination with chemotherapy

Three trials have compared the benefits of anti-EGFR mAbs and anti-VEGF bevacizumab in combination with chemotherapy in RAS WT mCRC and the results are mixed.

In the FIRE-3 trial, patients with mCRC were randomly assigned to FOLFIRI with either bevacizumab or cetuximab as first-line treatment [20, 39]. Patients who had pan-RAS WT tumor had significantly better objective response rates (76 vs. 65 %) and OS (33.1 vs. 25.9 months) with cetuximab compared with bevacizumab, while PFS were not different between groups (10.5 vs. 10.4 months). Grade 1–2 emesis, hypertension, abscesses, and bleeding were more frequent with bevacizumab, and grade 1–2 hypocalcemia, and grade 3–4 skin toxicity, infusion reactions, and hypomagnesemia were more common with cetuximab. The reason for longer OS, in the absence of a better PFS, is unclear. Patients were on protocol-specified therapy for 5 months and the survival curves did not diverge until 24 months, suggesting that subsequent therapies beyond first-line treatment, which were not detailed in the report, may be important.

In the phase II PEAK trial, FOLFOX plus panitumumab was compared with FOLFOX plus bevacizumab as first-line treatment of mCRC [84]. For patients with KRAS exon 2 WT tumors, OS was significantly better (34 vs. 24 months) with panitumumab, while PFS was similar. When only pan-RAS WT patients were included, PFS was significantly better with panitumumab (13 vs. 9.5 months) but the statistical significance of the difference in OS disappeared, although potentially clinically meaningful (41 vs. 29 months, $p = 0.06$).

The recently published phase III CALGB/SWOG 80405 trial, in which patients with KRAS exon 2 WT mCRC were randomly assigned to cetuximab or bevacizumab plus chemotherapy (FOLFOX or FOLFIRI) as first-line treatment, demonstrated that both OS (29.9 vs. 29 months) and PFS (10.4 vs. 10.8 months) were similar [69]. FOLFOX was chosen in more than 70% of patients in this study. When only pan-RAS WT patients were analyzed, objective response rates were significantly higher with cetuximab (69 vs. 54 %), while OS (32 vs. 31.2 months) and PFS (11.4 vs. 11.3 months) were similar in both arms [85]. In conclusion, whether it is preferable to add an anti-EGFR mAb rather than bevacizumab to first-line chemotherapy in RAS WT mCRC is unclear [**Table 1**]. Preferring an anti-EGFR mAb rather than bevacizumab appears to be reasonable for patients with symptomatic tumors, in which response rate is a clinically more important purpose or if the use of bevacizumab is contraindicated. In addition, anti-EGFR mAbs appear to be not superior to bevacizumab in second-line therapy and beyond. In a phase II study (SPIRITT trial), patients with KRAS WT mCRC were randomized to FOLFIRI plus bevacizumab or FOLFIRI plus panitumumab as second-line therapy after failure of first-line bevacizumab plus oxaliplatin-based chemotherapy. PFS was similar in both group (9.2 vs. 7.7 months) [86].

4.2.5. Simultaneous use of cetuximab/panitumumab and bevacizumab

Two trials evaluated the addition of an anti-EGFR mAb to chemotherapy plus bevacizumab as first-line treatment of mCRC. The PACCE trial compared the efficacy of adding panitumumab to first-line oxaliplatin- (n = 823) or irinotecan (n = 230)-based chemotherapy plus bevacizumab [87]. The panitumumab/oxaliplatin group had significantly worse PFS and OS. Similar detrimental effect of dual antibody therapy was also observed in the CAIRO2 trial, which compared first-line XELOX plus bevacizumab with or without cetuximab [88]. PFS was significantly worse with the addition of cetuximab even in patients with KRAS WT tumors. These results suggest that using bevacizumab and panitumumab/cetuximab is not appropriate, at least in the first-line setting.

5. Toxicity profile of the anti-EGFR mAbs

The most common adverse effects associated with cetuximab and panitumumab are fatigue, acneiform rash, nausea, electrolyte imbalances, and infusion reactions [89–91].

5.1. Skin toxicity

Anti-EGFR therapies are associated with a variety of cutaneous side effects. Acneiform rash is the most common skin toxicity and occurs in up to two-thirds of patients. Interestingly, severity of rash correlates with better response rates [89, 92, 93]. Moreover, the EVEREST trial suggests that cetuximab dose escalation gradually, even up to 500 mg/m^2 weekly, could safely increase response rates in patients who have no or a mild skin reaction within the first 3 weeks of therapy [94]. However, cetuximab dose escalation according to grade of early skin reactions is not a standard approach currently, since OS benefit could not be shown. Pruritus, another common cutaneous adverse effect of anti-EGFR mAbs, is more common with panitumumab (55% any grade) compared to cetuximab (18% any grade) [95].

5.2. Electrolyte disorders

Magnesium-wasting syndrome is observed in 22% of patients receiving anti-EGFR mAbs [90, 96] and consequent hypomagnesemia may be more prominent when oxaliplatin is used concomitantly [97]. Hypokalemia is another important electrolyte disorder observed in approximately 8% of patients receiving cetuximab [98]. Hypomagnesemia may lead to secondary hypocalcemia and refractory hypokalemia. Thus, serum levels of magnesium, potassium, and calcium should be monitored periodically during and for at least 8 weeks after anti-EGFR containing therapy.

5.3. Infusion reactions

Infusion reactions are more common with cetuximab (25%) compared with panitumumab (4%), and more frequently observed in some areas of the middle southeastern United States [91]. Most of the infusion reactions are severe and occur within 3 hours of the first infusion. Cetuximab infusion should not exceed 5 mL/minute and premedication with an H1 receptor antagonist is recommended. For patients who develop a severe reaction to cetuximab despite premedication, desensitization or switching to panitumumab may be considered. Given the lower rates of infusion reactions compared with cetuximab, routine premedication is not recommended prior to panitumumab infusion.

5.4. Venous thromboembolism

Although not common, anti-EGFR mAbs may increase the risk of venous thromboembolism, but not arterial thromboembolism, as shown in a meta-analysis [99].

6. Anti-EGFR mAbs for geriatric population

Approximately 70% of CRC cases develop over the age of 65 [100]. The efficacy and main principles of mCRC treatment in the elderly are similar to younger patients. However, organ function decline and comorbidities are more common in the elderly and make them more vulnerable to side effects of systemic cancer therapies.

Because the number of older patients enrolled in clinical trials is small and these patients usually have good performance status [101, 102], good quality evidence about safety and efficacy of anti-cancer treatments in the elderly is limited. The majority of elderly patients are neither fit nor frail, and there is no evidence to support or refute the benefit and safety of therapy. Individualized treatment decision according to functional status, comorbidities, toxicity profile of the drugs is essential in older patients.

Few data are available about the safety and efficacy of anti-EGFR mAbs in the elderly mCRC patients. However, only older age should not be considered as an absolute contraindication to use anti-EGFR mAbs in mCRC. A retrospective study including heavily pretreated KRAS WT mCRC patients older than 70 years (n = 56) demonstrated that addition of cetuximab to irinotecan was tolerable and beneficial in the elderly similar to younger patients [103]. Another study analyzed 305 elderly and 352 younger (<65 years old) mCRC patients receiving chemotherapy plus cetuximab. Efficacy and the prevalence of side effects was similar in older and younger patients [104]. In contrast, a phase II trial of capecitabine plus cetuximab as first-line treatment of mCRC demonstrated that rate of acneiform rash was higher in the elderly (n = 66) [105].

Panitumumab monotherapy provides similar PFS benefit in the elderly compared with younger patients and may be a well-tolerated first-line option for frail elderly patients with WT RAS mCRC, as shown in a phase II study [12, 106]. A retrospective study demonstrated that toxicity-related dose reductions for panitumumab were required in about one-fourth of frail elderly patients receiving first-line or second-line therapy for mCRC ($n = 40$) [107].

6.1. Anti-EGFR mAbs for patients with poor performance status

Regardless of age, individuals with a poor performance status (PS) (e.g., Eastern Cooperative Oncology Group [ECOG] PS ≥2, Karnofsky PS <60) usually cannot tolerate chemotherapy and have a poor prognosis [108]. However, particularly if PS decline is cancer related, patients with mCRC who have a PS of 2 should be considered for chemotherapy. FU or capecitabine alone, or cetuximab/panitumumab monotherapy (if RAS WT) are appropriate options for patients who are not candidates for combination chemotherapy including oxaliplatin or irinotecan because of their poor performance status.

6.2. Mechanisms of resistance to anti-EGFR treatment

Unfortunately, after a variable period of responsive phase, secondary resistance to anti-EGFR mAbs develop. Therefore, it is a clear priority to understand the molecular and cellular basis of primary and acquired resistance to cetuximab and panitumumab. The mutational status of the EGFR signaling effectors (KRAS, BRAF, or PIK3CA) appears to be the main components of resistance.

6.3. KRAS/NRAS/BRAF mutations

Prospective randomized studies showed that KRAS mutations are predictive of non-response to anti-EGFR based treatment [8–12, 18–20]. However, KRAS mutation status is not enough to select appropriate patients for anti-EGFR mAbs, because almost 60% of patients with KRAS WT mCRC also have poor response to anti-EGFR mAbs [34]. Mutations in KRAS outside of exon 2 and mutations in NRAS are also associated with lack of response to anti-EGFR mAbs [38]. Thus, all patients with newly diagnosed mCRC should be tested for RAS mutation status, as RAS mutation is the major cause of primary resistance to anti-EGFR mAbs.

BRAF oncogene encodes BRAF protein that is a member of RAS/RAF/MAPK pathway [109]. BRAF and KRAS mutations are mutually exclusive [110]. BRAF gene mutation (V600E) rate is 5–9% among patients with mCRC [111, 112]. Although BRAF mutation is a poor prognostic factor for mCRC, as shown in the CRYSTAL and PETACC-3 studies [57, 113], the use of BRAF as a predictive marker is unclear. BRAF mutation status does not predict the response to either panitumumab or cetuximab in the first-line treatment of mCRC, as demonstrated in the CRYSTAL and the PRIME studies [10, 57]. In contrast to the results in the first-line treatment, BRAF mutation is a predictor of resistance to anti-EGFR treatment in the second-line therapy or beyond [36, 50, 55].

Interestingly, vemurafenib, an orally administered BRAF V600 kinase inhibitor, has insufficient activity when used alone in BRAF-mutated mCRC patients [114]. Vemurafenib resistance in mCRC may be because of feedback activation of EGFR signaling [115, 116].

6.4. Hyperactivation of PI3K-PTEN axis

Although 41% of mCRC patients do not have RAS or BRAF mutation, they do not respond to anti-EGFR mAbs [55]. Oncogenic activation of the members of EGFR downstream pathways other than RAS/RAF/MAPK (e.g., PI3K/PTEN pathway) might be responsible for the resistance to anti-EGFR mAbs. It is well established that activating mutation in PI3KCA or inactivation of PTEN phosphates can deregulate PI3K signaling pathway [117].

Mutation in PI3KCA and loss of PTEN are associated with resistance to anti-EGFR mAbs [118–120]. BRAF negative, PTEN expressing, and PI3K non-expressing CRCs have higher response rate and longer PFS and OS than others, suggesting that PI3K expression and PTEN loss might be used as predictors of response to anti-EGFR mAbs in mCRC patients with WT KRAS [121].

The role of PI3K mutation on response to anti-EGFR mAbs in mCRC has been evaluated in a number of studies [40, 58, 118, 122, 123]. Two of these studies demonstrated that PI3KCA mutation and PTEN loss, which cause PI3K pathway activation, are significant predictors of resistance to anti-EGFR mAbs [118, 122]. In contrast, PI3KCA mutation was not associated with response to anti-EGFR mAbs in chemorefractory mCRC patients in another study [123]. PTEN inactivation is another predictor of resistance to anti-EGFR mAbs [118–120]. Moreover, PI3K expression and PTEN loss are also associated with decreased survival in addition to poor response to anti-EGFR mAbs [117].

Study	Year	Population	Patient number	Regimen	Median PFS (month)	p*	Median OS (month)	p*	Response rate (%)	p*
Reidy et al.[128]	2010	All	23	IMC-A12 (anti-IGF-1R antibody)	5.9	–	5.2	–	0	–
			21	IMC-A12 (anti-IGF-1R antibody) + Cetuximab	6.1		4.5		5	
		KRAS WT group	20	IMC-A12 (anti-IGF-1R antibody) + Cetuximab	9.4		10.9		0	

*95% confidence interval.
PFS, progression-free survival; OS, overall survival; All, all patients group; WT, wild type; MT, mutant type; N/A: not available; KRAS, KRAS exon 2, codons 12 and 13; anti-IGF-1R, insulin-like growth factor-1 receptor inhibitor.

Table 3. Selected phase II study of an insulin-like growth factor-1 receptor inhibitor for metastatic colorectal cancer refractory to cetuximab or panitumumab

6.5. Hyperexpression or hyperactivation of type 1 insulin-like growth factor receptor (IGF-1R)

The type 1 insulin-like growth factor receptor (IGF-1R) is a tyrosine kinase receptor that functions by activating downstream signaling pathways, including MAPK and PI3K/AKT. IGF-1R overexpression, which may cause neoplastic transformation of cultured cells, is present in several types of human tumors [124, 125], and its downregulation can inhibit the growth of tumor cells [126]. These findings make IGF-1R an attractive candidate as an anti-cancer therapeutic target. A previous study showed that combination therapy of mAbs targeting IGF-1R and EGFR results in further inhibition of CRC cell-line growth [127]. A phase II study evaluated the safety and the efficacy of human anti-IGF-1R mAb (either alone or in combination with cetuximab) in mCRC patients, and both treatment modalities were reported as insufficient in chemorefractory mCRC patients [128] [**Table 3**].

6.6. EGFR-tyrosine kinase inhibitors in mCRC

The orally active EGFR-tyrosine kinase inhibitors erlotinib and gefitinib prevent downstream signaling of the receptor and are inactive as monotherapy of mCRC [129, 130]. Promising results have been reported in phase II trials of erlotinib with capecitabine and oxaliplatin [131] and gefitinib plus FOLFOX in mCRC patients [132, 133]. However, randomized trials are required to evaluate the benefits of gefitinib or erlotinib in combination with chemotherapy by comparing chemotherapy alone.

7. Future perspectives

The mAbs targeting EGFR (cetuximab and panitumumab) have shown remarkable efficacy in the treatment of mCRCs. Despite the significance of KRAS mutations, the efficacy of anti-EGFR monoclonal antibodies in the 60–70% of mCRC patients with KRAS WT tumors is still limited, with response rates between 10 and 40% [134]. Similar to other targeted therapies, anti-EGFR drugs are active only in a fraction of patients and most of them subsequently become resistant to the treatment. Accordingly, two major challenges need to be addressed to optimize the efficacy of anti-EGFR therapies. The first is to identify the genetic alterations associated with the clinical response to anti-EGFR mAbs. The second is the elucidation of the molecular basis for primary or acquired resistance to these drugs. It seems likely that a comprehensive biomarker analysis will be required to identify the mCRC patients who will truly benefit from anti-EGFR mAbs.

Author details

Rumeysa Ciftci and Deniz Tural*

*Address all correspondence to: deniztural@gmail.com

Department of Medical Oncology, Bakirkoy Dr. Sadi Konuk Education and Research Hospital, Bakırkoy, İstanbul, Turkey

http://dx.doi.org/10.5772/62304

References

[1] Jemal A, Bray F, Center MM, Ferlay J, Ward E, Forman D. Global cancer statistics. CA Cancer J Clin. 2011;61:69–90.

[2] Jemal A, Siegel R, Ward E, Hao Y, Xu J, Thun MJ. Cancer statistics, 2009. CA Cancer J Clin 2009;59:225–249.

[3] Alberts SR, Wagman LD. Chemotherapy for colorectal cancer liver metastases. Oncologist 2008;13:1063–1073.

[4] Van Cutsem E, Nordlinger B, Adam R, Köhne CH, Pozzo C, Poston G, Ychou M, Rougier P; European Colorectal Metastases Treatment Group. Towards a pan-European consensus on the treatment of patients with colorectal liver metastases. Eur J Cancer. 2006 ; 42(14):2212–2221.

[5] Jäger E, Heike M, Bernhard H, Klein O, Bernhard G, Lautz D, Michaelis J, Meyer zum Büschenfelde KH, Knuth A. Weekly high-dose leucovorin versus low-dose leucovorin combined with fluorouracil in advanced colorectal cancer: results of a randomized multicenter trial. Study Group for Palliative Treatment of Metastatic Colorectal Cancer Study Protocol 1. J Clin Oncol. 1996;14(8):2274–2279.

[6] Masi G, Vasile E, Loupakis F, Cupini S, Fornaro L, Baldi G, Salvatore L, Cremolini C, Stasi I, Brunetti I, Fabbri MA, Puglisi M, Trenta P, Granetto C, Chiara S, Fioretto L, Allegrini G, CrinòL, Andreuccetti M, Falcone A. Randomized trial of two induction chemotherapy regimens in metastatic colorectal cancer: an updated analysis. J Natl Cancer Inst. 2011;103(1):21–30.

[7] Chibaudel B, Maindrault-Goebel F, Lledo G, Mineur L, AndréT, Bennamoun M, Mabro M, Artru P, Carola E, Flesch M, Dupuis O, Colin P, Larsen AK, Afchain P,Tournigand C, Louvet C, de Gramont A. Can chemotherapy be discontinued in unresectable metastatic colorectal cancer? The GERCOR OPTIMOX2 Study. J Clin Oncol. 2009;27(34):5727–5733.

[8] Van Cutsem E, Kohne CH, Hitre E, Zaluski J, Chang Chien CR, Makhson A, D'Haens G, Pinter T, Lim R, Bodoky G, Roh JK, Folprecht G, Ruff P, Stroh C, Tejpar S, Schlichting M, Nippgen J, Rougier P. Cetuximab and chemotherapy as initial treatment for metastatic colorectal cancer. N Engl J Med. 2009;360:1408–1417.

[9] Cunningham D, Humblet Y, Siena S, Khayat D, Bleiberg H, Santoro A, Bets D, Mueser M, Harstrick A, Verslype C, Chau I, Van Cutsem E. Cetuximab monotherapy and cetuximab plus irinotecan in irinotecan-refractory metastatic colorectal cancer. N Engl J Med. 2004;351:337–345.

[10] Douillard JY, Siena S, Cassidy J, Tabernero J, Burkes R, Barugel M, Humblet Y, Bodoky G, Cunningham D, Jassem J, Rivera F, Kocakova I, Ruff P, Blasinska-Morawiec M, Smakal M, Canon JL, Rother M, Oliner KS, Wolf M, Gansert J. Randomized, phase III trial of panitumumab with infusional fluorouracil, leucovorin, and oxaliplatin (FOL-

FOX4) versus FOLFOX4 alone as first-line treatment in patients with previously untreated metastatic colorectal cancer: the PRIME study. J Clin Oncol. 2010;28:4697–4705.

[11] Peeters M, Price TJ, Cervantes A, Sobrero AF, Ducreux M, Hotko Y, Andre T, Chan E, Lordick F, Punt CJ, Strickland AH, Wilson G, Ciuleanu TE, Roman L, Van Cutsem E, Tzekova V, Collins S, Oliner KS, Rong A, Gansert J. Randomized phase III study of panitumumab with fluorouracil, leucovorin, and irinotecan (FOLFIRI) compared with FOLFIRI alone as second-line treatment in patients with metastatic colorectal cancer. J Clin Oncol. 2010;28:4706–4713.

[12] Van Cutsem E, Peeters M, Siena S, Humblet Y, Hendlisz A, Neyns B, Canon JL, Van Laethem JL, Maurel J, Richardson G, Wolf M, Amado RG. Open-label phase III trial of panitumumab plus best supportive care compared with best supportive care alone in patients with chemotherapy-refractory metastatic colorectal cancer. J Clin Oncol. 2007;25:1658–1664.

[13] Cao Y, Tan A, Gao F, Liu L, Liao C, Mo Z. A meta-analysis of randomized controlled trials comparing chemotherapy plus bevacizumab with chemotherapy alone in metastatic colorectal cancer. Int J Colorectal Dis. 2009;24(6):677–685.

[14] Lenz HJ. Anti-EGFR mechanism of action: antitumor effect and underlying cause of adverse events. Oncology (Williston Park). 2006;20:5–13.

[15] Spano JP, Lagorce C, Atlan D, Milano G, Domont J, Benamouzig R, Attar A, Benichou J, Martin A, Morere JF, Raphael M, Penault-Llorca F, Breau JL, Fagard R, Khayat D, Wind P. Impact of EGFR expression on colorectal cancer patient prognosis and survival. Ann Oncol. 2005;16:102–108.

[16] Martinelli E, De Palma R, Orditura M, De Vita F, Ciardiello F. Anti-epidermal growth factor receptor monoclonal antibodies in cancer therapy. Clin Exp Immunol. 2009;158:1–9.

[17] Saif MW, Shah M. K-Ras mutations in colorectal cancer: a practice changing discovery. Clin Adv Hematol Oncol. 2009;7(1):45–53, 64.

[18] Bokemeyer C, Bondarenko I, Makhson A, Hartmann JT, Aparicio J, de Braud F, Donea S, Ludwig H, Schuch G, Stroh C, Loos AH, Zubel A, Koralewski P. Fluorouracil, leucovorin, and oxaliplatin with and without cetuximab in the first-line treatment of metastatic colorectal cancer. J Clin Oncol. 2009;27:663–671.

[19] Karapetis CS, Khambata-Ford S, Jonker DJ, O'Callaghan CJ, Tu D, Tebbutt NC, Simes RJ, Chalchal H, Shapiro JD, Robitaille S, Price TJ, Shepherd L, Au HJ, Langer C, Moore MJ, Zalcberg JR. K-ras mutations and benefit from cetuximab in advanced colorectal cancer. N Engl J Med. 2008;359:1757–1765.

[20] Heinemann V, von Weikersthal LF, Decker T, Kiani A, Vehling-Kaiser U, Al-Batran SE, Heintges T, Lerchenmuller C, Kahl C, Seipelt G, Kullmann F, Stauch M, Scheithauer W, Hielscher J, Scholz M, Muller S, Link H, Niederle N, Rost A, Hoffkes HG, Moehler

M, Lindig RU, Modest DP, Rossius L, Kirchner T, Jung A, Stintzing S. FOLFIRI plus cetuximab versus FOLFIRI plus bevacizumab as first-line treatment for patients with metastatic colorectal cancer (FIRE-3): a randomised, open-label, phase 3 trial. Lancet Oncol. 2014;15:1065–1075.

[21] de Macedo MP, de Melo FM, Ribeiro Jda S, de Mello CA, de Souza Begnami MD, Soares FA, Carraro DM, da Cunha IW. RAS mutations vary between lesions in synchronous primary colorectal cancer: testing only one lesion is not sufficient to guide anti-EGFR treatment decisions. Oncoscience. 2015;2(2):125–130.

[22] Knijn N, Mekenkamp LJ, Klomp M, Vink-Börger ME, Tol J, Teerenstra S, Meijer JW, Tebar M, Riemersma S, van Krieken JH, Punt CJ, Nagtegaal ID. KRAS mutation analysis: a comparison between primary tumours and matched liver metastases in 305 colorectal cancer patients. British Journal of Cancer. 2011;104:1020–1026.

[23] Ondrejka SL, Schaeffer DF, Jakubowski MA, Owen DA, Bronner MP. Does neoadjuvant therapy alter KRAS and/or MSI results in rectal adenocarcinoma testing? Am J Surg Pathol. 2011;35(9):1327–1330.

[24] Yang QH, Schmidt J, Soucy G, Odze R, Dejesa-Jamanila L, Arnold K, Kuslich C, Lash R. KRAS mutational status of endoscopic biopsies matches resection specimens. J Clin Pathol. 2012;65:604–607.

[25] Allegra CJ, Rumble RB, Hamilton SR, Mangu PB, Roach N, Hantel A, Schilsky RL. Extended RAS gene mutation testing in metastatic colorectal carcinoma to predict response to anti-epidermal growth factor receptor monoclonal antibody therapy: American Society of Clinical Oncology Provisional Clinical Opinion Update 2015. J Clin Oncol. 2015. pii: JCO.2015.63.9674.

[26] Ciardiello F, Tortora G. EGFR antagonists in cancer treatment. N Engl J Med. 2008;358:1160–1174.

[27] Greening DW, Lee ST, Ji H, Simpson RJ, Rigopoulos A, Murone C, Fang C, Gong S, O'Keefe G, Scott AM. Molecular profiling of cetuximab and bevacizumab treatment of colorectal tumours reveals perturbations in metabolic and hypoxic response pathways. Oncotarget. 2015;6(35):38166–38180.

[28] Scott AM, Wolchok JD, Old LJ. Antibody therapy of cancer. Nat Rev Cancer. 2012;12:278–287.

[29] Dahabreh IJ, Terasawa T, Castaldi PJ, Trikalinos TA. Systematic review: anti-epidermal growth factor receptor treatment effect modification by KRAS mutations in advanced colorectal cancer. Ann Intern Med. 2011;154(1):37–49.

[30] Tejpar S, Celik I, Schlichting M, Sartorius U, Bokemeyer C, Van Cutsem E. Association of KRAS G13D tumor mutations with outcome in patients with metastatic colorectal cancer treated with first-line chemotherapy with or without cetuximab. J Clin Oncol. 2012;30:3570–3577.

[31] Peeters M, Douillard JY, Van Cutsem E, Siena S, Zhang K, Williams R, Wiezorek J. Mutant KRAS codon 12 and 13 alleles in patients with metastatic colorectal cancer: assessment as prognostic and predictive biomarkers of response to panitumumab. J Clin Oncol. 2013;31:759–765.

[32] Mao C, Huang YF, Yang ZY, Zheng DY, Chen JZ, Tang JL. KRAS p.G13D mutation and codon 12 mutations are not created equal in predicting clinical outcomes of cetuximab in metastatic colorectal cancer: a systematic review and meta-analysis. Cancer. 2013;119:714–721.

[33] Schirripa M, Lonardi S, Cremolini C, et al. Phase II study of single-agent cetuximab in KRAS G13D mutant metastatic colorectal cancer (m CRC) (abstract). J Clin Oncol. 2014;32:5s, (suppl; abstr 3524). Abstract available online at: http://meetingli-brary.asco.org/content/130634-144 (Accessed on 12 June 2014).

[34] Linardou H, Dahabreh IJ, Kanaloupiti D, Siannis F, Bafaloukos D, Kosmidis P, Papa-dimitriou CA, Murray S. Assessment of somatic k-RAS mutations as a mechanism associated with resistance to EGFR-targeted agents: a systematic review and meta-analysis of studies in advanced non-small-cell lung cancer and metastatic colorectal cancer. Lancet Oncol. 2008;9:962–972.

[35] Normanno N, Rachiglio AM, Lambiase M, Martinelli E, Fenizia F, Esposito C, Roma C, Troiani T, Rizzi D, Tatangelo F, Botti G, Maiello E, Colucci G, Ciardiello F; CAPRI-GOIM investigators. Heterogeneity of KRAS, NRAS, BRAF and PIK3CA mutations in metastatic colorectal cancer and potential effects on therapy in the CAPRI GOIM trial. Ann Oncol. 2015; 26:1710–1714.

[36] Loupakis F, Ruzzo A, Cremolini C, Vincenzi B, Salvatore L, Santini D, Masi G, Stasi I, Canestrari E, Rulli E, Floriani I, Bencardino K, Galluccio N, Catalano V, Tonini G, Magnani M, Fontanini G, Basolo F, Falcone A, Graziano F. KRAS codon 61, 146 and BRAF mutations predict resistance to cetuximab plus irinotecan in KRAS codon 12 and 13 wild-type metastatic colorectal cancer. Br J Cancer. 2009;101:715–721.

[37] Peeters M, Kafatos G, Taylor A, Gastanaga VM, Oliner KS, Hechmati G, Terwey JH, van Krieken JH. Prevalence of RAS mutations and individual variation patterns among patients with metastatic colorectal cancer: a pooled analysis of randomised controlled trials. Eur J Cancer. 2015;51:1704–1713.

[38] Douillard JY, Oliner KS, Siena S, Tabernero J, Burkes R, Barugel M, Humblet Y, Bodoky G, Cunningham D, Jassem J, Rivera F, Kocakova I, Ruff P, Blasinska-Morawiec M, Smakal M, Canon JL, Rother M, Williams R, Rong A, Wiezorek J, Sidhu R, Patterson SD. Panitumumab-FOLFOX4 treatment and RAS mutations in colorectal cancer. N Engl J Med. 2013;369:1023–1034.

[39] Heinemann V, Fischer von Weikersthal L, Decker T. Analysis of KRAS/NRAS and BRAF mutations in FIRE-3: a randomized phase III study of FOLFIRI plus cetuximab or bevacizumab as first-line treatment for wild-type (WT) KRAS (exon 2) metastatic colorectal cancer (m CRC) patients (abstract). In:The 13th annual European Cancer

Congress (ECC); 28 September 2013; Amsterdam, the Netherlands. http://eccamsterdam2013.ecco-org.eu/Scientific-Programme/Searchable-Programme.aspx#anchor Scpr (Accessed: 2013-11-21).

[40] De Roock W, Claes B, Bernasconi D, De Schutter J, Biesmans B, Fountzilas G, Kalogeras KT, Kotoula V, Papamichael D, Laurent-Puig P, Penault-Llorca F, Rougier P, Vincenzi B, Santini D, Tonini G, Cappuzzo F, Frattini M, Molinari F, Saletti P, De Dosso S, Martini M, Bardelli A, Siena S, Sartore-Bianchi A, Tabernero J, Macarulla T, Di Fiore F, Gangloff AO, Ciardiello F, Pfeiffer P, Qvortrup C, Hansen TP, Van Cutsem E, Piessevaux H, Lambrechts D, Delorenzi M, Tejpar S. Effects of KRAS, BRAF, NRAS, and PIK3CA mutations on the efficacy of cetuximab plus chemotherapy in chemotherapy-refractory metastatic colorectal cancer: a retrospective consortium analysis. Lancet Oncol. 2010;11:753–762.

[41] Peeters M, Oliner KS, Price TJ. Analysis of KRAS/NRAS mutations in phase 3 study 20050181 of panitumumab (pmab) plus FOLFIRI versus FOLFIRI for second-line treatment (tx) of metastatic colorectal cancer (m CRC) (abstract). J Clin Oncol. 2014;32(suppl 3; abstr LBA387). http://meetinglibrary.asco.org/content/122548-143 (Accessed: 2014-03-25).

[42] Sorich MJ, Wiese MD, Rowland A, Kichenadasse G, Mc Kinnon RA, Karapetis CS. Extended RAS mutations and anti-EGFR monoclonal antibody survival benefit in metastatic colorectal cancer: a meta-analysis of randomized, controlled trials. Ann Oncol. 2015;26:13–21.

[43] Baker JB, Dutta D, Watson D, Maddala T, Munneke BM, Shak S, Rowinsky EK, Xu LA, Harbison CT, Clark EA, Mauro DJ, Khambata-Ford S. Tumour gene expression predicts response to cetuximab in patients with KRAS wild-type metastatic colorectal cancer. British Journal of Cancer. 2011;104:488–495.

[44] Lenz HJ, Van Cutsem E, Khambata-Ford S, Mayer RJ, Gold P, Stella P, Mirtsching B, Cohn AL, Pippas AW, Azarnia N, Tsuchihashi Z, Mauro DJ, Rowinsky EK. Multicenter phase II and translational study of cetuximab in metastatic colorectal carcinoma refractory to irinotecan, oxaliplatin, and fluoropyrimidines. J Clin Oncol. 2006;24(30): 4914–4921.

[45] Saltz LB, Meropol NJ, Loehrer PJSr, Needle MN, Kopit J, Mayer RJ. Phase II trial of cetuximab in patients with refractory colorectal cancer that expresses the epidermal growth factor receptor. J Clin Oncol. 2004;22(7):1201–1208.

[46] Chung KY, Shia J, Kemeny NE, Shah M, Schwartz GK, Tse A, Hamilton A, Pan D, Schrag D, Schwartz L, Klimstra DS, Fridman D, Kelsen DP, Saltz LB. Cetuximab shows activity in colorectal cancer patients with tumors that do not express the epidermal growth factor receptor by immunohistochemistry. J Clin Oncol. 2005;23(9):1803–1810.

[47] Hecht JR, Mitchell E, Neubauer MA, Burris HA3rd, Swanson P, Lopez T, Buchanan G, Reiner M, Gansert J, Berlin J. Lack of correlation between epidermal growth factor

receptor status and response to panitumumab monotherapy in metastatic colorectal cancer. Clin Cancer Res. 2010;16(7):2205–2213.

[48] Mitchell EP, Hecht JR, Baranda J, Malik I, Richards D, Reiner M, Stout S, Amado RG. Panitumumab activity in metastatic colorectal cancer (m CRC) patients with low or negative tumor epidermal growth factor receptor levels: an updated analysis (abstract). J Clin Oncol. 2007;25(18S):4082.

[49] Tsuchihashi Z, Khambata-Ford S, Hanna N, Jänne PA. Responsiveness to cetuximab without mutations in EGFR. N Engl J Med. 2005;353:208–209.

[50] Laurent-Puig P, Cayre A, Manceau G, Buc E, Bachet JB, Lecomte T, Rougier P, Lievre A, Landi B, Boige V, Ducreux M, Ychou M, Bibeau F, Bouche O, Reid J, Stone S, Penault-Llorca F. Analysis of PTEN, BRAF, and EGFR status in determining benefit from cetuximab therapy in wild-type KRAS metastatic colon cancer. J Clin Oncol. 2009;27:5924–5930.

[51] Moroni M, Veronese S, Benvenuti S, Marrapese G, Sartore-Bianchi A, Di Nicolantonio F, Gambacorta M, Siena S, Bardelli A. Gene copy number for epidermal growth factor receptor (EGFR) and clinical response to anti EGFR treatment in colorectal cancer: a cohort study. Lancet Oncol. 2005;6(5):279–286.

[52] Cappuzzo F, Varella-Garcia M, Finocchiaro G, Skokan M, Gajapathy S, Carnaghi C, Rimassa L, Rossi E, Ligorio C, Di Tommaso L, Holmes AJ, Toschi L, Tallini G, Destro A, Roncalli M, Santoro A, Jänne PA. Primary resistance to cetuximab therapy in EGFR FISH-positive colorectal cancer patients. Br J Cancer. 2008;99(1):83–89.

[53] Italiano A, Follana P, Caroli FX, Badetti JL, Benchimol D, Garnier G, Gugenheim J, Haudebourg J, Keslair F, Lesbats G, Lledo G, Roussel JF, Pedeutour F, François E. Cetuximab shows activity in colorectal cancer patients with tumors for which FISH analysis does not detect an increase in EGFR gene copy number. Ann Surg Oncol. 2008;15(2):649–654.

[54] Lochhead P, Kuchiba A, Imamura Y, Liao X, Yamauchi M, Nishihara R, Qian ZR, Morikawa T, Shen J, Meyerhardt JA, Fuchs CS, Ogino S. Microsatellite instability and BRAF mutation testing in colorectal cancer prognostication. J Natl Cancer Inst. 2013;105(15):1151–1156.

[55] Di Nicolantonio F, Martini M, Molinari F, Sartore-Bianchi A, Arena S, Saletti P, De Dosso S, Mazzucchelli L, Frattini M, Siena S, Bardelli A. Wild-type BRAF is required for response to panitumumab or cetuximab in metastatic colorectal cancer. J Clin Oncol. 2008;26:5705–5712.

[56] Bokemeyer C, Kohne C, Rougier P, Stroh C, Schlichting M, Van Cutsem E. Cetuximab with chemotherapy as first-line treatment for metastatic colorectal cancer: analysis of the CRYSTAL and OPUS studies according to KRAS and BRAF mutation status (abstract #3506). J Clin Oncol. 2010;28(15):3506.

[57] Van Cutsem E, Kohne CH, Lang I, Folprecht G, Nowacki MP, Cascinu S, Shchepotin I, Maurel J, Cunningham D, Tejpar S, Schlichting M, Zubel A, Celik I, Rougier P, Ciardiello F. Cetuximab plus irinotecan, fluorouracil, and leucovorin as first-line treatment for metastatic colorectal cancer: updated analysis of overall survival according to tumor KRAS and BRAF mutation status. J Clin Oncol. 2011;29:2011–2019.

[58] Mao C, Yang ZY, Hu XF, Chen Q, Tang JL. PIK3CA exon 20 mutations as a potential biomarker for resistance to anti-EGFR monoclonal antibodies in KRAS wild-type metastatic colorectal cancer: a systematic review and meta-analysis. Ann Oncol. 2012;23:1518–1525.

[59] Oden-Gangloff A, Di Fiore F, Bibeau F, Lamy A, Bougeard G, Charbonnier F, Blanchard F, Tougeron D, Ychou M, Boissière F, Le Pessot F, Sabourin JC, Tuech JJ, Michel P, Frebourg T. TP53 mutations predict disease control in metastatic colorectal cancer treated with cetuximab-based chemotherapy. Br J Cancer. 2009;100(8):1330–1335.

[60] Winder T, Zhang W, Yang D, Ning Y, Bohanes P, Gerger A, Wilson PM, Pohl A, Mauro DJ, Langer C, Rowinsky EK, Lenz HJ. Germline polymorphisms in genes involved in the IGF1 pathway predict efficacy of cetuximab in wild-type KRAS m CRC patients. Clin Cancer Res 2010;16(22):5591–602.

[61] Huang F, Xu LA, Khambata-Ford S. Correlation between gene expression of IGF-1R pathway markers and cetuximab benefit in metastatic colorectal cancer. Clin Cancer Res. 2012;18(4):1156–66.

[62] Garm Spindler KL, Pallisgaard N, Rasmussen AA, Lindebjerg J, Andersen RF, Crüger D, Jakobsen A. The importance of KRAS mutations and EGF61A > G polymorphism to the effect of cetuximab and irinotecan in metastatic colorectal cancer. Ann Oncol. 2009;20(5):879–84.

[63] Jonker DJ, O'Callaghan CJ, Karapetis CS, Zalcberg JR, Tu D, Au HJ, Berry SR, Krahn M, Price T, Simes RJ, Tebbutt NC, van Hazel G, Wierzbicki R, Langer C, Moore MJ. Cetuximab for the treatment of colorectal cancer. N Engl J Med. 2007; 357(20):2040–8.

[64] Au HJ, Karapetis CS, O'Callaghan CJ, Tu D, Moore MJ, Zalcberg JR, Kennecke H, Shapiro JD, Koski S, Pavlakis N, Charpentier D, Wyld D, Jefford M, Knight GJ, Magoski NM, Brundage MD, Jonker DJ. Health-related quality of life in patients with advanced colorectal cancer treated with cetuximab: overall and KRAS-specific results of the NCIC CTG and AGITG CO.17 Trial. J Clin Oncol. 2009;27(11):1822–8.

[65] Saltz L, Rubin M, Hochster H. Cetuximab (IMC-225) plus irinotecan is active in CPT-11-refractory colorectal cancer that expresses epidermal growth factor receptor (abstract 7). Proc Am Soc Clin Oncol. 2001;20:3a.

[66] Sobrero AF, Maurel J, Fehrenbacher L, Scheithauer W, Abubakr YA, Lutz MP, Vega-Villegas ME, Eng C, Steinhauer EU, Prausova J, Lenz HJ, Borg C, Middleton G, Kröning H, Luppi G, Kisker O, Zubel A, Langer C, Kopit J, Burris HA3rd. EPIC: phase III trial

of cetuximab plus irinotecan after fluoropyrimidine and oxaliplatin failure in patients with metastatic colorectal cancer. J Clin Oncol. 2008;26(14):2311–9.

[67] Maughan TS, Adams RA, Smith CG, Meade AM, Seymour MT, Wilson RH, Idziaszczyk S, Harris R, Fisher D, Kenny SL, Kay E, Mitchell JK, Madi A, Jasani B, James MD, Bridgewater J, Kennedy MJ, Claes B, Lambrechts D, Kaplan R, Cheadle JP, Investigators MCT. Addition of cetuximab to oxaliplatin-based first-line combination chemotherapy for treatment of advanced colorectal cancer: results of the randomised phase 3 MRC COIN trial. Lancet. 2011;377:2103–14.

[68] Tveit KM, Guren T, Glimelius B, Pfeiffer P, Sorbye H, Pyrhonen S, Sigurdsson F, Kure E, Ikdahl T, Skovlund E, Fokstuen T, Hansen F, Hofsli E, Birkemeyer E, Johnsson A, Starkhammar H, Yilmaz MK, Keldsen N, Erdal AB, Dajani O, Dahl O, Christoffersen T. Phase III trial of cetuximab with continuous or intermittent fluorouracil, leucovorin, and oxaliplatin (Nordic FLOX) versus FLOX alone in first-line treatment of metastatic colorectal cancer: the NORDIC-VII study. J Clin Oncol. 2012;30:1755–62.

[69] Venook AP, Niedzwiecki D, Lenz H-J, Innocenti F, Mahoney MR, O'Neil BH, Shaw JE, Polite BN, Hochster HS, Atkins JN, Goldberg RM, Mayer RJ, Schilsky RL, Bertagnolli MM, Blanke CD, (Alliance) Ca LGB. CALGB/SWOG 80405: Phase III trial of irinotecan/5-FU/leucovorin (FOLFIRI) or oxaliplatin/5-FU/leucovorin (m FOLFOX6) with bevacizumab (BV) or cetuximab (CET) for patients (pts) with KRAS wild-type (wt) untreated metastatic adenocarcinoma of the colon or rectum (MCRC). J Clin Oncol. 2014; 32:5s, 2014 (suppl; abstr LBA3).

[70] Folprecht G, Gruenberger T, Bechstein WO, Raab HR, Lordick F, Hartmann JT, Lang H,Frilling A, Stoehlmacher J, Weitz J, Konopke R, Stroszczynski C,Liersch T, Ockert D, Herrmann T, Goekkurt E, Parisi F, Köhne CH. Tumour response and secondary resectability of colorectal liver metastases following neoadjuvant chemotherapy with cetuximab: the CELIM randomised phase 2 trial. Lancet Oncol. 2010;11(1):38–47.

[71] Primrose J, Falk S, Finch-Jones M, Valle J, O'Reilly D, Siriwardena A, Hornbuckle J, Peterson M, Rees M, Iveson T, Hickish T, Butler R, Stanton L, Dixon E, Little L, Bowers M, Pugh S, Garden OJ, Cunningham D, Maughan T, Bridgewater J, Primrose J, Falk S, Finch-Jones M, et al. Systemic chemotherapy with or without cetuximab in patients with resectable colorectal liver metastasis: the new EPOC randomised controlled trial. Lancet Oncol. 2014;15(6):601–11.

[72] Van Cutsem E, Siena S, Humblet Y, Canon JL, Maurel J, Bajetta E, Neyns B, Kotasek D, Santoro A, Scheithauer W, Spadafora S, Amado RG, Hogan N, Peeters M. An open-label, single-arm study assessing safety and efficacy of panitumumab in patients with metastatic colorectal cancer refractory to standard chemotherapy. Ann Oncol. 2008;19(1):92–8.

[73] Amado RG, Wolf M, Peeters M, Van Cutsem E, Siena S, Freeman DJ, Juan T, Sikorski R, Suggs S, Radinsky R, Patterson SD, Chang DD. Wild-type KRAS is required for

panitumumab efficacy in patients with metastatic colorectal cancer. J Clin Oncol. 2008;26:1626–34.

[74] Price T, Peeters M, Kim TW, et al. ASPECCT: a randomized, multicenter, open-label, phase 3 study of panitumumab versus cetuximab for previously treated wild-type KRAS metastatic colorectal cancer (abstract). In: The 2013 European Cancer Congress; 29 September 2013; Amsterdam, the Netherlands, (abstract LBA18). http://eccamsterdam2013.ecco-org.eu/Scientific-Programme/Searchable-Programme.aspx#anchor Scpr (Accessed: 2013-11-21).

[75] Berlin J, Posey J, Tchekmedyian S, Hu E, Chan D, Malik I, Yang L, Amado RG, Hecht JR. Panitumumab with irinotecan/leucovorin/5-fluorouracil for first-line treatment of metastatic colorectal cancer. Clin Colorectal Cancer. 2007;6(6):427–32.

[76] Köhne CH, Hofheinz R, Mineur L, Letocha H, Greil R, Thaler J, Fernebro E, Gamelin E, Decosta L, Karthaus M. First-line panitumumab plus irinotecan/5-fluorouracil/leucovorin treatment in patients with metastatic colorectal cancer. J Cancer Res Clin Oncol. 2012; 138(1):65–72.

[77] Cohn AL, Shumaker GC, Khandelwal P, Smith DA, Neubauer MA, Mehta N, Richards D, Watkins DL, Zhang K, Yassine MR. An open-label, single-arm, phase 2 trial of panitumumab plus FOLFIRI as second-line therapy in patients with metastatic colorectal cancer. Clin Colorectal Cancer. 2011;10(3):171–7.

[78] AndréT, Blons H, Mabro M, Chibaudel B, Bachet JB, Tournigand C, Bennamoun M, Artru P, Nguyen S, Ebenezer C, Aissat N, Cayre A, Penault-Llorca F, Laurent-Puig P, de Gramont A; GERCOR. Panitumumab combined with irinotecan for patients with KRAS wild-type metastatic colorectal cancer refractory to standard chemotherapy: a GERCOR efficacy, tolerance, and translational molecular study. Ann Oncol. 2013;24(2): 412–9.

[79] Seymour MT, Brown SR, Middleton G, Maughan T, Richman S, Gwyther S, Lowe C, Seligmann JF, Wadsley J, Maisey N, Chau I, Hill M, Dawson L, Falk S, O'Callaghan A, Benstead K, Chambers P, Oliver A, Marshall H, Napp V, Quirke P. Panitumumab and irinotecan versus irinotecan alone for patients with KRAS wild-type, fluorouracil-resistant advanced colorectal cancer (PICCOLO): a prospectively stratified randomised trial. Lancet Oncol. 2013;14(8):749–59.

[80] Peeters M, Price TJ, Cervantes A, Sobrero AF, Ducreux M, Hotko Y, AndréT, Chan E, Lordick F, Punt CJ, Strickland AH, Wilson G, Ciuleanu TE, Roman L, Van Cutsem E, Tian Y, Sidhu R. Final results from a randomized phase 3 study of FOLFIRI {+/−} panitumumab for second-line treatment of metastatic colorectal cancer. Ann Oncol. 2014;25(1):107–16.

[81] Kohne C, Mineur L, Greil R, Letocha H, Thaler J, Hofheinz R, Fernebro E, Gamelin E, Wright L, Karthaus M. Primary analysis of a phase II study (20060314) combining first-

line panitumumab (pmab) with FOLFIRI in the treatment of patients (pts) with metastatic colorectal cancer (m CRC) [abstract]. J Clin Oncol. 2010;201:414.

[82] Price TJ, Peeters M, Kim TW, Li J, Cascinu S, Ruff P, Suresh AS, Thomas A, Tjulandin S, Zhang K, Murugappan S, Sidhu R. Panitumumab versus cetuximab in patients with chemotherapy-refractory wild-type KRAS exon 2 metastatic colorectal cancer (AS-PECCT): a randomised, multicentre, open-label, non-inferiority phase 3 study. Lancet Oncol. 2014;15:569–79.

[83] Vale CL, Tierney JF, Fisher D, Adams RA, Kaplan R, Maughan TS, Parmar MK, Meade AM. Does anti-EGFR therapy improve outcome in advanced colorectal cancer? A systematic review and meta-analysis. Cancer Treat Rev. 2012;38:618–25.

[84] Schwartzberg LS, Rivera F, Karthaus M, Fasola G, Canon JL, Hecht JR, Yu H, Oliner KS, Go WY. PEAK: a randomized, multicenter phase II study of panitumumab plus modified fluorouracil, leucovorin, and oxaliplatin (m FOLFOX6) or bevacizumab plus m FOLFOX6 in patients with previously untreated, unresectable, wild-type KRAS exon 2 metastatic colorectal cancer. J Clin Oncol. 2014;32(21):2240–7.

[85] Lenz H, Niedzwiecki D, Innocenti F, Blanke C, Mahony MR, O'Neil BH, Shaw JE, Polite B, Hochster H, Atkins J, Goldberg R, Mayer R, Schilsky RL, Bertagnolli M, Venook A. CALGB/SWOG 80405: PHASE III trial of irinotecan/5-FU/Leucovorin (FOLFIRI) or oxaliplatin/5-FU/leucovorin (m FOLFOX) with bevacizumab or cetuximab for patients with expanded ras analysis untreated metastatic adenocarcinoma of the colon or rectum (abstract 501O). Annals of Oncology. 2014;25(Supplement 5):v1–v41. In: The 2014 ESMO Congress, 27–30 September 2014. Madrid, Spain. https://www.webg-es.com/cslide/library/esmo/browse/search/r Bc#9faw03o W (Accessed: 04 December 2014).

[86] Hecht JR, Cohn A, Dakhil S, Saleh M, Piperdi B, Cline-Burkhardt M, Tian Y, Go WY. SPIRITT: a randomized, multicenter, phase II study of panitumumab with FOLFIRI and bevacizumab with FOLFIRI as second-line treatment in patients with unresectable wild type KRAS metastatic colorectal cancer. Clin Colorectal Cancer. 2015;14(2):72–80.

[87] Hecht JR, Mitchell E, Chidiac T, Scroggin C, Hagenstad C, Spigel D, Marshall J, Cohn A, Mc Collum D, Stella P, Deeter R, Shahin S, Amado RG. A randomized phase IIIB trial of chemotherapy, bevacizumab, and panitumumab compared with chemotherapy and bevacizumab alone for metastatic colorectal cancer. J Clin Oncol. 2009;27(5):672–80.

[88] Tol J, Koopman M, Cats A, Rodenburg CJ, Creemers GJ, Schrama JG, Erdkamp FL, Vos AH, van Groeningen CJ, Sinnige HA, Richel DJ, Voest EE, Dijkstra JR, Vink-Börger ME, Antonini NF, Mol L, van Krieken JH, Dalesio O, Punt CJ. Chemotherapy, bevacizumab, and cetuximab in metastatic colorectal cancer. N Engl J Med. 2009;360(6):563–72.

[89] Van Cutsem E, Humblet Y, Gelderblom H, Vermorken JB, Vire Ft, Glimelius B. Cetuximab dose-escalation study in patients with metastatic colorectal cancer with no or slight skin reactions on cetuximab standard dose treatment (EVEREST): pharmaco-

kinetics and efficacy data of a randomized study (abstract #237). In: The 4th annual ASCO Gastrointestinal Cancers Symposium. 20 January 2007. Orlando, FL.

[90] Schrag D, Chung KY, Flombaum C, Saltz L. Cetuximab therapy and symptomatic hypomagnesemia. J Natl Cancer Inst. 2005;97(16):1221–4.

[91] O'Neil BH, Allen R, Spigel DR, Stinchcombe TE, Moore DT, Berlin JD, Goldberg RM. High incidence of cetuximab-related infusion reactions in Tennessee and North Carolina and the association with atopic history. J Clin Oncol. 2007;25(24):3644–8.

[92] Peeters M, Siena S, Van Cutsem E, Sobrero A, Hendlisz A, Cascinu S, Kalofonos H, Devercelli G, Wolf M, Amado RG. Association of progression-free survival, overall survival, and patient-reported outcomes by skin toxicity and KRAS status in patients receiving panitumumab monotherapy. Cancer. 2009;115(7):1544–54.

[93] Berlin J, Van Cutsem E, Peeters M, Hecht JR, Ruiz R, Wolf M, Amado RG, Meropol NJ. Predictive value of skin toxicity severity for response to panitumumab in patients with metastatic colorectal cancer (m CRC): pooled analysis of five clinical trials (abstract). J Clin Oncol. 2007;25(18S):4134.

[94] Van Cutsem E, Tejpar S, Vanbeckevoort D, Peeters M, Humblet Y, Gelderblom H, Vermorken JB, Viret F, Glimelius B, Gallerani E, Hendlisz A, Cats A, Moehler M, Sagaert X, Vlassak S, Schlichting M, Ciardiello F. Intrapatient cetuximab dose escalation in metastatic colorectal cancer according to the grade of early skin reactions: the randomized EVEREST study. J Clin Oncol. 2012;30(23):2861–8.

[95] Ensslin CJ, Rosen AC, Wu S, Lacouture ME. Pruritus in patients treated with targeted cancer therapies: systematic review and meta-analysis. J Am Acad Dermatol. 2013;69(5):708–20.

[96] Tejpar S, Piessevaux H, Claes K, Piront P, Hoenderop JG, Verslype C, Van Cutsem E. Magnesium wasting associated with epidermal-growth-factor receptor-targeting antibodies in colorectal cancer: a prospective study. Lancet Oncol. 2007;8(5):387–94.

[97] Stintzing S, Fischhaber D, Mook C, Modest DP, Giessen C, Schulz C, Haas M, Boeck S, Michl M, Stemmler J, Laubender RP, Heinemann V. Clinical relevance and utility of cetuximab-related changes in magnesium and calcium serum levels. Anticancer Drugs. 2013;24(9):969–74.

[98] Cao Y, Liu L, Liao C, Tan A, Gao F. Meta-analysis of incidence and risk of hypokalemia with cetuximab-based therapy for advanced cancer. Cancer Chemother Pharmacol. 2010;66(1):37–42.

[99] Petrelli F, Cabiddu M, Borgonovo K, Barni S. Risk of venous and arterial thromboembolic events associated with anti-EGFR agents: a meta-analysis of randomized clinical trials. Ann Oncol. 2012;23(7):1672–9.

[100] van Eeghen EE, Bakker SD, van Bochove A, Loffeld RJ. Impact of age and comorbidity on survival in colorectal cancer. J Gastrointest Oncol. 2015;6(6):605–12.

[101] Hutchins LF, Unger JM, Crowley JJ, Coltman CAJr, Albain KS. Underrepresentation of patients 65 years of age or older in cancer-treatment trials. N Engl J Med. 1999;341(27): 2061–7.

[102] Murthy VH, Krumholz HM, Gross CP. Participation in cancer clinical trials: race-, sex-, and age-based disparities. JAMA. 2004;291(22):2720–6.

[103] Bouchahda M, Macarulla T, Spano JP, Bachet JB, Lledo G, Andre T, Landi B, Tabernero J, KarabouéA, Domont J, Levi F, Rougier P. Cetuximab efficacy and safety in a retrospective cohort of elderly patients with heavily pretreated metastatic colorectal cancer. Crit Rev Oncol Hematol. 2008;67(3):255–62.

[104] Jehn CF, Böning L, Kröning H, Possinger K, Lüftner D. Cetuximab-based therapy in elderly comorbid patients with metastatic colorectal cancer. Br J Cancer. 2012;106(2): 274–8.

[105] Sastre J, Grávalos C, Rivera F, Massuti B, Valladares-Ayerbes M, Marcuello E, Manzano JL, Benavides M, Hidalgo M, Díaz-Rubio E, Aranda E. First-line cetuximab plus capecitabine in elderly patients with advanced colorectal cancer: clinical outcome and subgroup analysis according to KRAS status from a Spanish TTD Group Study. Oncologist. 2012;17(3):339–45.

[106] Sastre J, Massuti B, Pulido G, Guillén-Ponce C, Benavides M, Manzano JL, Reboredo M, Rivera F, Grávalos C, Safont MJ, Martínez Villacampa M, Llovet P, Dotor E, Díaz-Rubio E, Aranda E. Spanish Cooperative Group for the Treatment of Digestive Tumours TT: first-line single-agent panitumumab in frail elderly patients with wild-type KRAS metastatic colorectal cancer and poor prognostic factors: a phase II study of the Spanish Cooperative Group for the Treatment of Digestive Tumours. Eur J Cancer. 2015;51(11):1371–80.

[107] Pietrantonio F, Cremolini C, Aprile G, Lonardi S, Orlandi A, Mennitto A, Berenato R, Antoniotti C, Casagrande M, Marsico V, Marmorino F,Cardellino GG, Bergamo F, Tomasello G, Formica V, Longarini R, Giommoni E, Caporale M, Di Bartolomeo M, Loupakis F, de Braud F. Pietrantonio F, Cremolini C, Aprile G, et al. Single-agent panitumumab in frail elderly patients with advanced RAS and BRAF wild-type colorectal cancer: challenging drug label to light up new hope. Oncologist. 2015;20(11): 1261–5.

[108] Crosara Teixeira M, Marques DF, Ferrari AC, Alves MF, Alex AK, Sabbaga J, Hoff PM, Riechelmann RP. The effects of palliative chemotherapy in metastatic colorectal cancer patients with an ECOG performance status of 3 and 4. Clin Colorectal Cancer. 2015;14(1):52–7.

[109] Wan PT, Garnett MJ, Roe SM, Lee S, Niculescu-Duvaz D, Good VM, Jones CM, Marshall CJ, Springer CJ, Barford D, Marais R, Cancer Genome P. Mechanism of activation of the RAF-ERK signaling pathway by oncogenic mutations of B-RAF. Cell. 2004;116:855–67.

[110] Benvenuti S, Sartore-Bianchi A, Di Nicolantonio F, Zanon C, Moroni M, Veronese S, Siena S, Bardelli A. Oncogenic activation of the RAS/RAF signaling pathway impairs the response of metastatic colorectal cancers to anti-epidermal growth factor receptor antibody therapies. Cancer Res. 2007;67:2643–8.

[111] Cutsem EV, Folprecht IL, Nowacki M, Barone C, Shchepotin I, Maurel J, Cunningham D, Celik I, Kohne C. Cetuximab plus FOLFIRI: Final data from the CRYSTAL study on the association of KRAS and BRAF biomarker status with treatment outcome. J Clin Oncol. 2010;28 (May 20 Supply):3570.

[112] Tol J, Nagtegaal ID, Punt CJ. BRAF mutation in metastatic colorectal cancer. N Engl J Med. 2009;361:98–9.

[113] Roth AD, Tejpar S, Delorenzi M, Yan P, Fiocca R, Klingbiel D, Dietrich D, Biesmans B, Bodoky G, Barone C, Aranda E, Nordlinger B, Cisar L, Labianca R, Cunningham D, Van Cutsem E, Bosman F. Prognostic role of KRAS and BRAF in stage II and III resected colon cancer: results of the translational study on the PETACC-3, EORTC 40993, SAKK 60–00 trial. J Clin Oncol. 2010;28:466–74.

[114] Kopetz S, Desai J, Chan E, Hecht JR, O'Dwyer PJ, Lee RJ, Nolop KB, Saltz L. PLX4032 in metastatic colorectal cancer patients with mutant BRAF tumors. J Clin Oncol. 2010; 28(Suppl:15s). abstract:3534.

[115] Prahallad A, Sun C, Huang S, Di Nicolantonio F, Salazar R, Zecchin D, Beijersbergen RL, Bardelli A, Bernards R. Unresponsiveness of colon cancer to BRAF(V600E) inhibition through feedback activation of EGFR. Nature. 2012;483:100–3.

[116] Corcoran RB, Ebi H, Turke AB, Coffee EM, Nishino M, Cogdill AP, Brown RD, Della Pelle P, Dias-Santagata D, Hung KE, Flaherty KT, Piris A, Wargo JA, Settleman J, Mino-Kenudson M, Engelman JA. EGFR-mediated re-activation of MAPK signaling contributes to insensitivity of BRAF mutant colorectal cancers to RAF inhibition with vemurafenib. Cancer Discov. 2012;2:227–35.

[117] Bardelli A, Siena S. Molecular mechanisms of resistance to cetuximab and panitumumab in colorectal cancer. J Clin Oncol. 2010;28:1254–61.

[118] Perrone F, Lampis A, Orsenigo M, Di Bartolomeo M, Gevorgyan A, Losa M, Frattini M, Riva C, Andreola S, Bajetta E, Bertario L, Leo E, Pierotti MA, Pilotti S. PI3KCA/PTEN deregulation contributes to impaired responses to cetuximab in metastatic colorectal cancer patients. Ann Oncol. 2009;20:84–90.

[119] Frattini M, Saletti P, Romagnani E, Martin V, Molinari F, Ghisletta M, Camponovo A, Etienne LL, Cavalli F, Mazzucchelli L. PTEN loss of expression predicts cetuximab efficacy in metastatic colorectal cancer patients. Br J Cancer. 2007;97:1139–45.

[120] Loupakis F, Pollina L, Stasi I, Ruzzo A, Scartozzi M, Santini D, Masi G, Graziano F, Cremolini C, Rulli E, Canestrari E, Funel N, Schiavon G, Petrini I, Magnani M, Tonini G, Campani D, Floriani I, Cascinu S, Falcone A. PTEN expression and KRAS mutations

on primary tumors and metastases in the prediction of benefit from cetuximab plus irinotecan for patients with metastatic colorectal cancer. J Clin Oncol. 2009;27:2622–9.

[121] Tural D, Batur S, Erdamar S, Akar E, Kepil N, Mandel NM, Serdengecti S. Analysis of PTEN, BRAF and PI3K status for determination of benefit from cetuximab therapy in metastatic colorectal cancer patients refractory to chemotherapy with wild-type KRAS. Tumour Biol. 2014;35:1041–9.

[122] Saridaki Z, Tzardi M, Papadaki C, Sfakianaki M, Pega F, Kalikaki A, Tsakalaki E, Trypaki M, Messaritakis I, Stathopoulos E, Mavroudis D, Georgoulias V, Souglakos J. Impact of KRAS, BRAF, PIK3CA mutations, PTEN, AREG, EREG expression and skin rash in >/= 2 line cetuximab-based therapy of colorectal cancer patients. PLo S One. 2011;6:e15980.

[123] Prenen H, De Schutter J, Jacobs B, De Roock W, Biesmans B, Claes B, Lambrechts D, Van Cutsem E, Tejpar S. PIK3CA mutations are not a major determinant of resistance to the epidermal growth factor receptor inhibitor cetuximab in metastatic colorectal cancer. Clin Cancer Res. 2009;15:3184–8.

[124] Kaleko M, Rutter WJ, Miller AD. Overexpression of the human insulin-like growth factor I receptor promotes ligand-dependent neoplastic transformation. Mol Cell Biol. 1990;10:464–473.

[125] Ouban A, Muraca P, Yeatman T, Coppola D. Expression and distribution of insulin-like growth factor-1 receptor in human carcinomas. Hum Pathol. 2003;34: 803–808.

[126] Hailey J, Maxwell E, Koukouras K, Bishop WR, Pachter JA, Wang Y. Neutralizing anti-insulin-like growth factor receptor 1 antibodies inhibit receptor function and induce receptor degradation in tumor cells. Mol Cancer Ther. 2002;1:1349–1353.

[127] Reinmuth N, Liu W, Fan F, Jung YD, Ahmad SA, Stoeltzing O, Bucana CD, Radinsky R, Ellis LM. Blockade of insulin-like growth factor I receptor function inhibits growth and angiogenesis of colon cancer. Clin Cancer Res. 2002;8:3259–69.

[128] Reidy DL, Vakiani E, Fakih MG, Saif MW, Hecht JR, Goodman-Davis N, Hollywood E, Shia J, Schwartz J, Chandrawansa K, Dontabhaktuni A, Youssoufian H, Solit DB, Saltz LB. Randomized, phase II study of the insulin-like growth factor-1 receptor inhibitor IMC-A12, with or without cetuximab, in patients with cetuximab- or panitumumab-refractory metastatic colorectal cancer. J Clin Oncol. 2010;28:4240–6.

[129] Townsley CA, Major P, Siu LL, Dancey J, Chen E, Pond GR, Nicklee T, Ho J, Hedley D, Tsao M, Moore MJ, Oza AM. Phase II study of erlotinib (OSI-774) in patients with metastatic colorectal cancer. Br J Cancer. 2006;94(8):1136–43.

[130] Rothenberg ML, La Fleur B, Levy DE, Washington MK, Morgan-Meadows SL, Ramanathan RK, Berlin JD, Benson AB3rd, Coffey RJ. Randomized phase II trial of the clinical and biological effects of two dose levels of gefitinib in patients with recurrent colorectal adenocarcinoma. J Clin Oncol. 2005;23(36):9265–74.

[131] Meyerhardt JA, Zhu AX, Enzinger PC, Ryan DP, Clark JW, Kulke MH, Earle CC, Vincitore M, Michelini A, Sheehan S, Fuchs CS. Phase II study of capecitabine, oxaliplatin, and erlotinib in previously treated patients with metastatic colorectal cancer. J Clin Oncol. 2006;24(12):1892–7.

[132] Kuo T, Cho CD, Halsey J, Wakelee HA, Advani RH, Ford JM, Fisher GA, Sikic BI. Phase II study of gefitinib, fluorouracil, leucovorin, and oxaliplatin therapy in previously treated patients with metastatic colorectal cancer. J Clin Oncol. 2005;23(24): 5613–9.

[133] Zampino MG, Magni E, Massacesi C, Zaniboni A, Martignetti A, Zorzino L, Lorizzo K, Santoro L, Boselli S, de Braud F. First clinical experience of orally active epidermal growth factor receptor inhibitor combined with simplified FOLFOX6 as first-line treatment for metastatic colorectal cancer. Cancer. 2007;110(4):752–8.

[134] Allegra CJ, Jessup JM, Somerfield MR, Hamilton SR, Hammond EH, Hayes DF, Mc Allister PK, Morton RF, Schilsky RL. American Society of Clinical Oncology provisional clinical opinion: testing for KRAS gene mutations in patients with metastatic colorectal carcinoma to predict response to anti-epidermal growth factor receptor monoclonal antibody therapy. J Clin Oncol. 2009;27(12):2091–6.

Chapter 18

Studies of Malaysian Plants in Prevention and Treatment of Colorectal Cancer

Yumi Z. H-Y. Hashim, Chris I. R. Gill, Cheryl Latimer,
Nigel Ternan and Phirdaous Abbas

Additional information is available at the end of the chapter

http://dx.doi.org/10.5772/62868

Abstract

Incidence rates vary 10-fold globally for colorectal cancer (CRC). Asia has lower rates than Western countries, but as the Western life-style becomes more prevalent in economically developing Asian countries, rates are increasing. Clinical therapy has improved over the last few decades, and national screening programmes are a proven and effective means of reducing mortality; chemoprevention through diet and life-style choices may provide additional value. Diet has strong associations with the aetiology of CRC, considerable epidemiological evidence exist that fruits and vegetables are associated with reduced risk of CRC. There is also extensive experimental evidence that phytochemicals from fruit and vegetables can modulate pathways of carcinogenesis. In this chapter, we consider Malaysia specifically, with its rich ethnopharmacological heritage and megabiodiversity; Malaysian natural compounds may be a source of potentially chemo-protective with relevance to CRC.

Keywords: colon cancer, in vitro, Malaysia, plants, anticancer

1. Introduction

Botanically, Malaysia is one of the most bio-diverse countries in the world with more than 23,000 plant species recorded [1]. Many components of these plants are traditionally used for flavour and fragrances as well as for medicinal purposes. In line with bio-prospecting trend to find new pharmaceutical lead compounds for medical applications; researchers from local academic and research institutions within Malaysia have initiated investigations of the bioactive properties of various native plants. In Malaysia, colorectal cancer is the second most frequent cancer after breast cancer [2]. The aim of this review is to collate data and conclusions from recent studies undertaken on indigenous Malaysian plants with a view toward prevention and/or treatment of colorectal cancer (CRC).

2. Epidemiology of CRC

The geographical distribution of CRC differs significantly (~10-fold) across the world with the highest incidence rates in Australia/New Zealand (age-specific rate; ASR 44.8 and 32.2 per 100,000 in men and women, respectively), North America (ASR 30.1 and 22.7 per 100,000), Europe (ASR 37.3 and 22.7 per 100,000), and Japan (ASR 42.1 and 23.5 per 100,000). The lowest incidence rates occur in West Africa (ASR 4.5 and 3.8 per 100,000) although in this case, under-reporting is likely due to incomplete coverage by registries [2].

The global rise of incidence and mortality rates attributable to cancer is likely due to the ageing population, with incidence predicted to increase to 22.2 million cases globally by 2030 [3]. The cancer pattern among countries exhibits a strong societal and economic influence, where countries with a low human development index (HDI) (composite measure of life expectancy, education, and gross domestic product per head) tend to have higher levels of infection-related cancers (i.e., cervical) compared to medium and high HDI countries where the cancer burden is more commonly related to reproductive, dietary, and hormonal factors (e.g., lung, breast, and colorectal) [3]. As such, it is clear that CRC incidence rates increase in accordance with a country's income [4].

Asia as a whole consists mainly of developing countries and as such, incidence rates of CRC (ASR 16.5 and 11.1 per 100,000 in men and women, respectively) are noticeably lower than for the mainly developed countries of Europe—both in terms of incidence and in mortality (**Table 1**). However, cancer incidence and mortality in Asia is likely to rise over the next 20 years, due in part to a rapid population expansion that will not be experienced by Western countries. This increase will clearly impact on the health care burden associated with cancer, and also quality of life across Asia as a whole. Ng and colleagues [4] recently considered the wide variation in cancer incidence and mortality across Asia with respect to cancer survival, defining it in terms of mortality to incidence ratios (MIR = 1 no effect on survival). Although cancer incidence is lower in Asia, cancer survival is higher in Western countries as the MIRs are lower. Moreover, while Eastern and Western Asia have a higher incidence of CRC compared to South-Eastern and South-Central Asia, the pattern for survival is reversed in that the latter two regions have poorer survival than Western and Eastern Asia [4]. In Malaysia (South Eastern Asia), CRC is the second most common malignancy after breast cancer, while incidence rates exceed that of China, cancer survival is similar. By contrast, in Japan, both incidence and survival are higher.

2.1. CRC pathogenesis

The majority of colorectal malignancies occur as sporadic forms that appear to arise from benign adenomatous polyps, with carcinomas emerging slowly over a period of 10–20 years [6–9]. Epidemiological data indicate that incidence and mortality rates of colorectal cancers

(CRC) are greatly influenced by age rather than by gender. The majority of cases are detected in individuals over the age of 60 [10], with 55% of cases occurring in more developed regions in contrast to 52% of all CRC deaths which occur in the less-developed regions of the world, reflecting poorer survival. For individuals diagnosed with CRC, it has been determined that the 5-year survival rate is approximately 50–60% [11] and that survival among CRC patient is improved if WCRF/AICR lifestyle guidelines on physical activity, body fatness, and diet are adhered to [12]. The age-dependent increase in CRC development is associated with a multi-step oncogenesis process and a number of histological stages, reflecting the accumulation of genetic errors in somatic cells over time. Sporadic CRC is currently thought to arise via 1 of 3 identified molecular pathways (Micro Satellite instability—MSI, Chromosomal Instability—CIN and CpG island methylator phenotype—CIMP) depending upon the individual's complement of gene alterations [13]. Conversely, the inheritance of germline mutations may also result in development of neoplasms at an early age, with approximately 5% of CRC cases being due to inherited single-gene syndromes such as familial adenomatous polyposis (FAP) and hereditary non-polyposis colorectal cancer (HNPCC) [14]. It is estimated that as much as 12–35% of colon cancers can be explained by heritable factors, but known single-nucleotide polymorphisms appear to explain only a small proportion of these [15].

The high degree of molecular heterogeneity present in CRC is reflected by the effectiveness of chemotherapeutic regimes; however, the clinical significance of the majority of these individual molecular alterations is still to be fully determined [16]. From a treatment perspective, early-stage CRC is managed by surgical resection and advanced CRC with a combination of chemotherapy and surgery. Most chemotherapeutic regimes use 5-Fluorouracil (5-FU) as the main cytotoxic agent and this is commonly administered in conjunction with oxaliplatin for adjuvant therapy for high-risk stage II/stage III CRC, and with either oxaliplatin or irinotecan for metastatic CRC. Furthermore, the addition of bevacizumab-based chemotherapy (a vascular endothelial growth factor (VEGF)-targeted agent) has proven to be more effective than cytotoxic chemotherapy alone for the treatment of metastatic CRC [17].

While there is no doubt that CRC treatments have advanced over the last decade, improvement in disease outcome has been more modest relative to the increase in treatment costs. Thus, population screening is an important and cost-effective strategy given the improved prognosis with early detection [18]. The pathogenesis of CRC makes it very well suited to population screening especially given the correlation between disease stage and mortality. It is clear that the detection and the removal of cancer precursors can reduce CRC incidence and mortality and effective detection of CRC allows for less invasive treatment with a better prognosis. As is to be expected, a large variation exists globally in the implementation of screening programmes both in terms of strategy used (organised vs opportunistic) and standards applied (diagnostic test, detection threshold), with implementation more common in Western countries [19]. Europe for the most part has implemented an organized screening programme, while the USA operates an opportunistic approach. In Asia, several countries have already developed organized programmes including Japan, Korea and, to a lesser extent, China. As yet, however, Malaysia has no organized screening in place. As cancer incidences are likely to continue to rise, screening programmes will necessarily become more of an issue for low resource countries. Moreover, as cancer pattern types change, there will arise a need to developed tailored approaches [19].

Region	Incidence		Mortality		5-year prevalence	
	Number	ASR (W)	Number	ASR (W)	Number	Prop
Australian/New Zealand	18887	38.2	5489	10	54266	245.4
Europe	447136	29.5	214866	12.5	1203943	192.3
North America	158169	26.1	63465	9.4	486650	172.9
Asia	607182	13.7	331615	7.2	1493520	47
Asian region						
Eastern Asia (EA)	421343	18.4	207716	8.4	1130066	87.1
Western Asia (WA)	27140	14.8	15306	8.4	62162	37.5
South Eastern Asia (SEA)	69016	12.5	43234	7.9	158845	35.7
South Central Asia (SCA)	89683	6.1	65359	4.4	142447	11.3
Country						
Australia	15869	38.4	4168	9	45622	245.8
Japan (EA)	112675	32.2	49345	11.9	384877	350.8
UK	40755	30.2	16202	10.7	104047	200.5
Malaysia (SEA)	4539	18.3	2300	9.4	9714	47
China (EA)	253427	14.2	139416	7.4	583054	52.7
Saudi Arabia (WA)	2047	11.6	1094	6.6	4486	22.3
India (SCA)	64332	6.1	48603	4.6	86650	9.8

Incidence and mortality data for all ages. Five-year prevalence for adult population only. ASR (W) and proportions per 100,000 persons per year. The ASR is a weighted mean of the age-specific rates. Adapted from [5].

Table 1. Incidence and mortality rates (estimated, all sexes) for colorectal cancer, globally and within Asia and selected regions.

2.2. Diet and CRC

The relatively recent increase in CRC incidence in Japan (Eastern Asia) and in urbanized regions of China (Eastern Asia) is of significant concern [20] and is thought to be due to the adoption of a more a Western lifestyle and diet [21]. Diet plays a central role in CRC pathogenesis, as those rich in saturated animal fat, and red meat (especially processed meat) [22] together with alcohol intake [23] and smoking [24] have been positively associated with colorectal neoplasia. Fruit and vegetable consumption is associated with a reduction in the risk of CRC [25], and this concept is supported by a large body of case-control studies, although results from cohort or prospective studies are less convincing [26]. Nevertheless, the protective effects of fruits and vegetables against colorectal cancer are attributed to the large number of

http://dx.doi.org/10.5772/62868

bioactive phytochemicals present within them [27], comprising mainly plant polyphenolic secondary metabolites [28] and plant structural and storage polysaccharides which make up dietary fiber [29, 30]. These various plant components or natural products are found within a range of indigenous Malaysian fruit and vegetables, and thus may potentially play a role in chemoprevention for CRC.

3. Natural product research in Malaysia

Natural products include a large and diverse group of substances produced by a variety of sources including marine organisms, bacteria, yeasts, fungi, and plants [31]. Research on natural products has focused primarily on the chemical properties, biosynthesis, and biological functions of secondary metabolites [32]. Natural products, in particular plants, have been used in traditional medicine and health practice. The World Health Organization has acknowledged traditional medicine as a contributor to achieve health care objectives [33] and Malaysia, blessed with its megabiodiversity and rich ethnopharmacological heritage, has been observed to elegantly capitalize on these attributes with a view toward boosting the wealth and wellness of its population [34].

In late 2010, the Malaysian government launched the Economic Transformation Programme (ETP), which focuses on 12 National Key Economic Areas (NKEAs). The Agriculture sector, under the purview of the Ministry of Agriculture (MoA) is one of the NKEA-identified areas where the Entry Point Project 1 (EPP1) is focused on high-value herbal products. The MoA has overseen the establishment of five R&D clusters, which focus on, respectively, discovery, crop production, and agronomy, standardization and product development, toxicology/pre-clinical and clinical studies, and processing technology. The initial phase of this EPP was focused on ensuring the supply of five main local herbs, namely Tongkat Ali (*Eurycoma longifolia* Jack), Misai Kucing (*Orthosiphon aristatus* (Blume) Miq.), Hempedu Bumi (*Andrographis paniculata* (Burm.f.) Nees), Dukung Anak (*Phyllanthus niruri* L.) and Kacip Fatimah (*Marantodes pumilum* (Blume) Kuntze (*syn. Labisia pumila* (Blume) Mez). Subsequently, six more herb species were added to the project, including Mengkudu (*Morinda citrifolia* L.), Roselle (*Hibiscus sabdariffa* L.), Ginger (*Zingiber officinale*), Mas Cotek (*Ficus deltoidea* Jack), Belalai Gajah (*Clinacanthus nutans* (Burm.f.) Lindau) and Pegaga (*Centella asiatica* (L.) Urb) [35]. In 2014, eight products developed through the EPP 1 underwent pre-clinical trials. It is estimated that commercialization of the identified herbs will contribute MYR2.2 billion to the Gross National Income (GNI) by 2020 [35].

In Malaysia, research on natural products including the EPP-listed local herbs described above is being undertaken by research centers and institutions of higher learning (**Table 2**). Nevertheless, research in this area is also being carried out by various independent research groups in the local academia.

Entities	Institutions
Advanced Medical and Dental Institute	Universiti Sains Malaysia (USM)
Atta-ur-Rahman Institute for Natural Product Discovery	Universiti Teknologi MARA (UiTM)
Bioresource and Drug Discovery Research Group (BDD), Faculty Science and Natural Resources (FSSA)	Universiti Malaysia Sabah (UMS)
Centre For Natural Products And Drug Research (CENAR)	Universiti Malaya (UM)
Drug Discovery and Development Research Group (under purview of the Natural Products Cluster)	Universiti Kebangsaan Malaysia (UKM)
Institute of Bioproduct Development (IBD)	Universiti Teknologi Malaysia
Laboratory of Natural products, Institute of Bioscience	Universiti Putra Malaysia (UPM)
Natural Medicine Products Centre (NMPC)	International Islamic University Malaysia (IIUM)
Natural Product and Drug Discovery Centre (NPDC)	Malaysian Institute of Pharmaceuticals and Nutraceuticals (IPharm)
Natural Product Lab, Institute of Marine Biotechnology	Universiti Malaysia Terengganu (UMT)
Natural Products Division	Forest Research Institute Malaysia (FRIM)

Table 2. Entities involved in natural product research and development in Malaysia.

4. Studies of the effect of Malaysian plants on colon cancer

It has been estimated that around 1200 medicinal plants have potential pharmaceutical value [1]. Many of these species have been scientifically investigated by researchers seeking to provide evidence of effectiveness toward different diseases such as cancer, diabetes, arthritis, heart diseases, and many others. However, work on the effects of Malaysian plants on colon cancer specifically has been very limited (**Tables 3** and **4**). Nonetheless, several observations may be made on work undertaken to date that allow trends to be identified for the future of such work.

It is clear that there is no focused approach on any particular species, and most of the studies were conducted at the early stage of screening for anti-cancer effects with little in the way of continued development thereafter. This work includes cytotoxicity screening of crude extracts or compounds derived from solvent fractions against several types of cancer using *in vitro* cell line-based experiments. While the species investigated are edible herbs and fruit plants, in several instances, the parts of the plant investigated may not be commonly consumed as food. For instance, Moghadamtousi et al. [36] studied the leaf of soursop plant, rather than the more commonly consumed fruits, while Aisha et al. [38] investigated the rind of mangosteen fruit instead of the flesh. To this end, selection of species seems to be based on ethnomedicinal evidence within local communities and capitalizing upon the novelty aspect in that the species (or parts of plants) have not been investigated by other groups. The use of inedible plant parts may be also be related to the zero waste and health to wealth concepts where all parts of plants are considered potential biomass to be exploited. As such, materials from inedible parts of plants may be more cost-effective to be used. Furthermore, the majority of studies appear to be "isolated studies" with lack of continuing development as stated above, which may perhaps be due to lack of funding and proper planning for future work including networking. The lack of funding may also correspond to lack of facilities and equipment required to do further in depth robust work.

Plant and part of plant used	Common name	Compound/ extract tested	Type of study	Details/IC_{50}	Reference
Annona muricata L. (Leaf)	Graviola, soursop; [a]durian belanda	Ethyl acetate extract	*In vitro* HCT 116, HT29 and CCD841 cell lines	*In vitro* cytotoxicity IC_{50} = 4.29 ± 0.24 μg/ml (HT29) IC_{50} = 3.91 ± 0.35 μg/ml (HCT116) IC_{50} = 34.24 ± 2.12 μg/ml (CCD841) 5-Fluorouracil (positive control) IC_{50} = 1.10 ± 0.11 μg/ml (HT29) IC_{50} = 0.90 ± 0.09 μg/ml (HCT116) The extract also showed cell cycle arrest at G_1, induction of apoptosis, anti-migration and anti-invasive effects.	[36]
Annona muricata L. (Leaf)	Graviola, soursop; [a]durian belanda	Ethyl acetate extract	*In vitro* HT29 and CCD 841 cell lines.	*In vitro* cytotoxicity HT29 IC_{50} = 5.72 ± 0.41 μg/ml (12 h) IC_{50} = 3.49 ± 0.22 μg/ml (24 h) IC_{50} = 1.62 ± 0.24 μg/ml (48 h) CCD 841 IC_{50} = 64.32 ± 3.76 μg/ml (12 h) IC_{50} = 47.10 ± 0.47 μg/ml (24 h) IC_{50} =32.51 ± 1.18 μg/ml (48 h)	[37]
			In vivo AOM-induced colon cancer in rats	Aberrant Crypt formation after 2 weekly injections of extract. 250 mg/kg = 61.2% inhibition 500 mg/kg = 72.5% inhibition 5-FU = 79.5% inhibition	
Garcinia mangostana (Fruit rind)	Mangosteen; [a]manggis	Xanthone (81% α-mangostin and 16% γ-	*In vitro* HCT 116 cell line *In vivo* Subcutaneous tumor of	*In vitro* cytotoxicity 1) IC_{50} = 6.5 ± 1.0 μg/ml 2) IC_{50} = 5.1 ± 0.2 μg/ml 3) IC_{50} = 7.2 ± 0.4 μg/ml IC_{50} of Cisplatin (positive	[38]

Plant and part of plant used	Common name	Compound/ extract tested	Type of study	Details/IC_{50}	Reference
		mangostin) from toluene extract of the fruit α-mangostin γ-mangostin)	HCT116 on nude mice	control) = 6.1 ± 0.2 μg/ml The extract also showed induction of apoptosis, anti-tumorigenicity and up-regulation of MAPK/ERK, c-Myc/Max, and p53 cell signalling pathways *In vivo* Xanthones extract caused significant growth inhibition of the subcutaneous tumor	
Garcinia mangostana (Fruit rind)	Mangosteen; [a]manggis	Hexane and ethyl acetate (Other extracts produced, butanol and methanol)	*In vitro* Caco-2 cell line (also tested on other cells KB and PBMC)	*In vitro* cytotoxicity IC_{50} = 13.0 ± 3.8 μg/ml (Hexane) IC_{50} = 8.1 ± 0.1 μg/ml (Ethyl acetate) IC_{50} of Tamoxifen positive control = 4.0 ± 0.4 μg/ml	[39]
Garcinia mangostana (Fruit rind)	Mangosteen; [a]manggis	α-mangostin β-mangostin γ-mangostin hexane extracts	*In vitro* DLD-1 cells	All three extracts showed anti-proliferative effects at 20 μM.	[40]

Table 3. Studies of anticancer effects of plant materials obtained from fruit trees in Malaysia.

Plant and part of plant used	Common name	Compound/extract tested	Type of study	Details/IC_{50}	References
Alpinia mutica (Rhizome)	[a]Tepus	Methanol and fractionated extracts (hexane, ethyl acetate and water)	*In vitro* HT 29 and HCT 116 cell line (also tested on other cell lines; KB, CasKi, MCF-7, A549 and MRC-5)	Hexane extracts showed IC_{50} of 36.1 ± 1.1 μg/ml (HCT116) and 47.4 ± 1.6 μg/ml (HT29) Ethyl acetate extracts showed IC_{50} of 20.4 ± 3.2 μg/ml (HCT116) and 24.2 ± 0.04 μg/ml (HT29) Methanol and water extracts showed IC_{50} of more than 100 μg/ml IC_{50} of doxorubicin (positive control) = 0.24 ± 0.04 μg/ml (HCT116) and 0.33 ± 0.03 μg/ml	[41]

Plant and part of plant used	Common name	Compound/extract tested	Type of study	Details/IC_{50}	References
				(HT29)	
Casearia capitellata (Leaf) *Baccaurea motleyana* (fruits and peel) *Phyllanthus pulcher* (Leaf, stem and root) *Strobilanthus crispus* (Leaf, flower)	[a]Simmilit matangi [a]Rambai [a]Naga buana [a]Pecah kaca/Pecah beling/ Pokok pecah/Jin batu/	Hexane, dichloromethane, ethyl acetate and methanol extracts, respectively	*In vitro* HT29 cell line (also tested on other cell lines; MCF-7, DU-145 and H460)	DCM extract of *P.pulcher* root showed the lowest IC_{50} among the extracts tested against HT29 cells (IC_{50} = 8.1 ± 0.5 μg/ml)	[42]
Curcuma mangga (Rhizome)	[a]Temu pauh/ Kunyit mangga	Crude methanol and fractionated extracts (hexane, ethyl acetate)	*In vitro* HT 29 and HCT 116 cell line(also tested on other cell lines; KB, CasKi, MCF-7, A549 and MRC-5)	Extracts showed the IC_{50} between 29.4 ± 0.2 and 36.8 ± 3.8 μg/ml against HCT116 cells Extracts showed the IC_{50} between 17.9 ± 0.3 and 22.0 ± 1.1 μg/ml against HT29 cells IC_{50} of doxorubicin (positive control) = 0.24 ± 0.04 μg/ml (HCT116) and 0.33 ± 0.03 μg/ml (HT29) Isolated compounds from the extracts also showed high cytotoxicity effects towards both cell lines (between 6.3 ± 0.26 and 14.9 ± 0.40 μg/ml) Several isolated compounds from the extracts also showed considerable cytotoxicity effects against the cancer cells	[43]
Curcuma mangga (Rhizome)	[a]Temu pauh/	Hexane and ethyl acetate extracts.	*In vitro* HT29 and CCD-18Co	*In vitro* cytotoxicity (72 h) Hexane: IC_{50} = 17.9 ± 1.2 μg/ml (HT29)	[44]

Plant and part of plant used	Common name	Compound/extract tested	Type of study	Details/IC_{50}	References
	Kunyit mangga			IC_{50} = 45.7 ± 1.0 μg/ml (CCD-18Co) Ethyl acetate: IC_{50} = 15.6 ± 0.8 μg/ml (HT29) IC_{50} = 46.5 ± 0.1 μg/ml (CCD-18Co)	
Pereskia bleo (Kunth) DC. (Cactaceae) (Leaf)	[a]Jarum tujuh bilah	Compounds from ethyl acetate fraction • Dihydroactini diolide • β-sitosterol • 2,4-di tert butyl phenol • α-tocopherol • Phytol	*In vitro* HCT 116 cell line (also tested on other cell lines; KB, CasKi, MCF-7, A549 and MRC-5)	Dihydroactinidiolide showed the lowest IC_{50} at 5 μg/ml against HCT116 cells Dihydroactinidiolide showed IC_{50} of 91.3 μg/ml against MRC-5 cells IC_{50} of doxorubicin (positive control) = 0.36 μg/ml (HCT116) and 0.55 μg/ml (MRC-5)	[45]
Piper betle (Leaf)	[a]Sirih	Aqueous extract	*In vitro* HCT 116 and HT29 cell lines	In the presence of the extract, a lower dosage of 5-FU is required to achieve the maximum drug effect in inhibiting the growth of HT29 cells. However, the extract did not significantly reduce 5-FU dosage in HCT116 cells	[46]
Strobilanthus crispus (part of plant used not stated)	[a]Pecah kaca/Pecah beling/ Pokok pecah/Jin batu/	Crude ethanol extract and fractions obtained from column chromatography	In vivo Sprague Dawley (SD) male rats *In vitro* HT29, CCD841	*S. crispus* ethanol extract protects against CRC formation (azoxymethane-induced aberrant crypt foci) in rats Exposure of HT29 and CCD-841 to extract and several fractions (tested between 0 and 500 μg/ml) induced a concentration dependent decrease in cell viability	[47]
Zingiber officinale (rhizome)	Ginger; [a]halia	Ginger: Water-based ultrasonic assisted extraction Honey: Packaged in plastic containers and	*In vitro* HT29 cell lines	*In vitro* cytotoxicity IC_{50} = 5.2 mg/ml (ginger alone) IC_{50} = 80 mg/ml (Gelam honey alone) The combinations of 3 and 4 mg/ml of ginger with 27 and 10 mg/ml	[48]

Plant and part of plant used	Common name	Compound/extract tested	Type of study	Details/IC_{50}	References
		sterilized using gamma radiation		of Gelam honey showed combination index (CI) values of 0.92 and 0.90, respectively, indicating synergistic effects. Cell death in response to the combined ginger and Gelam honey treatment was associated with the stimulation of early apoptosis	
Zingiber officinale (rhizome)	Ginger; [a]halia	Ethanol extract	*In vitro* HCT 116 and HT29 cell lines	Inhibition of proliferation IC_{50} (HCT116) = 496 ± 34.2 μg/ml IC_{50} (HT29) = 455 ± 18.6 μg/ml Induction of apoptosis at 500 μg/ml extract 35.05% (HCT116) and 19.81% (HT29) Ginger extract arrested HCT 116 and HT 29 cells at G0/G1 and G2/M phases with corresponding decreased in S-phase	[49]

[a]Local name in Malay language.
Cell lines: A549 (and human lung carcinoma cell line); CasKi (human cervical carcinoma cell line); CCD841 (normal human colon epithelial cell line); DU-145 (prostate cancer cell line); H460 (lung cancer cell line); HCT116 (colon cancer cell line); HT29 (colon cancer cell line); KB (human nasopharyngeal epidermoid carcinoma cell line); MCF-7 (hormone-dependent breast carcinoma cell line; MRC-5 (non-cancer human fibroblast cell line).

Table 4. Studies of anticancer effects of plant materials obtained herbs and spices in Malaysia.

Some species investigated for their effects against colon cancer in the listed studies have also been investigated for other biological effects. For example, prior to the report by Abdul Malek et al. [43], *Alpinia mutica* was previously reported to have inhibitory activity towards lipid oxidation [50] and anti-bacterial effects against *Bacillus subtilis* and methicillin-resistant *Staphylococcus aureus* (MRSA) [50] in addition to anti-platelet aggregation activities [51].

For *in vitro* work, two types of commercially available colon cancer cell lines, HT29 and HCT116, were used in the majority of studies. However, there is no consistency in the positive controls used in the empirical studies. Some studies include work on CCD841 normal human colon epithelial cells [36, 47], while others include work on 5-Fluorouracil [46, 47], doxorubicin [45], or cisplatin [38] as positive control. Cytotoxic screening results from the studies listed in **Table 3** and **Table 4** showed that effects on colon cancer were only moderate as compared to other cells lines tested. The follow-up study by Moghadamtousi et al. [37] demonstrated significant decreases in aberrant crypt foci counts in an AOM-induced CRC animal model supporting prior observation *in vitro*. The limited success of *in vitro* studies excluding the aforementioned study may explain the lack of in-depth studies on the effects of the extracts on colon cancer following the screening phase.

The colon cancer cell lines used in the studies differ in their origin, mutation status and metabolic requirements [52]. For example, HT29 cells utilize glucose through the pentose phosphate pathway [53], whereas HCT116 cells have higher requirements for glutamine [52, 54]. In terms of gene expression, HT29 is deficient in expression of p53 [55], while HCT116 cells possess mutations in PI3KCA and KRAS genes which confer constitutive activation of PI3K/AKT and KRAS pathways [56]. Since the two cells lines have different characteristics, the use of such cell lines in preliminary studies is substantial as it can set forth the mechanistic investigations on the effects of the plants against colon cancer.

Although the majority of work was *in vitro*-based preliminary work, Al-Henhena et al. [47] reported both *in vitro* and *in vivo* studies on *Strobilanthus crispus*. Meanwhile, some studies investigated the cytotoxic effects of not only the crude extracts and fractions, but also tested the isolated compounds [38, 40, 45]. Among the studies reported, the same group showed a more thorough investigation of the species selected. Other researchers have combined the selected species with other components to determine their combined effects on colon cancer cells. For instance, Ng et al. [46] looked at the potential effects of *Piper betle* leaf extract to reduce the 5-Fluorouracil dosage required to exert the same cytotoxicity in HT29 and HCT116 cells. Tahir et al. [48] studied the combined effects of *Zingiber officinale* extracts and Gelam honey on viability of HT29 cells. Some researchers have also studied the potential mechanism of the selected species beyond cytotoxicity tests. *Garcinia mangostana* rind extracts showed induction of apoptosis, anti-tumorigenicity, and upregulation of MAPK/ERK, c-Myc/Max, and p53 cell signaling pathways [38] while *Annona muricata* leaf extracts showed cell cycle arrest at G1, induction of apoptosis, anti-migration, and anti-invasive effects [36]. While the follow-up study by Moghadamtousi et al. [37] supports the previous *in vitro* observations with aberrant crypt foci counts significantly reduced by the treatment in an AOM induced CRC animal model. Taken together, studies on Malaysian plants against colon cancer are at different technological levels with, consequently, very limited data to enable a consensus to be made.

Compounding the lack of consensus and technical variability is the fact that choice of journals in which to publish is still very much dependent on funding; thus, publishing in the open access journals with high impact factors can only be afforded by certain groups of researchers. This clearly will have hampered the dissemination of research data as, while it may be beneficial for researchers to reach a wider audience at the early stage of work, this may correspond to having to publish in a low-cost, lower impact journals due to lack of funding. From another perspective, higher impact journals often require more conclusive data, which in turn means more experimental work—early stage work may not meet such journals' publication criteria and may be perceived to be low quality. Therefore, it would be more favorable to have a mechanism to help improve the dissemination of work in order to enhance the overall research and development in the subject area.

http://dx.doi.org/10.5772/62868

Based on the publications considered in **Tables 3** and **4**, it was also observed that authors did not always report the local names of species investigated. Since these are local plants that may not even have English names, it is to be recommended that this information is included together with full description of the species investigated. This could be one way to present the potential positive effects of the species to a wider scientific community thereby increasing the impact and scientific value of the work. Thus, the correct taxonomy including genus, species and family should be given for accuracy.

5. Conclusion

Some Malaysian plants that show anti-cancer effects towards colon cancer include *Alpinia mutica* (tepus), *Annona muricata* (soursop), *Baccaurea motleyana* (rambai), *Casearia capitellata* (simmilit mantangi), *Curcuma manga* (temu pauh), *Garcinia mangostana* (mangosteen), *Pereskia bleo* (Kunth) (jarum tujuh bilah), *Phyllanthus pulcher* (naga buana), *Strobilanthus crispus* (pecah kaca), *and Zingiber officinale* (ginger).

Nevertheless, much of the scientific evidence is preliminary at best despite the selection of plant species for study based upon ethnomedicinal practices. The introduction of the EPP by the Malaysian government is a commendable effort to raise the value of indigenous Malaysian plants in the pharmaceutical sector. However, a more concerted approach to the work is necessary including a comprehensive review of the existing data in order to fully exploit local plants toward prevention and treatment of colon cancer.

Acknowledgements

We wish to thank Dr. Rashidi Othman, Kulliyyah of Architecture and Environmental Design (KAED), International Islamic University Malaysia (IIUM) for his valuable comments.

Author details

Yumi Z. H-Y. Hashim[1*], Chris I. R. Gill[2], Cheryl Latimer[2], Nigel Ternan[2] and Phirdaous Abbas[1]

*Address all correspondence to: yumi@iium.edu.my

1 Department of Biotechnology Engineering, Kulliyyah of Engineering, International Islamic University Malaysia, Kuala Lumpur, Malaysia

2 School of Biomedical Sciences, Ulster University, Northern Ireland, United Kingdom

References

[1] Aman R. Tumbuhan Liar Berkhasiat Ubatan (Wild Plants with Medicinal Properties). Kuala Lumpur: Dewan Bahasa dan Pustaka; 2006. 12-14. ISBN: 9789836281517

[2] Ferlay J, Soerjomataram I, Dikshit R, Eser S, Mathers C, Rebelo M, Parkin DM, Forman D, Bray F. Cancer incidence and mortality worldwide: sources, methods and major patterns in GLOBOCAN 2012. Int J Cancer. 2015;136. doi:10.1002/ijc.29210

[3] Bray F, Jemal A, Grey N, Ferlay J, Forman D. Global cancer transitions according to the Human Development Index (2008–2030): a population-based study. Lancet Oncol. 2012;13(8):790–801. doi:10.1016/S1470-2045(12)70211-5

[4] Ng CJ, Teo CH, Abdullah N, Tan WP, Tan HM. Relationships between cancer pattern, country income and geographical region in Asia. BMC Cancer. 2015;15:613. doi:10.1186/s12885-015-1615-0

[5] WHO (World Health Organization). GLOBOCAN 2012 v1.0, Cancer Incidence and Mortality Worldwide: IARC CancerBase No. 11. [internet]. 2012. Available from: http://globocan.iarc.fr.[Accessed:2016-01-20]

[6] Peipins LA, Sandler RS. Epidemiology of colorectal adenomas. Epidemiol Rev. 1994;16(2):273–97.

[7] Kinzler KW, Vogelstein B. Lessons from hereditary colorectal cancer. Cell. 1996;87(2): 159–70. doi:10.1016/S0092-8674(00)81333-1

[8] Brenner H, Hoffmeister M, Stegmaier C, Brenner G, Altenhofen L, Haug U. Risk of progression of advanced adenomas to colorectal cancer by age and sex: estimates based on 840 149 screening colonoscopies. Gut. 2007;56(11):1585–9. doi:10.1136/gut.2007.122739

[9] Kuntz KM, Lansdorp-Vogelaar I, Rutter CM, Knudsen AB, van Ballegooijen M, Savarino JE, et al. A systematic comparison of microsimulation models of colorectal cancer: the role of assumptions about adenoma progression. Med Decis Mak. 2011;31(4):530–9. doi:10.1177/0272989X11408730

[10] Jemal A, Bray F, Center MM, Ferlay J, Ward E, Forman D. Global cancer statistics. CA Cancer J Clin. 2011;61(2):69–90. doi:10.3322/caac.20107

[11] WCRF. Food, nutrition and the prevention of cancer: a global perspective [comprehensive report]. World Cancer Research Fund/American Institute for Cancer Research, Washington, DC; 2006.

[12] Romaguera D, Ward H, Wark PA, Vergnaud AC, Peeters PH, van Gils CH, Ferrari P, Fedirko V, Jenab M, Boutron-Ruault MC, Dossus L, Dartois L, et al. Pre-diagnostic concordance with the WCRF/AICR guidelines and survival in European colorectal cancer patients: a cohort study. BMC Med. 2015;13:107. doi:10.1186/s12916-015-0332-5

[13] Carethers JM, Jung BH. Genetics and genetic biomarkers in sporadic colorectal cancer. Gastroenterology. 2015;149(5):1177–1190. doi:10.1053/j.gastro.2015.06.047

[14] Lang M, Gasche C. Chemoprevention of colorectal cancer. Dig Dis. 2015;33(1):58–67. doi:10.1159/000366037

[15] Jiao S, Peters U, Berndt S, Brenner H, Butterbach K, Caan BJ, et al. Estimating the heritability of colorectal cancer. Hum Mol Genet. 2014;23(14):3898–905. doi: 10.1093/hmg/ddu087

[16] Shiovitz S, Grady WM. Molecular markers predictive of chemotherapy response in colorectal cancer. Curr Gastroenterol Rep. 2015;17(2):431. doi:10.1007/s11894-015-0431-7

[17] Saltz LB, Clarke S, Diaz-Rubio E, et al. Bevacizumab in combination with oxaliplatin-based chemotherapy as first-line therapy in metastatic colorectal cancer: a randomized phase III study. J Clin Oncol. 2008;26:2013–9. doi:10.1200/JCO.2007.14.9930

[18] Lansdorp-Vogelaar I, Knudsen AB, Brenner H. Cost-effectiveness of colorectal cancer screening. Epidemiol Rev. 2011;33:88–100. doi:10.1093/epirev/mxr004

[19] Schreuders EH, Ruco A, Rabeneck L, Schoen RE, Sung JJ, Young GP, Kuipers EJ. Colorectal cancer screening: a global overview of existing programmes. Gut. 2015;64(10):1637–49. doi:10.1136/gutjnl-2014-309086

[20] Sung JJ, Ng SC, Chan FK, et al. An updated Asia Pacific Consensus Recommendations on colorectal cancer screening. Gut. 2015;64:121–32. doi:10.1136/gutjnl-2013-306503

[21] Sung JJ, Lau JY, Goh KL, Leung WK. Increasing incidence of colorectal cancer in Asia: implications for screening. Lancet Oncol. 2005;6:871–6. doi:10.1016/S1470-2045(05)70422-8

[22] Carr PR, Walter V, Brenner H, Hoffmeister M. Meat subtypes and their association with colorectal cancer: systematic review and meta-analysis. Int J Cancer. 2016;138(2):293–302. doi:10.1002/ijc.29423

[23] Fedirko V, Tramacere I, Bagnardi V, Rota M, Scotti L, Islami F, Negri E, Straif K, Romieu I, La Vecchia C. Alcohol drinking and colorectal cancer risk: an overall and dose-response meta-analysis of published studies. Ann Oncol. 2011;22:1958–1972. doi: 10.1093/annonc/mdq653

[24] Gong J, Hutter C, Baron JA, Berndt S, Caan B, Campbell PT, Casey G, Chan AT, Cotterchio M, Fuchs CS. A pooled analysis of smoking and colorectal cancer: timing of exposure and interactions with environmental factors. Cancer Epidemiol Biomark Prev. 2012;21:1974–1985. doi:10.1158/1055-9965.EPI-12-0692

[25] Bradbury KE, Appleby PN, Key TJ. Fruit, vegetable, and fiber intake in relation to cancer risk: findings from the European Prospective Investigation into Cancer and

Nutrition (EPIC). Am J Clin Nutr. 2014;100(Supplement 1):394S–8S. doi:10.3945/ajcn.113.071357

[26] Leenders M, Siersema PD, Overvad K, Tjønneland A, Olsen A, Boutron-Ruault M-C, et al. Subtypes of fruit and vegetables, variety in consumption and risk of colon and rectal cancer in the European Prospective Investigation into Cancer and Nutrition. Int J Cancer. 2015;137(11):2705–14. doi:10.1002/ijc.29640

[27] Li YH, Niu YB, Sun Y, Zhang F, Liu CX, Fan L, Mei QB. Role of phytochemicals in colorectal cancer prevention. World J Gastroenterol. 2015;21(31):9262–72. doi:10.3748/wjg.v21.i31.9262

[28] Núñez-Sánchez MA, González-Sarrías A, Romo-Vaquero M, García-Villalba R, Selma MV, Tomás-Barberán FA, García-Conesa MT, Espín JC. Dietary phenolics against colorectal cancer—from promising preclinical results to poor translation into clinical trials: pitfalls and future needs. Mol Nutr Food Res. 2015;59(7):1274–91. doi:10.1002/mnfr.201400866

[29] Fung KY, Cosgrove L, Lockett T, Head R, Topping DL. A review of the potential mechanisms for the lowering of colorectal oncogenesis by butyrate. Br J Nutr. 2012;108(5):820–31. doi:10.1017/S0007114512001948

[30] van Dijk M, Pot GK. The effects of nutritional interventions on recurrence in survivors of colorectal adenomas and cancer: a systematic review of randomised controlled trials. Eur J Clin Nutr. 2016. doi:10.1038/ejcn.2015.210. [Epub ahead of print]

[31] NCCIH (National Centre for Complementary and Integrative Health). [Internet]. 2015. Available from: https://nccih.nih.gov/grants/naturalproducts [Accessed: 2015-12-04]

[32] Editorial. All natural. Nat Chem Biol. 2007;3:351. doi:10.1038/nchembio0707-351

[33] WHO (World Health Organization). 1991. Report on the intercountry expert meeting of traditional medicine and primary health care. WHO-EMTRM/1-E/L/12.92/168, November 30–December 3, 1991, Cairo, Egypt.

[34] Akarasereenont P, Datiles MJR, Lumlerdkij N, Yaakob H, Prieto JM and Heinrich M. A South-East Asian Perspective on Ethnopharmacology. In: Heinrich M, Jager A, editors. Ethnopharmacology. Wiley-Blackwell; 2015. pp. 317–328. doi:10.1002/9781118930717.ch27

[35] Performance Management & Delivery Unit; PEMANDU. [Internet]. 2013. Available from http://etp.pemandu.gov.my/Agriculture-@-Agriculture_-_EPP_1-;_High-Value_Herbal_Products.aspx#sthash.YK0kpNR8.dpuf. [Accessed: 2015-12-04]

[36] Moghadamtousi SZ, Karimian H, Rouhollahi E, Paydar, Fadaeinasab M, Abdul Kadir H. *Annona muricata* leaves induce G1 cell cycle arrest and apoptosis through mitochondria-mediated pathway in human HCT-116 and HT-29 colon cancer cells. J Ethnopharmacol. 2014;156:277–289. doi:10.1016/j.jep.2014.08.011

[37] Moghadamtousi SZ, Rouhollahi E, Karimian H, Fadaeinasab M, Firoozinia M, Abdulla MA, Kadir HA. The chemopotential effect of *Annona muricata* leaves against azoxymethane-induced colonic aberrant crypt foci in rats and the apoptotic effect of acetogenin annomuricin E in HT-29 cells: a bioassay-guided approach. Plos One. 2015;10(4):e0122288. doi:10.1371/journal.pone.0122288

[38] Aisha AFA, Abu-Salah KM, Ismail Z, Majid AMSA. *In vitro* and *in vivo* anti-colon cancer effects of *Garcinia mangostana* xanthones extract. BMC Complement Altern Med. 2012;12(1):1–10. doi:10.1186/1472-6882-12-104

[39] Khonkarn R, Okonogi S, Ampasavate C, Anuchapreeda S. Investigation of fruit peel extracts as sources for compounds with antioxidant and antiproliferative activities against human cell lines. Food Chem Toxicol. 2010;48(8–9):2122–2129. doi:10.1016/j.fct.2010.05.014

[40] Matsumoto K, Akao Y, Ohguchi K, Ito T, Tanaka T, Iinuma M, Nozawa Y. Xanthones induce cell-cycle arrest and apoptosis in human colon cancer DLD-1 cells. Bioorganic Med Chem. 2005;13(21):6064–9. doi:10.1016/j.bmc.2005.06.065

[41] Abdul Malek SN, Phang CW, Ibrahim H, Abdul Wahab N, Sim KS. Phytochemical and cytotoxic investigations of *Alpinia mutica* rhizomes. Molecules. 2011;16:583–589. doi:10.3390/molecules16010583

[42] Ismail M, Bagalkotkar G, Iqbal S, Adamu HA. Anticancer properties and phenolic contents of sequentially prepared extracts from different parts of selected medicinal plant indigenous to Malaysia. Molecules. 2012;17:5745–5756. doi:10.3390/molecules17055745

[43] Abdul Malek SN, Lee GS, Hong SL, Yaacob H, Abdul Wahab N, Weber J-FF, Ali Shah SA. Phytochemical and cytotoxic investigations of *Curcuma mangga* rhizomes. Molecules. 2011;16:4539–4548. doi:10.3390/molecules16064539

[44] Hong GW, Hong SL, Lee GS, Yaacob H, Malek SNA. Non-aqueous extracts of *Curcuma mangga* rhizomes induced cell death in human colorectal adenocarcinoma cell line (HT29) via induction of apoptosis and cell cycle arrest at G0/G1 phase. Asian Pac J Trop Med. 2016;9(1):8–18. doi:10.1016/j.apjtm.2015.12.003

[45] Abdul Malek SN, Sim KS, Abdul Wahab N, Yaacob H. Cytotoxic components of *Pereskia bleo* (Kunth) DC. (Cactaceae) leaves. Molecules. 2009;14:1713–1724. doi:10.3390/molecules14051713

[46] Ng PL, Rajab NF, Then SM, Mohd Yusof YA, Wan Ngah WZ, Pin KY, Looi ML. *Piper betle* leaf extract enhances the cytotoxicity effect of5-fluorouracil in inhibiting the growth of HT29 and HCT116 colon cancer cells. J Zhejiang Univ Sci B Biomed Biotechnol. 2014;15:692–700. doi:10.1631/jzus.B1300303

[47] Al-Henhena N, Khalifa SAM, Poh YYR, Ismail S, Hamadi R, Shawter AN, Mohd Idris A, Azizan A, Al-Wajeeh NS, Abdulla MA, El-Seedi. Evaluation of chemopreventive

potential of *Strobilanthes crispus* against colon cancer formation *in vitro* and *in vivo*. BMC Complement Altern Med. 2015;15:419. doi:10.1186/s12906-015-0926-7

[48] Tahir AA, Sani NFA, Murad NA, Makpol S, Ngah WZW, Yusof YAM. Combined ginger extract & Gelam honey modulate Ras/ERK and PI3K/AKT pathway genes in colon cancer HT29 cells. Nutr J. 2015;14(1):1–10. doi:10.1186/s12937-015-0015-2

[49] Abdullah S, Zainal Abidin SA, Murad NA, Makpol S, Wan Ngah WZ, Mohd Yusof YA. Ginger extract (*Zingiber officinale*) triggers apoptosis and G0/G1 cells arrest in HCT 116 and HT 29 colon cancer cell lines. Afr J Biochem Res. 2010;4:134–142. ISSN: 1996-0778

[50] Mohamad H, Abas F, Permana D, Lajis NH, Alib AM, Sukaric MA, Hinc TYY, Kikuzakid H, Nakatanid N. DPPH free radical scavenger components from the fruits of *Alpinia rafflesiana* Wall. ex. Bak. (Zingiberaceae). Z. Naturforsch. 2004;59c:811–815.

[51] Jantan I, Pisar M, Sirat HM, Basar N, Jamil S, Ali RM, Jalil J. Inhibitory effects of compounds from Zingiberaceae species on platelet activating factor receptor binding. Phytother Res. 2004;18:1005–1007.

[52] Richard SM, Marignac MVL. Sensitization to oxaliplatin in HCT116 and HT29 cell lines by metformin and ribavirin and differences in response to mitochondrial glutaminase inhibition. J Cancer Res Ther. 2015;11:336–340. doi:10.4103/0973-1482.157317

[53] Vizán P, Alcarraz-Vizán G, Díaz-Moralli S, Solovjeva ON, Frederiks WM, Cascante M. Modulation of pentose phosphate pathway during cell cycle progression in human colon adenocarcinoma cell line HT29. Int J Cancer. 2009;124(12):2789–2796. doi:10.1002/ijc.24262

[54] Weinberg F, Hamanaka R, Wheaton WW, Weinberg S, Joseph J, Lopez M, et al. Mitochondrial metabolism and ROS generation are essential for Kras-mediated tumorigenicity. Proc Natl Acad Sci USA. 2010;107:8788–8793. doi:10.1073/pnas.1003428107

[55] Davidson D, Coulombe Y, Martinez Marignac V, Amrein L, Grenier J, Hodkinson K, et al. Irinotecan and DNA-PKcs inhibitors synergize in killing of colon cancer cells. Investig New Drugs. 2012;30:1248–56. doi:10.1007/s10637-010-9626-9

[56] Wang J, Kuropatwinski K, Hauser J, Ross MR, Zhou Y, Conway A, et al. Colon carcinoma cells harboring PIK3CA mutations display resistance to growth factor deprivation induced apoptosis. Mol Cancer Ther. 2007;6:1143–50. doi:10.1158/1535-7163.MCT-06-0555

Chapter 19

Adjuvant Systemic Therapy in Stage II and III Colon Cancer

Fatma Sen and Kezban Nur Pilancı

Additional information is available at the end of the chapter

http://dx.doi.org/10.5772/63208

Abstract

The prognosis of colon cancer is primarily determined through staging of the disease. After curative surgery, clinically occult micrometastases are thought to be the major source of disease recurrence. The main aim of postoperative systemic treatment is to eradicate micrometastases, thereby improving outcomes with an increased cure rate. Adjuvant systemic chemotherapy is indicated for patients with stage III colon cancer, as well as for patients with high-risk stage II colon cancer. Prognostic and predictive markers that identify heterogeneous groups are needed to implement tailored therapeutic strategies. Due to the lack of evidence of predictive value of multigene assays in terms of potential value of adjuvant chemotherapy, multigene assays should not be used to determine adjuvant therapy. The standard treatment for most patients with stage III disease is a combination of oxaliplatin with infusional and bolus 5-fluorouracil (5-FU) or with an oral agent such as capecitabine, which has equivalent results. Adjuvant therapy should not be administered to all patients with stage II colon cancer. High-risk stage II patients may be considered as an eligible group for adjuvant therapy after a complete discussion. There is no high level of evidence to use irinotecan-based combination chemotherapies in the adjuvant setting. The antiangiogenic agent bevacizumab in combination with standard adjuvant chemotherapy regimens also failed to improve outcomes, as did the EGFR agent cetuximab.

Keywords: Adjuvant, Chemotherapy, Colon cancer, Stage II, Stage III

1. Introduction

Colon cancer is heterogeneous in clinical behavior and in the molecular mechanisms underlying its pathogenesis. The prognosis of colon cancer is primarily determined by staging the disease. TNM is the main staging system in routine clinical practice [1]. In the adjuvant setting, TNM classification remains the only validated prognostic tool.

Nearly a quarter of the 93,090 new diagnoses of colon cancer per annum in the United States are predicted to be stage II disease, which is characterized by the absence of lymph node metastases (i.e., N0 disease), subdivided into IIA (invasion of T3 lesions through the muscularis propria into pericolorectal tissues) and IIB (T4a lesions, with direction invasion or adherence of the tumor to other organs or structures) [1, 2]. Five-year survival rates for stage II patients after surgery alone range from 72 to 85% [3].

Stage III disease includes colon cancer with any T and N1–2 and M0 [1]. According to TNM staging, patients with stage III disease have various long-term outcomes based on T and N stages at initial diagnosis. Tumors with T1–2 and N1 involvements are classified as stage IIIA and they result in 83% 5-year overall survival (OS) rates. Tumors with T3–4 and N1 involvements are staged as stage IIIB with 64% 5-year OS. Patients with stage IIIC colon cancer with any T and N2 involvement have the worst prognosis with 44% 5-year OS. Thus, approximately 40% of patients with stage III colon cancer experience disease recurrence and many lose the chance of cure during the course.

After curative surgery, clinically occult micrometastases are thought to be the major source of disease recurrence. Adjuvant therapy is administered with the fundamental aim of reducing any probability of disease recurrence and to annihilate micrometastases after the potentially curative resection of colon cancer. Despite many studies representing an augmentation of survival in patients with stage III (node-positive) colon cancer as a result of adjuvant systemic chemotherapy, its impact in resected stage II colon cancer still remains unproven in defiance of several related trials.

In this chapter, the principles of adjuvant systemic therapy in stage II and III colon cancers will be discussed with a review of the literature. Chemotherapy options will be discussed by using findings from clinical trials. Prognostic factors and potential predictive markers of possible benefit of adjuvant systemic therapy will be reviewed, and whether current knowledge in genetic expression profiling helps the physician during decision making will be highlighted.

2. Adjuvant systemic treatment in stage III colon cancer

(a) Fluorouracil with levamisole or leucovorin in stage III colon cancer

Up to the late 1980s, the role of systemic chemotherapy in the adjuvant setting was not established in colon cancer. In 1988, a systematic review of randomized controlled trials about adjuvant therapy of colorectal cancer was performed [4]. The findings of trials evaluating radiotherapy or chemotherapy were combined. Fluorouracil-containing regimens were shown to provide a small OS benefit (odds ratio [OR]: 0.83, 95% confidence interval [CI]: [0.70–0.98]). All other combinations of trials failed to demonstrate statistically significant OS benefit between treated and control patients.

The National Surgical Adjuvant Breast and Bowel Project (NSABP) has conducted several clinical trials on adjuvant chemotherapy and compared different adjuvant chemotherapy regimens or adjuvant chemotherapy versus surgery alone in patients with stage II and III colon cancer (**Table 1**). NSABP C-01 trial was the first adjuvant chemotherapy trial of NSABP conducted between November 1977 and February 1983 and included 1166 patients with stage II and III carcinomas of the colon [5]. Patients were randomized to one of three therapeutic categories: (1) no further treatment following curative resection (394 patients); (2) postoperative chemotherapy consisting of 5-fluorouracil (5-FU), semustine, and vincristine (379 patients); or (3) postoperative BCG (393 patients). A comparison between patients who received postoperative adjuvant chemotherapy and those treated with surgery alone indicated that there was an overall improvement in disease-free survival (DFS) ($P = 0.02$) and survival ($P = 0.05$) in favor of the chemotherapy-treated group. At 5 years of follow-up, patients treated with surgery alone were at 1.29-times the risk of developing a treatment failure and at 1.31-times the likelihood of dying compared with similar patients treated with combination adjuvant chemotherapy. The findings from this study were the first from a randomized prospective clinical trial to demonstrate that a significant DFS and survival benefit can be achieved with postoperative adjuvant chemotherapy in patients with stage II and III carcinomas of the colon who undergo curative resection.

Trial [reference number]	Stages included	Regimens	Number of patients	DFS	OS
NSABP C-01 [5]	II, III			**5-year DFS**	**5-year OS**
		(1) No adjuvant therapy	394		
		(2) 5-FU/semustine/ vincristine (MOF)	379	$P = 0.02$	$P = 0.05$
		(3) BCG	393		
NSABP C-02 [6]	All stages			**4-year DFS**	**4-year OS**
		(1) No adjuvant therapy	581	64%	73%
		(2) Portal vein infusion of 5-FU	577	74%	81%
				$P = 0.02$	$P = 0.07$
INT-0035 [7]	III			**3-year DFS**	**3-year OS**
		(1) No adjuvant therapy	315	<60%	47%

Trial [reference number]	Stages included	Regimens	Number of patients	DFS	OS
		(2) Levamisole	310	<60%	49%
		(3) 5-FU plus levamisole	304	>60%	60%
				$P < 0.0001$	$P = 0.0007$
NCCTG and Mayo Clinic by Laurie et al. [8]	II, III			**3-year DFS**	**3-year OS**
		(1) No adjuvant therapy	135		
		(2) Levamisole	130	$P = 0.05$	$P = 0.12$
		(3) 5-FU plus levamisole	136	$P = 0.003$	$P = 0.09$
NSABP C-03 [9]	II, III			**3-year DFS**	**3-year OS**
		(1) 5-FU/semustine /vincristine (MOF)	524	64%	77%
		(2) 5-FU plus leucovorin (LV) (5-FU/LV)	521	73%	84%
				$P = 0.0004$	$P = 0.003$
NSABP C-04 [10]	II, III			**5-year DFS**	**5-year OS**
		(1) 5-FU/LV	691	65%	74%
		(2) 5-FU plus levamisole	691	60%	70%
		(3) 5-FU/LV plus levamisole	696	55%	75%
NSABP C-05 [6]	II, III			4-year DFS	4-year OS
		(1) 5-FU/LV	1088	69%	80%
		(2) 5-FU/LV plus alpha-interferon	1088	70%	81%
				$P = 0.34$	$P = 0.41$
INT-0089 [11]	II, III			5-year DFS	5-year OS
		(1) 5-FU/LV Mayo Clinic	908	60	66
		(2) 5-FU/LV	910	58	66

http://dx.doi.org/10.5772/63208

Trial [reference number]	Stages included	Regimens	Number of patients	DFS	OS
		Roswell Park			
		(3) 5-FU plus levamisole for 6 months	802	55	64
		(4) 5-FU plus levamisole for 12 months	780	49	54
				$P > 0.05$	$P > 0.05$

DFS, disease-free interval; OS, overall survival.

Table 1. The randomized prospective clinical trials comparing adjuvant treatment with fluorouracil, fluorouracil/levamisole, or fluorouracil/leucovorin and surgery alone in patients with resected colon cancer.

In a randomized cooperative trial performed by Lauri et al., 401 eligible patients with resected stage II and III colorectal carcinoma were randomized to no adjuvant therapy or to adjuvant single-agent levamisole or to adjuvant levamisole plus fluorouracil (5-FU/levamisole). 5-FU/levamisole, and to a lesser extent single-agent levamisole, resulted in decreased cancer recurrence compared with no adjuvant therapy [8]. Both single-agent levamisole and 5-FU/levamisole regimens resulted in significant overall improvements in survival. These improvements reached borderline significance only for stage III patients treated with 5-FU/levamisole ($P = 0.03$). Adjuvant chemotherapy was found to be clinically safe.

In the INT-0035 trial, 5-FU/levamisole reduced the recurrence rate by 40% ($P < 0.0001$) and the death rate by 33% ($P = 0.0007$) in patients with stage III colon cancer. The regimen was found to be tolerable and patient compliance was excellent. There was no evidence of late adverse effects [7]. After these findings were reported, 5-FU/levamisole was recommended as adjuvant chemotherapy for patients with resected stage III colon cancer in a consensus meeting held by the National Institute of Health [12].

The results from the NSABP C-03 trial indicated that fluorouracil plus leucovorin (5-FU/LV) was an active treatment regimen for colon cancer in the adjuvant setting, which precipitated a head-to-head comparison between 5-FU/levamisole and 5-FU/LV [9]. In the landmark NSABP C-04 trial, more than 2000 patients with stage II and III colon cancer were randomized between treatment with 5-FU/LV, 5-FU/levamisole, or 5-FU/LV with levamisole [10]. In terms of DFS and OS, 5-FU/LV demonstrated superiority over 5-FU/levamisole as the standard-of-care adjuvant chemotherapy for patients with both stage II and III colon cancers.

In the randomized Intergroup 0089 trial (INT 0089), the efficacy of 5-FU/LV and 5-FU/levamisole as well as the two most common dose/schedules for the administration of 5-FU/LV, the Roswell Park (5-FU and high-dose LV) and the Mayo Clinic (5-FU and low-dose LV) regimens, were compared in patients with stage II and III patients [11]. The four treatment arms were 5-FU/levamisole (12-month protocol), 5-FU/high-dose LV (Roswell Park, 7 months),

5-FU/low-dose LV (Mayo, 6 months), and 5-FU/LV/levamisole (6 months). All treatment arms were found to be equivalent in terms of both 5-year DFS and OS with a median of 10 years. These results provided a choice for patient treatment schedules based on toxicities and other existing factors rather than on maximization of survival outcome [13].

The important messages from all these findings were as follows: (1) adjuvant 5-FU/LV administered for 6 months was equivalent to 5-FU/levamisole administered for 12 months, (2) two schedules of 5-FU/LV (Mayo Clinic for 6 months, Roswell Park for four cycles) showed different toxicity profiles but same efficacy, and (3) the incorporation of levamisole to 5-FU/LV did not improve long-term outcomes [14].

In stage III colon cancer, adjuvant systemic treatment became the standard treatment approach because it results in improvement in DFS and OS with an approximately 30% relative reduction in the risk of disease recurrence and a 20–30% relative reduction in mortality [6, 15].

(b) Oxaliplatin with 5-FU/LV in stage III colon cancer

The demonstration that adjuvant therapy with 5-FU/levamisole reduced the mortality rate among patients with stage III colon cancer prompted several trials, which established 6 months of treatment with 5-FU/LV as the standard adjuvant chemotherapy for stage III colon cancer. Furthermore, several cytotoxic agents investigated in the metastatic colorectal cancer setting were considered to hold promise for the adjuvant setting. Several phase III trials investigated potential roles of oxaliplatin and irinotecan in combination with 5-FU/LV in adjuvant setting after their successes in metastatic colorectal cancer [16–19]. In addition, an orally bioavailable prodrug of 5-FU, capecitabine, was introduced into the adjuvant setting and investigated for noninferiority to bolus 5-FU/LV (the Mayo Clinic regimen) [20]. Results from trials of these three agents helped shape the current treatment approaches (**Table 2**).

The Multicenter International Study of Oxaliplatin/5-FU/Leucovorin in the Adjuvant Treatment of Colon Cancer (MOSAIC) was a large-scale randomized controlled trial performed mainly in Europe, which assessed the efficacy and safety of FOLFOX4 as an adjuvant therapy [19]. One arm of study was the de Gramont Schedule [5-FU/LV regimen, which was a 2-h infusion of LV (200 mg/m^2), a 5-FU bolus (400 mg/m^2), and then a 22-h 5-FU infusion (600 mg/m^2) administered on two consecutive days every 14 days, for 12 cycles]. The FOLFOX4 was the other arm and consisted of the same 5-FU/LV regimen plus a 2-h infusion oxaliplatin (85 mg/m^2) on day 1, given simultaneously with LV. A significant improvement in 5-year DFS and 6-year OS was demonstrated in the FOLFOX4 group compared with the 5-FU/LV group. Ten-year follow-up results were recently reported [23]. The survival benefit of FOLFOX4 was maintained in patients with stage III colon cancer (10-year OS 67% in FOLFOX4 versus 59% in 5-FU/LV, hazard ratio [HR], 0.80; $P = 0.016$). Ten-year OS was similar in both treatment arms in stage II colon cancer (78% in FOLFOX4 versus 80% in 5-FU/LV).

In the NSABP C-07 trial, a total of 2409 eligible patients were randomized to either intravenous (iv) bolus 5-FU/LV (FU 500 mg/m^2 performed weekly for 6 weeks; LV 500 mg/m^2 iv weekly for 6 weeks of each 8-week cycle for three cycles) or 5-FU/LV plus oxaliplatin (FLOX, 85 mg/m^2 iv on days 1, 15, and 29 of each cycle) [24]. OS was found to be similar between treatment groups.

With 8-year median follow-up, FLOX remained superior for DFS (HR, 0.82; $P = 0.002$). The NSABP C-08 trial confirmed that modified sixth version of the FOLFOX regimen (mFOLFOX6) therapy was equivalent to FOLFOX4 therapy in terms of efficacy and safety [22]. Either adjuvant FOLFOX4 or mFOLFOX6 is routinely given as 12 courses (2 weeks per course).

Trial [reference number]	Stages included	Regimens	Number of patients		
NSABP C-07 [21]	II, III			**5-year DFS**	**5-year OS**
		(1) 5-FU/LV	1207	64%	78%
		(2) 5-FU/LV plus oxaliplatin (FLOX)	1200	69%	80%
				$P = 0.002$	$P = 0.08$
MOSAIC [15]	II, III			**6-year DFS**	**6-year OS**
		(1) Bolus plus continuous-infusion 5-FU/LV	1123	67%	76%
		(2) FOLFOX4	1123	73%	79%
				$P = 0.003$	$P = 0.046$
XELOXA [22]				5-year DFS	5-year OS
		(1) Bolus FU/FA		60%	74%
		(2) XELOX*		66%	78%
				$P = 0.0045$	$P = 0.148$

DFS, disease-free interval; OS, overall survival.
*XELOX was given as oxaliplatin 130 mg/m^2 on day 1 plus capecitabine 1000 mg/m^2 twice daily on days 1–14 every 3 weeks for 24 weeks). The bolus FU/FA was given as a standard adjuvant regimen (Mayo Clinic for 24 weeks or Roswell Park for 32 weeks).

Table 2. Clinical trials comparing fluoropyrimidines with fluoropyrimidine plus oxaliplatin-based combination regimens as adjuvant therapy in patients with stage III colon cancer.

The results of these randomized controlled phase III trials have led combination chemotherapy with FOLFOX to be the standard of care for resected stage III colon cancer [15, 19, 21, 24].

(c) Oral fluoropyrimidines with or without oxaliplatin in stage III colon cancer

Continuous 5-FU is administered via indwelling iv catheters in an infusion pump and carries the risk of some complications such as thrombosis, embolism, or infection. Thus, oral fluoropyrimidines were developed with the aim to avoid these complications while preserving the improved tolerability of continuous infusion. Capecitabine, uracil/tegafur (UFT), and S-1 are most the commonly investigated oral fluoropyrimidines in colon cancer. Capecitabine is absorbed intact through the intestinal wall. It is converted to FU after three sequential enzymatic reactions. Tumor cells contain higher levels of thymidine phosphorylase, which is the final requisite enzyme, than normal cells. This allows capecitabine to selectively accumulate in tumor cells and results in less toxicity or better tolerability.

In NSABP C-06 trial, three cycles of Roswell Park regimen (weekly bolus 5-FU/LV) were compared with five cycles of oral UFT/LV (300 mg/m^2/day with LV 90 mg/day for 4 weeks followed by a 1-week rest period) in 1608 patients with stage II and III colon cancer [25]. No difference was found between the two treatment arms in relapse-free survival (RFS), DFS, and OS. The toxicities and quality of life on the Functional Assessment of Cancer Therapy-Colorectal (FACT-C) instrument were not different between the two arms. Greater fatigue was experienced with UFT in one instrument, but three other instruments demonstrated greater convenience and lower prevalence of symptoms with UFT. A Japanese meta-analysis showed a reduced risk of recurrence (15%) and improved survival (11%) for adjuvant oral chemotherapy (usually UFT or carmofur plus mitomycin C) compared with surgery without chemotherapy in patients with resected stage I, II, and III colon cancers.

The efficacy of capecitabine in stage III colon cancer was assessed in the Xeloda in Adjuvant Colon Cancer Therapy (X-ACT) trial [20]. The 1987 patients with resected stage III colon cancer were randomized to receive either capecitabine (1250 mg/m^2 twice a day on days 1–14 every 3 weeks for a total of eight cycles) or the bolus 5-FU/LV (Mayo Clinic regimen consisted of 5-FU 425 mg/m^2 and LV 20 mg/m^2 given on days 1–5 as iv boluses every 4 weeks, for six cycles). The capecitabine was found to be at least as effective as 5-FU/LV. In fact, RFS was superior to capecitabine (3-year RFS: 65.5% versus 61.9%, HR, 0.86; P = 0.0407) and there was a trend toward better DFS (3-year DFS: 64.2% versus 60.6%; HR, 0.87; P = 0.0528) and OS (81.3% versus 77.6%; HR, 0.84; P = 0.0706). The required dose reductions were similar between the two treatment groups (42% capecitabine, 44% bolus 5-FU/LV). With the exception of hand-foot syndrome, capecitabine was generally better tolerated with fewer patients experiencing nausea and vomiting, mucositis, diarrhea, and leukopenia.

Although the data from the X-ACT study and NSABP C-06 demonstrated that oral fluoropyrimidine regimen was at least as effective as an iv regimen, UFT was not approved for commercial availability in the Unites States.

S-1 is an oral fluoropyrimidine consisting of tegafur, gimeracil, and oteracil. The antitumor effects of S-1 have been demonstrated in treating various gastrointestinal cancers including metastatic colon cancer when administered as monotherapy or in combination chemotherapy. A randomized phase III study from Japan investigated the efficacy of S-1 as adjuvant chemotherapy for curatively resected stage III colon cancer by evaluating its noninferiority to tegafur-uracil plus LV (UFT/LV) [26]. A total of 1518 patients aged 20–80 years were randomized to receive S-1 (80–120 mg/day on days 1–28 every 42 days; four courses) or UFT/LV (UFT, 300–600 mg/day, and LV, 75 mg/day on days 1–28 every 35 days; five courses). The 3-year DFS rate was 75.5% and 72.5% in the S-1 and UFT/LV group, respectively. The stratified HR for DFS in the S-1 group compared with the UFT/LV group was 0.85, demonstrating the noninferiority of S-1 (noninferiority stratified log-rank test, $P < 0.001$). In the subgroup analysis, no significant interactions were identified between the major baseline characteristics and the treatment groups. Thus, findings of this Japanese phase III trial confirmed noninferiority of S-1 in DFS at adjuvant setting of stage III colon cancer compared with UFT/LV.

In a multicenter, randomized trial NO16968 (XELOX in Adjuvant Colon Cancer Treatment [XELOXA]), capecitabine plus oxaliplatin (XELOX) was compared with bolus 5-FU/LV as an adjuvant therapy in patients with stage III colon cancer [22] (**Table 2**). XELOX was given as oxaliplatin 130 mg/m^2 on day 1 plus capecitabine 1000 mg/m^2 twice daily on days 1–14 every 3 weeks for 24 weeks). The bolus FU/FA was given as a standard adjuvant regimen (Mayo Clinic for 24 weeks or Roswell Park for 32 weeks). XELOX was superior to bolus FU/FA in terms of DFS with a HR of 0.80 (95% CI: [0.69–0.93]; $P = 0.0045$), corresponding to a 20% relative risk reduction. The 3-year DFS rates for XELOX and FU/FA were 70.9 and 66.5%, respectively. The 4-year and 5-year DFS rates in the XELOX group were 68.4 and 66.1%, respectively, compared with 62.3 and 59.8% in the FU/FA group, demonstrating that the superior efficacy of XELOX versus FU/FA was maintained over time, with increasing differences between study arms. The HR for OS for XELOX compared with FU/FA was 0.87 (95% CI: [0.72–1.05]; $P = 0.1486$). The 5-year OS for XELOX and FU/FA were 77.6% and 74.2%, respectively.

Adjuvant capecitabine with or without oxaliplatin versus 5-FU/LV with or without oxaliplatin has been directly compared in a pooled analysis [27]. In total, 8734 patients with resected stage III colon cancer from four randomized controlled trials (NSABP C-08, X-ACT, XELOXA, and AVANT) were evaluated in this pooled analysis. The adjuvant treatment regimens were XELOX (oxaliplatin and capecitabine), 5-FU/LV, capecitabine, FOLFOX-4, and mFOLFOX-6. DFS, RFS, and OS were found to be similar between patients treated with 5-FU/LV versus those treated with capecitabine in adjusted analyses. Multiple Cox regression analysis of OS revealed a significant interaction between oxaliplatin and fluoropyrimidine ($P = 0.014$). Post-relapse survival was similar in adjusted ($P = 0.23$) and unadjusted analyses ($P = 0.33$) for the comparison of XELOX or FOLFOX versus 5-FU/LV and was also similar for capecitabine-based regimens versus 5-FU/LV-based regimens (unadjusted $P = 0.26$). Thus, the combination therapy with oxaliplatin provided consistently improved outcomes without adversely affecting post-relapse survival in the adjuvant treatment of stage III colon cancer, irrespective of whether the fluoropyrimidine backbone was capecitabine or 5-FU/LV.

In another recent pooled analysis, a total of 12,233 patients, treated with adjuvant systemic treatment and enrolled to the randomized trials C-07, C-08, N0147, MOSAIC (Adjuvant Treatment of Colon Cancer), and XELOXA (adjuvant XELOX), were investigated to examine the impact of oxaliplatin and tumor-specific factors on the time course of recurrence and death [28]. The addition of oxaliplatin significantly reduced the risk of recurrence within the first 14 months post treatment for patients with stage II disease and within the first 4 years for patients with stage III disease. Oxaliplatin also significantly reduced the risk of death from 2 to 6 years post treatment for patients with stage III disease, with no differences in timing of outcomes between treatment groups (i.e., oxaliplatin did not simply postpone recurrence or death compared with 5-FU/LV). This pooled analysis also supported the addition of oxaliplatin to fluoropyrimidine-based adjuvant therapy in patients with stage III disease.

These data added to the existing evidence that oxaliplatin plus capecitabine or 5-FU/LV is the standard of care for the adjuvant treatment of stage III colon cancer and offers physicians' flexibility to treat patients according to the patients' overall physical performance and preference. The preferred oxaliplatin-fluoropyrimidine-based combination regimens are XELOX, FOLFOX4, FOLFOX6, FOLFOX7, XELOX, and FLOX.

(d) Irinotecan-based combination regimens

The efficacy of irinotecan in the adjuvant setting was evaluated in two large trials of patients with resected stage II/III colon cancer. In the trial performed in the United States, a 5-FU/LV bolus plus irinotecan regimen (IFL) was compared with 5-FU/LV bolus alone [18]. The IFL regimen was not shown to have superiority over 5-FU/LV-alone arm in terms of either DFS or OS. Furthermore, IFL resulted in significantly higher toxicity, including lethal toxicity. PETACC-3 was designed to compare 5-FU/LV/irinotecan (FOLFIRI) with 5-FU/LV in the adjuvant setting because IFL was demonstrated to be inferior to FOLFOX in patients with advanced colon cancer [11]. The 5-year DFS rate was found to be 56.7% with FOLFIRI and 54.3% with 5-FU/LV alone ($P = 0.106$). OS was similar between the two arms (5-year OS 73.6% versus 71.3%, respectively; log-rank $P = 0.094$). Thus, irinotecan should not be used in the standard management of stage II/III colon cancer.

3. Adjuvant systemic therapy in stage II colon cancer

It is remarkable that an OS and DFS benefit in the combined population compared with surgery alone could only be identified at a significant rate almost exclusively in patients with stage III disease in several trials of fluoropyrimidine-based chemotherapy that enrolled a mix of patients with stage II and III colon cancers [9, 29–32] (**Table 3**). On the other hand, some large trials that specifically delved into the benefit of fluoropyrimidine-based chemotherapy in patients with stage II disease failed to show a clear benefit for adjuvant chemotherapy [9, 33, 34]. In the INT-0035 trial, stage II and III patients were randomized into either 5-FU/levamisole administration or surgery alone [7]. The 7-year survival rate for the 5-FU/levamisole treatment group was 60.2% versus 47% for the surgery-alone group ($P = 0.0007$) among stage III patients, whereas the 7-year survival rate for stage II patients was 72% for both groups ($P = 0.83$). As a result, the study demonstrated a significant contribution of the adjuvant therapy to stage III patients, regardless of the small number ($n = 318$) of patients with stage II disease [7].

One of the most noteworthy several meta-analyses that assessed the benefit of adjuvant fluoropyrimidine-based chemotherapy in patients with resected stage II colon cancer is the International Multicenter Pooled Analysis of Colon Cancer Trials (IMPACT), which did not support the routine use of 5-FU/LV in all patients with stage II colon cancer [5, 13, 14]. The data pooled from 1016 patients with T3N0 disease enrolled in five similar trials of observation versus 5-FU/LV found a non-statistically significant improvement in EFS that favored chemotherapy (76% versus 73%; HR, 0.83), and 5-year OS was similar (82% versus 80%, HR, 0.86) [29].

The American Society of Clinical Oncology (ASCO) held a panel to provide recommendations through a literature-based meta-analysis conducted by the Ontario group regarding adjuvant therapy for patients with stage II colon cancer [35]. The Ontario group analysis included the comparison of 5-FU/LV versus observation for stage II colon cancer, 37 trials and 11 meta-analyses [36]. Chemotherapy was associated with a small but significant absolute improvement in DFS (5–10%) according to the results of this analysis, which failed to translate into a statistically significant difference in OS (risk ratio [RR] 0.87, 95% CI: [0.75–1.10], $P = 0.07$) [36]. These trials failed to support the routine use of adjuvant chemotherapy for stage II colon cancer, and the ASCO panel did not recommend the routine use of adjuvant chemotherapy for patients with stage II colon cancer due to the lack of significant improvement in OS.

	Patients	Regimens		5-year DFS		5-year OS	
Trial	Stage II/total	Control	Experimental arm	Control	Experimental arm	Control	Experimental arm
IMPACT 1	841/1493	Surgery alone	Surgery plus 5-FU and folinic acid	76%	79%	90%	88%
IMPACT 2	1016/1016	Surgery alone	Surgery plus 5-FU and leucovorin	73%	76%	80%	82%
INT-0035*	325/1296	Surgery alone	Surgery plus 5-FU and levamisole			72%	72%
NSABP	1565/4006	Surgery alone	Surgery plus combination chemotherapy**	NR	NR	75%	70%
Gill et al.	1440/3302	Surgery alone	Surgery plus 5-FU-based therapy***	72%	76%	80%	81%
ACCENT	6896/20898	Surgery plus FU/LV alone	Surgery plus 5-FU and oxaliplatin	NR	NR	67%	72%

ACCENT, Adjuvant Colon Cancer Endpoints; DFS, disease-free survival; IMPACT, International Multicenter Pooled Analysis of Colon Cancer Trials; INT-0035, intergroup study; NSABP, National Surgical Breast and Bowel Project; NR, not reported; OS, overall survival.
*7-year survival.
**Combination chemotherapy: semustine, vincristine, 5-FU, and perioperative 5-FU portal vein infusion.
***5-FU-based therapy: FU + leucovorin or FU + levamisole.

Table 3. Clinical trials of fluoropyrimidine-based adjuvant therapy for stage II colon cancer.

The ASCO panel further addressed the issue of adjuvant therapy for those stage II patients with high-risk features including inadequately sampled nodes, T4 lesion, perforation, or poorly differentiated histology. Although randomized trials failed to demonstrate an improvement in OS, the number of patients with high-risk stage II disease in these studies was considered inadequate to demonstrate benefit. Moreover, adjuvant therapy is considered reasonable for those patients with suboptimal lymph node examinations.

There are studies that indicated the benefits of adjuvant treatment in resected stage II colon cancer, including the NSABP study of fluorouracil-based adjuvant therapy trials for patients with stage II and III colon cancer from 1977 to 1990 [13, 34]. The data from these four combined studies, 41% of the patients in which had stage II (1565 patients) disease, indicated a 30% reduction in overall mortality for the stage II patients versus surgery alone [16]. The mortality reduction was 18% for stage II patients, which was greater than that observed for stage III patients regardless of the presence or absence of high-risk features, including the presence of obstruction, perforation, or extension to adjacent organs, having resulted in an absolute survival improvement of 5%; therefore, the NSABP recommended adjuvant chemotherapy for all stage II patients [37–39]. One of the studies that supported the NSABP study was a recent meta-analysis of 12 randomized controlled trials from 1985 to 2010 in which surgery alone was the control group, which found a significant benefit to adjuvant therapy in patients with stage II colon cancer [37]. A significant improvement in 5-year OS was associated with surgery combined with postoperative adjuvant chemotherapy for stage II colon cancer (HR, 0.81; 95% CI: [0.71–0.91]) and the 5-year DFS also favored the group of surgery combined with postoperative adjuvant chemotherapy for stage II colon cancer (HR, 0.86; 95% CI: [0.75–0.98]). An important reduction in risk of recurrence was found for stage II colon cancer in favor of postoperative adjuvant chemotherapy (RR, 0.82; 95% CI: [0.71–0.95]) [40].

The data of 3151 patients with stage II colon cancer who were considered to carry "usual" risk for recurrence were obtained from the Surveillance, Epidemiology, and End Results (SEER) Medicare database and analyzed. Stage II disease with usual risk was defined as tumors with a stage of T3N0 and without obstruction and perforation. The OS rate of the group administered with chemotherapy was 78% compared with 75% of the group not administered with chemotherapy [36]. The analysis confirmed that the findings in randomized studies of adjuvant therapy (e.g., IMPACT) were similar to those encountered in real-world practice with the improvement in OS with adjuvant therapy for patients with stage II colon cancer is at best 2–5%, which is a statistically insignificant improvement in OS with adjuvant therapy [36].

The QUASAR trial randomly assigned 3239 patients (2963 (91%) with stage II (node negative) disease and 2291 (71%) with colon cancer) with an "uncertain indication for adjuvant therapy" to chemotherapy with 5-FU/LV or with or without levamisole or observation following resection of colon or rectal cancer [41], which indicated a small but statistically significant survival benefit for patients with stage II disease treated with 5-FU/LV (HR, 0.86; 95% CI: [0.54–1.19]), 5-year survival 83.9% versus 81.5%). Nevertheless, patients with higher-risk disease may benefit more from adjuvant therapy because approximately 64% of patients had less than 12 lymph nodes sampled (the median number of lymph nodes examined was only six) in this study [42].

The benefit of oxaliplatin for stage II disease remains uncertain due to the scarcity of data available on the benefits of oxaliplatin-based adjuvant chemotherapy for patients with stage II disease. One of the most important trials in this respect is MOSAIC, which compared 6 months of adjuvant 5-FU/LV versus FOLFOX (oxaliplatin plus short-term infusional 5-FU and LV) in patients with resected stage II (40%) or III (60%) colon cancer [15]. Five-year DFS of patients with stage II cancer was slightly but not significantly higher than with FOLFOX (84% versus 80%, HR for recurrence 0.84, $P = 0.26$) [43]. After longer follow-up, no difference in 10-year OS was noted in the stage II subpopulation (79.5% versus 78.4%; HR, 1.00; $P = 0.98$) (21).

http://dx.doi.org/10.5772/63208

Colon cancer with high-risk features was defined as colon cancer with at least one of the following: stage T4, perforation, bowel obstruction, poor differentiation, and venous invasion (<10 lymph nodes examined). The patients with high-risk stage II disease who received FOLFOX did not have improved DFS or OS benefit compared with those who received infusional 5-FU/LV. Similar results were identified in the NSABP C-07 trial, which compared weekly oxaliplatin plus bolus 5-FU/LV (FLOX) to bolus 5-FU/LV in patients with stage II and III colon cancer [21].

Although most of these analyses showed that patients with stage II colon cancer do not have significantly better survival with adjuvant therapy, not all stage II patients are at equal risk. Patient/physician discussions individualized for the patient as well as explanations of the specific characteristics of the disease should be included in decision making for the use of adjuvant therapy in patients with stage II disease; prognosis and evidence related to the efficacy and possible toxicities associated with treatment should be centered on patient choice [38]. The oncologist should help the patient to make an informed decision by estimating the relative risk of recurrence and/or death with and without adjuvant chemotherapy and discussing the expected adverse effects of treatment. The possible benefit of adjuvant therapy is small as patients with average-risk stage II colon cancer have a very good prognosis. Although patients with stage II colon cancer and high-risk features have been considered more likely to benefit from adjuvant chemotherapy, currently it is known that many patients with high-risk features do not have recurrence, whereas some patients with average-risk features do. Thus, the current definition of high-risk stage II colon cancer is accepted as inadequate [39]. Moreover, there are no data points on features that are predictive of benefit from adjuvant chemotherapy and no data correlating risk features and selection of chemotherapy in patients with high-risk stage II disease.

Overall, the National Comprehensive Cancer Network (NCCN) panel found it reasonable to accept the relative benefit of adjuvant therapy in stage III disease as indirect evidence of benefit for stage II disease, particularly for those with high-risk features [39], which initiated efforts to use clinicopathologic and molecular features to select groups of patients with higher-risk stage II disease for a greater risk of recurrence who might benefit more from adjuvant chemotherapy.

Clinicopathologic features associated with a worse prognosis in patients with stage II disease are T4 primary [4, 44]; poorly differentiated histology (including signet ring and mucinous tumors) [45]; lymphovascular invasion (LVI) [40]; perineural invasion [40]; bowel obstruction or perforation [46, 47]; close, indeterminate, or positive margins; inadequately sampled lymph nodes (less than 13 in the surgical specimen) [48]; a high preoperative serum carcinoembryonic antigen (CEA) level [40, 49]; and occult nodal micrometastases as detected by molecular or immunohistochemical methods (**Table 4**). Expert groups such as ASCO [38], NCCN, and the European Society for Medical Oncology (ESMO) [50] have different definitions for high-risk early colon cancer.

Despite the adverse influence of the foregoing features on prognosis, there is subtle evidence to indicate that patients with any of these high-risk features are more prone to benefit from chemotherapy (i.e., factors associated with poorer prognosis are not necessarily predictive of chemotherapy response). The benefit of chemotherapy in higher-risk subsets of stage II disease has been examined by only a few studies [15, 32, 45, 51]. The next-generation Intergroup trial INT-0089 randomized 3759 patients with high-risk stage II (20% of accrual) and stage III patients to receive one of four combinations of 5-FU with LV and/or levamisole [7]. High-risk stage II disease was defined as those stage II patients with evidence of bowel obstruction, bowel perforation, or adherence to or invasion of adjacent organs or tumor perforation. The four combinations did not result in any difference among the high-risk stage II or the stage III patients. The 5-year OS rate ranged from 75 to 77% in the treated high-risk stage II patients and it was found to be comparable with the survival rate of the general population of stage II patients treated with surgery alone. It concludes an uncertainty as to whether this conventionally described high-risk group would have had a similar survival rate if no adjuvant therapy had been given [12]. While a more recent analysis of more than 24,847 patients with stage II colon cancer (75% had one or more poor prognostic features) from the SEER-Medicare database showed no 5-year survival benefit for adjuvant chemotherapy over observation, even in patients with stage II disease with one or more poor prognostic features (obstruction, perforation, emergency admission for surgery, T4 stage, resection of fewer than 12 lymph nodes, and poorly differentiated or undifferentiated histology) (HR, 1.03; 95% CI: [0.94–1.13]) [52].

1. Obstructed or perforated colon cancer
2. High-risk histology
3. LVI/extramural spread
4. Perineural invasion
5. Poorly differentiated tumor (grades 3–4)
6. T4 primary tumor
7. Inadequate lymph node sampling (<12)
8. Elevated preoperative CEA
9. 18q deletion
10. Indeterminate, close, or positive margin

Table 4. High-risk factors in patients with stage II colon cancer.

In the MOSAIC study, which assessed the effect of oxaliplatin (FOLFOX versus 5-FU/LV), there was a trend toward improved DFS with FOLFOX (82% versus 75%) in the subgroup of stage II patients with high-risk tumors (clinical T4, poorly differentiated, perforation, or obstruction (<10 nodes in the surgical specimen)) (**Table 4**). Although the OS was substantially the same in both groups (85% versus 83%, $P = 0.65$), the lack of a control group treated with surgery alone makes it impossible to identify whether these results are better than surgery alone [15].

The number of lymph nodes extracted is also very important to define high-risk stage II disease. An Intergroup 0089 trial (INT-0089) of high-risk, stage II and III colon cancer patients indicated

http://dx.doi.org/10.5772/63208

the number of lymph nodes analyzed as an independent prognostic variable [53]. Survival increased as the number of the analyzed lymph nodes increased, regardless of whether lymph nodes were found positive or negative ($P = 0.0001$ and $P = 0.0005$, respectively, for stage III and II disease). The American Joint Committee on Cancer and the College of American Pathologists recommended that at least 12 lymph nodes should be examined [32, 44]. The patient should be considered inadequately staged when fewer than 12 nodes are sampled and reported, in which case reexamination of the surgical specimen may be requested.

4. Monotherapy as adjuvant chemotherapy in colon cancer

Whenever any contraindication for combination chemotherapy with fluoropyrimidine and oxaliplatin exists, single-agent fluoropyrimidine could be an option as an adjuvant chemothErapy regimen. In contrast, there is no evidence to support use of oxaliplatin as a single agent in adjuvant setting. Additionally, irinotecan as single agent or irinotecan-based combination regimens should not be recommended for patients with stage III colon cancer as adjuvant systemic therapy.

5. Targeted agents in the adjuvant setting

Bevacizumab: In NSABP C-08 and AVANT, randomized phase III trials, the potential benefit of bevacizumab was evaluated in addition to oxaliplatin-based chemotherapy in patients with stage II and III colon cancer [54, 55]. The bevacizumab group had a significantly higher rate of toxicity including hypertension, wound complications, pain, proteinuria, and hand-foot syndrome, but bevacizumab in combination with chemotherapy did not provide a DFS or OS advantage over chemotherapy alone in the NSABP C-08 trial [54]. Bevacizumab also did not prolong DFS when added to adjuvant chemotherapy in resected stage III colon cancer with AVANT [56]. The DFS HR for bevacizumab-FOLFOX4 versus FOLFOX4 was 1.17 ($P = 0.07$), and for bevacizumab-XELOX versus FOLFOX4, it was 1.07 ($P = 0.44$). After a minimum follow-up of 60 months, the OS HR for bevacizumab-FOLFOX4 versus FOLFOX4 was 1.27 ($P = 0.02$), and for bevacizumab-XELOX versus FOLFOX4, it was 1.15 ($P = 0.21$). Thus, OS data suggested a potential detrimental effect with bevacizumab plus oxaliplatin-based adjuvant therapy in these patients.

Cetuximab: NCCTG NO147 and PETACC-8 trials investigated the possible role of cetuximab in the adjuvant setting [57, 58]. In NCCTG NO147, the potential benefit of cetuximab added to mFOLFOX6 in patients with resected stage III wild-type KRAS colon cancer was assessed. Three-year DFS for mFOLFOX6 alone was 74.6% versus 71.5% with the addition of cetuximab (HR, 1.21; $P = 0.08$) in patients with wild-type KRAS and 67.1% versus 65.0% (HR, 1.12; $P = 0.38$) in patients with mutated KRAS, with no significant benefit in any of the subgroups assessed. Among all patients, grade 3 or higher adverse events (72.5 versus 52.3%; OR, 2.4; $P < 0.001$) and failure to complete 12 cycles (33 versus 23%; OR, 1.6; $P < 0.001$) were significantly higher with cetuximab. Increased toxicity and greater detrimental differences in all outcomes were observed in patients aged 70 years or more [57]. In PETACC-8, whether the addition of cetuximab to standard adjuvant oxaliplatin, fluorouracil, and leucovorin chemotherapy (FOLFOX4) in patients with stage III colon cancer improved DFS was assessed [58]. In the experimental and control groups, DFS was similar in the intention-to-treat population and in patients with KRAS exon 2/BRAF wild-type (n = 984) or KRAS exon two-mutated tumors (n = 742).

On the basis of the available data, bevacizumab, cetuximab, or panitumumab should not be used in the adjuvant treatment of patients with curatively resected stage III colon cancer.

6. Molecular prognostic and predictive markers

Prognostic and predictive markers that identify heterogeneous groups are needed to implement tailored therapeutic strategies. There are several well-defined prognostic markers related to either patient or tumor, including grade of tumor, LVI, perineural invasion, lymphoid inflammatory response, positive surgical margins, bowel obstruction, and perforation [15]. These are well-defined parameters for patients with stage II colon cancer during decision making; however they are not used in patients with stage III colon cancer. The impact of tumor molecular factors on prognosis and the response to adjuvant chemotherapy in stage II and III disease is a current subject for ongoing studies [59–61].

(a) In stage II colon cancer

Allelic loss of chromosome 18q and microsatellite instability (MSI) in colon tumors are prognostic markers that may be employed to sift stage II patients in terms of risk and decide on who should receive adjuvant chemotherapy.

Allelic loss of chromosome 18q in colon tumors has been demonstrated to be a marker of poor prognosis [59] in an examination of 145 tumor samples for 18q loss. The 5-year survival rate was reported to be lower in patients with 18q loss than in those without 18q loss (54% versus 93%, respectively) [59].

Mismatch repair (MMR) genes may result in MMR protein deficiency and MSI if they are mutated or modified [60]. Approximately 15–20% of colorectal cancers have sporadic or inherited (Lynch syndrome) deficiency of an MMR protein, most commonly MLH1 or MSH2 [61], with tumors characteristically located proximally and a mucinous histology with tumor-infiltrating lymphocytes a better prognosis than do microsatellite-stable (MSS) tumors [62]. MSI (the biological footprint of DNA MMR deficiency) is an important piece of information to consider when deciding whether to use adjuvant chemotherapy in patients with stage II disease. MSI appearance seems to be related with a relative resistance to fluoropyrimidines.

Most (but not all) [63, 64] studies have shown that MSI or deficient mismatch repair (dMMR) is a marker of a more favorable outcome and a predictor of increased benefit from adjuvant therapy with a fluoropyrimidine alone in patients with stage II disease [65–67]. A retrospective study of 570 patients enrolled in three trials of 5-FU-based adjuvant therapy analyzed retrospectively tumor samples for MSI [65]. The 5-year survival rate was significantly better in patients with tumors that exhibited high-frequency MSI (88 versus 68.4%; $P = 0.004$) than those with tumors exhibiting microsatellite stability or low-frequency instability among patients who did not receive adjuvant therapy. Adjuvant chemotherapy improved the OS of patients with MSS tumors or tumors exhibiting low-frequency MSI ($P = 0.04$) but not those with high-frequency MSI. Even harm in terms of OS was suggested in patients treated with dMMR tumors [65]. In parallel, results from another retrospective study of pooled data from adjuvant trials by Sargent and George suggested that adjuvant 5-FU chemotherapy appeared to be destructive in patients with stage II disease in tumors characterized as dMMR [66]. In contrast to the findings of Sargent and George [66], a recent study of 1913 patients treated in the QUASAR study, a randomized comparison of 5-FU/LV and supportive care in stage II colon cancer, confirmed the prognostic significance of dMMR, but not its predictive capacity [42]. A recent study of patients in the CALGB 9581 and 89803 trials reached a similar conclusion [68]. MMR status was prognostic but not predictive of benefit or detrimental impact of adjuvant therapy in patients with stage II colon cancer.

It is not clear if oxaliplatin supplementation would overcome the lack of benefit from adjuvant 5-FU in patients with dMMR. Adjuvant chemotherapies with and without oxaliplatin have been examined on patients with dMMR tumors in retrospective analyses, among which one report noted a significant benefit from adding oxaliplatin to 5-FU/LV in patients with MSI tumors [69], whereas another suggested a lower rate of disease control with FOLFOX in patients with dMMR tumors compared with those with proficient mismatch repair (pMMR) tumors [70]. A preliminary report of a retrospective analysis of 433 patients with resected dMMR tumors (57% stage II) from several French centers was reported at the 2014 ASCO annual meeting [71]. Seventeen percent of the patients with stage II disease ($n = 41$) received adjuvant chemotherapy. Overall, 3-year RFS was 75% for surgery alone, 66% for FU alone, and 84% with FOLFOX. In the subgroup analysis, the benefit of FOLFOX compared with FU and surgery alone was significant for stage III disease (HR for relapse 0.38, 95% CI: [0.21–0.69]) with a tendency toward better results in patients with stage II disease (HR for relapse 0.14, 95% CI: [0.02–1.04]; $P = 0.05$). Tumor specimens characterized as MSI-high (MSI-H) are more common in stage II disease than in stage III disease according to the data from the PETACC-3 trial (22% versus 12%, respectively; $P < 0.0001$) [72]. The percentage of stage IV tumors characterized as MSI-H was only 3.5% [73] in another large-scale study. These results suggest that MSI-H tumors have a decreased likelihood to metastasize.

BRAF mutation in a patient with dMMR colorectal cancer is considered as a negative prognostic indicator, which is also supported by emerging data with a view that BRAF mutations are a negative prognostic factor among patients with pMMR and stage II colon cancer [72, 74, 75]. BRAF mutations were associated with poor OS in a combined analysis of 2299 patients enrolled in two NSABP trials that tested the value of adjuvant chemotherapy in patients with stage II or III colon cancer [76]. The 5-year survival rate was highest in patients with dMMR, BRAF wild-type tumors (90%) and worst in those with pMMR and BRAF-mutated tumors (69%). In a large population-based study of Samowitz et al., microsatellite-unstable tumors were associated with an excellent 5-year survival regardless of whether the V600E mutation was present or absent (76 and 75%, respectively), whereas for MSS tumors, the presence of a V600E mutation significantly worsened 5-year survival (17 versus 60%) [77]. Among patients with stage II MSS tumors, death risk was significantly higher in those with a BRAF mutation (four of 17 [24%] compared with 47 of 889 [5.3%], HR for death 4.88, 95% CI: [1.73–13.76]). In a preliminary report of data from the PETACC-3 adjuvant trial, which was conducted in patients with stage II or III colon cancer, a BRAF V600E mutation was a marker of poor RFS and OS in patients with MSS left-sided tumors, but not MSI-unstable or right-sided tumors [75]. Despite all these results, there still is not sufficient evidence to use BRAF mutation status to select patients among those with stage II colon cancer.

(b) In stage III colon cancer

In several studies, a subgroup of stage III disease, which has better prognosis similar with stage II disease, has been tried to be determined. Numerous studies, including a meta-analysis, have demonstrated that patients with dMMR colorectal cancer have better stage-independent survival relative to patients with pMMR [13]. Furthermore, a predictive role for MMR has been revealed by using data from randomized clinical trials of FU-based therapy versus surgery-only control [78]. The treatment benefit differed by MSI status. Patients with MSI-H and treated with FU-based therapy had a trend toward inferior outcomes compared with patients who were treated with surgery alone. In contrast, patients with MSI-H tumors had been reported to have similar outcomes with chemotherapy or appeared to receive a greater benefit from FU-based adjuvant treatment in other studies [63, 79].

A variety of other markers including 18q deletion, KRAS mutations, TP53, TGFBR2, DCC, and thymidylate synthase gene expression have been proposed to refine T- and N-based groups, but their integration into the clinical setting requires extensive validation of their relative value and optimal use [80]. In addition, there is lack of consensus in performing these markers, such as different antibodies used or different scoring methods, which makes their results incomparable. Colon cancer treatment guidelines do not recommend the use of predictive marker information during decision making because there is no strong evidence for a predictive marker regarding the benefit of adjuvant chemotherapy for stage III colon cancer.

7. Gene expression profiling during decision making of adjuvant chemotherapy in stage II and III colon cancer

After the discovery of numerous molecular features of cancer including gene expression profile, several molecular tests that provide important prognostic and predictive information were investigated to aid clinical decision making [39] (**Table 5**). Despite varying design and sample numbers of the validation analyses, all of these tests have been indicated to have prognostic value in independent patient series [81].

http://dx.doi.org/10.5772/63208

Assay	Gene signature
Oncotype DX Colon Cancer Assay (Genomic Health, Inc.)	12 genes (seven recurrence-risk genes and five reference genes)
ColoPrint colon cancer recurrence assay (Agendia)	18-gene expre ssion profile
ColDx microarray-based multigene assay	634 probe

Table 5. Gene expression assays in stage II colon cancer.

Genomic Health Inc. (Redwood City, CA, USA) has conducted four studies involving more than 1800 patients with stage II or stage III colon cancer; genomic profiling was performed to identify genes that predict recurrence in patients with colon cancer who were treated with surgery alone or surgery plus 5-FU/LV chemotherapy. By using the findings of these studies, the 12-gene colon cancer recurrence score (Oncotype DX Colon Cancer Assay) which quantifies the expression of seven recurrence-risk genes and five reference genes as a prognostic classifier of low, intermediate, or high likelihood of recurrence was designed [82]. This 12-gene assay's ability to predict recurrence rate was independently validated through the analysis of data from the prospective QUASAR trial [83] and through a separate analysis of data from the CALGB 9581 trial [84]. Recurrence at 3 years was, respectively, 12%, 18%, and 22% for the low-, intermediate-, and high-recurrence-risk groups [83].

The 12-gene recurrence score is the best documented and validated tool. In addition three other colon cancer recurrence score assays based upon microarray gene expression including one by Oh et al [85], one by Jiang et al [86], and the Almac microarrays ADXCRC provided added prognostic value. ColoPrint (Agendia, Amsterdam, the Netherlands) is a prognostic 18-gene signature and was identified on the basis of unbiased gene selection by searching the whole genome for genes that had the highest correlation to a tumor relapse event. This prognostic gene signature was validated in an independent set of 206 patients with stage I–III colon cancers and in 135 clinical samples of patients with stage II colon cancer, using a diagnostic microarray platform [87].

How the recurrence score should be integrated with other known prognostic markers for decisions regarding adjuvant chemotherapy is uncertain. Yothers et al. performed an independent, prospectively designed clinical validation study of recurrence score. Archival specimens were obtained from patients with stage II and III colon cancers who were randomized to receive 5-FU or 5-FU plus oxaliplatin in NSABP C-07 [88]. Continuous Recurrence Score predicted recurrence (HR for a 25-unit increase in score, 1.96, $P < 0.001$), as well as DFS (HR for a 25-unit increase in score, 1.60; $P < 0.001$) and OS (HR, 1.89; $P < 0.001$). After adjustment for stage, lymph nodes examined, MMR, grade, and treatment, and recurrence score were shown to predict recurrence risk ($P = 0.001$). Recurrence score did not have significant interaction with stage ($P = 0.90$) or age ($P = 0.76$). Relative benefit of oxaliplatin was found to be similar across the range of recurrence score (interaction $P = 0.48$); accordingly, absolute benefit of oxaliplatin increased with higher scores, most notably in patients with stage II and

IIIA/B diseases [88]. However, the authors underlined that the recurrence score was not predictive of oxaliplatin efficacy and did not directly identify patients who would or would not benefit from oxaliplatin treatment.

These genomic profiling tests may provide information about the level of risk of recurrence over other risk factors; thus they potentially have high prognostic value. Due to the lack of evidence of predictive value of multigene assays in terms of potential value of adjuvant chemotherapy, the NCCN panel does not recommend the use of multigene assays to determine adjuvant therapy [89]. ASCO guidelines do not address the use of this assay.

8. Impact of age and medical comorbidity on adjuvant treatment outcomes for stage III colon cancer

Adjuvant oxaliplatin plus capecitabine or 5-FU/LV (XELOX/FOLFOX) is the standard of care for stage III colon cancer; however, there is disagreement regarding oxaliplatin benefit in patients aged >70 years.

Recently, the efficacy and safety of adjuvant XELOX/FOLFOX versus 5-FU/LV were compared with respect to age and medical comorbidity using pooled data [56]. Individual data from patients with stage III colon cancer in four randomized, controlled trials (NSABP C-08, XELOXA, X-ACT, and AVANT) excluding bevacizumab-treated patients were analyzed. Patients were grouped by treatment, medical comorbidity (low versus high), or age (<70 versus ≥70 years) and compared for DFS, OS, and adverse events. Although benefits were modestly attenuated for patients aged ≥70 years, DFS benefits were demonstrated for XELOX/FOLFOX versus 5-FU/LV regardless of age or medical comorbidity. The OS was found to be improved in all groups. Grade 3/4 serious adverse event rates were comparable across cohorts and medical comorbidity scores and higher in patients aged ≥70 years. Oxaliplatin-relevant grade 3/4 adverse events, including neuropathy, were comparable across ages and medical comorbidity scores. Thus, the findings of this pooled analysis further supported the consideration of XELOX or FOLFOX as standard treatment options for the adjuvant management of stage III colon cancer in all age groups and in patients with comorbidities.

9. Optimal time to start adjuvant systemic therapy

Although no randomized trials have investigated the optimal time to initiate adjuvant systemic treatment, several retrospective studies in which the majority of patients had stage III disease demonstrated that a delay beyond 8 weeks resulted in shorter event-free survival and OS [73, 90, 91]. Starting 5–8 weeks post-surgery has not been shown to lead statistically significant decrease in OS compared with initiation within 4 weeks [73]. However, commencing beyond 8 weeks was associated with decreased OS compared with initiation within 8 weeks. Biagi et al. performed a systemic review and meta-analysis to define the optimal timing from surgery to initiation of adjuvant chemotherapy [92]. Ten eligible studies involving 15,410 patients (seven published articles, three abstracts) were identified. A meta-analysis of these demonstrated that a 4-week increase in time to adjuvant chemotherapy was associated with a significant decrease in both OS (HR, 1.14; 95% CI: [1.10–1.17]) and DFS (HR, 1.14; 95% CI: [1.10–1.18]).

The major limitation of this meta-analysis and majority of other studies is to include only studies with fluoropyrimidine-based adjuvant therapy. Currently, oxaliplatin in combination with fluoropyrimidine is preferred adjuvant regimens in stage III colon cancer. A population-based analysis was performed to investigate the effect of delay in initiating oxaliplatin-based chemotherapy on RFS and colon cancer-specific survival for stage III colon cancer [93]. At a median follow-up of 57.9 months, 5-year RFS was 70.9% (95% CI: [65.2–76.5]) for patients who began to receive adjuvant chemotherapy within 8 weeks and 72.1% (95% CI: [67.2–77]) for patients in whom adjuvant chemotherapy was started later than 8 weeks after surgery. Five-year cancer-specific survival was 82% (95% CI: [87.09–76.91]) and 82.8% (95% CI: [78.30–87.30]), respectively. In a multivariate analysis, delayed time to adjuvant chemotherapy was not found to have a prognostic significance on either RFS (HR, 1.08; $P = 0.609$) or cancer-specific survival (HR, 1.02; $P = 0.893$). Therefore, contrary to most existing data, which are primarily based on 5-FU-based adjuvant chemotherapy, delay of oxaliplatin-based adjuvant chemotherapy beyond 8 weeks did not appear to be associated with inferior outcomes.

Although recent evidence obtained from studies with oxaliplatin-based adjuvant chemotherapy and absence of data about the exact time when patients lose adjuvant systemic therapy, it is still concluded in international guidelines that adjuvant chemotherapy should be initiated as soon as it is practically feasible and ideally should not be delayed later than 8 weeks from surgery [94, 95].

10. Factors resulting in delay to start adjuvant chemotherapy

In a retrospective analysis, factors associated with starting treatment after 8 weeks were found to be older age, emergency resection, anastomotic leakage, referral to another hospital for adjuvant chemotherapy, and prolonged postoperative hospital admission [73]. A meta-analysis performed by Malietzis demonstrated that significant predictors of delayed initiation of adjuvant systemic treatment were age >75 years, marital status (single), low socioeconomic status, worse comorbidity status, low tumor grade, prolonged length of stay, and readmission [7]. Laparoscopy compared with open surgery was found to be a significant predictor of earlier initiation of adjuvant therapy.

The practice variation with respect to adherence to the NCCN recommendations within the National Cancer Date Base was evaluated in a recent study performed by Boland et al. [95]. The main purpose of that study was to examine the impact of adherence to guidelines on stage-specific survival outcomes in patients with stage III and high-risk stage II colon cancer, to identify factors associated with survival, and to identify subgroups of patients who may benefit from improved access to or delivery of cancer care. Male sex, insurance status other than private insurance such as Medicaid, other government insurance or lack of insurance, African

American race, lower household income, treatment at a community hospital, and treatment at an institution other than the hospital of diagnosis were found to be the main factors associated with increased risk of death both in patients with stage III disease and those with high-risk stage II disease.

In conclusion, oxaliplatin plus capecitabine or 5-FU/LV is the standard of care for the adjuvant treatment of stage III colon cancer (**Figure 1**). The preferred oxaliplatin-fluoropyrimidine-based combination regimes are XELOX, FOLFOX4, FOLFOX6, FOLFOX7, XELOX, and FLOX (**Table 6**). Whenever any contraindication for combination chemotherapy with fluoropyrimidine and oxaliplatin exists, single-agent fluoropyrimidine can be given as an adjuvant chemotherapy regimen (**Table 6**). During the decision making of adjuvant chemotherapy in stage II colon cancer patients, physicians should take into account the minimal potential improvement in OS of approximately 2–5% and the actual risk of mortality of 0.5–1%. High-risk stage II patients may be considered as an eligible group for adjuvant therapy after a complete discussion. Other factors, including MSI and 18q loss of heterozygosity, require further assessment to determine which combination of these is the most important and correlates best with therapeutic benefit. Making a treatment decision is not yet recommended according to the multigene assay. The new generation of adjuvant trials will help to determine if recently developed therapies will further improve the survival of this particular population. In stage II colon cancer treatment, the potential risks of adjuvant treatment and its benefit should be assessed and decision should be made on an individual patient basis.

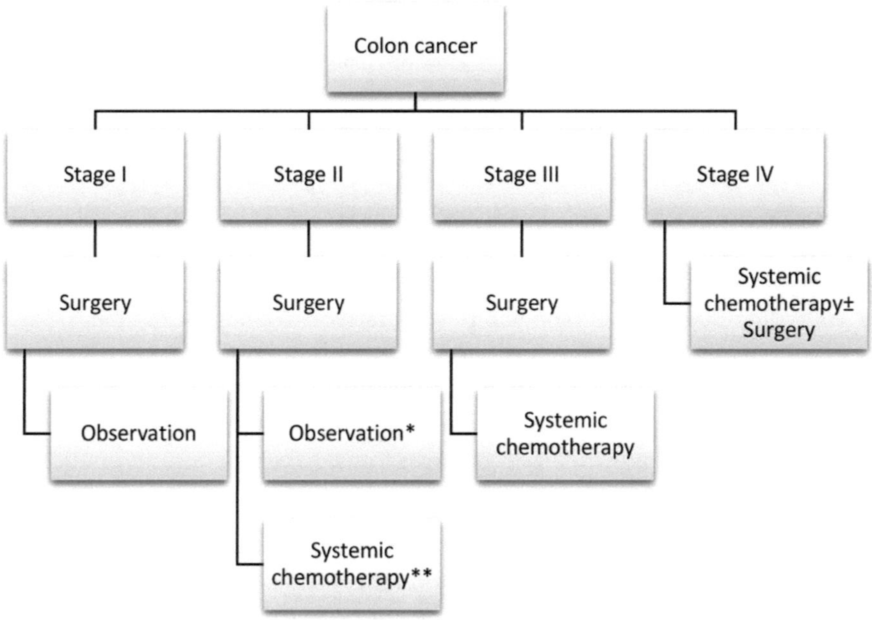

Figure 1 Algorithms for adjuvant systemic chemotherapy in colon cancer. *Observation is recommended to patients with T3N0 and dMMR or MSI-H colon cancer and without high-risk factors for systemic recurrence. **Systemic chemotherapy for 6 months after surgery is recommended for patients with high-risk factors for systemic recurrence.

Regimen	Drug	Route of administration	Dosage	Give on days of each cycle	Repeat every cycle	Total cycle
Fluorouracil-oxaliplatin-based combination regimens – preferred*						
FOLFOX4	Leucovorin	iv infusion	200 mg/m²	Days 1, 2	14 days	12 cycles
	Oxaliplatin	iv infusion	85 mg/m²	Day 1		
	5-FU	iv bolus	400 mg/m²	Days 1, 2		
	5-FU	iv 22 h infusion via pump	600 mg/m²	Days 1, 2		
FOLFOX6	Leucovorin	iv infusion	400 mg/m²	Day 1	14 days	12 cycles
	Oxaliplatin	iv infusion	85 mg/m²	Day 1		
	5-FU	iv bolus	400 mg/m²	Days 1, 2		
	5-FU	iv 22 h infusi on via pump	1200 mg/m²	Days 1, 2		
FOLFOX7	Leucovorin	iv infusion	400 mg/m²	Day 1	14 days	12 cycles
	Oxaliplatin	iv infusion	85 mg/m²	Day 1		
	5-FU	iv bolus	400 mg/m²	Day 1		
	5-FU	iv 22 h infu sion via pump	1200 mg/m²	Days 1, 2		
XELOX	Capec itabine Oxaliplatin	Oral iv infusion	850–1000 mg/m² twice daily 130 mg/m²	Days 1–14 Day 1	21 days	8 cycles
FLOX	5-FU	iv bolus	500 mg/m²	Days 1, 8, 15,	8 weeks	3 cycles
	Leucovorin	iv bolus	500 mg/m²	22, 29, 35	8 weeks	3 cycles
	Oxaliplatin	iv infusion	85 mg/m²	Days 1, 8, 15, 22, 29, 35 Days 1, 15, 29		
Fluoropyrimidines with or without leucovorin**						
Capeci tabine	Capeci tabine	Oral	1250 mg/m² twice daily	Days 1–14	21 days	8 cycles
5-FU/LV (Roswell Park regimen)	Leuco vorin 5-FU	iv infusion iv bolus	500 mg/m² 500 mg/m²	Days 1, 8, 15, 22, 29, 35 Days 1, 8, 15, , 29, 35	8 weeks	4 cycles
5-FU/LV (Mayo regimen)	Leuco vorin	iv bolus iv bolus	20 mg/m² 425 mg/m²	Days 1–5 Days 1–5	4 weeks	6 cycles

Regimen	Drug	Route of administration	Dosage	Give on days of each cycle	Repeat every cycle	Total cycle
	5-FU					
5-FU/LV	Leucovorin	iv bolus	400 mg/m^2	Day 1	14 days	12 cycles
(Modified de Gramont regimen)	5-FU	iv bolus	400 mg/m^2	Day 1		
	5-FU	iv 46 h infusion via pump	2400 mg/m^2	Day 1		

5-FU, 5-fluorouracil; iv, intravenous; LV, leucovorin.
*Fluorouracil-oxaliplatin-based combination regimens are preferred in all patients with stage III colon cancer and in selected patients with stage II colon cancer.
**Fluoropyrimidines with or without leucovorin should be given to patients who have a contraindication to oxaliplatin.

Table 6. Recommended chemotherapy regimens for patients with resected colon cancer.

Author details

Fatma Sen[1*] and Kezban Nur Pilancı[2]

*Address all correspondence to: fkaragoz_2000@yahoo.com

1 Division of Medical Oncology, Istanbul University, Institute of Oncology, Istanbul, Turkey

2 Division of Medical Oncology, Haseki Education and Research Hospital, İstanbul, Turkey

References

[1] Edge SB, Byrd DR, Compton CC, Fritz AG, Greene FL, Trotti A. AJCC cancer staging manual. 7th ed. New York, NY: Springer; 2010.

[2] Siegel RL, Miller KD, Jemal A. Cancer statistics, 2015. CA Cancer J Clin. 2015;65(1):5–29.

[3] O'Connell JB, Maggard MA, Ko CY. Colon cancer survival rates with the new American Joint Committee on Cancer sixth edition staging. J Natl Cancer Inst. 2004;96(19):1420–1425.

[4] Buyse M, Zeleniuch-Jacquotte A, Chalmers TC. Adjuvant therapy of colorectal cancer. Why we still don't know. JAMA. 1988;259(24):3571–3578.

[5] Wolmark N, Fisher B, Rockette H, Redmond C, Wickerham DL, Fisher ER, Jones J, Glass A, Lerner H, Lawrence W, Prager D, Wexler M, Evans J, Cruz A, Dimitrov N, Jochimsen

P, and Other NSABP InvestigatorsPostoperative adjuvant chemotherapy or BCG for colon cancer: results from NSABP protocol C-01. J Natl Cancer Inst. 1988;80(1):30–36.

[6] Wilkinson NW, Yothers G, Lopa S, Costantino JP, Petrelli NJ, Wolmark N. Long-term survival results of surgery alone versus surgery plus 5-FU/LV for stage II and stage III colon cancer: pooled analysis of NSABP C-01 through C-05. A baseline from which to compare modern adjuvant trials. Ann Surg Oncol. 2010;17(4):959–966.

[7] Moertel CG, Fleming TR, Macdonald JS, Haller DG, Laurie JA, Tangen CM, Ungerleider JS, Emerson WA, Tormey DC, Glick JH, Veeder MH, Mailliard JA. 5-FU/levamisole as effective adjuvant therapy after resection of stage III colon carcinoma: a final report. Ann Intern Med. 1995;122(5):321–326.

[8] Laurie JA, Moertel CG, Fleming TR, Wieand HS, Leigh JE, Rubin J, McCormack GW, Gerstner JB, Krook JE, Malliard J, Twito DI, Morton RF, Tschetter LK, Barlow JF. Surgical adjuvant therapy of large-bowel carcinoma: an evaluation of levamisole and the combination of levamisole and fluorouracil. The North Central Cancer Treatment Group and the Mayo Clinic. J Clin Oncol. 1989 Oct;7(10):1447–1456.

[9] Wolmark N, Rockette H, Fisher B, Wickerham DL, Redmond C, Fisher ER, Jones J, Mamounas EP, Ore L, Petrelli NJ, Spurr CL, Dimitrov N, Romond EH, Sutherland CM, Kardinal CH, DeFusco PA, Jochimsen P. The benefit of leucovorin-modulated fluorouracil as postoperative adjuvant therapy for primary colon cancer: results from National Surgical Adjuvant Breast and Bowel Project protocol C-03. J Clin Oncol. 1993;11(10):1879–1887.

[10] Wolmark N, Rockette H, Mamounas E, Jones J, Wieand S, Wickerham DL, Bear HD, Atkins JN, Dimitrov NV, Glass AG, Fisher ER, Fisher B. Clinical trial to assess the relative efficacy of fluorouracil and leucovorin, 5-FU/levamisole, and fluorouracil, leucovorin, and levamisole in patients with Dukes' B and C carcinoma of the colon: results from National Surgical Adjuvant Breast and Bowel Project C-04. J Clin Oncol. 1999;17(11):3553–3559.

[11] Haller DG, Catalano PJ, Macdonald JS, O'Rourke MA, Frontiera MS, Jackson DV, Mayer RJ. Phase III study of fluorouracil, leucovorin, and levamisole in high-risk stage II and III colon cancer: final report of Intergroup 0089. J Clin Oncol. 2005;23:8671–8678.

[12] NIH Consensus Conference Adjuvant therapy for patients with colon and rectal cancer. JAMA. 1990;264:1444–1450.

[13] Marshall JL, Haller DG, de Gramont A, Hochster HS, Lenz HJ, Ajani JA, Goldberg RM. Adjuvant therapy for stage II and III colon cancer: consensus report of the International Society of Gastrointestinal Oncology. Gastrointest Cancer Res. 2007;1(4):146–154.

[14] Lombardi L, Morelli F, Cinieri S, Santini D, Silvestris N, Fazio N, Orlando L, Tonini G, Colucci G, Maiello E. Adjuvant colon cancer chemotherapy: where we are and where we'll go. Cancer Treat Rev. 2010;36 Suppl 3:S34–S41.

[15] André T, Boni C, Navarro M, Tabernero J, Hickish T, Topham C, Bonetti A, Clingan P, Bridgewater J, Rivera F, de Gramont A. Improved OS with oxaliplatin, fluorouracil, and leucovorin as adjuvant treatment in stage II or III colon cancer in the MOSAIC trial. J Clin Oncol. 2009;27(19):3109–3116.

[16] de Gramont A, Figer A, Seymour M, Homerin M, Hmissi A, Cassidy J, Boni C, Cortes-Funes H, Cervantes A, Freyer G, Papamichael D, Le Bail N, Louvet C, Hendler D, de Braud F, Wilson C, Morvan F, Bonetti A. 5-FU/LV with or without oxaliplatin as first-line treatment in advanced colorectal cancer. J Clin Oncol. 2000;18:2938–2947.

[17] Goldberg RM. N9741: a phase III study comparing irinotecan to oxaliplatin-containing regimens in advanced colorectal cancer. Clin Colorectal Cancer. 2002;2:81.

[18] Saltz LB, Niedzwiecki D, Hollis D, Goldberg RM, Hantel A, Thomas JP, Fields ALA, Carver A, Mayer RJ. Irinotecan plus fluorouracil/leucovorin (IFL) versus fluorouracil/ leucovorin alone (FL) in stage III colon cancer (Intergroup trial CALGB C89803). 2004 ASCO Annual Meeting Proceedings. J Clin Oncol. 2004;22:14S (abstract 3500).

[19] André T, Boni C, Mounedji-Boudiaf L, Navarro M, Tabernero J, Hickish T, Topham C, Zaninelli M, Clingan P, Bridgewater J, Tabah-Fisch I, de Gramont A. Multicenter International Study of Oxaliplatin/5-FU/Leucovorin in the Adjuvant Treatment of Colon Cancer (MOSAIC) investigators oxaliplatin, fluorouracil, and leucovorin as adjuvant treatment for colon cancer. N Engl J Med. 2004;350(23):2343–2351.

[20] Twelves C, Wong A, Nowacki MP, Abt M, Burris H 3rd, Carrato A, Cassidy J, Cervantes A, Fagerberg J, Georgoulias V, Husseini F, Jodrell D, Koralewski P, Kröning H, Maroun J, Marschner N, McKendrick J, Pawlicki M, Rosso R, Schüller J, Seitz JF, Stabuc B, Tujakowski J, Van Hazel G, Zaluski J, Scheithauer W. Capecitabine as adjuvant treatment for stage III colon cancer. N Engl J Med. 2005;352:2696–2704.

[21] Kuebler JP, Wieand HS, O'Connell MJ, Smith RE, Colangelo LH, Yothers G, Petrelli NJ, Findlay MP, Seay TE, Atkins JN, Zapas JL, Goodwin JW, Fehrenbacher L, Ramanathan RK, Conley BA, Flynn PJ, Soori G, Colman LK, Levine EA, Lanier KS, Wolmark N. Oxaliplatin combined with weekly bolus fluorouracil and leucovorin as surgical adjuvant chemotherapy for stage II and III colon cancer: results from NSABP C-07. J Clin Oncol. 2007;25(16):2198–2204.

[22] Haller DG, Tabernero J, Maroun J, de Braud F, Price T, Van Cutsem E, Hill M, Gilberg F, Rittweger K, Schmoll HJ. Capecitabine plus oxaliplatin compared with fluorouracil and folinic acid as adjuvant therapy for stage III colon cancer. J Clin Oncol. 2011;29(11): 1465–1471.

[23] André T, de Gramont A, Vernerey D, Chibaudel B, Bonnetain F, Tijeras-Raballand A, Scriva A, Hickish T, Tabernero J, Van Laethem JL, Banzi M, Maartense E, Shmueli E, Carlsson GU, Scheithauer W, Papamichael D, Möehler M, Landolfi S, Demetter P, Colote S, Tournigand C, Louvet C, Duval A, Fléjou JF, de Gramont A. Adjuvant fluorouracil, leucovorin, and oxaliplatin in stage II to III colon cancer: updated 10-year

survival and outcomes according to BRAF mutation and mismatch repair status of the MOSAIC study. J Clin Oncol. 2015;33(35):4176–4187.

[24] Yothers G, O'Connell MJ, Allegra CJ, Kuebler JP, Colangelo LH, Petrelli NJ, Wolmark N. Oxaliplatin as adjuvant therapy for colon cancer: updated results of NSABP C-07 trial, including survival and subset analyses. J Clin Oncol. 2011;29(28):3768–3774.

[25] Wolmark N, Wieand S, Lembersky B, Colangelo L, Smith R, Pazdur R. A phase III trial comparing oral UFT to FULV in stage II and III carcinoma of the colon: results of NSABP protocol C-06. Proc Am Soc Clin Oncol. 2004;22:2 (abstract 3508).

[26] Yoshida M, Ishiguro M, Ikejiri K, Mochizuki I, Nakamoto Y, Kinugasa Y, Takagane A, Endo T, Shinozaki H, Takii Y, Mochizuki H, Kotake K, Kameoka S, Takahashi K, Watanabe T, Watanabe M, Boku N, Tomita N, Nakatani E, Sugihara K, ACTS-CC study group. S-1 as adjuvant chemotherapy for stage III colon cancer: a randomized phase III study (ACTS-CC trial). Ann Oncol. 2014;25(9):1743–1749.

[27] Schmoll HJ, Twelves C, Sun W, O'Connell MJ, Cartwright T, McKenna E, Saif M, Lee S, Yothers G, Haller D. Effect of adjuvant capecitabine or fluorouracil, with or without oxaliplatin, on survival outcomes in stage III colon cancer and the effect of oxaliplatin on post-relapse survival: a pooled analysis of individual patient data from four randomised controlled trials. Lancet Oncol. 2014;15(13):1481–1492.

[28] Shah MA, Renfro LA, Allegra CJ, André T, de Gramont A, Schmoll HJ, Haller DG, Alberts SR, Yothers G, Sargent DJ. Impact of patient factors on recurrence risk and time dependency of oxaliplatin benefit in patients with colon cancer: analysis from modern-era adjuvant studies in the adjuvant colon cancer end points (ACCENT) database. J Clin Oncol. 2016 pii: JCO630558.

[29] International Multicentre Pooled Analysis of B2 Colon Cancer Trials (IMPACT B2) Investigators. Efficacy of adjuvant fluorouracil and folinic acid in B2 colon cancer. J Clin Oncol. 1999;17(5):1356–1363.

[30] International Multicentre Pooled Analysis of Colon Cancer Trials (IMPACT) investigators. Efficacy of adjuvant fluorouracil and folinic acid in colon cancer. Lancet. 1995;345(8955):939–944.

[31] Zaniboni A, Labianca R, Marsoni S, Torri V, Mosconi P, Grilli R, Apolone G, Cifani S, Tinazzi A.GIVIO-SITAC 01: A randomized trial of adjuvant 5-fluorouracil and folinic acid administered to patients with colon carcinoma--long term results and evaluation of the indicators of health-related quality of life. Gruppo Italiano Valutazione Interventi in Oncologia. Studio Italiano Terapia Adiuvante Colon.Cancer. 1998 Jun 1;82(11):2135–44.

[32] O'Connell MJ, Mailliard JA, Kahn MJ, Macdonald JS, Haller DG, Mayer RJ, Wieand HS. Controlled trial of fluorouracil and low-dose leucovorin given for 6 months as post-operative adjuvant therapy for colon cancer. J Clin Oncol. 1997;15(1):246–250.

[33] Quasar Collaborative Group, Gray R, Barnwell J, McConkey C, Hills RK, Williams NS, Kerr DJ. Adjuvant chemotherapy versus observation in patients with colorectal cancer: a randomised study. Lancet. 2007;370(9604):2020–2029.

[34] Schippinger W, Samonigg H, Schaberl-Moser R, Greil R, Thödtmann R, Tschmelitsch J, Jagoditsch M, Steger GG, Jakesz R, Herbst F, Hofbauer F, Rabl H, Wohlmuth P, Gnant M, Thaler J, Austrian Breast and Colorectal Cancer Study Group. A prospective randomised phase III trial of adjuvant chemotherapy with 5-FU/LV in patients with stage II colon cancer. Br J Cancer. 2007;97(8):1021–1027.

[35] Figueredo A, Charette ML, Maroun J, Brouwers MC, Zuraw L. Adjuvant therapy for stage II colon cancer: a systematic review from the Cancer Care Ontario Program in evidence-based care's gastrointestinal cancer disease site group. J Clin Oncol. 2004;22(16):3395–3407.

[36] Schrag D, Rifas-Shiman S, Saltz L, Bach PB, Begg CB. Adjuvant chemotherapy use for medicare beneficiaries with stage II colon cancer. J Clin Oncol. 2002;20(19):3999–4005.

[37] Wu X, Zhang J, He X, Wang C, Lian L, Liu H, Wang J, Lan P. Postoperative adjuvant chemotherapy for stage II colorectal cancer: a systematic review of 12 randomized controlled trials. J Gastrointest Surg. 2012;16(3):646–655.

[38] Benson AB 3rd, Schrag D, Somerfield MR, Cohen AM, Figueredo AT, Flynn PJ, Krzyzanowska MK, Maroun J, McAllister P, Van Cutsem E, Brouwers M, Charette M, Haller DG. American Society of Clinical Oncology recommendations on adjuvant chemotherapy for stage II colon cancer. J Clin Oncol. 2004;22(16):3408–3419.

[39] Benson AB 3rd, Hamilton SR. Path toward prognostication and prediction: an evolving matrix. J Clin Oncol. 2011;29(35):4599–601.

[40] Quah HM, Chou JF, Gonen M, Shia J, Schrag D, Landmann RG, Guillem JG, Paty PB, Temple LK, Wong WD, Weiser MR. Identification of patients with high-risk stage II colon cancer for adjuvant therapy. Dis Colon Rectum. 2008;51(5):503–507.

[41] Mamounas E, Wieand S, Wolmark N, Bear HD, Atkins JN, Song K, Jones J, Rockette H. Comparative efficacy of adjuvant chemotherapy in patients with Dukes' B versus Dukes' C colon cancer: results from four National Surgical Adjuvant Breast and Bowel Project adjuvant studies (C-01, C-02, C-03, and C-04). J Clin Oncol. 1999;17(5):1349–1355.

[42] Hutchins G, Southward K, Handley K, Magill L, Beaumont C, Stahlschmidt J, Richman S, Chambers P, Seymour M, Kerr D, Gray R, Quirke P. Value of mismatch repair, KRAS, and BRAF mutations in predicting recurrence and benefits from chemotherapy in colorectal cancer. J Clin Oncol. 2011;29(10):1261–1270.

[43] Tournigand C, André T, Bonnetain F, Chibaudel B, Lledo G, Hickish T, Tabernero J, Boni C, Bachet JB, Teixeira L, de Gramont A. Adjuvant therapy with fluorouracil and oxaliplatin in stage II and elderly patients (between ages 70 and 75 years) with colon cancer: subgroup analyses of the Multicenter International Study of oxaliplatin,

fluorouracil, and leucovorin in the adjuvant treatment of colon cancer trial. J Clin Oncol. 2012;30(27):3353–3360.

[44] Taal BG, Van Tinteren H, Zoetmulder FA, NACCP group. Adjuvant 5-FU plus levamisole in colonic or rectal cancer: improved survival in stage II and III. Br J Cancer. 2001;85(10):1437–1443.

[45] Gill S, Loprinzi CL, Sargent DJ, Thomé SD, Alberts SR, Haller DG, Benedetti J, Francini G, Shepherd LE, Francois Seitz J, Labianca R, Chen W, Cha SS, Heldebrant MP, Goldberg RM. Pooled analysis of fluorouracil-based adjuvant therapy for stage II and III colon cancer: who benefits and by how much? J Clin Oncol. 2004;22(10):1797–1806.

[46] Faivre-Finn C, Bouvier-Benhamiche AM, Phelip JM, Manfredi S, Dancourt V, Faivre J. Colon cancer in France: evidence for improvement in management and survival.Gut. 2002;51(1):60–64.

[47] Chen HS, Sheen-Chen SM. Obstruction and perforation in colorectal adenocarcinoma: an analysis of prognosis and current trends. Surgery. 2000;127(4):370–376.

[48] Chang GJ, Rodriguez-Bigas MA, Skibber JM, Moyer VA. Lymph node evaluation and survival after curative resection of colon cancer: systematic review. J Natl Cancer Inst. 2007;99(6):433–441.

[49] Kim CW, Yoon YS, Park IJ, Lim SB, Yu CS, Kim JC. Elevation of preoperative s-CEA concentration in stage IIA colorectal cancer can also be a high-risk factor for stage II patients. Ann Surg Oncol. 2013 Sep;20(9):2914–2920.

[50] Schmoll HJ, Van Cutsem E, Stein A, Valentini V, Glimelius B, Haustermans K, Nordlinger B, van de Velde CJ, Balmana J, Regula J, Nagtegaal ID, Beets-Tan RG, Arnold D, Ciardiello F, Hoff P, Kerr D, Köhne CH, Labianca R, Price T, Scheithauer W, Sobrero A, Tabernero J, Aderka D, Barroso S, Bodoky G, Douillard JY, El Ghazaly H, Gallardo J, Garin A, Glynne-Jones R, Jordan K, Meshcheryakov A, Papamichail D, Pfeiffer P, Souglakos I, Turhal S, Cervantes A. ESMO Consensus Guidelines for management of patients with colon and rectal cancer. a personalized approach to clinical decision making. Ann Oncol. 2012;23(10):2479–2516.

[51] Artac M, Turhal NS, Kocer M, Karabulut B, Bozcuk H, Yalcin S, Karaagac M, Gündüz S, Isik N, Uygun K. Do high-risk features support the use of adjuvant chemotherapy in stage II colon cancer? A Turkish Oncology Group study. Tumori. 2014;100(2):143–148.

[52] O'Connor ES, Greenblatt DY, LoConte NK, Gangnon RE, Liou JI, Heise CP, Smith MA, Adjuvant chemotherapy for stage II colon cancer with poor prognostic features. J Clin Oncol. 2011;29(25):3381–3388.

[53] Le Voyer TE, Sigurdson ER, Hanlon AL, Mayer RJ, Macdonald JS, Catalano PJ, Haller DG. Colon cancer survival is associated with increasing number of lymph nodes

analyzed: a secondary survey of intergroup trial INT-0089. J Clin Oncol. 2003;21(15): 2912–2919.

[54] Allegra CJ, Yothers G, O'Connell MJ, Sharif S, Petrelli NJ, Lopa SH, Wolmark N. Bevacizumab in stage II-III colon cancer: 5-year update of the National Surgical Adjuvant Breast and Bowel Project C-08 trial. J Clin Oncol. 2013;31(3):359–364.

[55] de Gramont A, Van Cutsem E, Schmoll HJ, Tabernero J, Clarke S, Moore MJ, Cunningham D, Cartwright TH, Hecht JR, Rivera F, Im SA, Bodoky G, Salazar R, Maindrault-Goebel F, Shacham-Shmueli E, Bajetta E, Makrutzki M, Shang A, André T, Hoff PM. Bevacizumab plus oxaliplatin-based chemotherapy as adjuvant treatment for colon cancer (AVANT): a phase III randomised controlled trial. Lancet Oncol. 2012;13(12): 1225–1233.

[56] Haller DG, O'Connell MJ, Cartwright TH, Twelves CJ, McKenna EF, Sun W, Saif MW, Lee S, Yothers G, Schmoll HJ. Impact of age and medical comorbidity on adjuvant treatment outcomes for stage III colon cancer: a pooled analysis of individual patient data from four randomized, controlled trials. Ann Oncol. 2015;26(4):715–724.

[57] Alberts SR, Sargent DJ, Nair S, Mahoney MR, Mooney M, Thibodeau SN, Smyrk TC, Sinicrope FA, Chan E, Gill S, Kahlenberg MS, Shields AF, Quesenberry JT, Webb TA, Farr GH Jr, Pockaj BA, Grothey A, Goldberg RM. Effect of oxaliplatin, fluorouracil, and leucovorin with or without cetuximab on survival among patients with resected stage III colon cancer: a randomized trial. JAMA. 2012;307(13):1383–1393.

[58] Taieb J, Tabernero J, Mini E, Subtil F, Folprecht G, Van Laethem JL, Thaler J, Bridgewater J, Petersen LN, Blons H, Collette L, Van Cutsem E, Rougier P, Salazar R, Bedenne L, Emile JF, Laurent-Puig P, Lepage C, PETACC-8 Study Investigators. Oxaliplatin, fluorouracil, and leucovorin with or without cetuximab in patients with resected stage III colon cancer (PETACC-8): an open-label, randomised phase III trial. Lancet Oncol. 2014;15(8):862–873.

[59] Jen J, Kim H, Piantadosi S, Liu ZF, Levitt RC, Sistonen P, Kinzler KW, Vogelstein B, Hamilton SR. Allelic loss of chromosome 18q and prognosis in colorectal cancer. N Engl J Med. 1994;331(4):213–221.

[60] Markowitz SD, Bertagnolli MM. Molecular origins of cancer: molecular basis of colorectal cancer. N Engl J Med. 2009;361(25):2449–2460.

[61] Halvarsson B, Anderson H, Domanska K, Lindmark G, Nilbert M. Clinicopathologic factors identify sporadic mismatch repair-defective colon cancers. Am J Clin Pathol. 2008;129(2):238–244.

[62] French AJ, Sargent DJ, Burgart LJ, Foster NR, Kabat BF, Goldberg R, Shepherd L, Windschitl HE, Thibodeau SN. Prognostic significance of defective mismatch repair and BRAF V600E in patients with colon cancer. Clin Cancer Res. 2008;14(11):3408–3415.

[63] Elsaleh H, Joseph D, Grieu F, Zeps N, Spry N, Iacopetta B. Association of tumor site and sex with survival benefit from adjuvant chemotherapy in colorectal cancer. Lancet. 2000;355:1745–1750.

[64] Allegra CJ, Kim G, Kirsch IR. Microsatellite instability in colon cancer. N Engl J Med 2003;349(18):1774–1776.

[65] Ribic CM, Sargent DJ, Moore MJ, Thibodeau SN, French AJ, Goldberg RM, Hamilton SR, Laurent-Puig P, Gryfe R, Shepherd LE, Tu D, Redston M, Gallinger S. Tumor microsatellite-instability status as a predictor of benefit from fluorouracil-based adjuvant chemotherapy for colon cancer. N Engl J Med. 2003;349(3):247–257.

[66] Sargent DJ, George SL. Clinical trials data collection: when less is more. J Clin Oncol. 2010;28(34):5019–5021.

[67] Kim JE, Hong YS, Kim HJ, Kim KP, Lee JL, Park SJ, Lim SB, Park IJ, Kim CW, Yoon YS, Yu CS, Kim JC, Hoon KJ, Kim TW. Defective mismatch repair status was not associated with DFS and OS in stage II colon cancer treated with adjuvant chemotherapy. Ann Surg Oncol. 2015;22 Suppl 3:630–637.

[68] Bertagnolli MM, Redston M, Compton CC, Niedzwiecki D, Mayer RJ, Goldberg RM, Colacchio TA, Saltz LB, Warren RS. Microsatellite instability and loss of heterozygosity at chromosomal location 18q: prospective evaluation of biomarkers for stages II and III colon cancer – a study of CALGB 9581 and 89803. J Clin Oncol. 2011;29(23):3153–3162.

[69] Zaanan A, Cuilliere-Dartigues P, Guilloux A, Parc Y, Louvet C, de Gramont A, Tiret E, Dumont S, Gayet B, Validire P, Fléjou JF, Duval A, Praz F. Impact of p53 expression and microsatellite instability on stage III colon cancer DFS in patients treated by 5-FU/LV with or without oxaliplatin. Ann Oncol. 2010;21(4):772–780.

[70] Müller CI, Schulmann K, Reinacher-Schick A, Andre N, Arnold D, Tannapfel A, Arkenau H, Hahn SA, Schmoll SH, Porschen R, Schmiegel W, Graeven U, AIO Colorectal Study Group. Predictive and prognostic value of microsatellite instability in patients with advanced colorectal cancer treated with a fluoropyrimidine and oxaliplatin containing first-line chemotherapy. A report of the AIO Colorectal Study Group. Int J Colorectal Dis. 2008;23(11):1033–1039.

[71] Tougeron D, Sickerson G, LeComte T, Mouillet G, Trouilloud I, Coriat R, Aparicio T, Guetz GD, Lecaille C, Artru P, Cauchin E, Sefrioui D, Boussaha T, Ferru A, Taïeb J, Michel P, Karayan-Tapon L, Vernerey D, Bonnetain F, Zaanan A. Impact of adjuvant chemotherapy with 5-FU or FOLFOX in colon cancers with microsatellite instability. An AGEO multicenter study (abstract). J Clin Oncol. 2014;32(5s) (suppl, abstract): 3508.

[72] Roth AD, Tejpar S, Delorenzi M, Yan P, Fiocca R, Klingbiel D, Dietrich D, Biesmans B, Bodoky G, Barone C, Aranda E, Nordlinger B, Cisar L, Labianca R, Cunningham D, Van Cutsem E, Bosman F. Prognostic role of KRAS and BRAF in stage II and III resected colon cancer: results of the translational study on the PETACC-3, EORTC 40993, SAKK 60-00 trial. J Clin Oncol. 2010;28(3):466–74.

[73] Bos AC, van Erning FN, van Gestel YR, Creemers GJ, Punt CJ, van Oijen MG, Lemmens VE. Timing of adjuvant chemotherapy and its relation to survival among patients with stage III colon cancer. Eur J Cancer. 2015;51(17):2553–2561.

[74] Koopman M, Kortman GA, Mekenkamp L, Ligtenberg MJ, Hoogerbrugge N, Antonini NF, Punt CJ, van Krieken JH. Deficient mismatch repair system in patients with sporadic advanced colorectal cancer. Br J Cancer. 2009;100(2):266–273.

[75] Popovici VC, Budinska E, Roth A, Bosman F, Tejpar S, Delorenzi M. BRAF and KRAS mutations as additional risk factors in the context of clinical parameters of patients with colorectal cancer (abstract). J Cin Oncol. 2013;31 (suppl, abstract): 3522.

[76] Gavin PG, Colangelo LH, Fumagalli D, Tanaka N, Remillard MY, Yothers G, Kim C, Taniyama Y, Kim SI, Choi HJ, Blackmon NL, Lipchik C, Petrelli NJ, O'Connell MJ, Wolmark N, Paik S, Pogue-Geile KL. Mutation profiling and microsatellite instability in stage II and III colon cancer: an assessment of their prognostic and oxaliplatin predictive value. Clin Cancer Res. 2012;18(23):6531–6541.

[77] Samowitz WS, Sweeney C, Herrick J, Albertsen H, Levin TR, Murtaugh MA, Wolff RK, Slattery ML. Poor survival associated with the BRAF V600E mutation in microsatellite-stable colon cancers. Cancer Res. 2005;65(14):6063–6069.

[78] Popat S, Hubner R, Houlston RS. Systematic review of microsatellite instability and colorectal cancer prognosis. J Clin Oncol. 2005;23:609–618.

[79] Kim GP, Colangelo LH, Wieand HS, Paik S, Kirsch IR, Wolmark N, Allegra CJ, National Cancer Institute. Prognostic and predictive roles of high-degree microsatellite instability in colon cancer: a National Cancer Institute–National Surgical Adjuvant Breast and Bowel Project Collaborative Study. J Clin Oncol. 2007;25:767–772.

[80] Walther A, Johnstone E, Swanton C, Midgley R, Tomlinson I, Kerr D. Genetic prognostic and predictive markers in colorectal cancer. Nat Rev Cancer. 2009;9(7):489–499.

[81] Sveen A, Nesbakken A, Ågesen TH, Guren MG, Tveit KM, Skotheim RI, Lothe RA. Anticipating the clinical use of prognostic gene expression-based tests for colon cancer stage II and III: is Godot finally arriving? Clin Cancer Res. 2013;19(24):6669–6677.

[82] O'Connell MJ, Lavery I, Yothers G, Paik S, Clark-Langone KM, Lopatin M, Watson D, Baehner FL, Shak S, Baker J, Cowens JW, Wolmark N. Relationship between tumor gene expression and recurrence in four independent studies of patients with stage II/III colon cancer treated with surgery alone or surgery plus adjuvant fluorouracil plus leucovorin. J Clin Oncol. 2010;28(25):3937–3944.

[83] Gray RG, Quirke P, Handley K, Lopatin M, Magill L, Baehner FL, Beaumont C, Clark-Langone KM, Yoshizawa CN, Lee M, Watson D, Shak S, Kerr DJ. Validation study of a quantitative multigene reverse transcriptase-polymerase chain reaction assay for assessment of recurrence risk in patients with stage II colon cancer. J Clin Oncol. 2011;29(35):4611–4619.

[84] Venook AP, Niedzwiecki D, Lopatin M, Ye X, Lee M, Friedman PN, Frankel W, Clark-Langone K, Millward C, Shak S, Goldberg RM, Mahmoud NN, Warren RS, Schilsky RL, Bertagnolli MM. Biologic determinants of tumor recurrence in stage II colon cancer: validation study of the 12-gene recurrence score in cancer and leukemia group B (CALGB) 9581. J Clin Oncol. 2013;31(14):1775–1781.

[85] Oh SC, Park YY, Park ES, Lim JY, Kim SM, Kim SB, Kim J, Kim SC, Chu IS, Smith JJ, Beauchamp RD, Yeatman TJ, Kopetz S, Lee JS. Prognostic gene expression signature associated with two molecularly distinct subtypes of colorectal cancer. Gut. 2012;61(9): 1291–1298.

[86] Jiang Y, Casey G, Lavery IC, Zhang Y, Talantov D, Martin-McGreevy M, Skacel M, Manilich E, Mazumder A, Atkins D, Delaney CP, Wang Y. Development of a clinically feasible molecular assay to predict recurrence of stage II colon cancer. J Mol Diagn. 2008;10(4):346–354.

[87] Salazar R, Roepman P, Capella G, Moreno V, Simon I, Dreezen C, Lopez-Doriga A, Santos C, Marijnen C, Westerga J, Bruin S, Kerr D, Kuppen P, van de Velde C, Morreau H, Van Velthuysen L, Glas AM, Van't Veer LJ, Tollenaar R. Gene expression signature to improve prognosis prediction of stage II and III colorectal cancer. J Clin Oncol. 2011;29(1):17–24.

[88] Yothers G, O'Connell MJ, Lee M, Lopatin M, Clark-Langone KM, Millward C, Paik S, Sharif S, Shak S, Wolmark N. Validation of the 12-gene colon cancer recurrence score in NSABP C-07 as a predictor of recurrence in patients with stage II and III colon cancer treated with fluorouracil and leucovorin (FU/LV) and FU/LV plus oxaliplatin. J Clin Oncol. 2013;31(36):4512–4519.

[89] NCCN guidelines colon cancer, version 2.2016.

[90] Kennedy RD, Bylesjo M, Kerr P, Davison T, Black JM, Kay EW, Holt RJ, Proutski V, Ahdesmaki M, Farztdinov V, Goffard N, Hey P, McDyer F, Mulligan K, Mussen J, O'Brien E, Oliver G, Walker SM, Mulligan JM, Wilson C, Winter A, O'Donoghue D, Mulcahy H, O'Sullivan J, Sheahan K, Hyland J, Dhir R, Bathe OF, Winqvist O, Manne U, Shanmugam C, Ramaswamy S, Leon EJ, Smith WI Jr, McDermott U, Wilson RH, Longley D, Marshall J, Cummins R, Sargent DJ,Johnston PG,Harkin DP. Development and independent validation of a prognostic assay for stage II colon cancer using formalin-fixed paraffin-embedded tissue. J Clin Oncol. 2011;29(35):4620–4626.

[91] Klein M, Azaquoun N, Jensen BV, Gögenur I. Improved survival with early adjuvant chemotherapy after colonic resection for stage III colonic cancer: a nationwide study. J Surg Oncol. 2015;112(5):538–543.

[92] Biagi JJ, Raphael MJ, Mackillop WJ, Kong W, King WD, Booth CM. Association between time to initiation of adjuvant chemotherapy and survival in colorectal cancer: a systematic review and meta-analysis. JAMA. 2011;305(22):2335–2342.

[93] Kumar A, Peixoto RD, Kennecke HF, Renouf DJ, Lim HJ, Gill S, Speers CH, Cheung WY. Effect of adjuvant FOLFOX chemotherapy duration on outcomes of patients with stage III colon cancer. Clin Colorectal Cancer. 2015;14(4):262–268.

[94] Kountourakis P, Souglakos J, Gouvas N, Androulakis N, Athanasiadis A, Boukovinas I, Christodoulou C, Chrysou E, Dervenis C, Emmanouilidis C, Georgiou P, Karachaliou N, Katopodi O, Makatsoris T, Papakostas P, Pentheroudakis G, Pilpilidis I, Sgouros J, Tekkis P, Triantopoulou C, Tzardi M, Vassiliou V, Vini L, Xynogalos S, Xynos E, Ziras N, Papamichael D. Adjuvant chemotherapy for colon cancer: a consensus statement of the Hellenic and Cypriot Colorectal Cancer Study Group by the HeSMO. Ann Gastroenterol. 2016;29(1):18–23.

[95] Boland GM, Chang GJ, Haynes AB, Chiang YJ, Chagpar R, Xing Y, Hu CY, Feig BW, You YN, Cormier JN. Association between adherence to National Comprehensive Cancer Network treatment guidelines and improved survival in patients with colon cancer. Cancer. 2013;119(8):1593–1601.